CONTENTS

6th Edition

Understanding Nursing Research
Building an Evidence-Based Practice

Susan K. Grove, PhD, RN, ANP-BC, GNP-BC
Professor Emerita
College of Nursing
The University of Texas at Arlington
Arlington, Texas;
Adult Nurse Practitioner
Family Practice
Grand Prairie, Texas

Jennifer R. Gray, PhD, RN, FAAN
George W. and Hazel M. Jay Professor, College of Nursing
Associate Dean, College of Nursing
The University of Texas at Arlington
Arlington, Texas

Nancy Burns, PhD, RN, FCN, FAAN
Professor Emerita
College of Nursing
The University of Texas at Arlington
Arlington, Texas;
Faith Community Nurse
St. Matthew Cumberland Presbyterian Church
Burleson, Texas

ELSEVIER
SAUNDERS

3251 Riverport Lane
St. Louis, Missouri 63043

UNDERSTANDING NURSING RESEARCH: BUILDING
AN EVIDENCE-BASED PRACTICE, EDITION SIX

ISBN: 978-1-4557-7060-1

Executive Content Strategist: Lee Henderson
Content Development Manager: Billie Sharp
Content Development Specialist: Charlene Ketchum
Publishing Services Manager: Deborah L. Vogel
Project Manager: Bridget Healy
Design Direction: Maggie Reid

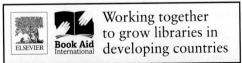

Working together to grow libraries in developing countries

www.elsevier.com • www.bookaid.org

Printed in China

Last digit is the print number: 9 8 7 6 5 4 3 2 1

CONTRIBUTOR

Diane Doran, RN, PhD, FCAHS
Professor Emerita
Lawrence S. Bloomberg Faculty of Nursing
University of Toronto
Toronto, Ontario
Revised Chapter 14

REVIEWERS

Lisa D. Brodersen, EdD, MA, RN
Professor, Coordinator of Institutional Research
    and Effectiveness
Allen College
Waterloo, Iowa

Sara L. Clutter, PhD, RN
Associate Professor of Nursing
Waynesburg University
Waynesburg, Pennsylvania

Jacalyn P. Dougherty, PhD, RN
Nursing Research Consultant
JP Dougherty LLC
Aurora, Colorado

**Joanne T. Ehrmin, RN, COA-CNS, PhD,
    MSN, BSN**
Professor
University of Toledo, College of Nursing
Toledo, Ohio

Betsy Frank, PhD, RN, ANEF
Professor Emerita
Indiana State University College of Nursing
    Health, and Human Services
Terre Haute, Indiana

Tamara Kear, PhD, RN, CNS, CNN
Assistant Professor of Nursing
Villanova University
Villanova, Pennsylvania

Sharon Kitchie, PhD, RN
Adjunct Instructor
Keuka College
Keuka Park, New York

Madelaine Lawrence, PhD, RN
Associate Professor
University of North Carolina at Wilmington
Wilmington, North Carolina

Robin Moyers, PhD, RN-BC
Nurse Educator
Carl Vinson VA Medical Center
Dublin, Georgia

Sue E. Odom, DSN, RN
Professor of Nursing
Clayton State University
Morrow, Georgia

Teresa M. O'Neill, PhD, APRN, RNC
Professor
Our Lady of Holy Cross College
New Orleans, Louisiana

Sandra L. Siedlecki, PhD, RN, CNS
Senior Nurse Scientist
Cleveland Clinic
Cleveland, Ohio

Sharon Souter, PhD, RN, CNE
Dean and Professor
University of Mary Hardin Baylor
Belton, Texas

Molly J. Walker, PhD, RN, CNS, CNE
Professor
Angelo State University
San Angelo, Texas

Cynthia Ward, DNP, RN-BC, CMSRN,
  ACNS-BC
Surgical Clinical Nurse Specialist
Carilion Roanoke Memorial Hospital
Roanoke, Virginia

Angela Wood, PhD, RN, Certified High-Risk
  Prenatal Nurse
Associate Professor and Chair
Department of Nursing
Carson-Newman University
Jefferson City, Tennessee

Fatma A. Youssef, RN, DNSc, MPH
Professor Emerita
Marymount University
School of Health Professions
Arlington, Virginia

To all nurses who change the lives of patients through applying the best research evidence.
—Susan, Jennifer, and Nancy

To my husband Jay Suggs who has provided me endless love and support during my development of research textbooks over the last 30 years.
—Susan

To my husband Randy Gray who is my love and my cheerleader.
—Jennifer

To my husband Jerry who has supported all of my academic endeavors through 58 years of marriage.
—Nancy

PREFACE

Research is a major force in nursing, and the evidence generated from research is constantly changing practice, education, and health policy. Our aim in developing this essentials research text, *Understanding Nursing Research: Building an Evidence-Based Practice*, is to create an excitement about research in undergraduate students. The text emphasizes the importance of baccalaureate-educated nurses being able to read, critically appraise, and synthesize research so this evidence can be used to make changes in practice. A major goal of professional nursing and health care is the delivery of evidence-based care. By making nursing research an integral part of baccalaureate education, we hope to facilitate the movement of research into the mainstream of nursing. We also hope this text increases student awareness of the knowledge that has been generated through nursing research and that this knowledge is relevant to their practice. Only through research can nursing truly be recognized as a profession with documented effective outcomes for the patient, family, nurse provider, and healthcare system. Because of this expanded focus on evidence-based practice (EBP), we have subtitled this edition *Building an Evidence-Based Practice.*

Developing a sixth edition of *Understanding Nursing Research* has provided us with an opportunity to clarify and refine the essential content for an undergraduate research text. The text is designed to assist undergraduate students in overcoming the barriers they frequently encounter in understanding the language used in nursing research. The revisions in this edition are based on our own experiences with the text and input from dedicated reviewers, inquisitive students, and supportive faculty from across the country who provided us with many helpful suggestions.

Chapter 1, Introduction to Nursing Research and Evidence-Based Practice, introduces the reader to nursing research, the history of research, and the significance of research evidence for nursing practice. This chapter has been revised to include the most relevant types of research synthesis being conducted in nursing—systematic review, meta-analysis, meta-synthesis, and mixed-methods systematic review. The discussion of research methodologies and their importance in generating an evidence-based practice for nursing has been updated and expanded to include the exploratory-descriptive qualitative research method. A discussion of the Quality and Safety Education for Nursing (QSEN) competencies and their link to research has been included in this edition. Selected QSEN competencies are linked to the findings from studies presented as examples throughout the text to increase students' understanding of the importance in delivering quality, safe health care to patients and families.

Chapter 2, Introduction to Quantitative Research, presents the steps of the quantitative research process in a concise, clear manner and introduces students to the focus and findings of quantitative studies. Extensive, recent examples of descriptive, correlational, quasi-experimental, and experimental studies are provided, which reflect the quality of current nursing research.

Chapter 3, Introduction to Qualitative Research, describes five approaches to qualitative research and the philosophies upon which they are based. These approaches include phenomenology, grounded theory, ethnography, exploratory-descriptive qualitative, and historical research. Data collection and analysis methods specific to qualitative research are discussed. Guidelines for reading and critically appraising qualitative studies are explained using examples of published studies.

Chapter 4, Examining Ethics in Nursing Research, provides an extensive discussion of the use of ethics in research and the regulations that govern the research process. Detailed content and current websites are provided to promote students' understanding of the Health Insurance Portability and Accountability Act (HIPAA), the U.S. Department of Health and Human Services Protection of Human Subjects, and the Federal Drug Administration regulations. Guidelines are provided to assist students in critically appraising the ethical discussions in published studies and to participate in the ethical review of research in clinical agencies.

Chapter 5, Research Problems, Purposes, and Hypotheses, clarifies the difference between a problem and a purpose. Example problem and purpose statements are included from current qualitative, quantitative, and outcome studies. Detailed guidelines are provided with examples to direct students in critically appraising the problems, purposes, hypotheses, and variables in studies.

Chapter 6, Understanding and Critically Appraising the Literature Review, begins with a description of the content and quality of different types of publications that might be included in a review. Guidelines for critically appraising published literature reviews are explored with a focus on the differences in the purpose and timing of the literature review in quantitative and qualitative studies. The steps for finding appropriate sources, reading publications, and synthesizing information into a logical, cohesive review are presented.

Chapter 7, Understanding Theory and Research Frameworks, briefly describes grand, middle range, physiological, and scientific theories as the bases for study frameworks. The purpose of a research framework is discussed with the acknowledgement that the framework may be implicit. Guidelines for critically appraising the study framework are presented as well. The guidelines are applied to studies with frameworks derived from research findings and from different types of theories.

Chapter 8, Clarifying Quantitative Research Designs, addresses descriptive, correlational, quasi-experimental, and experimental designs and criteria for critically appraising these designs in studies. The major strengths and threats to design validity are summarized in a table and discussed related to current studies. This chapter has been expanded to include an introduction to randomized controlled trials (RCT) and mixed-methods approaches being conducted by nurses.

Chapter 9, Examining Populations and Samples in Research, provides a detailed discussion of the concepts of sampling in research. Different types of sampling methods for both qualitative and quantitative research are described. Guidelines are included for critically appraising the sampling criteria, sampling method, and sample size of quantitative and qualitative studies.

Chapter 10, Clarifying Measurement and Data Collection in Quantitative Research, has been updated to reflect current knowledge about measurement methods used in nursing research. Content has been expanded and uniquely organized to assist students in critically appraising the reliability and validity of scales; precision and accuracy of physiologic measures; and the sensitivity, specificity, and likelihood ratios of diagnostic and screening tests.

Chapter 11, Understanding Statistics in Research, focuses on the theories and concepts of the statistical analysis process and the statistics used to describe variables, examine relationships, predict outcomes, and examine group differences in studies. Guidelines are provided for critically appraising the results and discussion sections of nursing studies. The results from selected studies are critically appraised and presented as examples throughout this chapter.

Chapter 12, Critical Appraisal of Quantitative and Qualitative Research for Nursing Practice, summarizes and builds on the critical appraisal content provided in previous chapters and offers direction for conducting critical appraisals of quantitative and qualitative studies. The guidelines for critically appraising qualitative studies have been significantly revised and simplified. This chapter also includes a current qualitative and quantitative study, and these two studies are critically appraised using the guidelines provided in this chapter.

Chapter 13, Building an Evidence-Based Nursing Practice, has been significantly updated to reflect the current trends in health care to provide evidence-based nursing practice. Detailed guidelines are provided for critically appraising the four common types of research synthesis conducted in nursing (systematic review, meta-analysis, meta-synthesis, and mixed-method systematic review). These guidelines were used to critically appraise current research syntheses to assist students in examining the quality of published research syntheses and the potential use of research evidence in practice. The chapter includes theories to assist nurses and agencies in moving toward EBP. Translational research is introduced as a method for promoting the use of research evidence in practice.

Chapter 14, Introduction to Outcomes Research, was significantly revised by Dr. Diane Doran, one of the leading authorities in the conduct of outcomes research. The goal of this chapter is to increase students' understanding of the impact of outcomes research on nursing and health care. Content and guidelines are provided to assist students in reading and critically appraising the outcomes studies appearing in the nursing literature.

The sixth edition is written and organized to facilitate ease in reading, understanding, and critically appraising studies. The major strengths of the text are as follows:

- State-of-the art coverage of EBP—a topic of vital importance in nursing.
- Balanced coverage of qualitative and quantitative research methodologies.
- Rich and frequent illustration of major points and concepts from the most current nursing research literature from a variety of clinical practice areas.
- Study findings implications for practice and link to QSEN competencies were provided.
- A clear, concise writing style that is consistent among the chapters to facilitate student learning.
- Electronic references and websites that direct the student to an extensive array of information that is important in reading, critically appraising, and using research knowledge in practice.

This sixth edition of *Understanding Nursing Research* is appropriate for use in a variety of undergraduate research courses for both RN and general students because it provides an introduction to quantitative, qualitative, and outcomes research methodologies. This text not only will assist students in reading research literature, critically appraising published studies, and summarizing research evidence to make changes in practice, but it also can serve as a valuable resource for practicing nurses in critically appraising studies and implementing research evidence in their clinical settings.

LEARNING RESOURCES TO ACCOMPANY *UNDERSTANDING NURSING RESEARCH*, 6TH EDITION

The teaching/learning resources to accompany *Understanding Nursing Research* have been expanded for both the instructor and student to allow a maximum level of flexibility in course design and student review.

Evolve Instructor Resources

A comprehensive suite of Instructor Resources is available online at http://evolve.elsevier.com/ Grove/understanding/ and consists of a Test Bank, PowerPoint slides, an Image Collection, Answer

Guidelines for the Appraisal Exercises provided for students, and new TEACH for Nurses Lesson Plans, which replace and enhance the Instructor's Manual provided for previous editions.

Test Bank

The Test Bank consists of approximately 550 NCLEX® Examination–style questions, including approximately 10% of questions in alternate item formats. Each question is coded with the correct answer, a rationale from the textbook, a page cross-reference, and the cognitive level in the new Bloom's Taxonomy (with the cognitive level from the original Bloom's Taxonomy in parentheses). The Test Bank is provided in ExamView and Evolve LMS formats.

PowerPoint Slides

The PowerPoint slide collection contains approximately 800 slides, now including seamlessly integrated Audience Response System Questions, images, and new Unfolding Case Studies. The PowerPoints have been simplified and converted into bulleted-list format (using less narrative). Content details in the slides have been moved as appropriate into the Notes area of the slides. New Unfolding Case Studies focus on practical EBP/PICO questions, such as a nurse on a unit needing to perform a literature search or to identify a systematic review or meta-analysis. Power-Point presentations are fully customizable.

Image Collection

The electronic Image Collection consists of all images from the text. This collection can be used in classroom or online presentations to reinforce student learning.

NEW TEACH for Nurses Lesson Plans

TEACH for Nurses is a robust, customizable, ready-to-use collection of chapter-by-chapter Lesson Plans that provide everything you need to create an engaging and effective course. Each chapter includes the following:
- Objectives
- Teaching Focus
- Key Terms
- Nursing Curriculum Standards
  - QSEN/NLN Competencies
  - Concepts
  - BSN Essentials
- Student Chapter Resources
- Instructor Chapter Resources
- Teaching Strategies
- In-Class/Online Case Study

Evolve Student Resources

The Evolve Student Resources include interactive Review Questions, a Research Article Library consisting of 10 full-text research articles, Critical Appraisal Exercises based on the articles in the Research Article Library, and new Printable Key Points.
- The interactive Review Questions (approximately 25 per chapter) aid the student in reviewing and focusing on the chapter material.

- The Research Article Library is an updated collection of 10 research articles, taken from leading nursing journals.
- The Critical Appraisal Exercises are a collection of application exercises, based on the articles in the Research Article Library, that help students learn to appraise and apply research findings. Answer Guidelines are provided for the instructor.
- New Printable Key Points provide students with a convenient review tool.

Study Guide

The companion Study Guide, written by the authors of the main text, provides both time-tested and innovative exercises for each chapter in *Understanding Nursing Research*, 6th Edition. Included for each chapter are a brief Introduction, a Key Terms exercise, Key Ideas exercises, Making Connections exercises, Exercises in Critical Analysis, and Going Beyond exercises. An integral part of the Study Guide is an appendix of three published research studies, which are referenced throughout. These three recently published nursing studies (two quantitative studies and one qualitative study) can be used in classroom or online discussions, as well as to address the Study Guide questions. The Study Guide provides exercises that target comprehension of concepts used in each chapter. Exercises — including fill-in-the-blank, matching, and multiple-choice questions — encourage students to validate their understanding of the chapter content. Critical Appraisal Activities provide students with opportunities to apply their new research knowledge to evaluate the quantitative and qualitative studies provided in the back of the Study Guide.

New to this edition are the following features: an increased emphasis on evidence-based practice; new Web-Based Activities, an increased emphasis on high-value learning activities, reorganized back-matter for quick reference, and quick-reference printed tabs.

- Increased emphasis on evidence-based practice: This edition of the Study Guide features an expanded focus on evidence-based practice (EBP) to match that of the revised textbook. This focus helps students who are new to nursing research see the value of understanding the research process and applying it to evidence-based nursing practice.
- Web-Based Activities: Each chapter now includes a Web-Based Activity section, to teach students to use the Internet appropriately for scholarly research and EBP.
- Increased high-value learning activities: The use of crossword puzzles has been reduced to allow room for the addition of learning activities with greater learning value.
- Back matter reorganized for quick reference: The "Answers to Study Guide Exercises" has been retitled "Answer Key" and not numbered as an appendix. Each of the three published studies are now separate appendix (three appendices total), rather than a single appendix. This simplifies cross referencing in the body of the Study Guide.
- Quick-reference printed tabs: Quick-reference printed tabs have been added to differentiate the Answer Key and each of the book's three published studies (four tabs total), for improved navigation and usability.

ACKNOWLEDGMENTS

Developing this essentials research text was a 2-year project, and there are many people we would like to thank. We want to extend a very special thank you to Dr. Diane Doran for her revision of Chapter 14 focused on outcomes research. We are very fortunate that she was willing to share her expertise and time so that students might have the most current information about outcomes research.

We want to express our appreciation to the Dean and faculty of The University of Texas at Arlington College of Nursing for their support and encouragement. We also would like to thank other nursing faculty members across the world who are using our book to teach research and have spent valuable time to send us ideas and to identify errors in the text. Special thanks to the students who have read our book and provided honest feedback on its clarity and usefulness to them. We would also like to recognize the excellent reviews of the colleagues, listed on the previous pages, who helped us make important revisions in the text.

In conclusion, we would like to thank the people at Elsevier who helped produce this book. We thank the following individuals who have devoted extensive time to the development of this sixth edition, the instructor's ancillary materials, student study guide, and all of the web-based components. These individuals include: Lee Henderson, Billie Sharp, Charlene Ketchum, Bridget Healy, Jayashree Balasubramaniam, and Vallavan Udayaraj.

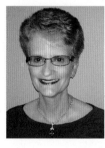 **Susan K. Grove**
PhD, RN, ANP-BC, GNP-BC

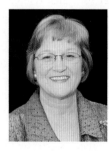 **Jennifer R. Gray**
PhD, RN, FAAN

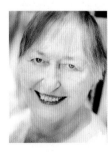 **Nancy Burns**
PhD, RN, FCN, FAAN

Introduction to Nursing Research and Evidence-Based Practice

CHAPTER OVERVIEW

LEARNING OUTCOMES

After completing this chapter, you should be able to:

1. Define research, nursing research, and evidence-based practice.
2. Describe the purposes of research in implementing an evidence-based practice for nursing.
3. Describe the past and present activities influencing research in nursing.
4. Discuss the link of Quality and Safety Education for Nurses (QSEN) to research.

5. Apply the ways of acquiring nursing knowledge (tradition, authority, borrowing, trial and error, personal experience, role modeling, intuition, reasoning, and research) to the interventions implemented in your practice.
6. Identify the common types of research— quantitative, qualitative, or outcomes— conducted to generate essential evidence for nursing practice.

7. Describe the following strategies for synthesizing healthcare research: systematic review, meta-analysis, meta-synthesis, and mixed-methods systematic review.
8. Identify the levels of research evidence available to nurses for practice.
9. Describe the use of evidence-based guidelines in implementing evidence-based practice.
10. Identify your role in research as a professional nurse.

KEY TERMS

Authority, p. 16
Best research evidence, p. 3
Borrowing, p. 16
Case study, p. 11
Clinical expertise, p. 4
Control, p. 8
Critical appraisal of research, p. 27
Deductive reasoning, p. 18
Description, p. 6
Evidence-based guidelines, p. 25
Evidence-based practice (EBP), p. 3

Explanation, p. 7
Gold standard, p. 25
Inductive reasoning, p. 18
Intuition, p. 18
Knowledge, p. 15
Mentorship, p. 18
Meta-analysis, p. 22
Meta-synthesis, p. 23
Mixed-methods systematic review, p. 23
Nursing research, p. 3
Outcomes research, p. 21
Personal experience, p. 17
Prediction, p. 7

Premise, p. 18
Qualitative research, p. 20
Qualitative research synthesis, p. 23
Quality and Safety Education for Nurses (QSEN), p. 15
Quantitative research, p. 19
Reasoning, p. 18
Research, p. 3
Role modeling, p. 17
Systematic review, p. 22
Traditions, p. 16
Trial and error, p. 17

Welcome to the world of nursing research. You may think it strange to consider research a *world*, but it is a truly new way of experiencing reality. Entering a new world means learning a unique language, incorporating new rules, and using new experiences to learn how to interact effectively within that world. As you become a part of this new world, you will modify and expand your perceptions and methods of reasoning. For example, using research to guide your practice involves questioning, and you will be encouraged to ask such questions as these:

• What is the patient's healthcare problem?
• What nursing intervention would effectively manage this problem in your practice?
• Is this nursing intervention based on sound research evidence?
• Would another intervention be more effective in improving your patient's outcomes?
• How can you use research most effectively in promoting an evidence-based practice (EBP)?

Because research is a new world to many of you, we have developed this text to facilitate your entry into and understanding of this world and its contribution to the delivery of quality, safe nursing care. This first chapter clarifies the meaning of nursing research and its significance in developing an evidence-based practice (EBP) for nursing. This chapter also explores the research accomplishments in the profession over the last 160 years. The ways of acquiring knowledge in nursing are discussed, and the common research methodologies used for generating research evidence for practice (quantitative, qualitative, and outcomes research) are introduced. The critical elements of evidence-based nursing practice are introduced, including strategies for synthesizing research evidence, levels of research evidence or knowledge, and evidence-based guidelines. Nurses' roles in research are described based on their level of education and their contributions to the implementation of EBP.

WHAT IS NURSING RESEARCH?

The word research means "to search again" or "to examine carefully." More specifically, research is a diligent, systematic inquiry, or study that validates and refines existing knowledge and develops new knowledge. Diligent, systematic study indicates planning, organization, and persistence. The ultimate goal of research is the development of an empirical body of knowledge for a discipline or profession, such as nursing.

Defining nursing research requires determining the relevant knowledge needed by nurses. Because nursing is a practice profession, research is essential to develop and refine knowledge that nurses can use to improve clinical practice and promote quality outcomes (Brown, 2014; Doran, 2011). Expert researchers have studied many interventions, and clinicians have synthesized these studies to provide guidelines and protocols for use in practice. Practicing nurses and nursing students, like you, need to be able to read research reports and syntheses of research findings to implement evidence-based interventions in practice and promote positive outcomes for patients and families. For example, extensive research has been conducted to determine the most effective technique for administering medications through an intramuscular (IM) injection. This research was synthesized and used to develop evidence-based guidelines for administering IM injections (Cocoman & Murray, 2008; Nicoll & Hesby, 2002).

Nursing research is also needed to generate knowledge about nursing education, nursing administration, healthcare services, characteristics of nurses, and nursing roles. The findings from these studies influence nursing practice indirectly and add to nursing's body of knowledge. Research is needed to provide high-quality learning experiences for nursing students. Through research, nurses can develop and refine the best methods for delivering distance nursing education and for using simulation to improve student learning. Nursing administration and health services studies are needed to improve the quality, safety, and cost-effectiveness of the healthcare delivery system. Studies of nurses and nursing roles can influence nurses' quality of care, productivity, job satisfaction, and retention. In this era of a nursing shortage, additional research is needed to determine effective ways to recruit individuals and retain them in the profession of nursing. This type of research could have a major impact on the quality and number of nurses providing care to patients and families in the future.

In summary, nursing research is a scientific process that validates and refines existing knowledge and generates new knowledge that directly and indirectly influences nursing practice. Nursing research is the key to building an EBP for nursing (Brown, 2014).

WHAT IS EVIDENCE-BASED PRACTICE?

The ultimate goal of nursing is an evidence-based practice that promotes quality, safe, and cost-effective outcomes for patients, families, healthcare providers, and the healthcare system (Brown, 2014; Craig & Smyth, 2012; Melnyk & Fineout-Overholt, 2011). Evidence-based practice (EBP) evolves from the integration of the best research evidence with clinical expertise and patients' needs and values (Institute of Medicine [IOM], 2001; Sackett, Straus, Richardson, Rosenberg, & Haynes, 2000). Figure 1-1 identifies the elements of EBP and demonstrates the major contribution of the best research evidence to the delivery of this practice. The best research evidence is the empirical knowledge generated from the synthesis of quality study findings to address a practice problem. Later, this chapter discusses the strategies used to synthesize research, levels of best research evidence, and sources for this evidence. A team of expert researchers, healthcare professionals, and sometimes policy makers and consumers will synthesize the best research evidence to develop

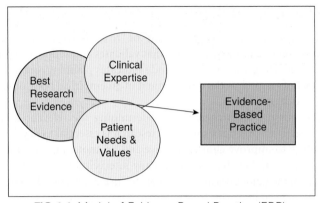

FIG 1-1 Model of Evidence-Based Practice (EBP).

standardized guidelines for clinical practice. For example, a team of experts conducted, critically appraised, and synthesized research related to the chronic health problem of hypertension (HTN) to develop an EBP guideline. Research evidence from this guideline is presented as an example later in this section.

Clinical expertise is the knowledge and skills of the healthcare professional who is providing care. The clinical expertise of a nurse depends on his or her years of clinical experience, current knowledge of the research and clinical literature, and educational preparation. The stronger the nurse's clinical expertise, the better is his or her clinical judgment in using the best research evidence in practice (Brown, 2014; Craig & Smyth, 2012). EBP also incorporates the needs and values of the patient (see Figure 1-1). The patient's need(s) might focus on health promotion, illness prevention, acute or chronic illness management, rehabilitation, and/or a peaceful death. In addition, patients bring values or unique preferences, expectations, concerns, and cultural beliefs to the clinical encounter. With EBP, patients and their families are encouraged to take an active role in the management of their health. It is the unique combination of the best research evidence being applied by expert nurse clinicians in providing quality, safe, and cost-effective care to a patient and family with specific health needs and values that results in EBP.

Extensive research is needed to develop sound empirical knowledge for synthesis into the best research evidence needed for practice. Findings from a single study are not enough evidence for determining the effectiveness of an intervention in practice. Research evidence from multiple studies are synthesized to develop guidelines, standards, protocols, algorithms (clinical decision trees), or policies to direct the implementation of a variety of nursing interventions. As noted earlier, a national guideline has been developed for the management of hypertension, *The Seventh Report of the Joint National Committee on Prevention, Detection, Evaluation, and Treatment of High Blood Pressure* (JNC 7). The complete JNC 7 guideline for the management of high blood pressure is available online at www.nhlbi.nih.gov/guidelines/hypertension (National Heart, Lung, and Blood Institute [NHLBI], 2003). In January of 2014, the American Society of Hypertension (ASH) and the International Society of Hypertension (ISH) published new clinical practice guidelines for the management of hypertension in the community (Weber et al, 2014). The JNC 7 guideline and the ASH and ISH clinical practice guideline identified the same classification system for blood pressure (Table 1-1). These guidelines include the classification of blood pressure as normal, prehypertension, hypertension stage 1, and hypertension stage 2. Both guidelines also recommend

TABLE 1-1 CLASSIFICATION OF BLOOD PRESSURE WITH NURSING INTERVENTIONS FOR EVIDENCE-BASED PRACTICE (EBP)				
CLASSIFICATION OF BLOOD PRESSURE (BP)			**NURSING INTERVENTIONS**[†]	
BP CATEGORY	**SYSTOLIC BP (mm Hg)***	**DIASTOLIC BP (mm Hg)***	**LIFESTYLE MODIFICATION**[‡]	**CARDIOVASCULAR DISEASE (CVD) RISK FACTORS EDUCATION**[§]
Normal	<120 *and*	<80	Encourage	Yes
Prehypertension	120-139 *or*	80-89	Yes	Yes
Stage 1 hypertension	140-159 *or*	90-99	Yes	Yes
Stage 2 hypertension	<160 *or*	<100	Yes	Yes

*Treatment is determined by the highest BP category, systolic or diastolic.
[†]Treat patients with chronic kidney disease or diabetes to BP goal of <130/80 mm Hg.
[‡]Lifestyle modification—balanced diet, exercise program, normal weight, and nonsmoker.
[§]CVD risk factors—hypertension; obesity (body mass index $\geq$ 30 kg/m^2), dyslipidemia, diabetes mellitus, cigarette smoking, physical inactivity, microalbuminuria, estimated glomerular filtration rate <60 mL/min, age (>55 years for men, >65 years for women), and family history of premature CVD (men <55 years, women <65 years).
Adapted from National Heart, Lung, and Blood Institute. (2003). *The seventh report of the Joint National Committee on Prevention, Detection, Evaluation, and Treatment of High Blood Pressure (JNC 7)*. Retrieved June 18, 2013 from, www.nhlbi. nih.gov/guidelines/hypertension/; and Weber, M. A., Schiffrin, E. L., White, W. B., Mann, S., Lindholm, L. H., Kenerson, J. G., et al. (2014). Clinical practice guidelines for the management of hypertension in the community: A statement by the American Society of Hypertension and the International Society of Hypertension. *Journal of Hypertension, 32*(1), 4-5.

life style modifications (balanced diet, exercise program, normal weight, and nonsmoker) and cardiovascular disease (CVD) risk factors (hypertension, obesity, dyslipidemia, diabetes mellitus, cigarette smoking, physical inactivity, microalbuminuria, and family history of premature CVD) education. You need to use an evidence-based guideline in monitoring your patients' blood pressure (BP) and educating them about lifestyle modifications to improve their BP and reduce their CVD risk factors (NHLBI, 2003; Weber et al., 2014).

The Eighth Joint National Committee (JNC 8) published "2014 Evidence-Based Guideline for the Management of High Blood Pressure in Adults" in December of 2013 (James et al. 2013). However, these guidelines currently lack the recognition of any national organization. Additional work is needed to ensure that the guidelines are approved by the NHLBI, ASH, the American Heart Association (AHA), and/or the American College of Cardiology (ACC). For this textbook, the evidence-based guidelines for management of hypertension presented in Table 1-1 are recommended for students and nurses to use in caring for their patients (Weber et al., 2014).

Figure 1-2 provides an example of the delivery of evidence-based nursing care to African American women with high BP. In this example, the best research evidence is classification of BP and education on lifestyle modification (LSM) and CVD risk factors based on the ASH (Weber et al., 2014) and JNC 7 (NHLBI, 2003) guidelines for management of high BP (see Table 1-1). These guidelines, developed from the best research evidence related to BP, LSM, and CVD risks monitoring and education, is translated by registered nurses and nursing students to meet the needs and values of African American women with high BP. The quality outcome of EBP in this example is women with a BP less than 140/90 mm Hg or referral for medication treatment (see Figure 1-2). A detailed discussion of how to locate, critically appraise, and use national standardized guidelines in practice is found in Chapter 13.

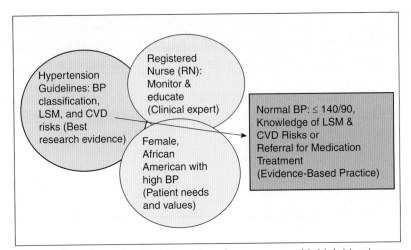

FIG 1-2 Evidence-based practice for African American women with high blood pressure (BP).

PURPOSES OF RESEARCH FOR IMPLEMENTING AN EVIDENCE-BASED NURSING PRACTICE

Through nursing research, empirical knowledge can be developed to improve nursing care, patient outcomes, and the healthcare delivery system. For example, nurses need a solid research base to implement and document the effectiveness of selected nursing interventions in treating particular patient problems and promoting positive patient and family outcomes. Also, nurses need to use research findings to determine the best way to deliver healthcare services to ensure that the greatest number of people receive quality, safe care. Accomplishing these goals will require you to locate EBP guidelines or to appraise critically, synthesize, and apply research evidence that provides a description, explanation, prediction, and control of phenomena in your clinical practice.

Description

Description involves identifying and understanding the nature of nursing phenomena and, sometimes, the relationships among them (Chinn & Kramer, 2011). Through research, nurses are able to (1) describe what exists in nursing practice; (2) discover new information; (3) promote understanding of situations; and (4) classify information for use in the discipline. Some examples of clinically important research evidence that have been developed from research focused on description include:

- Identification of the incidence and spread of infection in healthcare agencies
- Identification of the cluster of symptoms for a particular disease
- Description of the responses of individuals to a variety of health conditions and aging
- Description of the health promotion and illness prevention strategies used by a variety of populations
- Determination of the incidence of a disease locally (e.g., incidence of West Nile virus in Texas), nationally, and internationally (e.g., spread of bird flu).

Rush, Watts, and Janke (2013, p. 10) have conducted a qualitative study to describe "rural and urban older adults' perspectives of strength in their daily lives." (The types of research conducted in nursing—quantitative, qualitative, and outcomes—are discussed later in this chapter.) They noted the following in this study:

> "Nurses' strength enhancement efforts should raise older adults' awareness that strength is not an unlimited resource but needs to be constantly replenished.... Older adult participants described changes in strength that ranged from fluctuating daily changes to insidious, gradual declines and to drastic and unexpected losses.... Older adults' strategies for staying strong were consistent with their more holistic views of strength but may not be approaches nurses typically take into account. Although nurses need to give continued emphasis to promoting physical activity, they must also give equal attention to encouraging mental and social activities because of the important role they play for older adults staying strong." Rush et al., 2013, p. 15

The findings from this study provided nurses with descriptions of older adults' perspectives of strength and the strategies that they use to stay strong. You can use the findings from this study to encourage physical, mental, and social activities to assist older adults in staying strong. This type of research, focused on description, is essential groundwork for studies to provide explanations, predictions, and control of nursing phenomena in practice.

Explanation

Explanation clarifies the relationships among phenomena and identifies possible reasons why certain events occur. Research focused on explanation provides the following types of evidence essential for practice:
- Determination of assessment data (subjective data from the health history and objective data from the physical examination) that need to be gathered to address a patient's health need
- The link of assessment data to a diagnosis
- The link of causative risk factors or causes to illness, morbidity, and mortality
- Determination of the relationships among health risks, health behaviors, and health status
- Determination of links among demographic characteristics, disease status, psychosocial factors, and patients' responses to treatment.

For example, Manojlovich, Sidani, Covell, and Antonakos (2011) conducted an outcomes study to examine the links or relationships between a "nurse dose" (nurse characteristics and staffing) and adverse patient outcomes. The nurse characteristics examined were education, experience, and skill mix. The staffing variables included full-time employees, registered nurse (RN)-to-patient ratio, and RN hours per patient day. The adverse outcomes examined were methicillin-resistant *Staphylococcus aureus* (MRSA) infections and reported patient falls for a sample of inpatient adults in acute care units. The researchers found that the nurse characteristics and staffing variables were significantly correlated with MRSA infections and reported patient falls. Therefore the nursing characteristics and staffing were potential predictors of the incidence of MRSA infections and patient falls. This study illustrates how explanatory research can identify relationships among nursing phenomena that can be the basis for future research focused on prediction and control.

Prediction

Through prediction, one can estimate the probability of a specific outcome in a given situation (Chinn & Kramer, 2011). However, predicting an outcome does not necessarily enable one to modify or control the outcome. It is through prediction that the risk of illness or injury is identified and linked to possible screening methods to identify and prevent health problems. Knowledge generated from research focused on prediction is critical for EBP and includes the following:
- Prediction of the risk for a disease or injury in different populations
- Prediction of behaviors that promote health and prevent illness
- Prediction of the health care required based on a patient's need and values

Lee, Faucett, Gillen, Krause, and Landry (2013) conducted a quantitative study to examine the factors that were perceived by critical care nurses (CCNs) to predict the risk of musculoskeletal (MSK) injury from work. They found that greater physical workload, greater job strain, more frequent patient-handling tasks, and lack of a lifting team or devices were predictive of the CCNs' perceptions of risk of MSK injury. They recommended that "occupational health professionals, nurse managers, and nursing organizations should make concerted efforts to ensure the safety of nurses by providing effective preventive measures. Improving the physical and psychosocial work environment may make nursing jobs safer, reduce the risk of MSK injury, and improve nurses' perceptions of job safety" (Lee et al., 2013, p. 43). This predictive study isolated independent variables (physical workload, job strain, patient-handling tasks, and lack of lifting devices or teams) that were predictive of MSK injuries in CCNs. The variables identified in predictive studies require additional research to ensure that their manipulation or control results in quality outcomes for patients, healthcare professionals, and healthcare agencies (Creswell, 2014; Doran, 2011; Kerlinger & Lee, 2000).

Control

If one can predict the outcome of a situation, the next step is to control or manipulate the situation to produce the desired outcome. In health care, control is the ability to write a prescription to produce the desired results. Using the best research evidence, nurses could prescribe specific interventions to meet the needs of patients and their families (Brown, 2014; Craig & Smyth, 2012). The results of multiple studies in the following areas have enabled nurses to deliver care that increases the control over the outcomes desired for practice:

- Testing interventions to improve the health status of individuals, families, and communities
- Testing interventions to improve healthcare delivery
- Synthesis of research for development into EBP guidelines
- Testing the effectiveness of EBP guideline in clinical agencies

Extensive research has been conducted in the area of safe administration of IM injections. This research has been critically appraised, synthesized, and developed into evidence-based guidelines to direct the administration of medications by an IM route to infants, children, and adults in a variety of practice settings (Cocoman & Murray, 2008; Nicoll & Hesby, 2002). The EBP guideline for IM injections is based on the best research evidence and identifies the appropriate needle size and length to use for administering different types of medications, the safest injection site (ventrogluteal) for many medications, and the best injection technique to deliver a medication, minimize patient discomfort, and prevent physical damage (Cocoman & Murray, 2008; Greenway, 2004; Nicoll & Hesby, 2002; Rodger & King, 2000). Using the evidence-based knowledge for administering IM injections helps control the achievement of the following outcomes in practice: (1) adequate administration of medication to promote patient health; (2) minimal patient discomfort; and (3) no physical damage to the patient.

Broadly, the nursing profession is accountable to society for providing quality, safe, and cost-effective care for patients and families. Therefore the care provided by nurses must be constantly evaluated and improved on the basis of new and refined research knowledge. Studies that document the effectiveness of specific nursing interventions make it possible to implement evidence-based care that will produce the best outcomes for patients and their families. The quality of research conducted in nursing affects not only the quality of care delivered, but also the power of nurses in making decisions about the healthcare delivery system. The extensive number of clinical studies conducted in the last 50 years has greatly expanded the scientific knowledge available to you for describing, explaining, predicting, and controlling phenomena within your nursing practice.

HISTORICAL DEVELOPMENT OF RESEARCH IN NURSING

The development of research in nursing has changed drastically over the last 160 years and holds great promise for the twenty-first century. Initially, nursing research evolved slowly, from the investigations of Nightingale in the nineteenth century to the studies of nursing education in the 1930s and 1940s and the research of nurses and nursing roles in the 1950s and 1960s. From the 1970s through the 2010s, an increasing number of nursing studies that focused on clinical problems have produced findings that directly affected practice. Clinical research continues to be a major focus today, with the goal of developing an EBP for nursing. Reviewing the history of nursing research enables you to identify the accomplishments and understand the need for further research to determine the best research evidence for use in practice. Table 1-2 outlines the key historical events that have influenced the development of research in nursing.

TABLE 1-2 HISTORICAL EVENTS INFLUENCING THE DEVELOPMENT OF RESEARCH IN NURSING

YEAR	EVENT
1850	Florence Nightingale is recognized as the first nurse researcher.
1900	*American Journal of Nursing* is published.
1923	Teachers College at Columbia University offers the first educational doctoral program for nurses.
1929	First Master's in Nursing Degree is offered at Yale University.
1932	Association of Collegiate Schools of Nursing is organized to promote conduct of research.
1950	American Nurses Association (ANA) publishes study of nursing functions and activities.
1952	First research journal in nursing, *Nursing Research,* is published.
1953	Institute of Research and Service in Nursing Education is established.
1955	American Nurses Foundation is established to fund nursing research.
1957	Southern Regional Educational Board (SREB), Western Interstate Commission on Higher Education (WICHE), Midwestern Nursing Research Society (MNRS), and New England Board of Higher Education (NEBHE) are established to support and disseminate nursing research.
1963	*International Journal of Nursing Studies* is published.
1965	ANA sponsors the first nursing research conferences.
1967	Sigma Theta Tau International Honor Society of Nursing publishes *Image,* emphasizing nursing scholarship; now *Journal of Nursing Scholarship.*
1970	ANA Commission on Nursing Research is established.
1972	Cochrane published *Effectiveness and Efficiency,* introducing concepts relevant to evidence-based practice (EBP). ANA Council of Nurse Researchers is established.
1973	First Nursing Diagnosis Conference is held, which evolved into North American Nursing Diagnosis Association (NANDA).
1976	Stetler/Marram Model for Application of Research Findings to Practice is published.
1978	*Research in Nursing & Health* and *Advances in Nursing Science* are published.
1979	*Western Journal of Nursing Research* is published.
1980s-1990s	Sackett and colleagues developed methodologies to determine "best evidence" for practice.
1982-1983	Conduct and Utilization of Research in Nursing (CURN) Project is published.
1983	*Annual Review of Nursing Research* is published.

Continued

TABLE 1-2   HISTORICAL EVENTS INFLUENCING THE DEVELOPMENT OF RESEARCH IN NURSING—cont'd

YEAR	EVENT
1985	National Center for Nursing Research (NCNR) is established to support and fund nursing research.
1987	*Scholarly Inquiry for Nursing Practice* is published.
1988	*Applied Nursing Research* and *Nursing Science Quarterly* are published.
1989	Agency for Healthcare Policy and Research (AHCPR) is established and publishes EBP guidelines.
1990	*Nursing Diagnosis,* official journal of NANDA, is published; now *International Journal of Nursing Terminologies and Classifications.*
	ANA established the American Nurses Credentialing Center (ANCC), which implemented the Magnet Hospital Designation Program for Excellence in Nursing Services.
1992	*Healthy People 2000* is published by U.S. Department of Health and Human Services (U.S. DHHS).
	Clinical Nursing Research is published.
1993	NCNR is renamed the National Institute of Nursing Research (NINR) to expand funding for nursing research.
	Journal of Nursing Measurement is published.
	Cochrane Collaboration is initiated, providing systematic reviews and EBP guidelines (http://www.cochrane.org).
1994	*Qualitative Health Research* is published.
1999	AHCPR is renamed Agency for Healthcare Research and Quality (AHRQ).
2000	*Healthy People 2010* is published by U.S. DHHS.
	Biological Research for Nursing is published.
2001	Stetler publishes her model *Steps of Research Utilization to Facilitate Evidence-Based Practice.*
	Institute of Medicine (IOM) report *Crossing the Quality Chasm: A New Health System for the 21st Century* published, focusing on key healthcare issues of quality and safety.
2002	The Joint Commission revises accreditation policies for hospitals supporting evidence-based health care.
	NANDA becomes international—NANDA-I.
2003	IOM report *Health Professions Education: A Bridge to Quality* published, identifying six competencies essential for education of nurses and other health professionals.
2004	*Worldviews on Evidence-Based Nursing* is published.
2005	Quality and Safety Education for Nurses (QSEN) initiative for development of competencies for prelicensure and graduate education is developed.
2006	American Association of Colleges of Nursing (AACN) position statement on nursing research is published.
2007	QSEN website (http://qsen.org) is launched, featuring teaching strategies and resources to facilitate the attainment of the QSEN competencies.
2010	IOM report *The Future of Nursing: Leading Change* recommends that 80% of the nursing workforce be prepared at the baccalaureate level by the year 2020.
2011	NINR current strategic plan published.
	American Nurses Association (ANA) current research agenda is developed.
2013	Current QSEN competencies for prelicensure nurses available online at http://qsen.org/competencies/pre-licensure-ksas.
2013	*Healthy People 2020* available at U.S. DHHS website, http://www.healthypeople.gov/2020/topicsobjectives2020/default.aspx.
	AHRQ current mission and funding priorities available online (http://www.ahrq.gov/).
	NINR current mission and funding opportunities available online (http://www.ninr.nih.gov/).

Florence Nightingale

Nightingale (1859) is recognized as the first nurse researcher, with her initial studies focused on the importance of a healthy environment in promoting patients' physical and mental well-being. She studied aspects of the environment, such as ventilation, cleanliness, purity of water, and diet, to determine the influence on patients' health, which continue to be important areas of study today (Herbert, 1981). Nightingale is also noted for her data collection and statistical analyses, especially during the Crimean War. She gathered data on soldier morbidity and mortality rates and the factors influencing them and presented her results in tables and pie charts, a sophisticated type of data presentation for the period (Palmer, 1977). Nightingale was the first woman elected to the Royal Statistical Society (Oakley, 2010) and her research was highlighted in *Scientific American* (Cohen, 1984).

Nightingale's research enabled her to instigate attitudinal, organizational, and social changes. She changed the attitudes of the military and society about the care of the sick. The military began to view the sick as having the right to adequate food, suitable quarters, and appropriate medical treatment, which greatly reduced the mortality rate (Cook, 1913). Nightingale improved the organization of army administration, hospital management, and hospital construction. Because of Nightingale's research evidence and influence, society began to accept responsibility for testing public water, improving sanitation, preventing starvation, and decreasing morbidity and mortality rates (Palmer, 1977).

Nursing Research: 1900s through the 1970s

The *American Journal of Nursing* was first published in 1900 and, late in the 1920s and 1930s, case studies began appearing in this journal. A case study involves an in-depth analysis and systematic description of one patient or group of similar patients to promote understanding of healthcare interventions. Case studies are one example of the practice-related research that has been conducted in nursing over the last century.

Nursing educational opportunities expanded, with Teachers College at Columbia University offering the first educational doctoral program for nurses in 1923 and Yale University offering the first master's degree in nursing in 1929. In 1950 the American Nurses Association (ANA) initiated a 5-year study on nursing functions and activities. In 1959 the findings from this study were used to develop statements on functions, standards, and qualifications for professional nurses. During that time, clinical research began expanding as nursing specialty groups, such as community health, psychiatric-mental health, medical-surgical, pediatrics, and obstetrics, developed standards of care. The research conducted by the ANA and specialty groups provided the basis for the nursing practice standards that currently guide professional practice (Gortner & Nahm, 1977).

In the 1950s and 1960s nursing schools began introducing research and the steps of the research process at the baccalaureate level, and Master of Science in Nursing (MSN) level nurses were provided a background for conducting small replication studies. In 1953 the Institute for Research and Service in Nursing Education was established at Teachers College of Columbia University and began providing research experiences for doctoral students (Gortner & Nahm, 1977). The increase in research activities prompted the publication of the first research journal, *Nursing Research*, in 1952. The American Nurses Foundation was established in 1955 to fund nursing research projects. The Southern Regional Educational Board (SREB), Western Interstate Commission on Higher Education (WICHE), Midwestern Nursing Research Society (MNRS), and New England Board of Higher Education (NEBHE) were formed in 1957 to support and disseminate nursing research across the United States.

In the 1960s an increasing number of clinical studies focused on quality care and the development of criteria to measure patient outcomes. Intensive care units were developed, which promoted the investigation of nursing interventions, staffing patterns, and cost-effectiveness of care (Gortner & Nahm, 1977). An additional research journal, the *International Journal of Nursing Studies,* was published in 1963. In 1965 the ANA sponsored the first of a series of nursing research conferences to promote the communication of research findings and the use of these findings in clinical practice.

In the late 1960s and 1970s nurses were involved in the development of models, conceptual frameworks, and theories to guide nursing practice. The nursing theorists' work provided direction for future nursing research. In 1978, Chinn became the editor of a new journal, *Advances in Nursing Science,* which included nursing theorists' work and related research. Another event influencing research was the establishment of the ANA Commission on Nursing Research in 1970. In 1972 the commission established the Council of Nurse Researchers to advance research activities, provide an exchange of ideas, and recognize excellence in research. The commission also influenced the development of federal guidelines for research with human subjects and sponsored research programs nationally and internationally (See, 1977).

The communication of research findings was a major issue in the 1970s (Barnard, 1980). Sigma Theta Tau International, the Honor Society for Nursing, sponsored national and international research conferences, and chapters of this organization sponsored many local conferences to communicate research findings. Sigma Theta Tau first published *Image,* now entitled *Journal of Nursing Scholarship,* in 1967; it includes research articles and summaries of research conducted on selected topics. Stetler and Marram developed the first model in nursing to promote the application of research findings to practice in 1976. Two additional research journals were first published in the 1970s, *Research in Nursing & Health* in 1978 and the *Western Journal of Nursing Research* in 1979.

Professor Archie Cochrane originated the concept of evidence-based practice with a book he published in 1972, *Effectiveness and Efficiency: Random Reflections on Health Services.* Cochrane advocated the provision of health care based on research to improve its quality. To facilitate the use of research evidence in practice, the Cochrane Center was established in 1992 and the Cochrane Collaboration in 1993. The Cochrane Collaboration and Library house numerous resources to promote EBP, such as systematic reviews of research and evidence-based guidelines for practice (see later; also see the Cochrane Collaboration at http://www.cochrane.org).

In the 1970s the nursing process became the focus of many studies, with investigations of assessment techniques, nursing diagnoses classification, goal-setting methods, and specific nursing interventions. The first Nursing Diagnosis Conference, held in 1973, evolved into the North American Nursing Diagnosis Association (NANDA). In 2002 NANDA became international, known as NANDA-I. NANDA-I supports research activities focused on identifying appropriate diagnoses for nursing and generating an effective diagnostic process. NANDA's journal, *Nursing Diagnosis,* was published in 1990 and was later renamed the *International Journal of Nursing Terminologies and Classifications.* Details on NANDA-I can be found on their website (http://www.nanda.org).

Nursing Research: 1980s and 1990s

The conduct of clinical research was the focus of the 1980s, and clinical journals began publishing more studies. One new research journal was published in 1987, *Scholarly Inquiry for Nursing Practice,* and two in 1988, *Applied Nursing Research* and *Nursing Science Quarterly.* Although the body of empirical knowledge generated through clinical research increased rapidly in the 1980s, little of this knowledge was used in practice. During 1982 and 1983, the studies from a federally funded project, Conduct and Utilization of Research in Nursing (CURN), were published to facilitate the use of research to improve practice (Horsley, Crane, Crabtree, & Wood, 1983).

In 1983 the first volume of the *Annual Review of Nursing Research* was published (Werley & Fitzpatrick, 1983). These volumes include experts' reviews of research organized into four areas—nursing practice, nursing care delivery, nursing education, and the nursing profession. These summaries of current research knowledge encourage the use of research findings in practice and provide direction for future research. Publication of the *Annual Review of Nursing Research* continues today, with leading expert nurse scientists providing summaries of research in their areas of expertise. The increased research activities in nursing resulted in the publication of *Clinical Nursing Research* in 1992 and the *Journal of Nursing Measurement* in 1993.

Qualitative research was introduced in the late 1970s; the first studies appeared in nursing journals in the 1980s. The focus of qualitative research was holistic, with the intent to discover meaning and gain new insight and understanding of issues relevant to nursing. The number of qualitative researchers and studies expanded greatly in the 1990s, with qualitative studies appearing in most of the nursing research and clinical journals. In 1994 a journal focused on disseminating qualitative research, *Qualitative Health Research,* was first published.

Another priority of the 1980s was to obtain increased funding for nursing research. Most of the federal funds in the 1980s were designated for medical studies involving the diagnosis and treatment of diseases. However, the ANA achieved a major political victory for nursing research with the creation of the National Center for Nursing Research (NCNR) in 1985. The purpose of this center was to support the conduct and dissemination of knowledge developed through basic and clinical nursing research, training, and other programs in patient care research (Bauknecht, 1985). Under the direction of Dr. Ada Sue Hinshaw, the NCNR became the National Institute of Nursing Research (NINR) in 1993 to increase the status of nursing research and obtain more funding.

Outcomes research emerged as an important methodology for documenting the effectiveness of healthcare services in the 1980s and 1990s. This effectiveness research evolved from the quality assessment and quality assurance functions that originated with the professional standards review organizations (PSROs) in 1972. In 1989 the Agency for Healthcare Policy and Research (AHCPR) was established to facilitate the conduct of outcomes research (Rettig, 1991). AHCPR also had an active role in communicating research findings to healthcare practitioners and was responsible for publishing the first clinical practice guidelines. These guidelines included a synthesis of the best research evidence, with directives for practice developed by healthcare experts in various areas. Several of these evidence-based guidelines were published in the 1990s and provided standards for practice in nursing and medicine. The Healthcare Research and Quality Act of 1999 reauthorized the AHCPR, changing its name to the Agency for Healthcare Research and Quality (AHRQ). This significant change positioned the AHRQ as a scientific partner with the public and private sectors to improve the quality and safety of patient care.

Building on the process of research utilization, physicians, nurses, and other healthcare professionals focused on the development of EBP for health care during the 1990s. A research group led by Dr. David Sackett at McMaster University in Canada developed explicit research methodologies to determine the "best evidence" for practice. David Eddy first used the term *evidence-based* in 1990, with the focus on providing EBP for medicine (Craig & Smyth, 2012; Sackett et al., 2000). The American Nurses Credentialing Center (ANCC) implemented the Magnet Hospital Designation Program for Excellence in Nursing Services in 1990, which emphasized EBP for nursing. The emphasis on EBP in nursing resulted in more biological studies and randomized controlled trials (RCTs) being conducted and led to the publication of *Biological Research for Nursing* in 2000.

Nursing Research: in the Twenty-First Century

The vision for nursing research in the twenty-first century includes conducting quality studies using a variety of methodologies, synthesizing the study findings into the best research evidence, and using this research evidence to guide practice (Brown, 2014; Craig & Smyth, 2012; Melnyk & Fineout-Overholt, 2011). EBP has become a stronger focus in nursing and healthcare agencies over the last 15 years. In 2002, The Joint Commission (formerly called the Joint Commission on Accreditation of Healthcare Organizations), responsible for accrediting healthcare organizations, revised the accreditation policies for hospitals to support the implementation of evidence-based health care. To facilitate the movement of nursing toward EBP in clinical agencies, Stetler (2001) developed her Research Utilization to Facilitate EBP Model (see Chapter 13 for a description of this model). The focus on EBP in nursing was supported with the initiation of the *Worldviews on Evidence-Based Nursing* journal in 2004.

The American Association of Colleges of Nursing (AACN), established in 1932 to promote the quality of nursing education, revised their position statement on nursing research in 2006 to provide future directions for the discipline. To ensure an effective research enterprise in nursing, the discipline must (1) create a research culture, (2) provide high-quality educational programs (baccalaureate, master's, practice-focused doctorate, research-focused doctorate, and postdoctorate) to prepare a workforce of nurse scientists, (3) develop a sound research infrastructure, and (4) obtain sufficient funding for essential research (AACN, 2006). The complete AACN position statement on nursing research can be found online at http://www.aacn.nche.edu/publications/position/nursing-research. In 2011 the ANA published a research agenda compatible with the AACN (2006) research position statement.

The focus of healthcare research and funding has expanded from the treatment of illness to include health promotion and illness prevention. *Healthy People 2000* and *Healthy People 2010*, documents published by the U.S. Department of Health and Human Services (U.S. DHHS, 2000), have increased the visibility of health promotion goals and research. *Healthy People 2020* information is now available at the U.S. DHHS (2013) website http://www.healthypeople.gov/2020/. Some of the new topics covered by *Healthy People 2020* include adolescent health, blood disorders and blood safety, dementias (including Alzheimer's Disease), early and middle childhood, genomics, global health, healthcare-associated infections, lesbian, gay, bisexual, and transgender health, older adults, preparedness, sleep health, and social determinants of health. In the next decade, nurse researchers will have a major role in the development of interventions to promote health and prevent illness in individuals, families, and communities.

The AHRQ is the lead agency supporting research designed to improve the quality of health care, reduce its cost, improve patient safety, decrease medical errors, and broaden access to essential services. AHRQ (2013) conducts and sponsors research that provides evidence-based information on healthcare outcomes, quality, cost, use, and access. This research information is needed to promote effective healthcare decision making by patients, clinicians, health system executives, and policy makers. The AHRQ (2013) website (http://www.ahrq.gov) provides the most current information on this agency and includes current guidelines for clinical practice.

Current Actions of the National Institute of Nursing Research

The mission of the National Institute of Nursing Research (NINR) is to "promote and improve the health of individuals, families, communities, and populations. The Institute supports and conducts clinical and basic research and research training on health and illness across the lifespan to build the scientific foundation for clinical practice, prevent disease and disability, manage and eliminate symptoms caused by illness, and improve palliative and end-of-life care"

(NINR, 2013). The NINR is seeking expanded funding for nursing research and is encouraging a variety of methodologies (quantitative, qualitative, and outcomes research) to be used to generate essential knowledge for nursing practice. The NINR (2013) website (http://ninr.nih.gov) provides the most current information on the institute's research funding opportunities and supported studies. The strategic plan for the NINR (2011) is available online at https://www.ninr.nih.gov/sites/www.ninr.nih.gov/files/ninr-strategic-plan-2011.pdf.

Linking Quality and Safety Education for Nursing Competencies and Nursing Research

In 2001 the Institute of Medicine (IOM) published a report, *Crossing the Quality Chasm: A New Health System for the 21st Century,* that emphasized the importance of quality and safety in the delivery of health care. In 2003 the IOM published a report, *Health Professions Education: A Bridge to Quality,* which identified the six competency areas essential for inclusion in nursing education to ensure that students were able to deliver quality, safe care. Specific competencies were identified for the following six areas: patient-centered care, teamwork and collaboration, evidence-based practice, quality improvement, safety, and informatics. The Quality and Safety Education for Nurses (QSEN) initiative is focused on developing the requisite knowledge, skills, and attitude (KSA) statements for each of the competencies for pre-licensure and graduate education. The QSEN initiative has been funded since 2005 by the Robert Wood Johnson Foundation.

The QSEN Institute website (http://qsen.org), launched in 2007, features teaching strategies and resources to facilitate the accomplishments of the QSEN competencies in nursing educational programs. The most current competencies for the prelicensure educational programs can be found online at http://qsen.org/competencies/pre-licenrue-ksas (QSEN, 2013; Sherwood & Barnsteiner, 2012). The EBP competency is defined as "integrating the best current evidence with clinical expertise and patient/family preferences and values for delivery of optimal health care" (QSEN, 2013). Undergraduate nursing students need to be skilled in critical appraisal of studies, use of appropriate research evidence in practice, adherence to institutional review board (IRB) guidelines, and appropriate data collection. Diffusion of the QSEN competencies across nursing educational programs is a major focus for educators who are shaping students' learning experiences and outcomes based on these competencies (Barnsteiner, Disch, Johnson, McGuinn, Chappell, & Swartwout, 2013). In this text, the QSEN competencies are linked to relevant research content and the findings from selected studies. Your expanded knowledge of research is an important part of your developing an EBP and is necessary to attain the QSEN competencies.

ACQUIRING KNOWLEDGE IN NURSING

Acquiring knowledge in nursing is essential for the delivery of quality, safe patient and family nursing care. Some key questions about knowledge include the following: What is knowledge? How is knowledge acquired in nursing? Is most of nursing's knowledge based on research?

Knowledge is essential information, acquired in a variety of ways, that is expected to be an accurate reflection of reality and is incorporated and used to direct a person's actions (Kaplan, 1964). During your nursing education, you acquire an extensive amount of knowledge from your classroom and clinical experiences. You learn to synthesize, incorporate, and apply this knowledge so that you can practice as a nurse.

The quality of your nursing practice depends on the quality of the knowledge that you acquire. Therefore you need to question the quality and credibility of new information that you hear or read. For example, what are the sources of knowledge that you are acquiring during your nursing education? Are the nursing interventions taught based more on research or tradition? Which interventions are based on research, and which need further study to determine their effectiveness?

Nursing has historically acquired knowledge through traditions, authority, borrowing, trial and error, personal experience, role modeling, intuition, and reasoning. However, in the last 20 years, most nursing texts include content that is based on research evidence, and most faculty members support their lectures and educational strategies with study findings. This section introduces different ways of acquiring knowledge in nursing.

Traditions

Traditions include "truths" or beliefs based on customs and trends. Nursing traditions from the past have been transferred to the present by written and oral communication and role modeling, and they continue to influence the practice of nursing. For example, some of the policy and procedure manuals in hospitals contain traditional ideas. Traditions can positively influence nursing practice because they were developed from effective past experiences. However, traditions also can narrow and limit the knowledge sought for nursing practice. For example, nursing units are frequently organized and run according to set rules or traditions that may not be efficient or effective. Often these traditions are neither questioned nor changed because they have existed for years and are frequently supported by those with power and authority. Nursing's body of knowledge needs to be more evidence-based than traditional if nurses are to have a powerful impact on patient outcomes.

Authority

An authority is a person with expertise and power who is able to influence opinion and behavior. A person is given authority because it is thought that she or he knows more in a given area than others. Knowledge acquired from an authority is illustrated when one person credits another as the source of information. Nurses who publish articles and books or develop theories are frequently considered authorities. Students usually view their instructors as authorities, and clinical nursing experts are considered authorities within the clinical practice setting. It is important that nurses with authority teach and practice based on research evidence versus being based on customs and traditions.

Borrowing

Some nursing leaders have described part of nursing's knowledge as information borrowed from disciplines such as medicine, sociology, psychology, physiology, and education (McMurrey, 1982). Borrowing in nursing involves the appropriation and use of knowledge from other fields or disciplines to guide nursing practice. Nursing has borrowed in two ways. For years, some nurses have taken information from other disciplines and applied it directly to nursing practice. This information was not integrated within the unique focus of nursing. For example, some nurses have used the medical model to guide their nursing practice, thus focusing on the diagnosis and treatment of disease. This type of borrowing continues today as nurses use advances in technology to become highly specialized and focused on the detection and treatment of disease. The second way of borrowing, which is more useful in nursing, involves integrating information from other disciplines within the focus of nursing. For example, nurses borrow knowledge from other disciplines such as psychology and sociology, but integrate this knowledge in their holistic care of patients and families experiencing acute and chronic illnesses.

Trial and Error

Trial and error is an approach with unknown outcomes that is used in a situation of uncertainty in which other sources of knowledge are unavailable. Because each patient responds uniquely to a situation, there is uncertainty in nursing practice. Hence nurses must use trial and error in providing nursing care. However, this trial and error approach frequently involves no formal documentation of effective and ineffective nursing actions. With this strategy, knowledge is gained from experience, but often it is not shared with others. The trial and error approach to acquiring knowledge also can be time-consuming because you may implement multiple interventions before finding one that is effective. There also is a risk of implementing nursing actions that are detrimental to a patient's health. If studies are conducted on nursing interventions, selection and implementation of interventions need to be based on scientific knowledge rather than on trial and error.

Personal Experience

Personal experience involves gaining knowledge by being personally involved in an event, situation, or circumstance. Personal experience enables the nurse to gain skills and expertise by providing care to patients and families in clinical settings. Learning that occurs from personal experience enables the nurse to cluster ideas into a meaningful whole. For example, you may read about giving an IM injection or be told how to give an injection in a classroom setting, but you do not know how to give an injection until you observe other nurses giving injections to patients and actually give several injections yourself.

The amount of personal experience affects the complexity of a nurse's knowledge base. Benner (1984) conducted a phenomenological qualitative study to identify the levels of experience in the development of clinical knowledge and expertise, and these include (1) novice, (2) advanced beginner, (3) competent, (4) proficient, and (5) expert. Novice nurses have no personal experience in the work they are to perform, but have some preconceptions and expectations about clinical practice that they acquired during their education. These preconceptions and expectations are challenged, refined, confirmed, or refuted by personal experience in a clinical setting. The advanced beginner nurse has just enough experience to recognize and intervene in recurrent situations. For example, the advanced beginner is able to recognize and intervene in managing patients' pain. Competent nurses are able to generate and achieve long-range goals and plans because of years of personal experience. The competent nurse also can use her or his personal knowledge to take conscious, deliberate actions that are efficient and organized. From a more complex knowledge base, the proficient nurse views the patient as a whole and as a member of a family and community. The proficient nurse recognizes that each patient and family responds differently to illness and health. The expert nurse has an extensive background of experience and is able to identify accurately and intervene skillfully in a situation. Personal experience increases the ability of the expert nurse to grasp a situation intuitively, with accuracy and speed.

Benner's qualitative research (1984) provided an increased understanding of how knowledge is acquired through personal experience. As you gain clinical experience during your educational program and after you graduate, you will note your movement through these different levels of knowledge.

Role Modeling

Role modeling is learning by imitating the behaviors of an expert. In nursing, role modeling enables the novice nurse to learn through interactions with or examples set by highly competent, expert nurses. Role models include admired teachers, expert clinicians, researchers, or those who inspire others through their example. An intense form of role modeling is mentorship, in which the expert nurse serves as a teacher, sponsor, guide, and counselor for the novice nurse. The knowledge gained through personal experience is greatly enhanced by a quality relationship with a role model or mentor. Many new graduates enter internship programs provided by clinical agencies so that expert nurses can mentor them during the novice's first few months of employment.

Intuition

Intuition is an insight into or understanding of a situation or event as a whole that usually cannot be explained logically (Grove, Burns, & Gray, 2013). Because intuition is a type of knowing that seems to come unbidden, it may also be described as a "gut feeling" or "hunch." Because intuition cannot easily be explained scientifically, many people are uncomfortable with it. Some even think that it does not exist. However, intuition is not the lack of knowing; rather, it is a result of deep knowledge (Benner, 1984). This knowledge is so deeply incorporated that it is difficult to bring it to the surface consciously and express it in a logical manner. Some nurses can intuitively recognize when a patient is experiencing a health crisis. Using this intuitive knowledge, these nurses can assess the patient's condition, intervene, and contact the physician as needed for medical intervention.

Reasoning

Reasoning is the processing and organizing of ideas to reach conclusions. Through reasoning, people are able to make sense of their thoughts, experiences, and research evidence (Grove et al., 2013). This type of logical thinking is often evident in the oral presentation of an argument, in which each part is linked to reach a logical conclusion. The science of logic includes inductive and deductive reasoning. Inductive reasoning moves from the specific to the general; particular instances are observed and then combined into a larger whole or a general statement (Chinn & Kramer, 2011). An example of inductive reasoning follows.

PARTICULAR INSTANCES

A headache is an altered level of health that is stressful.

A terminal illness is an altered level of health that is stressful.

GENERAL STATEMENT

Therefore it can be induced that all altered levels of health are stressful.

Deductive reasoning moves from the general to the specific or from a general premise to a particular situation or conclusion (Chinn & Kramer, 2011). A premise or proposition is a statement of the proposed relationship between two or more concepts. An example of deductive reasoning follows.

PREMISES

All humans experience loss.

All adolescents are humans.

CONCLUSION

Therefore it can be deduced that all adolescents experience loss.

In this example, deductive reasoning is used to move from the two general premises about humans and adolescents to the conclusion that "All adolescents experience loss." However, the conclusions generated from deductive reasoning are valid only if they are based on valid premises. Research is a means to test and confirm or refute a premise or proposition so that valid premises can be used as a basis for reasoning in nursing practice.

ACQUIRING KNOWLEDGE THROUGH NURSING RESEARCH

Acquiring knowledge through traditions, authority, borrowing, trial and error, personal experience, role modeling, intuition, and reasoning is important in nursing. However, these ways of acquiring knowledge are inadequate in providing an EBP (Brown, 2014; Craig & Smyth, 2012). The knowledge needed for practice is specific and holistic, as well as process-oriented and outcomes-focused. Thus a variety of research methods are needed to generate this knowledge. This section introduces quantitative, qualitative, and outcomes research methods that are used to generate empirical knowledge for nursing practice. These research methods are essential to generate evidence for the following specific goals of the nursing profession (AACN, 2006; ANA, 2011; NINR, 2013):

- Promoting an understanding of patients' and families' experiences with health and illness (a common focus of qualitative research)
- Implementing effective nursing interventions to promote patient health (a common focus of quantitative research)
- Providing quality, safe, and cost-effective care within the healthcare system (a common focus of outcomes research)

Introduction to Quantitative and Qualitative Research

Quantitative and qualitative research methods complement each other because they generate different types of knowledge that are useful in nursing practice. Familiarity with these two types of research will help you identify, understand, and critically appraise these studies. Quantitative and qualitative research methodologies have some similarities; both require researcher expertise, involve rigor in implementation of studies, and generate scientific knowledge for nursing practice. Some of the differences between the two methodologies are presented in Table 1-3.

Most of the studies conducted in nursing have used quantitative research methods. Quantitative research is a formal, objective, systematic process in which numerical data are used to obtain information about the world. The quantitative approach toward scientific inquiry emerged from a branch of philosophy called logical positivism, which operates on strict rules of logic, truth, laws, and predictions. Quantitative researchers hold the position that "truth" is absolute and that a single reality can be defined by careful measurement. To find truth, the researcher must be objective, which means that values, feelings, and personal perceptions cannot enter into the measurement of reality. Quantitative research is conducted to test theory by describing variables (descriptive research), examining relationships among variables (correlational research), and determining cause and effect interactions between variables (quasi-experimental and experimental research;

TABLE 1-3 CHARACTERISTICS OF QUANTITATIVE AND QUALITATIVE RESEARCH METHODS		
CHARACTERISTIC	**QUANTITATIVE RESEARCH**	**QUALITATIVE RESEARCH**
Philosophical origin	Logical positivism	Naturalistic, interpretive, humanistic
Focus	Concise, objective, reductionistic	Broad, subjective, holistic
Reasoning	Logistic, deductive	Dialectic, inductive
Basis of knowing	Cause and effect relationships	Meaning, discovery, understanding
Theoretical focus	Tests theory	Develops theory and frameworks
Researcher involvement	Control	Shared interpretation

Grove et al., 2013; Shadish, Cook, & Campbell, 2002). Chapter 2 describes the different types of quantitative research and the quantitative research process.

Qualitative research is a systematic, subjective approach used to describe life experiences and situations and give them meaning (Munhall, 2012). This research methodology evolved from the behavioral and social sciences as a method of understanding the unique, dynamic, holistic nature of humans. The philosophical base of qualitative research is interpretive, humanistic, and naturalistic and is concerned with understanding the meaning of social interactions by those involved (Standing, 2009). Qualitative researchers believe that truth is complex and dynamic and can be found only by studying people as they interact with and in their sociohistorical settings (Creswell, 2014; Munhall, 2012). Nurses' interest in conducting qualitative research began in the late 1970s. Currently, an extensive number of qualitative studies are being conducted that use various qualitative research methods. Qualitative research is conducted to promote an understanding of human experiences and situations and develop theories that describe these experiences and situations. Because human emotions are difficult to quantify (i.e., assign a numerical value to), qualitative research seems to be a more effective method of investigating emotional responses than quantitative research (see Table 1-3). Chapter 3 describes the different types of qualitative research.

Types of Quantitative and Qualitative Research

Several types of quantitative and qualitative research have been conducted to generate nursing knowledge for practice. These types of research can be classified in a variety of ways. The classification system for this book is presented in Box 1-1 and includes the most common types of quantitative and qualitative research conducted in nursing. The quantitative research methods are classified into four categories—descriptive, correlational, quasi-experimental, and experimental (Grove et al., 2013; Kerlinger & Lee, 2000; Shadish et al., 2002; see Chapter 2).

- Descriptive research explores new areas of research and describes situations as they exist in the world.
- Correlational research examines relationships and is conducted to develop and refine explanatory knowledge for nursing practice.

BOX 1-1   CLASSIFICATION OF RESEARCH METHODS PRESENTED IN THIS TEXTBOOK

Quantitative Research
Descriptive
Correlational
Quasi-experimental
Experimental

Qualitative Research
Phenomenological
Grounded theory
Ethnographic
Exploratory-descriptive qualitative
Historical

Outcomes Research

- Quasi-experimental and experimental studies determine the effectiveness of nursing interventions in predicting and controlling the outcomes desired for patients and families.
  The qualitative research methods included in this text are phenomenological, grounded theory, ethnographic, exploratory-descriptive, and historical research (see Box 1-1).
- Phenomenological research is an inductive descriptive approach used to describe an experience as it is lived by an individual, such as the lived experience of chronic pain.
- Grounded theory research is an inductive research technique used to formulate, test, and refine a theory about a particular phenomenon. Grounded theory research initially was described by Glaser and Strauss (1967) in their development of a theory about grieving.
- Ethnographic research was developed by the discipline of anthropology for investigating cultures through an in-depth study of the members of the culture. Health practices vary among cultures, and these practices need to be recognized in delivering care to patients, families, and communities.
- Exploratory-descriptive qualitative research is conducted to address an issue or problem in need of a solution and/or understanding. Qualitative nurse researchers use this methodology to explore an issue or problem area using varied qualitative techniques, with the intent of describing the topic of interest and promoting understanding.
- Historical research is a narrative description or analysis of events that occurred in the remote or recent past. Through historical research, past mistakes and accomplishments are examined to facilitate an understanding of and an effective response to present situations (Fawcett & Garity, 2009; Marshall & Rossman, 2011; Munhall, 2012; see Chapter 3).

Introduction to Outcomes Research

The spiraling cost of health care has generated many questions about the quality and effectiveness of healthcare services and patient outcomes related to these services. Consumers want to know what services they are purchasing and whether these services will improve their health. Healthcare policy makers want to know whether the care is cost-effective and of high quality. These concerns have promoted the conduct of outcomes research, which focuses on examining the results of care and determining the changes in health status for the patient (Doran, 2011; Rettig, 1991). Some essential areas that require investigation through outcomes research include the following: (1) patient responses to nursing and medical interventions; (2) functional maintenance or improvement of physical, mental, and social functioning for the patient; (3) financial outcomes achieved with the provision of healthcare services; and (4) patient satisfaction with the health outcomes, care received, and healthcare providers (Doran, 2011). Nurses are playing an active role in conducting outcomes research by participating in multidisciplinary research teams that examine the outcomes of healthcare services. This knowledge provides a basis for improving the quality of care that nurses deliver in practice. Chapter 14 includes a description of outcomes research and provides guidelines for critically appraising these types of studies.

UNDERSTANDING BEST RESEARCH EVIDENCE FOR PRACTICE

EBP involves the use of the best research evidence to support clinical decisions in practice. Best research evidence was previously defined as a summary of the highest quality, current, empirical knowledge in a specific area of health care that has been developed from a synthesis of quality studies (quantitative, qualitative, and outcomes) in that area. As a nurse, you make numerous clinical decisions each day that affect the health outcomes of your patients. By using the best research evidence available, you can make quality clinical decisions that will improve patients' and families' health outcomes. This section was developed to expand your understanding of the concept of best research evidence for practice by providing the following: (1) a description of the strategies used to synthesize research evidence; (2) a model of the levels of research evidence available; and (3) a link of the best research evidence to evidence-based guidelines for practice.

Strategies Used to Synthesize Research Evidence

The synthesis of study findings is a complex, highly structured process that is best conducted by at least two or even a team of expert researchers and healthcare providers. There are various types of research synthesis, and the type of synthesis conducted varies based on the quality and types of research evidence available. The quality of the research evidence available in an area is dependent on the number and validity or credibility of the studies that have been conducted in an area. The types of research commonly conducted in nursing (see earlier) are quantitative, qualitative, and outcomes. The research synthesis processes used to summarize knowledge varies for quantitative and qualitative research.

Research evidence in nursing and health care is synthesized by using the following processes: (1) systematic review; (2) meta-analysis; (3) meta-synthesis; and (4) mixed-methods systematic review. Depending on the quantity and strength of the research findings available, nurses and healthcare professionals use one or more of these four synthesis processes to determine the current best research evidence in an area. Table 1-4 identifies the processes used in research synthesis, the purpose of each synthesis process, the types of research included in the synthesis (sampling frame), and the analytical techniques used to achieve the synthesis of research evidence (Craig & Smyth, 2012; Higgins & Green, 2008; Sandelowski & Barroso, 2007; Whittemore, 2005). Table 1-4 is also included in the inside front cover of this textbook.

A systematic review is a structured, comprehensive synthesis of the research literature to determine the best research evidence available to address a healthcare question. A systematic review involves identifying, locating, appraising, and synthesizing quality research evidence for expert clinicians to use to promote an EBP (Craig & Smyth, 2012; Higgins & Green, 2008). Teams of expert researchers, clinicians, and sometimes students conduct these reviews to determine the current best knowledge for use in practice. Systematic reviews are also used in the development of national and international standardized guidelines for managing health problems such as acute pain, hypertension, and depression. Standardized guidelines are made available online, published in articles and books, and presented at conferences and professional meetings. Some common sources for these standardized guidelines are presented at the end of this chapter. The process for critically appraising systematic reviews is discussed in Chapter 13.

A meta-analysis is conducted to combine or pool the results from previous quantitative studies into a single statistical analysis that provides one of the highest levels of evidence about an intervention's effectiveness (Andrel, Keith, & Leiby, 2009; Craig & Smyth, 2012; Grove et al., 2013; Higgins & Green, 2008). Qualitative studies do not produce statistical findings and cannot be included in a meta-analysis. Some of the strongest evidence for using an intervention in practice is generated from a meta-analysis of multiple, controlled quasi-experimental and experimental studies. In addition, a meta-analysis can be performed on correlational studies to determine the type (positive or negative) or strength of relationships among selected variables (see Table 1-4). Because meta-analyses involve statistical analysis to combine study results, it is possible to be objective rather than subjective when synthesizing research evidence. Many systematic reviews conducted to generate evidence-based guidelines include meta-analyses. The process for critically appraising a meta-analysis is discussed in Chapter 13.

TABLE 1-4	**PROCESSES USED TO SYNTHESIZE RESEARCH EVIDENCE**		
SYNTHESIS PROCESS	**PURPOSE OF SYNTHESIS**	**TYPES OF RESEARCH INCLUDED IN THE SYNTHESIS (SAMPLING FRAME)**	**TYPE OF ANALYSIS FOR ACHIEVING SYNTHESIS**
Systematic review	Use of specific, systematic methods to identify, select, critically appraise, and synthesize research evidence to address a particular problem in practice (Craig & Smyth, 2012; Higgins & Green, 2008)	Usually includes quantitative studies with similar methodology, such as randomized controlled trials (RCTs); can also include meta-analyses focused on an area of the practice problem	Narrative and statistical
Meta-analysis	Synthesis or pooling of the results from several previous studies using statistical analysis to determine the effect of an intervention or strength of relationships (Higgins & Green, 2008)	Includes quantitative studies with similar methodology, such as quasi-experimental and experimental studies focused on the effect of an intervention or correlational studies focused on relationships	Statistical
Meta-synthesis	Systematic compilation and integration of qualitative studies to expand understanding and develop a unique interpretation of the studies' findings in a selected area (Barnett-Page & Thomas, 2009; Finfgeld-Connett, 2010; Sandelowski & Barroso, 2007)	Uses original qualitative studies and summaries of qualitative studies to produce the synthesis	Narrative
Mixed-methods systematic review	Synthesis of findings from individual studies conducted with a variety of methods (quantitative, qualitative, and mixed-methods) to determine the current knowledge in an area (Higgins & Green, 2008)	Synthesis of a variety of quantitative, qualitative, and mixed-methods studies	Narrative

Qualitative research synthesis is the process and product of systematically reviewing and formally integrating the findings from qualitative studies (Sandelowski & Barroso, 2007). The process for synthesizing qualitative research is still evolving, and a variety of synthesis methods have appeared in the literature (Barnett-Page & Thomas, 2009; Finfgeld-Connett, 2010; Higgins & Green, 2008). In this text, the concept of meta-synthesis is used to describe the process for synthesizing qualitative research. Meta-synthesis is defined as the systematic compilation and integration of qualitative study results to expand understanding and develop a unique interpretation of study findings in a selected area. The focus is on interpretation rather than on combining study results, as with quantitative research synthesis (see Table 1-4). The process for critically appraising a meta-synthesis is discussed in Chapter 13.

Over the last 10 to 15 years, nurse researchers have conducted mixed-methods studies that include quantitative and qualitative research methods (Creswell, 2014). In addition, determining the current research evidence in an area might require synthesizing quantitative and qualitative studies. Higgins and Green (2008) refer to this synthesis of quantitative, qualitative, and mixed-methods studies as a mixed-methods systematic review (see Table 1-4). Mixed-methods systematic reviews might include a variety of study designs, such as qualitative research and quasi-experimental, correlational, and/or descriptive studies (Higgins & Green, 2008). Some researchers have conducted syntheses of quantitative and/or qualitative studies, termed *integrative reviews of research.* The value of these reviews depends on the standards used to conduct them. The process for critically appraising a mixed-method systematic review is discussed in Chapter 13.

Levels of Research Evidence

The strength or validity of the best research evidence in an area depends on the quality and quantity of the studies that have been conducted in an area. Quantitative studies, especially experimental studies such as the RCT, provide the strongest research evidence (see Chapter 8). Also, the replication or repeating of studies with similar methodology increases the strength of the research evidence generated. The levels of the research evidence are a continuum, with the highest quality of research evidence at one end and weakest research evidence at the other (Brown, 2014; Craig & Smyth, 2012; Melnyk & Fineout-Overholt, 2011; Figure 1-3). The systematic research reviews and meta-analyses of high-quality experimental studies provide the strongest or best research

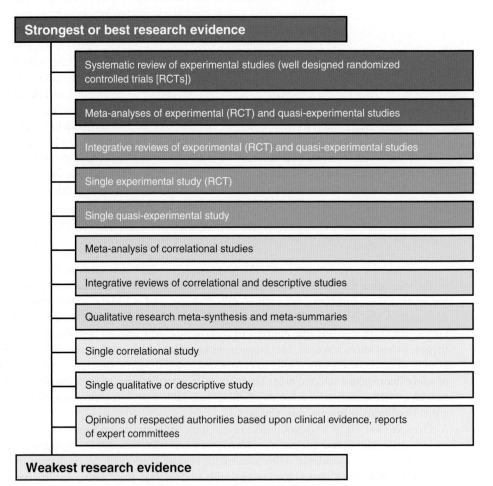

FIG 1-3 Levels of Research Evidence.

evidence for use by expert clinicians in practice. Meta-analyses and integrative reviews of quasi-experimental, experimental, and outcomes studies also provide very strong research evidence for managing practice problems. Mixed-methods systematic reviews and meta-syntheses provide quality syntheses of quantitative, qualitative, and/or mixed-methods studies. Correlational, descriptive, and qualitative studies often provide initial knowledge, which serves as a basis for generating quasi-experimental and outcomes studies (see Figure 1-3). The weakest evidence comes from expert opinions, which can include expert clinicians' opinions or the opinions expressed in committee reports. When making a decision in your clinical practice, be sure to base that decision on the best research evidence available.

The levels of research evidence identified in Figure 1-3 (also included in the front cover of this text) will help you determine the quality of the evidence that is available for practice. The best research evidence generated from systematic reviews, meta-analyses, meta-syntheses, and mixed-methods systematic reviews is used to develop standardized, evidence-based guidelines for use in practice.

Introduction to Evidence-Based Guidelines

Evidence-based guidelines are rigorous, explicit clinical guidelines that have been developed based on the best research evidence available in that area. These guidelines are usually developed by a team or panel of expert clinicians (nurses, physicians, pharmacists, and other health professionals), researchers, and sometimes consumers, policy makers, and economists. The expert panel works to achieve consensus on the content of the guideline to provide clinicians with the best information for making clinical decisions in practice. There has been a dramatic growth in the production of evidence-based guidelines to assist healthcare providers in building an EBP and improving healthcare outcomes for patients, families, providers, and healthcare agencies.

Every year, new guidelines are developed, and some of the existing guidelines are revised based on new research evidence. These guidelines have become the gold standard (or standard of excellence) for patient care, and nurses and other healthcare providers are encouraged to incorporate these standardized guidelines into their practice. Many of these evidence-based guidelines have been made available online by national and international government agencies, professional organizations, and centers of excellence. When selecting a guideline for practice, be sure that the guideline was developed by a credible agency or organization and that the reference list reflects the synthesis of extensive number of studies.

An extremely important source for evidence-based guidelines in the United States is the National Guideline Clearinghouse (NGC), initiated in 1998 by the AHRQ. The NGC started with 200 guidelines and has expanded to more than 1400 evidence-based guidelines (see http://www.guideline.gov). Another excellent source of systematic reviews and evidence-based guidelines is the Cochrane Collaboration and Library in the United Kingdom, which can be accessed at http://cochrane.org. Professional nursing organizations, such as the Oncology Nursing Society (http://www.ons.org) and National Association of Neonatal Nurses (http://www.nann.org), have also developed evidence-based guidelines for nursing practice. Their websites will introduce you to some of evidence-based guidelines that exist nationally and internationally. Chapter 13 provides you with direction when critically appraising the quality of an evidence-based guideline and implementing that guideline in your practice.

WHAT IS YOUR ROLE IN NURSING RESEARCH?

Generating a scientific knowledge base with implementation in practice requires the participation of all nurses in various research activities. Some nurses are developers of research and conduct studies to generate and refine the knowledge needed for nursing practice (Grove et al., 2013). Others are consumers of research and use research evidence to improve their nursing practice. The AACN (2006) and ANA (2010a, 2010b) have published statements about the roles of nurses in research. Whatever their education or position, all nurses have roles in research; some ideas about these roles are presented in Figure 1-4. The research role that a nurse assumes usually expands with his or her advanced education, expertise, and career path. Nurses with associate degrees usually have limited education about the research process and critical appraisal of studies, so they are not included in Figure 1-4.

Nurses with a Bachelor of Science in Nursing (BSN) degree are knowledgeable about the research process and have skills in reading and critically appraising studies. They assist with the implementation of evidence-based guidelines, protocols, algorithms, and policies in practice. In addition, these nurses might provide valuable assistance in identifying research problems and collecting data for studies. The QSEN (2013) competencies identify such knowledge and skills as being essential for prelicensure students.

Nurses with a Master of Science in Nursing (MSN) have the educational preparation to appraise critically and synthesize findings from studies to revise or develop protocols, algorithms, or policies for use in practice (see Figure 1-4). They also have the ability to identify and critically appraise the quality of evidence-based guidelines developed by national organizations. Advanced practice nurses and nurse administrators have the ability to lead healthcare teams in making essential changes in nursing practice and in the healthcare system based on current research evidence. Most MSN programs provide an opportunity for students to conduct a thesis or research study under the direction of a faculty mentor and thesis committee. However, most students do not complete

Educational Preparation	Research Functions
BSN	Read and critically appraise studies. Use best research evidence in practice with guidance. Assist with research problem identification and data collection.
MSN	Critically appraise and synthesize studies to develop and revise protocols, algorithms, and policies for practice. Implement best research evidence in practice. Collaborate in research projects and provide clinical expertise for research.
DNP	Participate in the development of national evidence-based guidelines. Develop, implement, critically appraise, and revise as needed protocols, policies, and evidence-based guidelines used in clinical agencies. Conduct clinical studies, usually in collaboration with other nurse researchers.
PhD	Major role in conducting independent research and contributing to the empirical knowledge generated in a selected area of nursing. Obtain initial funding for research. Coordinate research teams of BSN, MSN, and DNP nurses.
Post-Doctorate	Assume a full researcher role with a funded program of research. Lead and/or participate in nursing and interdisciplinary research teams. Identified as experts in their areas of research. Mentor PhD-prepared nurse researchers.

FIG 1-4 Nurses' participation in research at various levels of education.

the thesis option of their program. Therefore MSN-prepared nurses could identify problems requiring research and sometimes conduct studies but usually do so in collaboration with other nurse scientists (AACN, 2006; ANA 2010a, 2010b).

The doctorate in nursing can be practice-focused (doctor of nursing practice [DNP]) or research-focused (doctor of philosophy [PhD]). DNPs are educated to have the highest level of clinical expertise, with the ability to translate scientific knowledge for use in practice. These doctorally prepared nurses have advanced research and leadership knowledge to develop, implement, evaluate, and revise evidence-based guidelines, protocols, algorithms, and policies for practice (Clinton & Sperhac, 2006). In addition, DNP-prepared nurses have the expertise to conduct and/or collaborate with clinical studies focused on translating evidence-based interventions into practice.

PhD-prepared nurses assume a major role in the conduct of research and generation of nursing knowledge in a selected area of interest (see Figure 1-4). These nurse scientists often coordinate research teams that include DNP-, MSN-, and BSN-prepared nurses to facilitate the conduct of quality studies in a variety of healthcare agencies. The postdoctorate-prepared nurse usually assumes a full-time researcher role and has a funded program of research. They lead interdisciplinary teams of researchers and sometimes conduct studies in multiple settings. These scientists are often identified as experts in selected areas of research and provide mentoring of new PhD-prepared researchers (AACN, 2006).

The following chapters in this text have been developed to expand your understanding of quantitative, qualitative, and outcomes research processes and increase your ability to appraise studies critically. A **critical appraisal of research** involves careful examination of all aspects of a study to judge its strengths, limitations, meaning, and significance. You will also be provided assistance in identifying and implementing the best research evidence in practice. We think that you will find that nursing research is an exciting adventure that holds much promise for the future practice of nursing. We hope that this text will increase your understanding of research and the research process and facilitate your implementation of an EBP as a nurse.

KEY CONCEPTS

- Research is defined as diligent, systematic inquiry to validate and refine existing knowledge and develop new knowledge.
- Nursing research is defined as a scientific process that validates and refines existing knowledge and generates new knowledge that directly and indirectly influences nursing practice.
- Evidence-based practice is the conscientious integration of best research evidence with clinical expertise and patient needs and values in the delivery of quality, safe, and cost-effective health care.
- The purposes of research in nursing include description, explanation, prediction, and control of phenomena in practice.
- Nightingale was the first nurse researcher who developed empirical knowledge to improve practice in the nineteenth century.
- The conduct of clinical research continues to be a major focus in the twenty-first century, with the goal of developing an evidence-based practice for nursing.
- Knowledge is acquired in nursing in a variety of ways, including tradition, authority, borrowing, trial and error, personal experience, role modeling, intuition, reasoning and, most importantly, research.

- The Quality and Safety Education for Nurses (QSEN) initiative is focused on developing the requisite knowledge, skills, and attitudes (KSAs) of students needed to attain the required QSEN prelicensure competencies.
- The QSEN (2013) evidence-based practice competency area is defined as "integrating the best current evidence with clinical expertise and patient/family preferences and values for delivery of optimal health care".
- Quantitative research is a formal, objective, systematic process using numerical data to obtain information about the world. This research method is used to describe, examine relationships, and determine cause and effect.
- Qualitative research is a systematic, subjective approach used to describe life experiences and give them meaning. Knowledge generated from qualitative research will provide meaning and understanding of specific emotions, values, life experiences, and historical events.
- A third research method is outcomes research, which focuses on examining the end results of care and determining the changes needed in health status for the patient and healthcare system.
- Research evidence in nursing is synthesized using the following processes: (1) systematic review; (2) meta-analysis; (3) meta-synthesis; and (4) mixed-methods systematic review.
- A systematic review is a structured, comprehensive synthesis of quantitative studies in a particular healthcare area to determine the best research evidence available for expert clinicians to use to promote an evidence-based practice.
- Meta-analysis is a type of study that statistically combines or pools the results from previous studies into a single quantitative analysis that provides one of the highest levels of evidence for an intervention's efficacy.
- Meta-synthesis involves the systematic compilation and integration of qualitative studies to expand understanding and develop a unique interpretation of the findings in a selected area.
- Mixed-methods systematic review is the synthesis of findings from individual studies conducted with a variety of methods (quantitative, qualitative, and mixed-methods) to determine the current knowledge in an area.
- The levels of research evidence are a continuum, with the highest quality of research evidence at one end and weakest research evidence at the other. Systematic research reviews and meta-analyses of quality experimental studies provide the strongest or best research evidence for practice (see Figure 1-3).
- Evidence-based guidelines are rigorous, explicit clinical guidelines that have been developed based on the best research evidence available in that area.
- Nurses with a BSN, MSN, doctoral degree (DNP and PhD), and postdoctorate education have clearly designated roles in research based on the breadth and depth of the research knowledge gained during their educational programs and their clinical expertise.

REFERENCES

Agency for Healthcare Research and Quality (AHRQ), (2013). *Research tools and data.* Rockville, Maryland: Author. Retrieved June 18, 2013, from, http://www.ahrq.gov/research/index.html.

American Association of Colleges of Nursing (AACN), (2006). *AACN position statement on nursing research.* Washington, DC: AACN. Retrieved June 17, 2013, from, http://www.aacn.nche.edu/publications/position/nursing-research.

American Nurses Association (ANA), (2011). *American Nurses Association research agenda.* Washington, DC: Author. Retrieved June 17, 2013 from, http://nursingworld.org/MainMenuCategories/ThePracticeofProfessionalNursing/Improving-Your-Practice/Research-Toolkit/ANA-Research-Agenda/Research-Agenda-.pdf.

American Nurses Association, (2010a). *Nursing: Scope and standards of practice* (2nd ed.). Washington, DC: Author.

American Nurses Association, (2010b). *Nursing's social policy statement: The essence of the profession* (2nd ed.). Washington, DC: Author.

Andrel, J. A., Keith, S. W., & Leiby, B. E. (2009). Meta-analysis: A brief introduction. *Clinical and Translational Science, 2*(5), 374–378.

Barnard, K. E. (1980). Knowledge for practice: Directions for the future. *Nursing Research, 29*(4), 208–212.

Barnett-Page, E., & Thomas, J. (2009). Methods for the synthesis of qualitative research: A critical review. *BMC Medical Research Methodology, 9*, 59. http://dx.doi.org/ 10.1186/147-2288-9-59.

Barnsteiner, J., Disch, J., Johnson, J., McGuinn, K., Chappell, K., & Swartwout, E. (2013). Diffusing QSEN competencies across schools of nursing: The AACN/ RWJF faculty development institutes. *Journal of Professional Nursing, 29*(2), 68–74.

Bauknecht, V. L. (1985). Capital commentary: NIH bill passes, includes nursing research center. *American Nurse, 17*(10), 2.

Benner, P. (1984). *From novice to expert: Excellence and power in clinical nursing practice.* Menlo Park, CA: Addison-Wesley.

Brown, S. J. (2014). *Evidence-based nursing: The research-practice connection* (3rd ed.). Sudbury, MA: Jones & Bartlett.

Chinn, P. L., & Kramer, M. K. (2011). *Integrated theory and knowledge development in nursing* (8th ed.). St. Louis: Mosby Elsevier.

Clinton, P., & Sperhac, A. M. (2006). National agenda for advanced practice nursing: The practice doctorate. *Journal of Professional Nursing, 22*(1), 7–14.

Cocoman, A., & Murray, J. (2008). Intramuscular injections: A review of best practice for mental health nurses. *Journal of Psychiatric and Mental Health Nursing, 15*(5), 424–434.

Cohen, B. (1984). Florence Nightingale. *Scientific American, 250*(3), 128–137.

Cook, E. (1913). *The life of Florence Nightingale.* (Vol. 1). London, England: Macmillan.

Craig, J., & Smyth, R. (2012). *The evidence-based practice manual for nurses* (3rd ed.). Edinburgh, Scotland: Churchill Livingstone Elsevier.

Creswell, J. W. (2014). *Research design: Qualitative, quantitative and mixed methods approaches* (4th ed.). Thousand Oaks, CA: Sage.

Doran, D. M. (2011). *Nursing sensitive outcomes: The state of the science* (2nd ed.). Sudbury, MA: Jones & Bartlett.

Fawcett, J., & Garity, J. (2009). *Evaluating research for evidence-based nursing practice.* Philadelphia: F. A. Davis.

Finfgeld-Connett, D. (2010). Generalizability and transferability of meta-synthesis research findings. *Journal of Advanced Nursing, 66*(2), 246–254.

Glaser, B. G., & Strauss, A. L. (1967). *The discovery of grounded theory: Strategies for qualitative research.* Chicago: Aldine.

Gortner, S. R., & Nahm, H. (1977). An overview of nursing research in the United States. *Nursing Research, 26*(1), 10–33.

Greenway, K. (2004). Using the ventrogluteal site for intramuscular injection. *Nursing Standard, 18*(25), 39–42.

Grove, S. K., Burns, N., & Gray, J. R. (2013). *The practice of nursing research: Appraisal, synthesis, and generation of evidence* (7th ed.). Philadelphia, PA: Elsevier Saunders.

Herbert, R. G. (1981). *Florence Nightingale: Saint, reformer or rebel?* Malabar, FL: Robert E. Krieger.

Higgins, J. P. T., & Green, S. (2008). *Cochrane handbook for systematic reviews of interventions.* West Sussex, England: Wiley-Blackwell and The Cochrane Collaboration.

Horsley, J. A., Crane, J., Crabtree, M. K., & Wood, D. J. (1983). *Using research to improve nursing practice: A guide. CURN project.* New York: Grune & Stratton.

Institute of Medicine, (2001). *Crossing the quality chasm: A new health system for the 21st century.* Washington, DC: National Academy Press.

James, P. A., Oparil, S., Carter, B. L., Cushman, W. C., Denison-Himmelfard, C., Handler, J., et al. (2013). 2014 *evidence-based guidelines for the management of high blood pressure in adults: Report from the panel members appointed to the Eight Joint National Committee (JNC 8). JAMA,* E1–E14. Dec 18; [e-pub ahead of print]. Retrieved January 5, 2014 from, http:// dx.doi.org/10.1001/jama.2013.284427.

Kaplan, A. (1964). *The conduct of inquiry; Methodology for behavioral science.* San Francisco: Chandler.

Kerlinger, F. N., & Lee, H. B. (2000). *Foundations of behavioral research* (4th ed.). Fort Worth, TX: Harcourt College Publishers.

Lee, S., Faucett, J., Gillen, M., Krause, N., & Landry, L. (2013). Risk perception of musculoskeletal injury among critical care nurses. *Nursing Research, 62*(1), 36–44.

Manojlovich, M., Sidani, S., Covell, C. L., & Antonakos, C. L. (2011). Nurse dose: Linking staffing variables to adverse patient outcomes. *Nursing Research, 60*(4), 214–220.

Marshall, C., & Rossman, G. B. (2011). *Designing qualitative research* (5th ed.). Thousand Oaks, CA: Sage.

McMurrey, P. H. (1982). Toward a unique knowledge base in nursing. *Image, 14*(1), 12–15.

Melnyk, B. M., & Fineout-Overholt, E. (2011). *Evidence-based practice in nursing and healthcare: A guide to best practice* (2nd ed.). Philadelphia: Lippincott, Williams, & Wilkins.

Munhall, P. L. (2012). *Nursing research: A qualitative perspective* (5th ed.). Sudbury, MA: Jones & Bartlett.

National Heart, Lung, and Blood Institute, (2003). *The seventh report of the Joint National Committee on Prevention, Detection, Evaluation, and Treatment of High Blood Pressure (JNC 7)*. Retrieved June 11, 2013 from, www.nhlbi.nih.gov/guidelines/hypertension.

National Institute of Nursing Research, (2011). *Bringing science to life: NINR strategic plan*. Retrieved June 17, 2013 from, https://www.ninr.nih.gov/sites/www.ninr.nih.gov/files/ninr-strategic-plan-2011.pdf.

National Institute of Nursing Research, (2013). *About the NINR*. Retrieved June 18, 2013 from, http://www.ninr.nih.gov/aboutninr/.

Nicoll, L. H., & Hesby, A. (2002). Intramuscular injections: An integrative research review and guideline for evidence-based practice. *Applied Nursing Research, 16* (2), 149–162.

Nightingale, F. (1859). *Notes on nursing: What it is, and what it is not*. Philadelphia: Lippincott.

Oakley, K. (2010). Nursing by the numbers. *Occupational Health, 62*(4), 28–29.

Palmer, I. S. (1977). Florence Nightingale: Reformer, reactionary, researcher. *Nursing Research, 26*(2), 84–89.

Quality, Safety Education for Nurses (QSEN), (2013). *Pre-licensure knowledge, skills, and attitudes (KSAs)*. Retrieved February 17, 2013 from, http://qsen.org/competencies/pre-licensure-ksas/.

Rettig, R. (1991). History, development, and importance to nursing of outcomes research. *Journal of Nursing Quality Assurance, 5*(2), 13–17.

Rodger, M. A., & King, L. (2000). Drawing up and administering intramuscular injections: A review of the literature. *Journal of Advanced Nursing, 31*(3), 574–582.

Rush, K. L., Watts, W. E., & Janke, R. (2013). Rural and urban older adults' perspectives of strength in their daily lives. *Applied Nursing Research, 26*(1), 10–16.

Sackett, D. L., Straus, S. E., Richardson, W. S., Rosenberg, W., & Haynes, R. B. (2000). *Evidence-based medicine: How to practice and teach EBM* (2nd ed.). London: Churchill Livingstone.

Sandelowski, M., & Barroso, J. (2007). *Handbook for synthesizing qualitative research*. New York: Springer.

See, E. M. (1977). The ANA and research in nursing. *Nursing Research, 26*(3), 165–171.

Shadish, W. R., Cook, T. D., & Campbell, D. T. (2002). *Experimental and quasi-experimental designs for generalized causal inference*. Chicago: Rand McNally.

Sherwood, G., & Barnsteiner, J. (2012). *Quality and safety in nursing: A competency approach to improving outcomes*. Ames, IA: Wiley-Blackwell.

Standing, M. (2009). A new critical framework for applying hermeneutic phenomenology. *Nurse Researcher, 16*(4), 20–30.

Stetler, C. B. (2001). Updating the Stetler model of research utilization to facilitate evidence-based practice. *Nursing Outlook, 49*(6), 272–279.

U.S. Department of Health and Human Services, (U.S. DHHS) (2000). *Healthy people 2010: Understanding and improving health*. Washington, DC: U.S. Department of Health and Human Services.

U.S. Department of Health and Human Services, (U.S. DHHS) (2013). *Healthy people 2020: Topics and objectives*. Retrieved June 18, 2013 from, http://www.healthypeople.gov/2020/topicsobjectives2020/default.aspx.

Weber, M. A., Schiffrin, E. L., White, W. B., Mann, S., Lindholm, L. H., Kenerson, J. G., et al. (2014). Clinical practice guidelines for the management of hypertension in the community: A statement by the American Society of Hypertension and the International Society of Hypertension. *Journal of Hypertension, 32*(1), 3–15.

Werley, H. H., & Fitzpatrick, J. J. (1983). *Annual review of nursing research* (Vol. 1). New York: Springer.

Whittemore, R. (2005). Combining evidence in nursing research: Methods and implications. *Nursing Research, 54*(1), 56–62.

CHAPTER 2

Introduction to Quantitative Research

LEARNING OUTCOMES

After completing this chapter, you should be able to:

1. Define terms relevant to the quantitative research process—*basic research, applied research, rigor,* and *control*.
2. Compare and contrast the problem-solving process, nursing process, and research process.
3. Identify the steps of the quantitative research process in descriptive, correlational, quasi-experimental, and experimental published studies.
4. Read quantitative research reports.
5. Conduct initial critical appraisals of quantitative research reports.

KEY TERMS

Abstract, p. 51
Analyzing a research report, p. 55

Applied research, p. 35
Assumptions, p. 42

Basic research, p. 35
Bias, p. 37

What do you think of when you hear the word research? Frequently, the idea of experimentation or study comes to mind. Typical features of an experiment include randomizing subjects into groups, collecting data, and conducting statistical analyses. You may think of researchers conducting a study to determine the effectiveness of an intervention, such as determining the effectiveness of a walking exercise program on body mass index (BMI) of patients with type 2 diabetes. These ideas are associated with quantitative research. Quantitative research includes specific steps that are detailed in research reports. Reading and critically appraising quantitative studies require learning new terms, understanding the steps of the quantitative research process, and applying a variety of analytical skills.

This chapter provides an introduction to quantitative research to help develop expertise in reading and understanding quantitative research reports. Relevant terms are defined, and the problem-solving and nursing processes are presented to provide a background for understanding the quantitative research process. The steps of the quantitative research process are introduced, and a descriptive correlational study is presented as an example to promote understanding of the process. Also included are a discussion of the critical thinking skills needed for reading research reports and guidelines for conducting an initial critical appraisal of these quantitative research reports. The chapter concludes with the identification of the steps of the research process from published quasi-experimental and experimental studies, with an initial critical appraisal of these studies.

WHAT IS QUANTITATIVE RESEARCH?

Quantitative research is a formal, objective, rigorous, systematic process for generating numerical information about the world. Quantitative research is conducted to describe new situations, events, or concepts; examine relationships among variables; and determine the effectiveness of treatments or interventions on selected health outcomes in the world. Some examples include:
1. Describing the spread of flu cases each season and their potential influence on local and global health (descriptive study)
2. Examining the relationships among the variables—for example, minutes watching television per week, minutes playing video games per week, and body mass index (BMI) of a school-age child (correlational study)

3. Determining the effectiveness of calcium with vitamin D_3 supplements on the bone density of adults (quasi-experimental study).

The classic experimental designs to test the effectiveness of treatments were originated by Sir Ronald Fisher (1935). He is noted for adding structure to the steps of the quantitative research process with ideas such as the hypothesis, research design, and statistical analysis. Fisher's studies provided the groundwork for what is now known as experimental research.

Throughout the years, a number of other quantitative approaches have been developed. Campbell and Stanley (1963) developed quasi-experimental approaches to study the effects of treatments under less controlled conditions. Karl Pearson (Porter, 2004) developed statistical approaches for examining relationships between variables, which were used in analyzing data when correlational research was conducted. The fields of sociology, education, and psychology are noted for their development and expansion of strategies for conducting descriptive research. A broad range of quantitative research approaches is needed to develop the empirical knowledge for building evidence-based practice (EBP) in nursing (Brown, 2014; Craig & Smyth, 2012). EBP is introduced in Chapter 1 and detailed in Chapter 13. EBP is essential for promoting quality, safe outcomes for patients and families, nursing education and practice, and the healthcare system (Doran, 2011; Quality and Safety Education for Nurses [QSEN], 2013; Sherwood & Barnsteiner, 2012). Understanding the quantitative research process is essential for meeting the QSEN (2013) competencies for undergraduate nursing students, which are focused on patient-centered care, teamwork and collaboration, EBP, quality improvement (QI), safety, and informatics. This section introduces you to the different types of quantitative research and provides definitions of terms relevant to the quantitative research process.

Types of Quantitative Research

Four common types of quantitative research are included in this text:
- Descriptive
- Correlational
- Quasi-experimental
- Experimental

The type of quantitative research conducted is influenced by the current knowledge of a research problem. When little knowledge is available, descriptive studies often are conducted. As the knowledge level increases, correlational, quasi-experimental, and experimental studies are conducted.

Descriptive Research

Descriptive research is the exploration and description of phenomena in real-life situations. It provides an accurate account of characteristics of particular individuals, situations, or groups (Brown, 2014; Fawcett & Garity, 2009; Kerlinger & Lee, 2000). Descriptive studies are usually conducted with large numbers of subjects or study participants, in natural settings, with no manipulation of the situation. Through descriptive studies, researchers discover new meaning, describe what exists, determine the frequency with which something occurs, and categorize information in real-world settings. The outcomes of descriptive research include the identification and description of concepts, identification of possible relationships among concepts, and development of hypotheses that provide a basis for future quantitative research.

Correlational Research

Correlational research involves the systematic investigation of relationships between or among variables. When conducting this type of study, researchers measure selected variables in a sample and then use correlational statistics to determine the relationships among the study variables.

Using correlational analysis, the researcher is able to determine the degree or strength and type (positive or negative) of a relationship between two variables. The strength of a relationship varies, ranging from −1 (perfect negative correlation) to +1 (perfect positive correlation), with 0 indicating no relationship (Grove, 2007).

A positive relationship indicates that the variables vary together; that is, both variables increase or decrease together. For example, research has shown that the more people smoke, the more lung damage they experience. A negative relationship indicates that the variables vary in opposite directions; thus as one variable increases, the other will decrease (Grove, Burns, & Gray, 2013). For example, research has shown as the number of smoking pack-years (number of years smoked times the number of packs smoked per day) increases, people's life spans usually decrease, demonstrating a negative relationship. The primary intent of correlational studies is to **explain the nature of relationships in the real world, not to determine cause and effect**. The focus of correlational research is on describing relationships, not testing the effectiveness of interventions. However, the relationships identified with correlational studies are the means for generating hypotheses to guide quasi-experimental and experimental studies that do focus on examining cause and effect relationships.

Quasi-Experimental Research

The purpose of quasi-experimental research is to examine causal relationships or determine the effect of one variable on another. Thus these studies involve implementing a treatment or intervention and examining the effects of this intervention using selected methods of measurement (Shadish, Cook, & Campbell, 2002). In nursing research, a treatment is an intervention implemented by researchers to improve the outcomes of clinical practice. For example, a treatment of a swimming exercise program might be implemented to improve the balance and muscle strength of older women with osteoarthritis. Quasi-experimental studies differ from experimental studies by the level of control achieved by the researcher. These studies usually lack a certain amount of control over the manipulation of the treatment, management of the setting, and/or selection of the subjects. When studying human behavior, especially in clinical settings, researchers frequently are unable to select the subjects randomly or manipulate or control certain variables related to the treatment, subjects, or the setting. As a result, nurse researchers conduct more quasi-experimental studies than experimental studies. Control is discussed in more detail later in this chapter.

Experimental Research

Experimental research is an objective, systematic, highly controlled investigation conducted for the purpose of predicting and controlling phenomena in nursing practice. In an experimental study, causality between the independent (treatment) and dependent (outcome) variables is examined under highly controlled conditions (Shadish et al., 2002). Experimental research is the most powerful quantitative method because of the rigorous control of variables. The three main characteristics of experimental studies are the following: (1) controlled manipulation of at least one treatment variable (independent variable); (2) exposure of some of the subjects to the treatment (experimental group) and no exposure of the remaining subjects (control group); and (3) random assignment of subjects to the control or experimental group. Random selection of subjects and the conduct of the study in a laboratory or research facility strengthen control in an experimental study. The degree of control achieved in experimental studies varies according to the population studied, variables examined, and environment of the study.

Defining Terms Relevant to Quantitative Research

Understanding quantitative research requires comprehension of the following important terms—*basic research, applied research, rigor,* and *control.* These terms are defined in the following sections, with examples provided from published studies.

Basic Research

Basic research is sometime referred to as pure research. It includes scientific investigations conducted for the pursuit of knowledge for knowledge's sake or for the pleasure of learning and finding truth (Miller & Salkind, 2002). Basic scientific investigations seek new knowledge about health phenomena, with the hope of establishing general scientific principles. The purpose of basic research is to generate and refine theory; thus the findings frequently are not directly useful in practice (Wysocki, 1983). Basic nursing research might include laboratory investigations with animals or humans to promote further understanding of physiological functioning, genetic and inheritable disorders, and pathological processes. These studies might focus on increasing our understanding of oxygenation, perfusion disorders, fluid and electrolyte imbalances, acid-base status, immune system disorders, eating and exercise patterns, sleeping disorders, and pain and comfort status.

You might conduct an initial critical appraisal of quantitative studies and identify whether basic or applied research was conducted. Sharma, Ryals, Gajewski, and Wright (2010) conducted a basic study to determine the effect of aerobic exercise on analgesia and neurotropin-3 synthesis on chronic pain using female mice. The researchers noted that the literature and nurses in clinical practice supported using aerobic exercise to reduce pain and improve functioning in those with chronic pain, but the molecular basis for the positive actions of exercise was not clearly understood. Sharma et al. (2010) conducted a basic experimental study; the steps of this study are provided as an example at the end of this chapter.

Sharma and colleagues' (2010) study demonstrates the importance of laboratory research to increase our understanding of the effects of treatments on cellular pathological processes. Basic research using animals is often conducted to provide an increased understanding of the genetics of health problems and establish a basis for further human research in this area. A major force in genetic research is the National Human Genome Research Institute (NHGRI, 2013), which plans and conducts a broad program of laboratory research to increase our understanding of human genetic makeup, genetics of diseases, and potential gene therapy. This basic research provides a basis for conducting applied "clinical research to translate genomic and genetic research into a greater understanding of human genetic disease, and to develop better methods for the detection, prevention, and treatment of heritable and genetic disorders" (NHGRI, 2013).

Applied Research

Applied research is also called practical research, which includes scientific investigations conducted to generate knowledge that will directly influence or improve clinical practice. The purpose of applied research is to solve problems, make decisions, and/or predict or control outcomes in real-life practice situations. The findings from applied studies can also be invaluable to policy makers as a basis for making changes to address health and social problems. Many of the studies conducted in nursing are applied studies because researchers have chosen to focus on clinical problems and the testing of nursing interventions to improve patient outcomes. Applied research also is used to test theory and validate its usefulness in clinical practice (Fawcett & Garity, 2009). Researchers often examine the new knowledge discovered through basic research for its usefulness in practice by applied research, making these approaches complementary.

Pinto, Hickman, Clochesy, and Buchner (2013) conducted an applied study to determine the effectiveness of an avatar-based, depression, self-management technology intervention in treating depressive symptoms in young adults. This intervention is called "Electronic Self-Management Resource Training for Mental Health" (eSMART-MH). "eSMART-MH is a novel avatar-based depression self-management intervention in which young adults interact with virtual healthcare providers and a virtual health coach in a virtual primary care environment to practice effective communication about depression symptoms and receive tailored behavioral feedback" (Pinto et al., 2013, p. 46). The researchers found that the eSMART-MH intervention demonstrated initial efficacy and was developmentally appropriate for depression self-management in young adults. These applied study findings, combined with the findings of additional studies in this area, have the potential to generate important knowledge for the delivery of evidence-based care to young adults experiencing depression. The greater the rigor and control implemented in these types of applied studies, the higher the quality of the research evidence developed for practice.

Rigor in Quantitative Research

Rigor is the striving for excellence in research; it requires discipline, adherence to detail, strict accuracy, and precision. A rigorously conducted quantitative study has precise measuring tools, a representative sample, and a tightly controlled study design. Critically appraising the rigor of a study involves examining the reasoning and precision used in conducting the study. Logical reasoning, including deductive and inductive reasoning (see Chapter 1), is essential to the development of quantitative studies (Chinn & Kramer, 2011). The research process, discussed later in this chapter, includes specific steps that are rigorously developed with meticulous detail and are logically linked in descriptive, correlational, quasi-experimental, and experimental studies.

Another aspect of rigor is precision, which encompasses accuracy, detail, and order. Precision is evident in the concise statement of the research purpose and detailed development of the study design. However, the most explicit example of precision is the measurement or quantification of the study variables. For example, a researcher might use a cardiac monitor to measure and record the heart rate of subjects into a database during an exercise program, rather than palpating a radial pulse for 30 seconds and recording it on a data collection sheet.

Control in Quantitative Research

Control involves the imposing of rules by researchers to decrease the possibility of error, thereby increasing the probability that the study's findings are an accurate reflection of reality. The rules used to achieve control in research are referred to as design. Thus quantitative research includes various degrees of control, ranging from uncontrolled to highly controlled, depending on the type of study (Table 2-1). Descriptive and correlational studies are rigorously conducted but are often designed with minimal researcher control because subjects are examined as they exist in their natural setting, such as home, work, school, or health clinic.

Quasi-experimental studies focus on determining the effectiveness of a treatment (independent variable) in producing a desired outcome (dependent variable) in a partially controlled setting. Thus these studies are conducted with more control of extraneous variables, selection of subjects and settings, and development and implementation of the treatment or intervention (see Table 2-1). However, experimental studies are the most highly controlled type of quantitative research conducted to examine the effect of interventions on dependent variables. Experimental studies often are conducted on subjects in experimental units in healthcare agencies or on animals in laboratory settings, such as the study by Sharma and associates (2010), which used mice

TABLE 2-1	CONTROL IN QUANTITATIVE RESEARCH	
TYPE OF QUANTITATIVE RESEARCH	**RESEARCHER CONTROL OF INTERVENTION AND EXTRANEOUS VARIABLES**	**RESEARCH SETTING**
Descriptive	No intervention Limited or no control of extraneous variables	Natural or partially controlled setting
Correlational	No intervention Limited or no control of extraneous variables	Natural or partially controlled setting
Quasi-experimental	Controlled intervention Rigorous control of extraneous variables	Partially controlled setting
Experimental	Highly controlled intervention and extraneous variables	Research unit or laboratory setting

to examine the effects of aerobic exercise on chronic pain (see Table 2-1). The following elements are areas for control in quantitative studies:

- Extraneous variables
- Sampling process
- Selection of setting
- Development and implementation of the study intervention

Extraneous Variables

Through control, the researcher can reduce the influence of extraneous variables. Extraneous variables exist in all studies and can interfere with obtaining a clear understanding of the relationships among the study variables. For example, if a study focused on the effect of relaxation therapy on the perception of incisional pain, the researchers would have to control the extraneous variables, such as type of surgical incision and time, amount, and type of pain medication administered after surgery, to prevent their influence on the patient's perception of pain. Selecting only patients with abdominal incisions who are hospitalized and receiving only one type of pain medication intravenously after surgery would control some of these extraneous variables. Controlling extraneous variables enables researchers to determine the effects of an intervention or treatment on study outcomes more accurately.

Sampling

Sampling is a process of selecting participants who are representative of the population being studied. Random sampling usually provides a sample that is representative of a population because each member of the population is selected independently and has an equal chance, or probability, of being included in the study. In quantitative research, random and nonrandom samples are used. A randomly selected sample is very difficult to obtain in nursing research, so quantitative studies often are conducted with nonrandom samples. To increase the control and rigor of a study and decrease the potential for bias (slanting of findings away from what is true or accurate), the subjects who are initially selected with a nonrandom sampling method are often randomly assigned to the treatment group or the control (no treatment) group in quasi-experimental and experimental studies. For example, Pinto and co-workers (2013) initially obtained their sample of young adolescents using a nonrandom convenience sampling method. However, the study design was strengthened by the random assignment of these adolescents to receive the avatar-based, depression, self-management intervention (experimental group) or standard care of education on healthy living (comparison or control group).

Research Settings

The setting is the location in which a study is conducted. There are three common settings for conducting research—natural, partially controlled, and highly controlled (see Table 2-1). A natural setting, or field setting, is an uncontrolled, real-life situation or environment. Conducting a study in a natural setting means that the researcher does not manipulate or change the environment for the study. Descriptive and correlational studies often are conducted in natural settings. A partially controlled setting is an environment that the researcher has manipulated or modified in some way. An increasing number of nursing studies are occurring in partially controlled settings to limit the effects of extraneous variables on the study outcomes. A highly controlled setting is an artificially constructed environment developed for the sole purpose of conducting research. Laboratories, research or experimental centers, and test units in hospitals or other healthcare agencies are highly controlled settings in which experimental studies are often conducted. This type of setting reduces the influence of extraneous variables, which enables the researcher to examine the effect of one variable on another accurately. Chapter 9 presents a more detailed discussion of samples and settings.

Study Interventions

Quasi-experimental and experimental studies examine the effect of an independent variable or intervention on a dependent variable or outcome. More intervention studies are being conducted in nursing to establish an EBP. Controlling the development and implementation of a study intervention increases the validity of the study design and credibility of the findings. A study intervention needs to be (1) clearly and precisely developed, (2) consistently implemented, and (3) examined for effectiveness through quality measurement of the dependent variables. The detailed development of a quality intervention and the consistent implementation of this intervention are known as intervention fidelity (Grove et al., 2013; Morrison, et al., 2009). Chapter 8 provides guidelines for critically appraising interventions in studies.

PROBLEM-SOLVING AND NURSING PROCESSES: BASIS FOR UNDERSTANDING THE QUANTITATIVE RESEARCH PROCESS

Research is a process, and it is similar in some ways to other processes. Therefore the background acquired early in nursing education in problem solving and the nursing process also is useful in research. A process includes a purpose, series of actions, and goal. The purpose provides direction for the implementation of a series of actions to achieve an identified goal. The specific steps of the process can be revised and re-implemented to reach the endpoint or goal. Table 2-2 links the steps of the problem-solving process, nursing process, and research process. Relating the research process to the problem-solving and the nursing processes may be helpful in understanding the steps of the quantitative research process.

Comparing Problem Solving with the Nursing Process

The problem-solving process involves the systematic collection of data to identify a problem, difficulty, or dilemma; determination of goals related to the problem; identification of possible approaches or solutions to achieve those goals (plan); implementation of the selected solutions; and evaluation of goal achievement (Chinn & Kramer, 2011). Problem solving frequently is used in daily activities and nursing practice. For example, you use problem solving when you select your clothing, decide where to live, or turn a patient with a fractured hip.

The nursing process is a subset of the problem-solving process. The steps of the nursing process are assessment, diagnosis, plan, implementation, evaluation, and modification (see Table 2-2). Assessment involves the collection and interpretation of subjective data (health history) and

TABLE 2-2   COMPARISON OF THE PROBLEM-SOLVING PROCESS, NURSING PROCESS, AND RESEARCH PROCESS

PROBLEM-SOLVING PROCESS	NURSING PROCESS	RESEARCH PROCESS
Data collection	**Assessment** Data collection (objective and subjective data) Data interpretation	**Knowledge of nursing world** Clinical experiences Literature review
Problem definition	**Nursing diagnosis**	**Problem and purpose identification**
Plan Setting goals Identifying solutions	**Plan** Setting goals Planning interventions	**Methodology** Design Sample Measurement methods Data collection Data analysis
Implementation	**Implementation**	**Implementation**
Evaluation and revision	**Evaluation and modification**	**Outcomes, communication, and synthesis of study findings to promote evidence-based nursing practice**

objective data (physical exam) for the development of nursing diagnoses. These diagnoses guide the remaining steps of the nursing process, just as the step of identifying the problem directs the remaining steps of the problem-solving process. The planning step in the nursing process is the same as in the problem-solving process. Both processes involve implementation (putting the plan into action) and evaluation (determining the effectiveness of the process). If the process is ineffective, nurses need to review all steps and revise (modify) them as necessary to achieve quality outcomes for the patient and family (Wilkinson, 2012). Nurses implement the nursing process until the problems and diagnoses are resolved, and the identified goals are achieved.

Comparing the Nursing Process with the Research Process

The nursing process and research process have important similarities and differences. The two processes are similar because they both involve abstract critical thinking and complex reasoning. These processes help identify new information, discover relationships, and make predictions about phenomena. In both processes, information is gathered, observations are made, problems are identified, plans are developed (methodology), and actions are taken (data collection and analysis). Both processes are reviewed for effectiveness and efficiency—the nursing process is evaluated, and outcomes are determined in the research process (see Table 2-2). Implementing the two processes expands and refines the user's knowledge. With this growth in knowledge and critical thinking, the user can implement increasingly complex nursing processes and studies.

The research and nursing processes also have definite differences. Knowledge of the nursing process will assist you in understanding the research process. However, the research process is more complex than the nursing process and involves the rigorous application of a variety of research methods (Grove et al., 2013). The research process also has a broader focus than that of the nursing process, in which the nurse focuses on a specific patient and family. During the quantitative research process, the researcher focuses on large groups of individuals, such as a population of patients with hypertension. In addition, researchers must be knowledgeable about the world of nursing to identify problems that require study. This knowledge comes from clinical and other personal experiences and by conducting a review of the literature.

The theoretical underpinnings of the research process are much stronger than those of the nursing process. All steps of the research process are logically linked to each other, as well as to the theoretical foundations of the study. The conduct of research requires greater precision, rigor, and control than what are needed in the implementation of the nursing process. The outcomes from research frequently are shared with a large number of nurses and other healthcare professionals through presentations and publications. In addition, the outcomes from several studies can be synthesized to provide sound evidence for nursing practice (Melnyk & Fineout-Overholt, 2011).

IDENTIFYING THE STEPS OF THE QUANTITATIVE RESEARCH PROCESS

The **quantitative research process** involves conceptualizing a research project, planning and implementing that project, and communicating the findings. Figure 2-1 identifies the steps of the quantitative research process that are usually included in a research report. The figure illustrates the logical flow of the process as one step builds progressively on another. The steps of the quantitative research process are briefly introduced here; Chapters 4 to 11 discuss them in more detail. The descriptive correlational study conducted by Dickson, Howe, Deal, and McCarthy (2012) on the relationships of work, self-care, and quality of life in a sample of older working adults

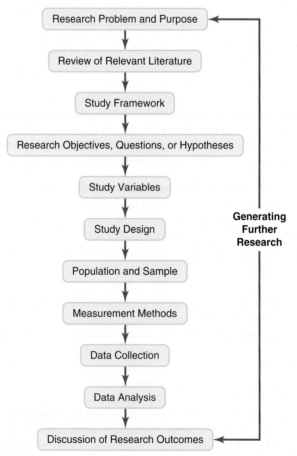

FIG 2-1 Steps of the Quantitative Research Process.

with cardiovascular disease (CVD) is used as an example to introduce the steps of the quantitative research process.

Research Problem and Purpose

A research problem is an area of concern in which there is a gap in the knowledge needed for nursing practice. The problem statement in a study usually identifies an area of concern for a particular population that requires investigation. Research is then conducted to generate essential knowledge that addresses the practice concern, with the ultimate goal of developing sound research evidence for nursing practice (Brown, 2014; Craig & Smyth, 2012). The research problem is usually broad and could provide the basis for several studies. The research purpose is generated from the problem and identifies the specific focus or goal of the study. The focus of a quantitative study might be to identify, describe, or explain a situation; predict a solution to a situation; or control a situation to produce positive outcomes in practice. The purpose includes the variables, population, and often the setting for the study. Chapter 5 presents a detailed discussion of the research problem and purpose.

♦ RESEARCH EXAMPLE

Problem and Purpose

Research Study Excerpt

Dickson and colleagues (2012) clearly expressed their study research problem and purpose in the following study excerpts. The problem of older workers with CVD affects millions of people and the need for additional research is identified. The purpose is focused on the concern identified in the problem and clearly indicates that the goal of the study is to describe and examine relationships among variables important to working individuals with CVD.

Research Problem

"According to the Bureau of Labor Statistics (2008), the American workforce is aging. By 2015, the number of workers aged 55 years or more will reach 31.2 million, a 72% increase from 2000. As a result, health problems associated with the aging process, such as cardiovascular disease (CVD), present new health and safety challenges for older workers. More than 3.5 million workers have CVD.... However, older workers with CVD are 3 times more likely to report work limitations than those without CVD.... Older workers with CVD also report increased rates of absenteeism and longer periods of disability from work. Furthermore, within 6 years after a recognized heart attack, approximately 22% of men and 46% of the women report being disabled from work (American Heart Association, 2005).... For the large segment of the American workforce with CVD, self-care that entails adhering to treatment regimens while working and managing symptoms is critical to their quality of life.... Few studies exist to guide clinicians in supporting ongoing employment among patients with CVD." Dickson et al., 2012, pp. 6-7

Research Purpose

"Therefore, the purpose of this study was to examine the self-care behaviors of adherence to medication, diet, exercise, and symptom monitoring of older workers with CVD, and explore the relationships among job characteristics (job demands, job control, and workplace support), self-care, and quality of life." Dickson et al., 2012, p. 7

Review of Relevant Literature

Researchers conduct a review of relevant literature to generate a picture of what is known and not known about a particular problem and to document why a study needs to be conducted. Relevant literature includes only those sources that are pertinent to or highly important in providing the in-depth knowledge needed to study a selected problem (Fawcett & Garity, 2009). Often, the literature

direct the conduct of the studies and the interpretation of findings (Grove et al., 2013). Chapter 5 provides guidelines for critically appraising the objectives, questions, and hypotheses in research reports.

Dickson and associates (2012) developed the following two specific aims:

"1. To describe adherence to common self-care practices of older workers with CVD

2. To examine how job-level factors explain variation in self-care adherence behaviors and quality of life, taking into account common illness characteristics (depression and physical functioning)" Dickson et al., 2012, p. 7

Study Variables

The research purpose and objectives, questions, or hypotheses identify the variables to be examined in a study. Variables are concepts at various levels of abstraction that are measured, manipulated, or controlled in a study. More concrete concepts, such as temperature, weight, or blood pressure, are referred to as variables in a study. More abstract concepts, such as creativity, empathy, or social support, sometimes are referred to as research concepts.

Researchers operationalize the variables or concepts in a study by identifying conceptual and operational definitions. A conceptual definition provides a variable or concept with theoretical meaning (Grove et al., 2013), and it comes from a theorist's definition of the concept or is developed through concept analysis. The conceptual definitions of variables provide a link from selected concepts in the study framework to the study variables. Researchers develop an operational definition so that the variable can be measured or manipulated in a study. The knowledge gained from studying the variable will increase understanding of the theoretical concept from the study framework that the variable represents (see Chapter 7 for a more detailed discussion of concepts and frameworks). Chapter 5 provides a more extensive discussion of study variables.

Dickson and co-workers (2012) clearly identified the following study variables in their research purpose and aims: job-level factors or characteristics, quality of life, self-care adherence behaviors, and common illness characteristics of depression and physical functioning. Clear conceptual definitions were provided for the variables of self-care adherence behaviors and job-level factors or characteristics but not for the other variables of quality of life and illness characteristics of depression and physical functioning. All study variables were operationally defined, with clearly identified measurement methods for the variables. The conceptual and operational definitions for self-care adherence behaviors and job-level factor variables are provided as an example.

DEFINITIONS OF STUDY VARIABLES

Self-Care Adherence Behaviors
Conceptual Definition
"Self-care, conceptualized as a naturalistic decision-making process, is situation- and content-specific and influenced by the person's knowledge about and experience with decision making in the particular context, the person's skill to act on the decision made, and the compatibility of the decision and action with the person's values [see Figure 2-2] that determine the self-care adherence behaviors for older adults with CVD." Dickson et al., 2012, p. 6

Operational Definition
"In this study, measurement of self-care focused on the adherence to commonly recommended behaviors ... and was assessed using the Specific Adherence Survey from the Medical Outcomes study.

The specific Adherence Survey consists of eight CVD-pertinent questions that assess adherence to medication, diet, exercise, symptom monitoring, and alcohol and cigarette use over the prior 4-week period.... In addition, individuals who reported a history of chronic angina or history of myocardial infarction also completed the Self-Care of Heart Disease Index (SCHDI), a new instrument based on the established Self-Care of Heart Failure Index." Dickson et al., 2012, p. 8

Job-Level Factors
Conceptual Definition
Job-level factors or characteristics influencing the self-care of workers with CVD include job demands, job control, and workplace support.

Operational Definition
"The Job Content Questionnaire (JCQ) was used to assess job-related factors of job demands, job control, and workplace support.... The JCQ consists of 27 items that constitute five scales: job control, psychologic demands, physical demands, support (supervisor and co-worker support), and job insecurity." Dickson et al., 2012, p. 8

Study Design

Research design is a blueprint for the conduct of a study that maximizes control over factors that could interfere with the study's desired outcome. The type of design directs the selection of a population, procedures for sampling, methods of measurement, and plans for data collection and analysis. The choice of research design depends on what is known and not known about the research problem, the researcher's expertise, the purpose of the study, and the intent to generalize the findings.

Sometimes the design of a study indicates that a pilot study was conducted. A pilot study is often a smaller version of a proposed study, and researchers frequently conduct these to refine the study sampling process, treatment, or measurement of variables (Hertzog, 2008). For example, researchers might conduct pilot studies in a manner similar to the proposed study using similar subjects, the same setting, the same treatment, the same measurement methods, and the same data collection and analysis techniques to determine their quality. Chapter 8 presents a basis for critically appraising designs in research reports.

Designs have been developed to meet unique research needs as they emerge; thus, a variety of descriptive, correlational, quasi-experimental, and experimental designs have been generated over time. In descriptive and correlational studies, no treatment is administered, so the purposes of these study designs include improving the precision of measurement, describing what exists, and clarifying relationships that provide a basis for quasi-experimental and experimental studies. Quasi-experimental and experimental study designs usually involve treatment and control groups, and focus on achieving high levels of control, as well as precision in measurement (see Table 2-1). A study's design usually is in the methodology section of a research report. Dickson and colleagues (2012) conducted a descriptive correlational study with a typical descriptive design and a predictive correlational design. The descriptive part of the design provided a basis for describing the study variables of self-care adherence behaviors, job-level factors, quality of life, depression, and physical functioning for older adults with CVD. The predictive correlation part of the design focused on examining the relationships among the study variables and the use of job-level factors to predict self-care adherence behaviors, which were then included with depression and physical functioning to predict quality of life.

Population and Sample

The population is all elements (individuals, objects, or substances) that meet certain criteria for inclusion in a study (Kerlinger & Lee, 2000). A sample is a subset of the population selected for a particular study, and the members of a sample are the subjects or participants. Sampling was introduced earlier in this chapter, and Chapter 9 provides a background for critically appraising populations, samples, and settings in research reports.

The following excerpt identifies the sampling method, sample size, population, setting, sampling criteria, and sample characteristics for the study conducted by Dickson and associates (2012). This study included a quality description of the sampling process and a power analysis discussion, which is often conducted to determine an adequate sample size for a study (Grove et al., 2013). The sample characteristics were presented in a table and in narrative in the article.

"a . . . convenience sample [sampling method] of 129 adults (>age 45) with CVD [sample size and population] enrolled from outpatient settings associated with a large urban medical center [setting]. . . . Individuals were eligible to participate if they met the following inclusion criteria: (1) diagnosis related to the cardiovascular system (hypertension, coronary heart disease, e.g., myocardial infarction and angina, cardiac arrhythmia, valve disease, heart failure; stroke, peripheral vascular disease, or hyperlipidemia; (2) age 45 years or older; and (3) employed within the past year. Individuals were excluded from participating if they were unable or unwilling to provide informed consent, were unable to read or write in English, or had been unemployed for the prior year [inclusion and exclusion sampling criteria].

A sample of 129 adults with CVD (female 56%, African American 36.5%; mean age 59.2 ± 8.83 years) participated in the study. Seventy-nine percent were actively employed at the time of the study (average hours worked per week 29.29 ± 19.07). Employment in a service job was the most common occupation reported. Hypertension was reported in 43% of the sample; 34% had coronary heart disease (prior myocardial infarction, angina, or heart failure) [sample characteristics]." Dickson et al., 2012, pp. 7, 9

Measurement Methods

Measurement is the process of "assigning numbers to objects (or events or situations) in accord with some rule" (Kaplan, 1964, p. 177). A component of measurement is instrumentation, which is the application of specific rules to the development of a measurement method or instrument (Grove et al., 2013). An instrument is selected to measure a specific variable in a study. The numerical data generated with an instrument may be at the nominal, ordinal, interval, or ratio level of measurement. The level of measurement, with nominal being the lowest form of measurement and ratio being the highest, determines the type of statistical analysis that can be performed on the data. Chapter 10 introduces you to the concept of measurement, describes different types of measurement methods, and provides direction to appraise measurement techniques in studies critically.

Dickson and co-workers (2012) measured self-care adherence to commonly recommended behaviors using the Specific Adherence Survey from the Medical Outcomes study and the SCHDI. (These instruments were mentioned earlier in the operational definition of self-care.) The following study excerpt identified the scales and questionnaires used to measure the other study variables. The researchers provided quality descriptions of the measurement methods used in their study and indicated that these methods were commonly used in other studies and found to be reliable (consistent measurement) and valid (accurate in measuring a variable).

"Quality of life was measured in two ways. Health-related quality of life (HRQOL) was measured using the MacNew Heart Disease Heart-Related Quality of Life questionnaire. This valid and reliable instrument has been used extensively in CVD research to evaluate how quality of life is affected by one's heart disease and treatment.... A general measure of quality of life was also assessed using a single question—'How do you rate your quality of life?'—rated on a four-point Likert scale of 1 = poor to 4 = very good....

The Job Content Questionnaire (JCQ) was used to assess job-related factors of job demands, job control, and workplace support. This instrument is widely used in organization of work research and has demonstrated adequate reliability across many work groups....

Depression was measured by the Patient Health Questionnaire (PHQ)-9, a brief measure that has been used as a provisional diagnostic tool for major or minor depression in addition to depressive symptoms.... Physical functioning was assessed by the Duke Activity Status Index (DAS), which measures the individual's ability to perform a range of specific daily activities and has been used in studies of CVD and other chronic conditions." Dickson et al., 2012, p. 8

Data Collection

Data collection is the precise, systematic gathering of information relevant to the research purpose or the specific objectives, questions, or hypotheses of a study. To collect data, the researcher must obtain permission from the setting or agency in which the study will be conducted. Researchers must also obtain consent from all study participants to indicate their willingness to be in the study. Frequently, the researcher asks the study participants to sign a consent form, which describes the study, promises them confidentiality, and indicates that they can withdraw from the study at any time. The research report should document permission from an agency to conduct a study and consent of the study participants (see Chapter 4).

During data collection, investigators use a variety of techniques for measuring study variables, such as observation, interview, questionnaires, scales, and biological measures. In an increasing number of studies, nurses are measuring physiological and pathological variables using high-technology equipment. Researchers collect and systematically record data on each subject, organizing the data in a way that facilitates computer entry (see Chapter 10 for more details on critically appraising data collection in a study). Data collection is usually described in the methodology section of a research report under the subheading of "Procedures."

Dickson and colleagues (2012) clearly covered their data collection process in the following excerpt regarding procedures:

"After approval from the appropriate institutional review boards, participants were recruited from outpatient programs that serve employed populations through the delivery of medical care, employee health, and occupational health programs in a large urban population. Flyers promoting the study were available to individuals who visited the participating settings. A research assistant trained in the study recruitment and enrollment protocol was available during scheduled clinic hours to facilitate enrollment, obtain written informed consent, and complete data collection. Individuals received a non-coercive incentive of $20 for survey completion." Dickson et al., 2012, pp. 7-8

Data Analysis

Data analysis reduces, organizes, and gives meaning to the data. Analysis techniques conducted in quantitative research include descriptive and inferential analyses (see Chapter 11) and some sophisticated, advanced analysis techniques. Investigators base their choice of analysis techniques primarily on the research objectives, questions, or hypotheses, and level of measurement achieved by the measurement methods. Often research reports indicate the analysis techniques that were used in the study, and this content is covered prior to the study results. You can find the outcomes of the data analysis process in the results section of the research report; this section is best organized by the research objectives, questions, or hypotheses of the study.

Dickson and associates (2012) clearly identified the analysis techniques used in their study in the following excerpt. The "Results" section of their study described the study outcomes and clearly presented the results in figure, tables, and narrative.

Data Analysis

"Standard descriptive statistics of central tendency and dispersion were used to describe the sample. Relationships among physical functioning, depression, job-level factors of job demands (psychologic and physical), job control, workplace support (supervisor and co-worker) and job insecurity, adherence, and quality of life were analyzed using appropriate correlational methods. The student t-test and analysis of variance compared differences in the groups (e.g., employment status, gender, and race) with respect to adherence and quality of life...."

Results

"...There was significant correlation of the SCHDI self-care maintenance scale and the Specific Adherence Survey ($r=.614$, $p<.001$).... Older individuals had better self-care adherence practices. An independent sample t-test comparing the Specific Adherence Survey score by age category found a significant difference.... Depression was associated with poorer adherence to treatment recommendations ($r=-.313$, $p=.001$). Individuals with higher levels of physical functioning reported better adherence ($r=.281$, $p=.002$)....

Increased psychologic job demands were negatively associated with adherence ($r=-.31$, $p=.002$), but the relationship between physical job demands and adherence was not significant.... Better adherence was reported by those with increased job control ($r=.244$, $p=.016$) and workplace support (coworker support $r=.267$, $p=.002$; supervisor support $r=.291$, $p=.001$)." Dickson et al., 2012, pp. 8-9

Dickson and colleagues also conducted regression analyses to predict self-care adherence behaviors and quality of life. Regression analysis is a common technique used in nursing studies for making predictions. More details on regression analysis are presented in Chapter 11; the regression results from this study are discussed in that chapter.

Discussion of Research Outcomes

The results obtained from data analyses require interpretation to be meaningful. Interpretation of research outcomes involves examining the results from data analysis, identifying study limitations, exploring the significance of the findings, forming conclusions, generalizing the findings, considering the implications for nursing, and suggesting further studies. The study outcomes are usually presented in the discussion section of the research report. Limitations are restrictions in a study methodology and/or framework that may decrease the credibility and generalizability of the findings. A generalization is the extension of the conclusions made based on the research findings from the sample studied to a larger population. The study conclusions provide a basis for the implications of the findings for practice and identify areas for further research. Study outcomes are discussed in detail toward the end of Chapter 11. Dickson and associates (2012) provided the following quality discussion of their study outcomes:

Discussion

"To our knowledge, this is the first study to explore the complex relationship between job characteristics and adherence among older workers with CVD. We found that although most individuals reported taking medications, few consistently adhered to other self-care behaviors commonly recommended for patients with CVD.... Our results suggest that increased job demands and low job control may be reasons for the diminished adherence to routinely recommended self-care behaviors that has been found in older workers with CVD.... Our finding that depression and physical functioning are related to adherence among older workers with CVD is also an important contribution.... In addition, employment status among chronically ill adults is strongly linked to quality of life [study findings].... To our knowledge, the relationship between adherence and age is a unique finding that requires further investigation because the proportion of America's workforce aged more than 55 years is growing rapidly [suggestion for further research]."

Limitations

"... The new SCHDI used to describe self-care maintenance and management had marginal reliability and requires further psychometric validation. Few individuals in our sample reported symptoms, so we were unable to explore the relationship among job-level factors to individual response to symptoms. This is an important area for future research because others have found that lack of job flexibility, long work hours, and fear of discrimination have been identified as reasons that individuals with acute coronary symptom delay seeking treatment when experiencing chest pain symptoms during work hours.

... [We] used a convenience sample of working adults; therefore, we were unable to examine the influence of specific organizational policies and practices.... Further testing of the model [Figure 2-2] that includes the interaction of the work organization and job-level factors on self-care and health is warranted.

Our sample included a range of CVD diagnosis with varying levels of self-care requirements and treatment complexity. The sample size was not sufficient to examine differences across different diagnoses (e.g., hypertension compared with stroke). Furthermore CVD diagnosis was self-reported, which is a limitation [this section covered limitations and suggestions for further research]...."

Conclusions

"The results of this exploratory study are an important step to address the 2009 American Heart Association's policy statement on worksite wellness program for CVD prevention [conclusion].... Research to develop and test interventions to foster worksite programs that facilitate self-care behaviors among older workers with CVD is needed. Research efforts should include the objective measurement of adherence and self-care [suggested further research]. Programs that target general self-care such as diet and exercise, as well as more complex self-care (e.g., after myocardial infarction or those with heart failure), are indicated to address the needs across the working population. Nurses with expertise in occupational health are well suited to champion these efforts [implications for practice]." Dickson et al., 2012, p. 10-12

READING RESEARCH REPORTS

Understanding the steps of the research process and learning new terms related to those steps will assist you in reading research reports. A **research report** summarizes the major elements of a study and identifies the contributions of that study to nursing knowledge. Research reports are presented at professional meetings and conferences and are published online and in print journals and books. These reports often are difficult for nursing students and new graduates to read and to apply the knowledge in practice. Maybe you have had difficulty locating research articles or understanding the content of these articles. We would like to help you overcome some of these barriers and assist you in understanding the research literature by (1) identifying sources that publish research reports, (2) describing the content of a research report, and (3) providing tips for reading the research literature.

Sources of Research Reports

The most common sources for nursing research reports are professional journals. Research reports are the major focus of several nursing research journals, identified in Table 2-3. Two journals in particular, *Applied Nursing Research* and *Clinical Nursing Research,* focus on communicating research findings to practicing nurses. These journals usually include less detail on the framework, methodology, and statistical results of a study and more on discussion of the findings and implications for practice. The journal *Worldviews on Evidence-Based Nursing* focuses on innovative ideas for using evidence to improve patient care globally.

Many of the nursing clinical specialty journals also place a high priority on publishing research findings. Table 2-3 identifies some of the clinical journals in which research reports constitute a major portion of the journal content. More than 100 nursing journals are published in the United States, and most of them include research articles. The findings from many studies are now communicated through the Internet as journals are placed online; selected websites include the most current healthcare research. How to search for quality research sources is described in detail in Chapter 6.

TABLE 2-3	RESEARCH AND CLINICAL JOURNALS PROVIDING IMPORTANT SOURCES OF RESEARCH REPORTS
RESEARCH JOURNALS	**CLINICAL JOURNALS**
Advances in Nursing Science	*American Journal of Alzheimer's Care & Related Disorders and Research*
Applied Nursing Research	*Birth*
Biological Research for Nursing	*Cardiovascular Nursing*
Clinical Nursing Research	*Computers in Nursing*
International Journal of Nursing Studies	*Heart & Lung*
Journal of Nursing Research	*Issues in Comprehensive Pediatric Nursing*
Journal of Nursing Scholarship	*Issues in Mental Health Nursing*
Nursing Research	*International Journal of Nursing Terminologies and Classifications*
Nursing Science Quarterly	*Journal of Child and Adolescent Psychiatric and Mental Health Nursing*
Qualitative Health Research	*Journal of Continuing Education in Nursing*
Qualitative Nursing Research	*Journal of Holistic Nursing*
Research in Nursing & Health	*Journal of National Black Nurses' Association*
Scholarly Inquiry for Nursing Practice	*Journal of Nursing Education*
World Views on Evidence-Based Nursing	*Journal of Pediatric Nursing: Nursing Care of Children and Families*
	Journal of Transcultural Nursing
	Maternal-Child Nursing Journal
	Public Health Nursing
	Rehabilitation Nursing
	The Diabetes Educator

Content of Research Reports

At this point, you may be overwhelmed by the seeming complexity of a research report. You will find it easier to read and comprehend these reports if you understand each of the component parts. A research report often includes six parts: (1) abstract, (2) introduction, (3) methods, (4) results, (5) discussion, and (6) references. These parts are described in this section and the study by Twiss and co-workers (2009), which examined the effects of an exercise intervention on the muscle strength and balance of breast cancer survivors with bone loss, is presented as an example.

Abstract Section

The report usually begins with an abstract, which is a clear, concise summary of a study (Crosby, 1990; Grove et al., 2013). Abstracts range from 100 to 250 words and usually include the study purpose, design, setting, sample size, major results, and conclusions. Researchers hope that their abstracts will convey the findings from their study concisely and capture your attention so that you will read the entire report. Usually, four major content sections of a research report follow the abstract: introduction, methods, results, and discussion. Box 2-1 outlines the content covered in each of these sections. It is also briefly discussed in the following sections.

BOX 2-1   MAJOR SECTIONS OF A RESEARCH REPORT

Introduction
Statement of the problem, with background and significance
Statement of the purpose
Brief literature review
Identification of the framework
Identification of the research objectives, questions, or hypotheses (if applicable)

Methods
Identification of the research design
Description of the treatment or intervention (if applicable)
Description of the sample and setting
Description of the methods of measurement (including reliability and validity)
Discussion of the data collection process

Results
Description of the data analysis procedures
Presentation of results in tables, figures, or narrative organized by the purpose(s) and/or objectives, questions, or hypotheses

Discussion
Discussion of major findings
Identification of the limitations
Presentation of conclusions
Implications of the findings for nursing practice
Recommendations for further research

⚡ RESEARCH EXAMPLE

Abstract

Research Study Excerpt

Twiss and colleagues (2009) developed the following clear, comprehensive abstract, which conveys the critical information about their quasi-experimental study and includes the study's clinical relevance. However, the abstract might be considered a little long at 325 words.

"Purpose

... (a) to determine if 110 postmenopausal breast cancer survivors (BCS) with bone loss who participated in 24 months of strength and weight training (ST) exercises had improved muscle strength and balance and had fewer falls compared to BCS who did not exercise; and (b) to describe type and frequency of ST exercises; adverse effects of exercises; and participants' adherence to exercise at home, at fitness centers, and at 36-month follow-up.

Design

Findings reported are from a federally funded multi-component intervention study of 223 postmenopausal BCS with either osteopenia or osteoporosis who were randomly assigned to exercise ($n=110$) or comparison ($n=113$) groups.

Methods

Time points for testing outcomes were baseline, 6, 12, and 24 months into the intervention. Muscle strength was tested using Biodex Velocity Spectrum Evaluation and dynamic balance using Timed Backward Tandem Walk. Adherence to exercises was measured using self-report of number of prescribed sessions attended and participants' reports of falls.

Findings

Mean adherence over 24 months was 69.4%. Using generalized estimating equation (GEE) analyses, compared to participants not exercising, participants who exercised for 24 months had significantly improved hip flexion ($p=.011$), hip extension ($p=.0006$), knee flexion ($p=.0001$), knee extension ($p=.0018$), wrist flexion ($p=.031$), and balance ($p=.010$). Gains in muscle strength were 9.5% and 28.5% for hip flexion and extension, 50.0% and 19.4% for wrist flexion and extension, and 21.1% and 11.6% for knee flexion and extension. Balance improved by 39.4%. Women who exercised had fewer falls, but difference in number of falls between the two groups was not significant.

Conclusions

Many postmenopausal BCS with bone loss can adhere to a 24 month ST exercise intervention, and exercises can result in meaningful gains in muscle strength and balance.

Clinical Relevance

More studies are needed for examining relationships between muscle strength and balance in postmenopausal BCSs with bone loss and their incidence of falls and fractures." Twiss et al., 2009, p. 20

Introduction Section

The introduction section of a research report identifies the nature and scope of the problem being investigated and provides a case for the conduct of the study. You should be able to identify the significance of conducting the study clearly to generate knowledge for nursing practice. Twiss and colleagues' (2009) study was significant because an estimated 182,460 women in the United States are diagnosed with breast cancer each year, and these women are at risk for osteoporosis because of their cancer therapies. An exercise intervention could be an effective way to increase their muscle strength and balance and decrease falls. The purpose of this study was clearly stated in the abstract.

Depending on the type of research report, the literature review and framework may be separate sections or part of the introduction. The literature review documents the current knowledge of the problem investigated and includes the sources used to develop the study and interpret the findings. For example, Twiss and co-workers (2009) summarized the literature in a background section that included research in the areas of ST exercises, adherence to exercise, adverse effects of exercise, muscle strength, balance, and falls. A research report also needs to include a framework, but only about half of the published studies identify one. They (Twiss et al., 2009) did not identify a framework for their study. The inclusion of a physiological framework that focused on the impact of exercise on the physiological function of the musculoskeletal system would have strengthened this study. The relationships in the framework provide a basis for the formulation of hypotheses to be tested in quasi-experimental and experimental studies.

Investigators often end the introduction by identifying the objectives, questions, or hypotheses that they used to direct the study. However, their study (Twiss et al.. 2009) lacked a framework, and no hypotheses were developed to direct this quasi-experimental study.

Methods Section

The methods section of a research report describes how the study was conducted and usually includes the study design, treatment (if appropriate), sample, setting, measurement methods, and data collection process. This section of the report needs to be presented in enough detail so that the reader can critically appraise the adequacy of the study methods to produce reliable findings.

Twiss and co-workers (2009) provided extensive coverage of their study methodology. The design was clearly identified as a multisite, randomized controlled trial (RCT). They also included the subsection sample, which described the population, sampling method, sample criteria, sample size, attrition, and reasons for withdrawing from the study. Institutional approval for the conduct of this study and consent of the participants and their physicians were also discussed in this subsection. A subsection setting was included, which clearly indicated the sites where the study was conducted.

ST exercises was another subsection and provided a detailed description of the exercise intervention and how it was implemented in this study. A protocol for the intervention was also included in a table in the article. Measures was another subsection of the study methodology that detailed the quality of the measurement methods used to measure the dependent variables of muscle strength, balance, falls, adherence to the exercise sessions, and any adverse effects from the exercise. The measurements used in this study were identified previously in the study abstract. The methods section concluded with a subsection of statistical analysis that detailed the analytical techniques used to analyze the study data.

Results Section

The results section presents the outcomes of the statistical tests used to analyze the study data and significance of these outcomes. The research purpose or objectives, questions, and hypotheses formulated for the study are used to organize this section. Researchers identify the statistical analyses conducted to address the purpose or each objective, question, or hypothesis, and present the specific results obtained from the analyses in tables, figures, or narrative of the report (Grove et al., 2013). Focusing more on the summary of the study results and their significance than on the statistical results can help reduce the confusion that may be caused by the numbers.

Twiss and colleagues (2009) had a findings section that might have been more clearly labeled as "Results." This section began with a description of the sample; sample characteristics were presented in a table. The study results were organized by the study variables of adverse effects of exercises, adherence to exercises, muscle strength and balance, and falls. As indicated in the abstract, the study results were significant for all study variables except falls.

Discussion Section

The discussion section ties together the other sections of the research report and gives them meaning. This section includes the major findings, limitations of the study, conclusions drawn from the findings, implications of the findings for nursing, and recommendations for further research.

Twiss and associates (2009) discussed their findings in detail and compared and contrasted them with the findings of previous research studies. They also included a separate section in the study, "Limitations," which included the following: participants were not obtaining sufficient vitamin D, stronger intervention fidelity was needed, self-report of adherence often results in an overestimation of true levels of adherence, a lack of test-retest reliability for the investigator-developed instruments used in the study, and the small number of minority women who completed the study were not representative of this Midwestern state.

The discussion section also included a subsection, "Conclusions," that presented the implications for practice and identified the future studies needed. The conclusions drawn from a research project can be useful in at least three different ways. First, you can implement the intervention or treatment tested in a study with patients to improve their care and promote a positive health outcome. Second, reading research reports might change your view of a patient's situation or provide greater insight into the situation. Finally, studies heighten your awareness of the problems experienced by patients and assist you in assessing and working toward solutions for these problems. Twiss and co-workers (2009) also provided a clinical resources section; this included websites with research evidence about osteoporosis, breast cancer, and BCS support that would be useful for practice.

References Section

A references section that includes all sources cited in the research report follows the discussion section. The reference list includes the studies, theories, and methodology resources that provided a basis for the conduct of the study. These sources provide an opportunity to read about the research problem in greater depth. We strongly encourage you to read the Twiss and colleagues' (2009) article to identify the sections of a research report and examine the content in each of these sections. These researchers detailed a rigorously conducted quasi-experimental study, provided findings that are supportive of previous research, and identified conclusions that provide sound evidence to direct the care of patients who are BCSs with bone loss.

Tips for Reading Research Reports

When you start reading research reports, you may be overwhelmed by the new terms and complex information presented. We hope that you will not be discouraged but will see the challenge of examining new knowledge generated through research. You probably will need to read the report slowly two or three times. You can also use the glossary at the end of this book to review the definitions of unfamiliar terms. We recommend that you read the abstract first and then the discussion section of the report. This approach will enable you to determine the relevance of the findings to you personally and to your practice. Initially your focus should be on research reports that you believe can provide relevant information for your practice.

Reading a research report requires the use of a variety of critical thinking skills, such as skimming, comprehending, and analyzing, to facilitate an understanding of the study (Wilkinson, 2012). Skimming a research report involves quickly reviewing the source to gain a broad overview of the content. Try this approach. First, familiarize yourself with the title and check the author's name. Next, scan the abstract or introduction and discussion sections. Knowing the findings of the study will provide you with a standard for evaluating the rest of the article. Then read the major headings and perhaps one or two sentences under each heading. Finally, reexamine the conclusions and implications for practice from the study. Skimming enables you to make a preliminary judgment about the value of a source and whether to read the report in depth.

Comprehending a research report requires that the entire study be read carefully. During this reading, focus on understanding major concepts and the logical flow of ideas within the study. You may wish to highlight information about the researchers, such as their education, current positions, and any funding they received for the study. As you read the study, steps of the research process might also be highlighted. Record any notes in the margin so that you can easily identify the problem, purpose, framework, major variables, study design, treatment, sample, measurement methods, data collection process, analysis techniques, results, and study outcomes. Also record any creative ideas or questions you have in the margin of the report.

We encourage you to highlight the parts of the article that you do not understand and ask your instructor or other nurse researchers for clarification. Your greatest difficulty in reading the research report probably will be in understanding the statistical analyses. Information in Chapter 11 should help you understand the analyses included in studies. Basically, you must identify the particular statistics used, results from each statistical analysis, and meaning of the results. Statistical analyses describe variables, examine relationships among variables, or determine differences among groups. The study purpose or specific objectives, questions, or hypotheses indicate whether the focus is on description, relationships, or differences. Therefore you need to link each analysis technique to its results and then to the study purpose or objectives, questions, or hypotheses presented in the study.

The final reading skill, analyzing a research report, involves determining the value of the report's content. Break the content of the report into parts, and examine the parts in depth for accuracy, completeness, uniqueness of information, and organization. Note whether the steps of the research process build logically on each other or whether steps are missing or incomplete. Examine the discussion section of the report to determine whether the researchers have provided a critical argument for using the study findings in practice. Using the skills of skimming, comprehending, and analyzing while reading research reports will increase your comfort with studies, allow you to become an informed consumer of research, and expand your knowledge for making changes in practice. These skills for reading research reports are essential for conducting a comprehensive critical appraisal of a study. Chapter 12 focuses on the guidelines for critically appraising quantitative and qualitative studies.

PRACTICE READING QUASI-EXPERIMENTAL AND EXPERIMENTAL STUDIES

Knowing the sections of the research report—Introduction, Methods, Results, and Discussion (see Box 2-1)—provides a basis for reading research reports of quantitative studies. You can apply the critical thinking skills of skimming, comprehending, and analysis to your reading of the sample quasi-experimental and experimental studies provided here. Being able to read research reports and identify the steps of the research process should enable you to conduct an initial critical appraisal of a report. Throughout this text, you'll find boxes, entitled "Critical Appraisal Guidelines," which provide questions you will want to consider in your critical appraisal of various research elements or steps. This chapter concludes with initial critical appraisals of a quasi-experimental study and an experimental study using the guidelines provided.

? INITIAL CRITICAL APPRAISAL GUIDELINES

Quantitative Research

The following questions are important in conducting an initial critical appraisal of a quantitative research report:
1. What type of quantitative study was conducted—descriptive, correlational, quasi-experimental, or experimental?
2. Can you identify the following sections in the research report—Introduction, Methods, Results, and Discussion—as identified in Box 2-1?
3. Were the steps of the study clearly identified? Figure 2-1 identifies the steps of the quantitative research process.
4. Were any of the steps of the research process missing?

Quasi-Experimental Study

The purpose of quasi-experimental research is to examine cause and effect relationships among selected independent and dependent variables. Researchers conduct quasi-experimental studies in nursing to determine the effects of nursing interventions or treatments (independent variables) on patient outcomes (dependent variables; Shadish et al., 2002). Artinian and associates (2007) conducted a quasi-experimental study to determine the effects of nurse-managed telemonitoring (TM) on the blood pressure (BP) of African Americans. The steps for this study are illustrated with excerpts from the research report.

⚡ RESEARCH EXAMPLE

Steps of the Research Process in a Quasi-Experimental Study

Research Study Excerpt

1. Introduction

Research Problem

"Nearly one in three, or approximately 65 million adults in the United States have hypertension, defined as (a) having systolic blood pressure (SBP) of 140 mmHg or higher or diastolic blood pressure (DBP) of at least 90 mm Hg or higher, (b) taking antihypertensive medication, or (c) being told at least twice by a physician or other health professional about having high blood pressure (BP) (American Heart Association [AHA], 2005; AHA Statistics Committee and Stroke Statistics Subcommittee [AHASC], 2006; Fields et al., 2004). ... Estimated direct and indirect costs associated with hypertension total $63.5 billion (AHA, 2005).... The crisis of high BP (HBP) is particularly apparent among African Americans; their prevalence of HBP is among the highest in the world. ... Unless healthcare professionals can improve care for individuals with hypertension, approximately two thirds of the population will continue to have uncontrolled BP and face other major health risks (Chobanian et al., 2003).... There is a need to test alternative treatment strategies." Artinian et al., 2007, pp. 312-313

Research Purpose

"The purpose of this randomized controlled trial with urban African Americans was to compare usual care (UC) only with BP telemonitoring (TM) plus UC to determine which leads to greater reduction in BP from baseline over 12 months of follow-up, with assessments at 3, 6, and 12 months postbaseline." Artinian et al., 2007, p. 313

Literature Review

The literature review for this study included relevant, current studies that summarized what is known about the impact of TM on BP. The sources were current and ranged in publication dates from 1998 to 2005, with most of the studies published in the last 5 years. The study was accepted for publication on May 31, 2007 and published in the September/October 2007 issue of *Nursing Research*. Artinian and associates (2007, p. 314) summarized the current knowledge about the effect of TM on BP by stating that,

"Although promising, the effects of TM on BP have been tested in small, sometimes nonrandomized, samples, with one study suggesting that patients may not always adhere to measuring their BP at home. The influence of TM on BP control warrants further study."

Framework

Artinian and co-workers (2007) developed a model that identified the theoretical basis for their study. The model is presented in Figure 1 of this example (Figure 2-3) and indicates that

"Nurse-managed TM is an innovative strategy that may offer hope to hypertensive African Americans who have difficulty accessing care for frequent BP checks. . . . In other words, TM may lead to a reduction in opportunity costs or barriers for obtaining follow-up care by minimizing the contextual risk factors that interfere with frequent health care visits. . . . Combined with information about how to control hypertension, TM may both help individuals gain conscious control over their HBP and contribute to feelings of confidence for carrying out hypertension self-care actions. . . . Home TM appeared to contribute to individuals' increased personal control and self-responsibility for managing their BP, which ultimately led to improved BP control." Artinian et al., 2004; Artinian, Washington, & Templin, 2001

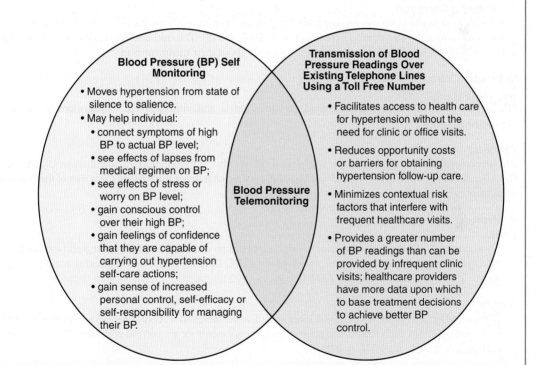

FIG 2-3 Theoretical basis for the effects of telemonitoring on blood pressure. (From Artinian, N. T., Flack, J. M., Nordstrom, C. K., Hockman, E. M., Washington, O. G. M., Jen, K. C., & Fathy, M. [2007]. Effects of nurse-managed telemonitoring on blood pressure at 12-month follow-up among urban African Americans. *Nursing Research, 56*(5), 313.)

The framework for this study was based on tentative theory that was developed from the findings of previous research by Artinian and colleagues (2001, 2004) and other investigators. This framework provides a basis for interpreting the study findings and giving them meaning.

Continued

⚔ RESEARCH EXAMPLE—cont'd

Hypothesis Testing

"H1: Individuals who participate in UC plus nurse-managed TM will have a greater reduction in BP from base-line at 3-, 6-, and 12-month follow-up than would individuals who receive UC only." Artinian et al., 2007, p. 317

Variables

The independent variable was a TM program and the dependent variables were systolic and diastolic BP (SBP and DBP). Only the TM program and SBP are defined with conceptual and operational definitions. The conceptual definitions are derived from the study framework and the operational definitions are often found in the methods section, under measurement methods and intervention headings.

Independent Variable: Telemonitoring Program
Conceptual Definition

TM program is an innovative strategy that may offer hope to hypertensive African Americans to reduce their opportunity costs and barriers for obtaining follow-up care for BP management (Artinian et al., 2007).

Operational Definition

TM "refers to individuals self-monitoring their BP at home, then transmitting the BP readings over existing telephone lines using a toll-free number" (Artinian et al., 2007, p. 313). The readings were reviewed by the care providers, with immediate feedback provided to the patients about their treatment plan.

Dependent Variable: Systolic Blood Pressure
Conceptual Definition

SBP is an indication of the patient's blood pressure control and ultimately the management of his or her hypertension.

Operational Definition

The outcome of SBP was measured with an electronic BP monitor (Omron HEM-737 Intellisense, Omron Health Care, Bannockburn, IL; Artinian et al., 2007). The SBP was the first number recorded on the screen of the Omron BP equipment.

2. Methods
Design

"A randomized, two-group, experimental, longitudinal design was used. The treatment group received nurse-managed TM and the control group received enhanced UC. Data were collected at baseline and 3-, 6-, and 12-month follow-ups." Artinian et al., 2007, p. 314

Sample

"African Americans with hypertension [population] were recruited through free BP screenings offered at community centers, thrift stores, drugstores, and grocery stores located on the east side of Detroit" [natural settings]. Artinian et al., 2007, p. 315

The sampling criteria for including and excluding subjects from the study were detailed and provided a means of identifying patients with hypertension. The sample size was 387 (194 in the TM group and 193 in the usual care [UC] group), with a 13% attrition or loss of subjects over the 12-month study. The subjects' recruitment and participation in the study are detailed in a figure in the article (see Artinian et al., 2007, p. 316).

Intervention

Artinian and associates (2007) detailed the nurse-managed TM intervention in their research article (pp. 315-316). LifeLink Monitoring (Bearsville, NY) was used to provide the TM services for this study. The researchers also described the enhanced UC that was received by the experimental and control groups.

Outcome Measurement

The BP was measured with the electronic Omron BP monitor.

"... [A]fter a 5-minute rest period, at least two BPs were measured, and the average of all was used for analyses. Participants wore unrestrictive clothing and sat next to the interviewer's table, their feet on the floor;
their back supported; and their arm abducted, slightly flexed, and supported at heart level by the smooth, firm
surface of a table." Artinian et al., 2007, pp. 316-317

Data Collection

"Most of the data were collected during 2-hour structured face-to-face interviews and brief physical exams,
which were conducted by trained interviewers in a private room at one of the project-affiliated neighborhood
community centers. Mailed postcards provided interview appointment reminders 1 week before the scheduled interview; telephone call reminders were made the evening before the interview. ... Participants were
compensated $25.00 after the completion of each interview." Artinian et al., 2007, p. 316

The study was approved by the Wayne State University Human Investigation Committee and all participants
signed consent forms indicating their willingness to be subjects in the study.

3. Results

"The hypothesis was supported partially by the data. Overall, the TM intervention group had a greater
reduction in SBP (13.0 mm Hg) than the UC group did (7.5 mm Hg; $t = -2.09$, $p = .04$) from baseline
to the 12-month follow-up. Although the TM intervention group had a greater reduction in the DBP
(6.3 mm Hg) compared with the UC group (4.1 mm Hg), the differences were not statistically significant
($t = -1.56$, $p = .12$)." Artinian et al., 2007, pp. 317-318

4. Discussion

"The nurse-managed TM group experienced both clinically and statistically significant reductions in SBP
(13.0 mm Hg) and clinically significant reductions in DBP (6.3 mm Hg) over a 12-month monitoring period
[study conclusions]. ... The BP reductions achieved here are important results, which, if maintained over
time, could improve care and outcomes significantly for urban African Americans with hypertension. ... This
may mean that an individual could avoid starting a drug regimen or may achieve BP control using a one-drug
regimen rather than a two-drug regimen and thus be at risk for fewer medication side effects [implications of
the findings for nursing practice]. ... Future research needs to determine if this intervention effect maintained
over time leads to reducing the number of complications associated with uncontrolled BP and if it leads to
reducing the number of drugs necessary to achieve BP control." Artinian et al., 2007, pp. 320-321

Initial Critical Appraisal

Quasi-Experimental Study

Artinian and colleagues (2007) presented a clear, concise, and comprehensive report of their quasi-experimental
study of the effect of TM on BP in urban African Americans. These researchers also clearly organized their research
article using the four major sections— Introduction, Methods, Results, and Discussion. Each section clearly detailed
the steps of the quantitative research process and no steps of the research process were omitted.

The findings from this applied study do have implications for practice because this nurse-managed TM intervention significantly affected BP in a population with a high incidence of hypertension. Based on Artinian and colleagues' (2001, 2007, 2004) research and the research of others that documented the importance of home BP
monitoring, a scientific statement from the American Heart Association, American Society of Hypertension,
and Preventive Cardiovascular Nurses Association recommended the use of and reimbursement for home BP monitoring (Pickering, et al., 2008). Artinian was a member of the group making this recommendation about home BP
monitoring. For more information about the home BP monitoring recommendation, you can view the American
Heart Association (2011) website at http://my.americanheart.org/professional/General/Call-to-Action-on-Use-
and-Reimbursement-for-Home-Blood-Pressure-Monitoring_UCM_423866_Article.jsp.

Experimental Study

The purpose of experimental research is to examine cause and effect relationships between independent and dependent variables under highly controlled conditions. The planning and implementation of experimental studies are highly controlled by the researcher, and often these studies are conducted in a laboratory setting on animals or objects. Few nursing studies are purely experimental. Sharma and co-workers (2010) conducted an experimental study of the effects of aerobic exercise on analgesia and neurotropin-3 synthesis in an animal model of chronic widespread pain. This study was introduced earlier in the discussion of basic research. We encourage you to read this study, identify the sections of the research report (see Box 2-1), determine the steps of the quantitative research process, and then compare your findings with those presented in this section.

RESEARCH EXAMPLE

Steps of the Research Process in an Experimental Study

Research Study Excerpt

1. Introduction

Research Problem

"Present literature and clinical practice provide strong support for the use of aerobic exercise in reducing pain and improving function for individuals with chronic musculoskeletal pain syndromes. However, the molecular basis for positive actions of exercise remains poorly understood. Recent studies suggest that neurotropin-3 (NT-3) may act in an analgesic fashion in various pain states...

Chronic widespread pain is complex and poorly understood and affects about 12% of the adult population in developed countries. Many laboratory animal models of pain have been produced to mimic human painful conditions. The acid model used in the present study is a noninflammatory muscle pain model and is considered to mirror some aspects of human fibromyalgia and other related syndromes that display referred hypersensitivity to mechanical stimuli. . . . To date, no animal studies have evaluated the effect of exercise on muscular hypersensitivity." Sharma et al., 2010, pp. 714-715

Research Purpose

"The purpose of the present study was to examine the effects of moderate-intensity aerobic exercise on pain-like behavior and NT-3 in an animal model of widespread pain." Sharma et al., 2010, p. 714

Review of Literature

The research report of Sharma and colleagues (2010) was received on May 25, 2009, accepted for publication January 17, 2010, and published in 2010 in the journal of *Physical Therapy* (see the References for a complete citation of this study). The review of literature in this study is current because the sources cited in the study were published from 1987 through 2007, and most of the sources were published in the last 5 years (2002-2007). The literature review included a synthesis of relevant studies, as indicated in the following study excerpt.

"In recent years, evidence has emerged concerning the role of NT-3 as a pain modulator for thermal, mechanical, and inflammatory hyperalgesia. Previous studies from our laboratory revealed that increased levels of NT-3 (either genetically overexpressed or delivered intramuscularly) abolished mechanical hypersensitivity that developed in response to intramuscular acid injections. If exercise increases NT-3 synthesis and NT-3 reduces cutaneous and thermal hyperalgesia, the next logical step is to test whether exercise-induced analgesia can be achieved in a muscular pain model." Sharma et al., 2010, p. 715

Framework

Sharma and associates (2010) did not clearly identify a framework for their study, but the study seemed to be based on the physiological effects of exercise on NT-3 and deep tissue hyperalgesia in an animal model of pain. The focus was on providing a possible molecular basis for exercise training in reducing muscular pain. A clearly stated framework identifies the theoretical relationships or propositions that guide the development of study hypotheses for quasi-experimental and experimental studies. No hypotheses were identified to direct the conduct of this study. The study framework is also important for the interpretation of research findings and making them meaningful to nursing practice.

Variables

The independent or treatment variable was exercise training, and the dependent or outcome variables included cutaneous and deep tissue hyperalgesia, NT-3 synthesis, and NT-3 protein levels. The intervention exercise training and the outcome variables of NT-3 synthesis and NT-3 protein levels are conceptually and operationally defined as examples. The complete research report provides much more detail on the intervention implemented, measurement of the dependent variables of cutaneous and deep tissue hyperalgesia with behavioral testing, and measurement of NT-3 synthesis and NT-3 protein levels using biochemical assays.

Independent Variable: Exercise Training
Conceptual Definition

The independent variable was not clearly conceptually defined in the study but might be defined as aerobic exercise implemented to determine the cellular effects on widespread muscle pain in an animal model.

Operational Definition

"Two six-lane, motorized treadmills were used for exercise training. The exercise training intervention was implemented 5 days per week for 3 weeks" (Sharma et al., 2010, p. 716).

Dependent Variables: NT-3 Synthesis and NT-3 Protein Levels
Conceptual Definition

These dependent variables were not clearly defined conceptually but might be defined as biochemical assays that indicate the cellular response of skeletal muscles to exercise in an animal model.

Operational Definitions

"Levels of NT-3 messenger RNA (mRNA) and protein in skeletal muscles were measured using standard measures of quantitative real-time polymerase chain reaction (PCR) and enzyme-linked immunosorbent assay (ELISA), respectively." Sharma et al, 2010, p. 717

2. Methods

Sharma and co-workers (2010) clearly described the ethical approval of their study, selection of the mice for the study, and laboratory setting for conducting the study.

"All experiments were approved by the Institutional Animal Care and Use Committee of the University of Kansas Medical Center and adhered to the university's animal care guidelines. Forty CF-1 female mice (weight=25 g) were used to examine the effects of moderately intense exercise on primary (muscular) and secondary (cutaneous) hyperalgesia and NT-3 synthesis. Because women develop widespread pain syndromes at a greater rate than age-matched men, hyperalgesia was induced in female mice. The mice were exposed to 12-hour light-dark cycle and had access to food and water ad libitum. The mice received two 20-µl injections of either acidic saline ... or normal saline ... 2 days apart into the right gastrocnemius muscle to induce chronic widespread hyperalgesia or pain-like behavior." Sharma et al., 2010, p. 715

Continued

RESEARCH EXAMPLE—cont'd

Experimental Design

Initially, the mice were randomly assigned to the acidic saline injection (experimental) group or the normal saline injection (placebo) group. Five days after inducing hyperalgesia with acidic saline injections into the right limb, the animals were further assigned to an exercise or no-exercise group, as follows: experimental with exercise ($n = 10$), experimental without exercise group ($n = 10$), placebo with exercise group ($n = 10$), and placebo without exercise group ($n = 10$). Sharma and colleagues (2010) included a strong, four-group experimental design to control the effects of the injection (placebo group receiving saline injection versus experimental group receiving acidic saline), as well as the effects of the exercise training (no exercise versus exercise training groups). The dependent variables were measured preinjection, postinjection, and 2 weeks postinjection to determine the changes following the injections and exercise training.

Measurements

Sharma and associates (2010) provided detailed descriptions of the measurement of the dependent variables cutaneous and deep tissue hyperalgesia with behavior testing. The NT-3 sensitivity and NT-3 protein levels were measured with biochemical assays that were previously identified in the operational definitions of the variables.

3. Results

"Moderate-intensity aerobic exercise reduced cutaneous and deep tissue hyperalgesia induced by acidic saline and stimulated NT-3 synthesis in skeletal muscle. The increase in NT-3 was more pronounced at the protein level compared with the messenger ribonucleic acid (mRNA) expression. In addition, the increase in NT-3 protein was significant in the gastrocnemius muscle but not in the soleus muscle, suggesting that exercise can preferentially target NT-3 synthesis in specific muscle types." Sharma et al., 2010, p. 714

4. Discussion

Sharma and co-workers (2010) discussed their research findings and linked them to previous research. The researchers stressed that the results are limited to animal models and cannot be generalized to humans experiencing chronic pain. Thus further human studies were recommended to determine the intensity of exercise needed to decrease pain symptoms and improve physical functioning in individuals with chronic pain. The researchers closed with the following conclusions and suggestions for further research.

"We have demonstrated that moderate-intensity exercise training did not cure but significantly reduced cutaneous and deep tissue mechanical hypersensitivity induced by acidic saline injections. This finding is consistent with the findings of human studies, as exercise does not reverse the painful condition but rather decreases pain and improves function. The data also demonstrate an increase in activity-dependent NT-3 levels in selected peripheral tissues. Based on emerging views about the analgesic properties of NT-3, it is plausible to suggest that the decrease in mechanical hypersensitivity following exercise may be due in part, to elevated levels of NT-3 protein. However, the mechanism by which NT-3 modulates mechanoreceptors is still unknown and remains to be investigated." Sharma et al., 2010, p. 724

Initial Critical Appraisal

Experimental Study

Sharma and colleagues (2010) presented a complex, comprehensive report of their experimental study of the effects of aerobic exercise on analgesia and NT-3 synthesis and protein levels in female mice. They also clearly organized their article using the four major sections—Introduction, Methods, Results, and Discussion. Each section clearly detailed the specific steps of the quantitative research process. This experimental study provides basic knowledge about the biological processes of mice exposed to chronic pain and provides a basis for applied human research to examine the effects of aerobic exercise on chronic widespread pain, such as the pain experienced by patients with fibromyalgia. The study would have been strengthened by including a framework and hypothesis to direct its implementation and discussion of findings.

KEY CONCEPTS

- Quantitative research is the traditional research approach in nursing; it includes descriptive, correlational, quasi-experimental, and experimental types of research.
- Basic, or pure, research is a scientific investigation that involves the pursuit of knowledge for knowledge's sake, or for the pleasure of learning and finding truth.
- Applied, or practical, research is a scientific investigation conducted to generate knowledge that will directly influence or improve clinical practice.
- Conducting quantitative research requires rigor and control.
- A comparison of the problem-solving process, nursing process, and research process shows the similarities and differences in these processes and provides a basis for understanding the research process.
- The quantitative research process involves conceptualizing a research project, planning and implementing that project, and communicating the findings. The steps of the quantitative research process are briefly introduced in this chapter.
- The research problem is an area of concern in which there is a gap in the knowledge needed for nursing practice. The research purpose is generated from the problem and identifies the specific goal or focus of the study.
- The review of relevant literature is conducted to generate a picture of what is known and unknown about a particular topic and provides a rationale for why the study needs to be conducted.
- The study framework is the theoretical basis for a study that guides the development of the study and enables the researcher to link the findings to nursing's body of knowledge.
- Research objectives, questions, and/or hypotheses are formulated to bridge the gap between the more abstractly stated research problem and purpose and the study design and plan for data collection and analysis.
- Study variables are concepts at various levels of abstraction that are measured, manipulated, or controlled in a study.
- Research design is a blueprint for conducting a study that maximizes control over factors that could interfere with the study's desired outcomes.
- The population is all the elements that meet certain criteria for inclusion in a study. A sample is a subset of the population that is selected for a particular study; the members of a sample are the subjects or study participants.
- Measurement is the process of assigning numerical values to objects, events, or situations in accord with some rule. Methods of measurement are identified to measure each of the variables in a study.
- The data collection process involves the precise and systematic gathering of information relevant to the research purpose or the objectives, questions, or hypotheses of a study.
- Data analyses are conducted to reduce, organize, and give meaning to the data and address the research purpose and/or objectives, questions, or hypotheses.
- Research outcomes include the findings, limitations, generalization of findings, conclusions, implications for nursing, and suggestions for further research.
- The content of a research report includes six parts—abstract, introduction, methods, results, discussion, and references.
- Reading research reports involves skimming, comprehending, and analyzing the report.
- The guidelines for conducting an initial critical appraisal of a quantitative study are provided.
- Examples of initial critical appraisals are provided for a quasi-experimental study and an experimental study.

REFERENCES

American Heart Association, (2005). *Heart disease and stroke statistics—2005 update.* Dallas, TX: Author.

American Heart Association (AHA). (2011). *Call to action on use and reimbursement for home blood pressure monitoring.* Retrieved July 1, 2013 from, http://my.americanheart.org/professional/General/Call-to-Action-on-Use-and-Reimbursement-for-Home-Blood-Pressure-Monitoring_UCM_423866_Article.jsp.

American Heart Association Statistics Committee and Stroke Statistics Subcommittee. (AHASC). (2006). Heart disease and stroke statistics—2006 update. *Circulation, 113*(6), e85–e152.

Artinian, N. T., Flack, J. M., Nordstrom, C. K., Hockman, E. M., Washington, O. G. M., Jen, K. C., et al. (2007). Effects of nurse-managed telemonitoring on blood pressure at 12-month follow-up among urban African Americans. *Nursing Research, 56*(5), 312–322.

Artinian, N., Washington, O., Klymko, K., Marbury, C., Miller, W., & Powell, J. (2004). What you need to know about home blood pressure telemonitoring, but may not know to ask. *Home Healthcare Nurse, 22*(10), 680–686.

Artinian, N., Washington, O., & Templin, T. (2001). Effects of home telemonitoring and community-based monitoring on blood pressure control in urban African Americans: A pilot study. *Heart & Lung, 30*(3), 191–199.

Bodenheimer, T., Lorig, K., Holman, H., & Grumbach, K. (2002). Patient self-management of chronic disease in primary care. *Journal of the American Medical Association, 288*(19), 2469–2475.

Brown, S. J. (2014). *Evidence-based nursing: The research-practice connection* (3rd ed.). Sudbury, MA: Jones & Bartlett.

Bureau of Labor Statistics. (2008). *Spotlight on statistics: Older workers.* Retrieved September 28, 2008 from, http://www.bls.gov.

Campbell, D. T., & Stanley, J. C. (1963). *Experimental and quasi-experimental designs for research.* Chicago: Rand McNally.

Chinn, P. L., & Kramer, M. K. (2011). *Integrated theory and knowledge development in nursing* (8th ed.). St. Louis: Elsevier Mosby.

Chobanian, A., Bakris, G., Black, H., Cushman, W., Green, L., Izzo, J., Jr., et al. (2003). Seventh report of the Joint National Committee on Prevention, Detection, Evaluation, and Treatment of High Blood Pressure. *Hypertension, 42*(6), 1206–1252.

Craig, J., & Smyth, R. (2012). *The evidence-based practice manual for nurses* (3rd ed.). Edinburgh: Churchill Livingstone Elsevier.

Crosby, L. J. (1990). The abstract: An important first impression. *Journal of Neuroscience Nursing, 22*(3), 192–194.

Dickson, V. V., Howe, A., Deal, J., & McCarthy, M. M. (2012). The relationship of work, self-care, and quality of life in a sample of older working adults with cardiovascular disease. *Heart & Lung, 41*(1), 5–14.

Doran, D. M. (2011). *Nursing outcomes: The state of the science* (2nd ed.). Canada: Jones & Bartlett Learning.

Fawcett, J., & Garity, J. (2009). *Evaluating research for evidence-based nursing practice.* Philadelphia: F. A. Davis.

Fields, L., Burt, V., Cutler, J., Hughers, J., Roccella, E., & Sorlie, P. (2004). The burden of adult hypertension in the United States 1999–2000: A rising tide. *Hypertension, 44*(4), 398–404.

Fisher, R. A. Sir, (1935). *The designs of experiments.* New York: Hafner.

Grove, S. K. (2007). *Statistics for health care research: A practical workbook.* St. Louis: Saunders Elsevier.

Grove, S. K., Burns, N., & Gray, J. R. (2013). *The practice of nursing research: Appraisal, synthesis, and generation of evidence* (7th ed.). St. Louis: Saunders.

Hertzog, M. A. (2008). Considerations in determining sample size for pilot studies. *Research in Nursing & Health, 31*(2), 180–191.

Kaplan, A. (1964). *The conduct of inquiry: Methodology for behavioral science.* San Francisco: Chandler.

Kerlinger, F. N., & Lee, H. B. (2000). *Foundations of behavioral research* (4th ed.). Fort Worth, TX: Harcourt.

Melnyk, B. M., & Fineout-Overholt, E. (2011). *Evidence-based practice in nursing and health care: A guide to best practice* (2nd ed.). Philadelphia: Lippincott, Williams & Wilkins.

Miller, D. C., & Salkind, N. J. (2002). *Handbook of research design and social measurement* (5th ed.). Newbury Park, CA: Sage.

Morrison, D. M., Hoppe, M. J., Gillmore, M. R., Kluver, C., Higa, D., & Wells, E. A. (2009). Replicating an intervention: The tension between fidelity and adaptation. *AIDS Education and Prevention, 21*(2), 128–140.

National Human Genome Research Institute, *An overview of the division of intramural research,* (2013) Retrieved July 1, 2013 from, http://www.genome.gov/10001634.

National Institute of Occupational Safety and Health (NIOSH), (2008). *Work organization and stress-related disorders.* Retrieved July 1, 2013 from, http://www.cdc.gov/niosh/programs/workorg/emerging.html.

Pickering, T. G., Miller, N. H., Ogedegbe, G., Krakoff, L. R., Artinian, N. T., & Goff, D. (2008). Call to action on use and reimbursement for home blood pressure monitoring: A joint scientific statement from the American Heart Association, American Society of Hypertension, and Preventive Cardiovascular Nurses Association. *Journal of Cardiovascular Nursing, 23*(4), 299–323.

Pinto, M. D., Hickman, R. L., Clochesy, J., & Buchner, M. (2013). Avatar-based depression self-management technology: Promising approach to improve depressive symptoms among young adults. *Applied Nursing Research, 26*(1), 45–48.

Porter, T. M. (2004). *Karl Pearson: The scientific life in a statistical age.* Oxfordshire, United Kingdom: Princeton University Press.

Quality and Safety Education for Nurses (QSEN). *Pre-licensure knowledge, skills, and attitudes (KSAs).* (2013) Retrieved July 1, 2013 from, http://qsen.org/competencies/pre-licensure-ksas/.

Riegel, B., & Dickson, V. A. (2008). A situation-specific theory of heart failure self-care. *Journal of Cardiovascular Nursing, 23*(3), 190–196.

Shadish, W. R., Cook, T. D., & Campbell, D. T. (2002). *Experimental and quasi-experimental designs for generalized causal inference.* Chicago: Rand McNally.

Sharma, N. K., Ryals, J. M., Gajewski, B. J., & Wright, D. E. (2010). Aerobic exercise alters analgesia and neurotropin-3 synthesis in an animal model of chronic widespread pain. *Physical Therapy, 90*(5), 714–725.

Sherwood, G., & Barnsteiner, J. (2012). *Quality and safety in nursing: A competency approach to improving outcomes.* Ames, IA: Wiley-Blackwell.

Twiss, J. J., Waltman, N. L., Berg, K., Ott, C. D., Gross, G. J., & Lindsey, A. M. (2009). An exercise intervention for breast cancer survivors with bone loss. *Journal of Nursing Scholarship, 41*(1), 20–27.

Weijman, I., Ros, W., Rutten, G., Schaufeli, W., Schabracq, M., & Winnubst, J. (2005). The role of work-related and personal factors in diabetes self-management. *Patient Education and Counseling, 59*(1), 87–96.

Wilkinson, J. M. (2012). *Nursing process and critical thinking* (5th ed.). Upper Saddle River, NJ: Pearson.

Wysocki, A. B. (1983). Basic versus applied research: Intrinsic and extrinsic considerations. *Western Journal of Nursing Research, 5*(3), 217–224.

LEARNING OUTCOMES

After completing this chapter, you should be able to:

1. Contrast the characteristics of qualitative research with the characteristics of quantitative research.
2. Describe five qualitative research approaches—phenomenological research, grounded theory research, ethnography, exploratory-descriptive qualitative research, and historical research.
3. Describe the intended outcome of each qualitative approach.
4. Describe four ways that data may be collected in a qualitative study.
5. Describe strategies used by qualitative researchers to increase the credibility and transferability of their findings.
6. Compare how data collected in an interview might be different from data collected in a focus group.
7. Critically appraise the collection, analysis, and interpretation of data of qualitative studies.

KEY TERMS

Qualitative research is a systematic approach used to describe experiences and situations from the perspective of the person in the situation. The researcher analyzes the words of the participant, finds meaning in the words, and provides a description of the experience that promotes deeper understanding of the experience. You may empathize with a family member whose loved one has had a heart transplant, for example, but have a limited appreciation for the perceptions of the family member. How does your understanding change when you read the words of a family member who has lived the experience? "On the day doctor said he [son] needed a transplant, my world collapsed. I was depressed, feeling bad, bad, bad. Then I said: My son is going to need me. I can't get sick. Then I found my strength in that." (Sadala, Stolf, Bocchi, & Bicudo, 2013, p.123). Because caring about and wanting to help people are motivations for being a nurse, nurses value qualitative research for the insight that it can provide. Qualitative research can generate rich descriptions of the experiences of patients and families that increase nurses' understanding of the best ways to intervene and be supportive. As a result, qualitative findings make a distinct contribution to evidence-based practice (Brown, 2014; Munhall, 2012).

This chapter introduces the values supporting qualitative research and presents an overview of five qualitative perspectives commonly conducted in nursing—phenomenological research, grounded theory research, ethnographic research, exploratory-descriptive qualitative research, and historical research. An example of each type of study is described. You are introduced to some of the more common methods used to collect, analyze, and interpret qualitative data. This content provides a background for you to use in reading and comprehending published qualitative studies, critically appraising qualitative studies, and applying study findings to your practice.

VALUES OF QUALITATIVE RESEARCHERS

Qualitative researchers describe perspectives on various phenomena. Phenomena are the experiences that comprise the lives of humans. An experience is considered unique to the individual, time, and context, which is why qualitative researchers describe a phenomenon from the perspective of the persons who are experiencing the phenomenon. Qualitative researchers seek to provide a holistic picture of phenomena guided by the following beliefs:
1. There are multiple, constructed realities because meaning is subjective (created by individuals) and intersubjective (created by groups) (Munhall, 2012; Oliver, 2012).

2. Knowledge is co-constructed by the persons involved in an interaction.
3. Human behavior, such as words and actions, are choices influenced by the past and present, as well as by the physical, psychological, and social contexts of the behavior or experience (Oliver, 2012).
4. Time and context influence individual and group perspectives.

The reasoning process used in qualitative research involves putting pieces together perceptually to make wholes. From this process, meaning is produced. Because perception varies with the individual, many different meanings are possible (Munhall, 2012). The findings from a qualitative study lead to an understanding of a phenomenon in a particular situation and are not generalized in the same way as a quantitative study. The meanings that emerge provide an initial picture or theory of the phenomenon being studied. To move beyond the initial view, qualitative researchers must remain open to different descriptions or explanations of the phenomenon during data analysis and interpretation. The **rigor** or strength of a qualitative study is the extent to which the identified meanings represent the perspectives of the participants accurately. Rigorous qualitative methods can ensure that the researcher maintains an open perspective on the phenomenon.

RIGOR IN QUALITATIVE RESEARCH

Scientific rigor is valued because the findings of rigorous studies are seen as being more credible and of greater worth. Studies are critically appraised as a means of judging rigor. Rigor is defined differently for qualitative research because the desired outcome is different from the desired outcome for quantitative research (Grove, Burns, & Gray, 2013). Rigor is assessed in relation to the detail built into the design of the qualitative study, carefulness of data collection, and thoroughness of analysis. Qualitative researchers are expected to maintain an open mind and allow the meaning to be revealed, even if the meaning is not what was anticipated (Munhall, 2012). The qualitative researcher is expected to provide sufficient information in the published report so that the reader can critically appraise the dependability and confirmability of the study (Petty, Thomson, & Stew, 2012). Studies that are dependable and confirmable can be said to have truth, value, or credibility. The findings of a qualitative study cannot be generalized but may be applied "in other contexts or with other participants" (Petty et al., 2012, p. 382). The extent to which the findings of a qualitative study are dependable, confirmable, credible, and transferable is the degree of rigor that the study has. Chapter 12 has more information about how to determine whether a study is dependable, confirmable, credible, and transferable.

QUALITATIVE RESEARCH APPROACHES

Each of these five approaches is based on a philosophical orientation that influences the interpretation of the data. For each approach, whether phenomenology, grounded theory, ethnography, exploratory-descriptive qualitative research, or historical research, it is critical to understand the philosophy on which the method is based. Each approach is discussed in relation to its philosophical orientation and intended outcome. A nursing study is provided to illustrate each methodology. Deciding which qualitative approach to use depends on the research question and purpose of the study (Bolderston, 2012).

Qualitative Studies

The following questions can be asked to appraise the qualitative approach of a study critically:
1. Was the clinical or practice problem that the study addressed a significant problem?
2. What was the research problem that the study was designed to address?
3. What was the purpose of the study? Did the researcher clearly state the purpose? Is the purpose of the study consistent with using a qualitative research design?
4. Did the researcher identify the qualitative research approach used in the study?
5. Were the methods consistent with the qualitative research approach and its philosophical orientation?
6. Are the results consistent with the qualitative research approach used?

Phenomenological Research
Philosophical Orientation

Phenomenology refers to both a philosophy and a group of research methods congruent with the philosophy that guide the study of experiences or phenomena (Dowling & Cooney, 2012). Phenomenologists view the person as integrated with the environment. The world shapes the person, and the person shapes the world. The broad research question that phenomenologists ask is, "What is the meaning of one's lived experience?" Being a person is self-interpreting; therefore, the only reliable source of information to answer this question is the person (Mapp, 2008). Understanding human behavior or experience, which is a central concern of nursing, requires that the person interpret the action or experience for the researcher; the researcher then interprets the explanation provided by the person.

Phenomenologists differ in their philosophical beliefs. Nursing phenomenological researchers usually base their study design on Husserl or Heidegger, whose views of the person and the world differ (Petty et al., 2012). Each of these philosophical perspectives supports a specific type of phenomenological research.

Husserl's view is that the focus is on the phenomenon itself and the meaning-laden statements in the data that capture the essence or true meaning of what the participant perceives and experiences (Dowling & Cooney, 2012). The meaning-laden statements are analyzed to discover the structure within the phenomenon. Husserl's philosophy supports descriptive phenomenological research, whose purpose is to describe experiences as they are lived, or in phenomenological terms, to capture the "lived experience" of study participants. To describe lived experiences, according to Husserl, researchers must bracket or set aside their own biases and preconceptions to describe the phenomenon in a naïve way (Dowling & Cooney, 2012).

Heidegger argued that it was impossible to set aside one's preconceptions and understand the world naively. He believed that phenomenological researchers describe how participants have interpreted their experiences (Converse, 2012) and interpret the data, looking for the hidden meaning (Dowling & Cooney, 2012). The interpretative approach, consistent with Heidegger's philosophy, involves analyzing the data and presenting a rich word picture of the phenomenon as interpreted by the researcher.

Hermeneutics is one type of interpretive phenomenological research method that is congruent with Heidegger's philosophical perspective and is being used by nurse researchers (Dowling & Cooney, 2012). Hermeneutics involves textual analysis that begins with a naïve reading of the texts (Flood, 2010). Transcripts of interviews and published documents are the texts analyzed by nurse researchers. From these naïve readings, the researcher identifies sub-themes and

✗ . themes that are examined in light of the study's research questions. As the text, themes, and relevant literature are integrated, a description of the phenomenon as interpreted is produced.

Phenomenology's Outcome

✗ . The purpose of phenomenological research is to provide a thorough description of a lived experience. Some researchers will summarize their findings with a written summary that combines the findings into a thorough description or an exemplar of the experience.

RESEARCH EXAMPLE

Phenomenological Study

Research Study

Trollvik, Nordbach, Silen, and Ringsberg (2011) conducted a phenomenological study of the lived experience of children, ages 7 to 10 years, who had asthma. Two of the authors conducted 15 individual interviews with the participants, who were recruited from children hospitalized for asthma. Conducting qualitative research with children can be challenging because they may lack the cognitive ability to reflect on their experiences. To provide additional data and another means of communication, the participants were asked to draw a picture of a situation that they described in their interview. The pictures provided validation of the interview transcript and "provided a deeper understanding of their life world and their inner thoughts" (Trollvik et al., 2011, p. 301).

From the interview transcripts, the researchers identified five subthemes that were found to form two clusters of meaning (themes). The first was fear of exacerbations. The children described realizing when their symptoms were worsening as being not able to breathe, feeling tired, and fearing that they would lose control, especially when the symptoms occurred at night. The children could not predict to what extent they could participate in activities with their friends. The second theme was fear of being ostracized. Because asthma limited their activities at times, the children were sometimes excluded or could not participate fully in physical activities with their friends. Not wanting to be seen as "different," the children sometimes continued an activity, even though their symptoms were worsening. They struggled with feelings of loneliness and tried to limit the number of people who knew about their diagnosis (Trollvik et al., 2011).

Critical Appraisal

Trollvik and colleagues (2011) provided information that supported the significance of the clinical problem of childhood asthma by noting that asthma is the most common childhood disease, can be life-threatening, and affects physical activity and growth (significance). The research problem was that few studies of children's perspective of living with asthma had been done (research problem). The study's purpose was consistent with using a qualitative approach, and the researchers clearly identified phenomenology as the approach used. The methods used to collect data (interviews and pictures drawn by the children) and analyze the data were explicit and consistent with phenomenology and its philosophical orientation. In the report, the researchers connected the children's drawings to the themes and connected the themes to direct quotes of the participants to provide a rich description of the experience of living with asthma. The process of linked sources of data to themes increased the confirmability of the study's findings. Also included in the report were the study's strengths and weaknesses, the acknowledgment of which strengthened the study's credibility. Another strength was that they used an additional data source (pictures) because children may lack the cognitive and verbal skills for full expression of their perspectives.

Grounded Theory Research

Grounded theory research is an inductive technique that emerged from the discipline of sociology. The term grounded means the theory developed from the research has its roots in the data from which it was derived. Most scholars base the grounded theory methodology on symbolic interaction theory. George Herbert Mead (Mead, 1934), a social psychologist, developed symbolic interaction theory, which involves exploring how people define reality and how their beliefs are related to their actions. Reality is created by attaching meanings to situations. Meaning is expressed in such symbols as words, religious objects, patterns of behavior, and clothing. These symbolic meanings are the basis for actions and interactions. However, symbolic meanings are different for each individual, and we cannot completely know the symbolic meanings for another individual. In social life, meanings are shared by groups and are communicated to new members through social-ization processes. Group life is based on consensus and shared meanings. Interaction may lead to redefining a meaning or constructing new meanings. The grounded theory researcher seeks to understand the interaction between self and group from the perspective of those involved.

Grounded theory has been used most frequently to study areas in which little previous research has been conducted and to gain a new viewpoint in familiar areas of research. Through their inter-views to understand the perspectives of persons who were dying, Glaser and Strauss (1967) devel-oped grounded theory research as a method and published a book describing it as a qualitative method. Nurses were attracted to the method because of its applicability to the life experiences of persons with health problems and its potential for developing explanations of human behavior (Wuerst, 2012). Nurse researchers continue to use grounded theory methods to study a wide range of topics, such as the coping processes of persons with cancer (Chen & Chang, 2012), the conva-lescence of survivors of intensive care a year after discharge (Ågård, Egerod, Tønnesen, & Lomborg, 2012), and troubled dating relationships of adolescents (Martsolf, Draucker, Bednarz, & Lea, 2011).

Intended Outcome

Fully developed grounded theory studies result in theoretical frameworks with relational state-ments between concepts. Some grounded theorists provide a diagram displaying the interactions among the social processes that were identified. For example, Fenwick, Chaboyer, and St. John (2012) conducted a grounded theory study of the decision-making processes used by persons to manage persistent pain. They found that persistent pain resulted in disruption of the known self. The overall process of self-management was identified as "transforming the deciding self" with three subprocesses: "degenerating self, disconnecting self, and preserving self" (p. 57). Their diagram (Table 3-1) also identified the conditions influencing the disruption of self and actions and consequences of the subprocesses. Based on their theory, nurses can recognize the type of deci-sion making being used by a patient and have a context for intervening to move the patient to a more productive type of decision making.

TABLE 3-1 INTERACTIONS AMONG SOCIAL PROCESSES

RELATED THEMES	→	ACTIONS	→	CONSEQUENCES
		Degenerating Self		
Fearing alterations to the norm Depleting personal energies Struggling for the will to live	→	Impulsive decision making	→	Susceptible decision maker
		Disconnecting Self		
Cure chasing Wavering self-confidence Limiting self-confidence	→	Bargaining decision making	→	Adaptive decision maker
		Preserving Self		
Monitoring the self Building boundaries Partnering with others	→	Judicious decision making	→	Expert decision making

Adapted from Figure 3 of Fenwick, C., Chaboyer, W., & St John, W. (2012). Decision-making processes for the self-management of persistent pain: A grounded theory study. *Contemporary Nurse, 42* (1), 53-66.

RESEARCH EXAMPLE

Grounded Theory Study

Research Study Excerpt

Many nursing programs have integrated high-fidelity simulation into the learning activities of their curriculum to promote the confidence, knowledge, and skills of student nurses. Despite the studies conducted related to simulation, Walton, Chute, and Ball (2011) argued that the teaching method lacked theoretical support. They conducted a grounded theory study to "gain understanding of how students learn with simulation and to identify basic social processes and supportive teaching strategies" (p. 300). Based on their experiences as faculty and their review of the literature, they presented four research questions to guide the study.

"The research questions that were addressed in this qualitative research study are as follows: (a) How do students learn using simulation? (b) What is the process of learning with simulations from the students' perspective? (c) What faculty teaching styles promote learning? and (d) How can faculty support students during simulation?" Walton et al., 2011, p. 300

Walton and co-workers interviewed 16 senior-level nursing students and analyzed the interview data over 1 year. Their analyses identified the stages through which nursing students moved as they took on their professional roles.

"Negotiating the Role of the Professional Nurse was the core category, which included the following five phases: (I) feeling like an imposter, (II) trial and error, (III) taking the role seriously, (IV) transference of skills and knowledge, and (V) professionalization. Figure 3-1 is a conceptual model of 'negotiating the role of the professional nurse.' The boxes represent each of the phases, subcategories, and corresponding faculty strategies." Walton et al., 2011, p. 301

Students described the first phase of feeling like an imposter in terms of uncomfortable feelings. "Fear and anxiety were seen in various degrees throughout each phase of 'negotiating the role of the professional nurse'. . . . The students felt uncomfortable and fearful at the uncertainty of simulated scenarios" (Walton et al., 2011, p. 302). As the students became more secure in what they knew in phase II, "they started to practice by volunteering to demonstrate the tasks with faculty or peers". . . and "appreciated gentle correction in their quest for improvement" (pp. 303, 304). Several students commented on practicing skills and responses to patient situations in their minds as they tried to gain the maximum benefit from their time in the simulation laboratory. As they continued to develop, students reported that they began to see themselves as team leaders and were able to assist other students. "Their uncertainty and anxiety decreased during this transition as they demonstrated understanding of their role. They assimilated the role of the professional nurse by growing in independence, advocating for clients, integrating into the healthcare team, and looking for life direction. . . . They looked at what specialty fit with their lifestyle and personal needs, as well as how they viewed themselves as professional nurses" (pp. 306-307).

The initial findings of Walton and colleagues (2011) were validated by two focus groups of students who had not participated in the interviews. The students in the focus groups added the teaching behaviors that they perceived to be supportive to each phase of the transition to professional nurse.

Critical Appraisal

Walton and associates (2011) indicated the significance of the practice problem by stating that simulation as a teaching method is being used worldwide, with limited theoretical understanding of the process that makes it effective. They identified the qualitative research approach to be grounded theory, which is consistent with the need for learning about social processes. They collected data through interviews and focus groups, coded the data to reveal the themes, and provided direct quotes from students to support each subcategory in the transition process to professional nurse. Each subcategory was clearly linked to a phase of the transition process. The researchers acknowledged their biases related to simulation. The rigor of the study was also supported by the validation of the interview findings by seeking input from additional students in focus groups. The transferability of the findings is limited somewhat because the study was conducted at a religiously affiliated school of nursing with students who were primarily white.

Implications for Quality and Safety in Nursing Education

To protect the safety of patients and ensure high-quality care, newly graduated nurses must internalize the role of the professional nurse and participate as part of a healthcare team (Quality and Safety Education for Nurses [QSEN], 2013; Sherwoood & Barnsteiner, 2012). Walton and co-workers (2011) provided a road map for this transition (see Figure 3-1).

Phases	Subcategories	Faculty Strategies

Phase I
 	
Feeling like an Imposter
	- Anticipatory socialization
	- Wanting specific instruction
	- Feeling disorganized
	- Feeling uncomfortable & anxious
	- Joking around
	- Wanting more structure
	-Struggling with spontaneity
		Welcoming students
		Validating students' feelings:
		    Afraid, disorganized, overwhelmed
		Acknowledging that anxiety is normal
		    Performance, equipment, testing
		    It is okay to make errors
		Providing orientation, rules, dress code
		Demonstrating several times
		Explain expectations, debriefing

Phase II **Trial and Error**	- Practicing, repetition, verbalizing - Joking to mask fear - Replaying scenario in head/minds - Reviewing errors–unsure of the role - Self-reflecting & self-forgiving - Mentoring other students	Encouraging repetition & practice Joking around is part of process Okay to make errors Give positive feedback on what students are doing correctly May need to re-demonstrate Debriefing with gentleness
Phase III **Taking the Role Seriously**	- Defining the scenario as real - Deciding to learn, getting into the role - Using nurse speak - Routinization - Building perspective in role of the nurse - Developing team leadership skills - Learning to analyze - Starting to pull it all together	Dressing the role in scrubs or lab coat Using nurse vocabulary Role modeling expectations Role modeling team skills Avoiding isolation of students Encouraging team building

Phase IV
 	
Transference
	- Emerging human perspective in clinical
	- Feeling confident in the role
	    Skills, problem solving
	- Socialization of the role
	- Failing skill or making errors
	    Disappointment, devastation
	    Lack of confidence, cycle of fear
	- Rebuilding confidence
		Talking about abnormal or extreme
		    patient response and coping with
		    causing pain
		Learning from errors
		Allowing students to debrief each
		scenario, Providing positive feedback first
		Asking questions: How could we improve?
		Demonstrating immense patience

Phase V **Professional-ization**	- Growing in the role - Advocating for clients - Integrating into the healthcare team - Looking into life direction–type of nursing	Developing collegial relationship Assisting students with visualizing goals Addressing students as "nurses" Promoting client advocacy Providing high-level simulations Avoiding interruptions in simulations

FIG 3-1 Phases of negotiating the role of the professional nurse. (From Walton, J., Chute, E., & Ball, L. [2011]. Negotiating the role of the professional nurse: The pedagogy of simulation: A grounded theory study. *Journal of Professional Nursing, 27*[5], 299-310.)

Ethnographic Research

Ethnographic research was developed by anthropologists as a method to study cultures through immersion in the culture over time. The word ethnography means "portrait of a people." Anthropologists study a people's origins, past ways of living, and ways of surviving through time—in other words, their culture. Culture is the focus of ethnography. Early ethnography researchers studied primitive, foreign, or remote cultures (Savage, 2006). Such studies enabled the researcher who spent a year or longer in another culture to acquire new perspectives about a specific people, including their ways of living, believing, and adapting to changing environmental circumstances. This reflects the emic approach, one of studying behaviors from within the culture that recognizes the uniqueness of the individual (Ponterotto, 2005). The emic view from inside the culture is the typical goal of ethnography. The etic approach involves studying behavior from outside the culture and examining similarities and differences across cultures. Etic approaches are more frequently used by anthropologists or sociologists in contrast to nurses, who tend to use an emic approach. Nurses, however, may not observe a culture over months or years, but may observe an organizational culture for a shorter time to learn about the culture of a hospital or healthcare organization. This type of study is called a focused ethnography (Savage, 2006). Observations shorter than months or years are appropriate when the research question is narrower, and the scope of the study is limited to a specific place or organization.

The philosophical perspective of ethnographic research is based in anthropology and recognizes that culture is material and nonmaterial. Material culture consists of all created or constructed aspects of culture, such as buildings used for cultural events, symbols of the culture, family traditions, networks of social relations, and the beliefs reflected in social and political institutions. Symbolic meaning, social customs, and beliefs—components of the nonmaterial culture—may be apparent in a different culture only over time, but are essential elements of cultures. Cultures also have ideals that people hold as desirable, even though they do not always live up to these standards. Anthropologists and nurse ethnographers seek to discover the multiple parts of a culture and determine how these parts are interrelated. A picture of the culture as a whole becomes clearer.

The nurse who increased the visibility of ethnography within nursing was Madeline Leininger, who earned her doctoral degree in anthropology. The fieldwork for her degree was a year that she spent in Papua New Guinea. From this experience, she developed the Sunshine Model of Transcultural Nursing Care, which identifies aspects of culture to consider when communicating with patients and families of another culture (Leininger, 1988). Nurses use Leininger's Theory of Transcultural Nursing (Leininger, 2002) in practice by assessing multiple aspects of the patient, family, and their environment, including religion, societal norms, economic status, country of origin, ethnic subgroup, and beliefs about illness and healing. This theory has led to an ethnographic research strategy for nursing, termed ethnonursing research. Ethnonursing research "focuses mainly on observing and documenting interactions with people [and] how these daily life conditions and patterns are influencing human care, health, and nursing care practices" (Leininger, 1985, p. 238). However, a number of nurse anthropologists not associated with the ethnonursing orientation are also providing important contributions to nursing's body of knowledge (Roper & Shapiro, 2000).

The ethnographic researcher must become very familiar with the culture being studied by observing the culture, actively participating in it, and interviewing members of the culture. The process of becoming immersed in a culture involves being in the culture and gaining increasing familiarity with aspects of the culture, such as language, sociocultural norms, traditions, and other social dimensions, including family, communication patterns (verbal and nonverbal), religion, work patterns, and expression of emotion. Through immersion, the ethnographic researcher becomes increasingly accepted into the culture. Although ethnographic researchers must be actively involved in the culture they are studying, they must avoid "going native," which would interfere with data collection and analysis. In going native, the researcher becomes a part of the culture and loses the ability to observe clearly (Roberts, 2009).

Intended Outcome

The ethnographer prepares a written report based on the analysis of the culture. Depending on the initial research question, the researcher may propose strategies to increase the cultural acceptability of a health intervention, encourage health promotion behaviors, or improve the quality of care that is being delivered in an organization. For example, a group of nurse researchers conducted an ethnographic study of family presence when their loved ones were being weaned from mechanical ventilation (Happ et al., 2007). They collected data by watching the family members of 30 patients during weaning and described their "active engagement in the observation and interpretation" of the patient's status as surveillance (p. 51). The researchers recommended that the typography of family member behaviors they developed "could enhance the dialogue about family-centered care and guide future research on family needs and presence in the ICU" (p. 56).

◢ RESEARCH EXAMPLE

Ethnographic Research

Research Study Excerpt

In another example, Portacolone (2013) was concerned about older adults living alone and conducted an ethnography that involved collecting data over several years about older adults as individuals, relationships between the older adult and institutions in the community, and the larger social problems affecting the person. To collect the data in an unobtrusive manner, Portacolone served as a *Meals on Wheels* volunteer, delivering meals to older adults living at home. She also conducted interviews with a purposive sample of 47 older adults living alone and additional interviews with officials who worked with agencies providing services to older adults.

"Most of the encounters occurred in the informants' home. During the encounter, I engaged in any activity suggested by the informant: this comprised eating and drinking, watching TV, looking at pictures, talking with their friends or home care aides, doing yoga, singing, or walking. As I spent time with each informant, I found the time to ask questions related to their experience of living alone. Their answers were recorded in an audio-recorder and transcribed verbatim. To capture the fresh observations and reflections spurred by each encounter, field notes were written soon after leaving the premises" (Portacolone, 2013, p.168).

The researcher described how the notion of precariousness began to emerge.

"As I was listening to their account, I often felt the sense of ground failing beneath my feet. I translated these impressions in my own words as 'precariousness.' One informant in particular—Paul, a 92-year retiree—strongly gave me the essence of this sensation, which I then re-encountered—in different shapes and flavors—in other informants. The more informants I encountered, the more this image took shape. The word precariousness, as already mentioned, evokes a sense of insecurity and uncertainty stemming from the vanishing of resources from multiple angles" (Portacolone, 2013, p. 169).

Portacolone (2013) examined the data at the micro level, focusing on the individual, and provided stories and examples of precariousness. At the meso level of analysis, the older adult interacted with his or her family and multiple community organizations and institutions. Families were described as not always being able to provide consistent support because of distance, work responsibilities, and strained relationships. The resources that organizations provided required effort on the part of the older adult to obtain information and arrange to receive services. At the macro level, the values that older adults in the United States place on independence and

Continued

RESEARCH EXAMPLE—cont'd

individualism were viewed as patriotic and embedded in the larger culture. "Individuation feeds precariousness as the number of challenges faced by older solo dwellers compound, physical and mental resources decrease, income remains fixed or decreases, and older solo dwellers see themselves as the sole [person] responsible for their situation" (p. 172). Portacolone (2013) offers interdependence as a viable alternative to independence that would "decrease the need of older adults to prove to the outside world that they can make it alone. Within this new paradigm, older adults living alone will not be afraid to ask for help, as they will be aware that doing so will not lead to a forced move into an institution" (p. 173).

Critical Appraisal

The Portacolone (2013) study is significant because of the increasing numbers of older persons living alone, although no statistics about the number of older persons living alone were included. Usually, the researcher would have included statistics as evidence supporting the significance of the study. However, because the study report was published in the *Journal of Aging,* the researcher may have assumed that readers were most likely aware of these statistics. The research problem and purpose of the study were consistent with the ethnographic method, which was identified in the abstract as the approach of the study. The methods were developed to be consistent with ethnography and its philosophical orientation.

Portacolone's (2013) observations occurred over extended periods of time, which allowed identification of impressions that were validated through additional observations. The number and depth of interviews also strengthened the findings. Sufficient quotes and specific examples were provided as evidence of the researcher's conclusions. Because of the rigorous methods used, the study was high quality, but with two identified weaknesses. The first was that the researcher did not identify her own age, cultural background, and potential biases. The second more serious weakness was the omission of any discussion about obtaining institutional review board (IRB) approval and informed consent from the participants.

Implications for Practice

Older persons living alone recognized that their situation was precarious and that events beyond their control could result in not being able to continue living alone (Portacolone, 2013). The essential resources of financial stability and physical health were interrelated and carefully managed to maintain their living situation. Nurses in hospitals, clinics, and homecare need to recognize that the older person may not ask for help for fear of an outside authority determining the person can no longer live at home. As a result, nurses may need to be sensitive to these concerns when offering additional services to older persons living alone.

QSEN Implications

Teams of healthcare professionals collaborate to provide patient-centered care (Sherwood & Barnsteiner, 2012). Nurses and social workers can use the findings of this study as they work together to address the physical and social needs of older adults living alone.

Exploratory-Descriptive Qualitative Research

As you read qualitative study reports, you may find that some researchers did not identify a particular approach to their study, such as phenomenology or grounded theory. Some researchers have described their studies as being naturalistic inquiry, descriptive, or just qualitative. For example, Letourneau and colleagues (2011) designed their study to "describe service providers' understanding of the impact and dynamics of IPV [intimate partner violence] . . . and the unique needs, resources, barriers, and desired supports of these mothers" (p. 194). Nowak and Stevens (2011) indicated the purpose of their "qualitative, descriptive" study with parents who had experienced fetal loss as being "to identify and describe factors associated with this high-risk population" (p. 123). Researchers design qualitative studies such as these to obtain information needed to develop a program or intervention for a specific group of patients. Usually, the researchers are exploring a new topic or describing a situation, so we have chosen to label these studies as exploratory-descriptive qualitative research (Grove et al., 2013). Studies consistent with this approach are not a specific type of research; rather, they are studies conducted for a specific purpose that do not fit into another of the categories (Sandelowski, 2000, 2010).

Philosophical Orientation

Exploratory-descriptive qualitative studies are developed to provide information and insight into clinical or practice problems. Qualitative studies are often developed to address problems in practice but approach the problem differently. The philosophical orientation of exploratory-descriptive qualitative research may vary, depending on the purpose of the study, but often the researcher has a pragmatic orientation (McCready, 2010). The pragmatic researcher is in search of useful information and practical solutions (Creswell, 2013) and designs studies to understand what works (Houghton, Hunter, & Meskell, 2012). Letourneau and associates (2011) were concerned about the needs of families that had been affected by IPV and the extent to which the care and services being provided met the needs of their clients. The study provided the information on which a solution could be based.

Intended Outcome

A well-designed, exploratory-descriptive qualitative study answers the research question. The purpose of the study is achieved, and the researchers have the information they need to address the situation or patient concern that was the focus of the study. The findings of the study are applied to the practice problem that instigated the inquiry. In the study of Letourneau and co-workers (2011), for example, the researchers reported that service providers recognized internalizing and externalizing behaviors of children in families affected by IPV. The service providers also described the instrumental, informational, emotional, and affirmational support needed by women affected by IPV. These findings could be applied to refining the services provided to families affected by IPV.

⚡ RESEARCH EXAMPLE

Exploratory-Descriptive Qualitative study

As noted, Nowak and Stevens (2011) addressed another social problem in their exploratory-descriptive qualitative study. In a region with a high fetal mortality rate, they identified the research problem to be a need for more information about "the circumstances and contexts in which individuals experience loss" (p. 123).

"Women who had experienced a fetal or infant loss were recruited using purposive sampling technique.... [D]ata from fetal losses as early as 14 weeks were also collected due to the disproportionate number of losses that occurred between 14 and 19 weeks of gestation.... The sample consisted of four African American, four White, and three Hispanic women. Of the men that participated, one was African American, two were White, and one was Hispanic. Average time from death to interview was 3 months after fetal deaths and 6 months for infant deaths.... After obtaining informed consent, the researcher conducted a tape-recorded interview of 1 to 3 hours duration (Nowak & Stevens, 2011, p. 123).

The tape recordings were transcribed and the transcriptions were verified prior to data analysis. "Each interview was read several times. Thoughts and themes that emerged with each reading were recorded in a narrative fashion as journal entries (Bloomberg & Volpe, 2008).... Themes were grouped into broad categories that represented the final analysis results... We defined *vigilance* as 'doing everything possible to help this baby make it' by being continually alert and responsive despite poverty, healthcare inequity, and stress" (Nowak & Stevens, 2011, p. 124). The researchers continued

Continued

by describing vigilance that occurred in "environments of violence, poverty, and stress" and supported the theme with quotes from interviews (p. 124). Vigilance also was described "in the context of early pregnancy," "in sensing change in their bodies," "in sensing change in their babies," and "in findings answers" (pp. 125-127).

"The importance of vigilance in parents' experiences in fetal and infant mortality was a key finding in the current study. The finding has been infrequently reported in the literature. Participants shared stories that demonstrated their vigilance in early pregnancy, as well as later when they sensed negative changes in themselves or their babies. They were vigilant because of prior losses and were vigilant in finding answers to their losses when explanations of their babies' deaths were not clear.... Despite their desire for healthy pregnancies and healthy infants, the many life challenges that the study participants experienced may have contributed to their risk for fetal and infant loss" (Nowak & Stevens, 2011, p. 128).

Critical Appraisal

The researchers described fetal infant loss in a specific community. As is appropriate for qualitative studies, the sample of 15 parents was purposively selected because of their experiences with the phenomenon of interest. Thus, the sample size and sampling method were appropriate for a qualitative study. The structured interview guide was included, as well as an explanation of how the researchers used open-ended questions to elicit more information. The poignant quotes that were included provided glimpses into the experiences of the participants so that readers could recognize and empathize with the parents' experiences of fetal and infant losses. The findings were discussed in the context of existing literature, with the researchers noting the contribution of these findings to the literature. The study report could have been stronger if the researchers had included additional information about protection of human subjects, such as referral to psychosocial supports to address the continuing emotional impact of the loss and to community resources to remedy the social conditions that may have contributed to the losses experienced by the parents.

Implications for Practice

By recognizing the effects of poverty, violence, and inadequate access to care, nurses who provide care during times of fetal and infant loss can be more sensitive to the efforts made by the women and their partners to prevent the loss. Referrals can be made to address these issues, as appropriate.

Historical Research

Historical research examines events of the past. Many historians believe that the greatest value of historical knowledge is increased self-understanding; in addition, historical knowledge provides nurses with an increased understanding of their profession. Connolly and Gibson (2011) connected the topic of their historical study, the role of nurses in children with tuberculosis (TB) from 1900 to 1935, to the roles nurses need to assume today to change current healthcare policy. Thompson and Keeling (2012) described in depth how nurses were involved in preventing infant mortality between 1884 and 1925.

Philosophical Orientation

The major assumption of historical philosophy is that lessons can be learned from the past. Historians study the past through oral and written reports and artifacts, searching for patterns that can lead to generalizations. For example, to answer the question—"What causes epidemics?"—a historian could search throughout history for commonalities in various epidemics and develop a theoretical explanation of their causes. The philosophy of history is a search for wisdom in which the historian examines what has been, what is, and what ought to be. Historical philosophers have attempted to identify a developmental scheme for history to explain events and structures as elements of the same social process. Some nurses who conduct historical research have studied nurses and their roles at critical turning points in the profession. Historical nurse researchers believe that nursing as a profession has a history that must be transmitted to those entering the profession as part of their socialization process. Other historical nurse researchers have identified events in health care with the intent of encouraging the readers of the report to learn from the successes and failures of the past.

Historical researchers may collect data by interviewing people with knowledge of events, especially for more recent events. For example, a historical researcher studying army nursing during deployments to Vietnam during the 1970s could interview nurses who served there, because some of them are still living. The interview of a person who played a role in the historical event is considered a primary source of data. Other primary sources are documents written by the person being studied. For example, a diary kept by a nurse while she was deployed to a war zone would be a primary source for the study. Before using it as a source of data, the researcher would confirm with the author that the diary was an authentic document. If the author was not alive, the researcher would seek evidence to confirm authorship. Once documents are authenticated, the researcher would rely more heavily on them as primary sources. However, people who lived at the same time or those who heard stories of that time may provide information to provide breadth and depth to the description that the researcher is developing. These people are secondary sources of data. When primary sources are few or inaccessible, historical researchers rely on secondary sources. The researcher studying army nurses in Vietnam in the 1970s might interview military veterans who received care from the nurses, review newspaper articles from the time, and read army documents used to prepare nurses entering the military at that time. The secondary sources may confirm, expand, or provide an opposite viewpoint to what is available from the primary sources.

Intended Outcome

Historical researchers provide a description of a series of events, a chronology of factors that affected the topic of interest. Reports from historical studies are written differently than reports for other types of studies in that they include limited information about the methods used and have a greater focus on the story being told. Some historical researchers publish a book of their findings rather than publishing them in a journal article. Studies using this approach provide exemplars of nurses who changed health care by their leadership in a specific social or political time and place. The findings of other historical studies have inspired nurses to address current social and political issues and have provided insight into environmental forces that shaped events affecting health care at different times in history.

⑤ RESEARCH EXAMPLE

Historical Research

Research Study Excerpt

Connolly and Gibson (2011) conducted a historical study of tuberculosis, race, and children to describe "nurses' efforts at early twentieth century pediatric TB prevention and treatment in one state, Virginia" (p. 231). To support the study's purpose, they linked the study to current healthcare legislation and changes.

"What can history contribute to our understanding of 21st century children's health care? . . .There are several reasons for doing so. First, much research on children's health lacks a meaningful historical dimension. But the values, norms, policies, and institutions that template pediatric nursing today are all predicated on
Continued

decisions made in the past. As such, a better understanding of the negotiations and debates that shaped contemporary practice and policy can facilitate a more meaningful consideration of how best to deliver health care today and in the future." Connolly & Gibson, 2011, p. 231

As is typical with reports of historical studies, the researchers do not describe their methods in the report. They delineated the period of interest, 1900 to 1935, and the specific disease, TB, in the context of society in the state of Virginia. A pervasive reality of that time was racism and the resulting segregation. "In Virginia, because public health reform was intricately bound to a value system that sought to reinforce the state's existing racial and class hierarchy, nurses, physicians, and others practiced within a framework that restricted their options" (Connolly & Gibson, 2011, p. 232). They described the result of the societal values in terms of a health disparity using government statistics. "Nationwide, non-White youngsters between the ages of 5 and 14 years died of TB at a rate of 155 per 100,000, compared to 23 per 100,000 TB death for White children" (Rogers, 1917, p. 231).

Within the temporal and geographic context, Connolly and Gibson (2011) explored the responses of nurses in public health institutions to TB as a threat to the public:

"Many of the early 20th century anti-TB initiatives designed by Virginians were led by, or crafted with heavy input from, public health nurses.... Richmond's Nurses Settlement was founded in 1900 to provide nursing care to the sick poor and incorporated in 1902 as the Instructive Visiting Nurse Association (IVNA), with the explicit goal of bringing nursing care to people in their homes. The nurses themselves funded the operation, donating their own money and garnering support from private charities and the public health department. In Norfolk, the King's Daughters Visiting Nurse program (a nondenominational Christian women's organization) also responded to the needs of Black patients when, in 1910, they hired their first Black nurse to care for 'Negro women and children.' The perceived need was so great for the services of this nurse that another Black nurse was hired within the first 3 months (Norfolk City Union of the King's Daughters Annual Report for 1910)." Connolly & Gibson, 2011, p. 233

By using a timeline with key events (see Figure 3-2), Connolly and Gibson (2011) provided a visual representation of changes that occurred over time. They described the transition from TB treatment to prevention, which led to the creation of a "*preventorium* for those children not yet sick with TB" (p. 235). Agnes Dillon Randolph, a public health nurse with political connections, was credited with identifying a way to fund prevention through the sale of Christmas seals. "In an effort to fund as many preventoria and other TB programs as possible, the National Tuberculosis Association (NTA) worked with local officials like Randolph to make sure that its annual Christmas Seal campaign was a lucrative community and a national event" (Knopf, 1922, p. 235).

The researchers concluded the report by emphasizing the lessons from 1900 to 1935 that can be applied today.

"Perhaps the most important legacy of Virginia's public health nurses is one that we can use today. Unwilling to be trapped by conventional wisdom, the patterns of the past, or accept the status quo, they drew on all of the resources they could muster to innovate new models of health care. So, too, can today's nurses challenge historical precedent to improve the well-being of all Americans." Connolly & Gibson, 2011, p. 237

Critical Appraisal

The abstract is a clear, succinct summary of the study and its results.

"Drawing on a wealth of primary documents, this historical research describes nurses' efforts regarding early 20th century pediatric tuberculosis care in Virginia. Virginia nurses played a leadership role in designing a template for children's care. Ultimately, however, their legacy is a mixed one. They helped forge a system funded by a complicated, poorly coordinated, race- and class-based mix of public and private support that is now delivered through an idiosyncratic web of community, state, and federal programs. However, they also took courageous action, and their efforts improved the lives of many children. By so doing, they helped invent pediatric nursing" (Connolly & Gibson, 2011, p. 230).

Connolly and Gibson (2011) began their report by explicitly stating the study's relevance to current changes in health care. Another strength is the use of primary sources. Of the 52 sources cited in the report, 28 were published between 1900 and 1935. For example, the researchers documented the veracity of their findings by citing annual reports of organizations providing care, diaries of children who lived in preventoria, government reports, and other original documents that are part of historical collections in libraries. To understand the context better, the researchers also provided information from secondary sources, such as books and articles by historians. The timeline the researchers developed (see Figure 3-2) was a clear way to summarize and portray the critical events they described.

The report is appropriately written as a chronology but could have been strengthened by contrasting the positive and negative aspects of the nurses' legacy throughout the body, instead of only in the abstract. Also, the perspectives of black nurses and children seem to be missing from the report.

Implications for Practice

The courageous actions of Agnes Dillon Randolph and Nannie Minor, the only other nurse named in the report, can inspire nurses today to take a stand against discrimination and injustice in the distribution of health care.

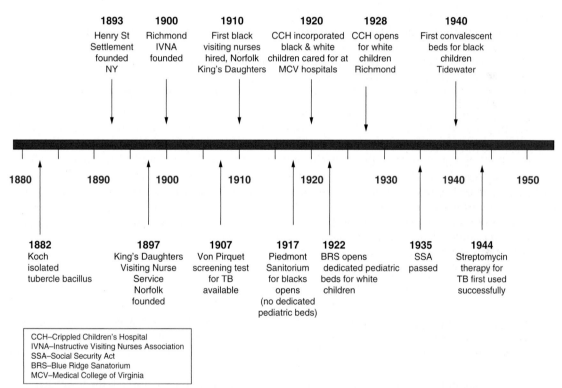

FIG 3-2 Landmark moments in pediatric TB prevention in Virginia. (From Connolly, C., & Gibson, M. [2011]. The "White Plague" and color: Children, race, and tuberculosis in Virginia 1900-1935. *Journal of Pediatric Nursing, 26,* 230-238.)

QUALITATIVE RESEARCH METHODOLOGIES

This section presents a detailed description of the methods commonly used in conducting qualitative studies. In some ways, the methods used are no different from those used in quantitative studies. The researcher must select a topic, state the problem or question, justify the significance of the study, design the study, identify sources of data, such as subjects, gain access to those sources of data, recruit subjects, gather data, describe, analyze, and interpret the data, and develop a written report of the results and findings. There are, however, methods unique to qualitative studies and sometimes to specific types of qualitative research. An understanding of some of the unique methods used by qualitative researchers will help you appreciate the efforts involved in conducting such a study.

This section describes how participants (subjects) are selected and how data are collected, managed, and analyzed. The methods used to ensure rigor in qualitative research also are explored.

Selection of Participants

Subjects in qualitative studies are referred to as participants because the researcher and participants carry out the study cooperatively. The researcher recruits participants because of their particular knowledge, experience, or views related to the study (Munhall, 2012).

Researcher-Participant Relationships

One of the important differences between quantitative and qualitative research lies in the degree of involvement of the researcher with the participants of the study. This involvement, considered to be a source of bias in quantitative research, is thought by qualitative researchers to be a critical element of the research process. The nature of the researcher-participant relationship has an impact on the collection and interpretation of data (Maxwell, 2014). The researcher creates a respectful relationship with each participant, which includes being honest and open about the purpose and methods of the study. The researcher's aims and means need to be negotiated with the participants and honor their perspectives and values (Grove et al., 2013; Maxwell, 2014; Munhall, 2012). In various degrees, the researcher influences the people being studied and, in turn, is influenced by them. Thus the researcher must have their support and confidence to complete the research. The researcher's personality is a key factor in qualitative research. Skills in empathy and intuition are cultivated; the researcher must become closely involved in the subject's experience to interpret it. It is necessary for researchers to be open to the perceptions of the participants, rather than to attach their own meaning to the experience.

Researcher-participant relationships in qualitative studies may be brief when data collection occurs once in an interview or focus group. Phenomenology and grounded theory studies may involve one or two interviews, although researcher-participant relationships may extend over time when the study design involves repeated interviews to study a lived experience or process over time.

Ethnographic studies require special attention to the researcher-participant relationship. The ethnographic researcher observes behavior, communication, and patterns within groups in specific cultures. The researcher may form close bonds with participants who are key informants, persons with extensive knowledge and influence in a culture. The relationships among the researcher and participants can become complex, especially in ethnography studies in which the researcher lives for an extended time in the culture being studied.

DATA COLLECTION METHODS

✗. The data in most qualitative research studies are "the participant's thoughts, ideas, and perceptions" (Bolderston, 2012, p. 68). The most common data collection methods used in the types of qualitative studies discussed in this chapter are interviewing participants, conducting focus groups, observing participants, and examining written text. These methods, as they are used in qualitative studies, are described in the following sections in some detail; examples from the literature are provided.

Interviews

Differences exist between interviews conducted for a qualitative study and those conducted for a quantitative study. In quantitative studies, researchers structure interviews to collect subject responses to questionnaires or surveys (see Chapter 10). Interviews in qualitative studies range from semistructured interviews (fixed set of questions, no fixed responses) to unstructured interviews (open-ended questions, with probes). Probes are queries made by the researcher to obtain more information from the participant about a particular interview question.

For unstructured interviews, also called open-ended interviews, the initial statement or question may be "Tell me about a time that you received bad news about a diagnostic test" or "After your diagnosis, how did you learn about diabetes?" Although the researcher defines the focus of the interview, there may be no fixed sequence of questions. The questions addressed in interviews tend to change as the researcher gains insights from previous interviews and observations. Respondents are allowed, and even encouraged, to raise important issues the researcher may not have addressed.

The researcher's goal is to obtain an authentic insight into the participant's experiences. Although data may be collected in a single interview, dialogue between researcher and participant may continue at intervals across weeks or months and provide rich data for analysis. Use of recurring interviews allows the researcher to explore an evolving process (Munhall, 2012) and allows the researcher-participant relationship to develop. As the relationship develops and trust grows, the participant may reveal the emotional and value-laden aspects of the process more freely.

The purpose of the interview may vary, depending on the type of qualitative approach. Interviews in a phenomenology study may have one main question, with follow-up questions used as needed to elicit the participant's perspective on the phenomenon. Interviews in grounded theory studies are similar in that only one or two questions may be asked, but the follow-up questions will focus on the social processes of the phenomenon. In an exploratory-descriptive qualitative study, the interviewer may ask more structured questions to achieve the purpose of the study. Historical researchers may interview people who were participants in or observers of events that occurred in the past. The focus of the interview may be to validate available information about the event, uncover details previously not known about the event, or obtain views about the event from those who were not heard from previously. Interviews can also be used to construct the participants' biographies. The personal histories of a number of persons can be used to understand the evolving history of a region or institution.

Some strategies used to record information from interviews include writing notes during the interview, writing detailed notes immediately after the interview, and recording the interview. Video may be recorded, as well as audio. For example, audio recordings were used to record telephone interviews of hospital administrators to describe the mental health services provided for female veterans in Veterans Affairs Medical Centers across the United States (MacGregor, Hamilton, Oishi, & Yano, 2011). Telephone interviews were the most feasible way to collect data in this study.

Interviews should be arranged for a time and private place convenient for the participant. Interviews may be held in the participant's home, clinic office, public library meeting room, or restaurant. A place where the interview is less likely to be interrupted and the participant feels secure is more helpful. Meeting in a clinic, for example, may not be appropriate if the interview involves describing the care being received. A person living with an infection caused by the human immunodeficiency virus (HIV) may not want to be interviewed in a place where he or she might be seen by friends or family. You also want a place that is quiet enough to allow for effective audio recording.

⁇ CRITICAL APPRAISAL GUIDELINES

Interviews in Qualitative Studies

When critically appraising studies in which data were collected by interview, address the following questions:

1. Were the strategies used to recruit the participants and obtain informed consent described in the research report?
2. Did the researchers report the length of the interviews? The length of the interviews are usually reported as a range of time.
3. Did the report include information on the questions and prompts used to facilitate the interview?
4. Does the length of the interviews seem adequate for the number and type of research questions? For example, if the researcher indicated that the interviews ranged in length from 10 to 30 minutes and the researcher asked each participant five open-ended questions, you might raise a concern about whether the participants had enough time to provide in-depth answers.

🔊 RESEARCH EXAMPLE

Interview

Research Study Excerpt

McDermott-Levy (2011) conducted interviews in her study of Arab-Muslim female students in a baccalaureate nursing program in the United States. She prepared an initial question and probing questions to elicit descriptions of their experiences of living and studying in the United States.

"The women participated in individual audiotaped interviews in a private conference room at the University. This ensured privacy of the students' responses, which facilitated openness.... The women were asked open-ended questions related to their experience of being Arab-Muslim women living and studying nursing in the United States.... Each interview was conducted in English and lasted from 1-1.5 hours. The interviews were conducted in English because the participants had a trusting relationship with the English-speaking investigator and were successful in their academic program for 12 months prior to data collection." McDermott-Levy, 2011, p. 269

Critical Appraisal

The researcher described the context and the length of the interviews and provided the rationale for the decisions that were made. The length of the interview allowed adequate time for substantive responses to be provided. One concern was that the researcher who conducted the interviews was the students' academic advisor. Because Oman culture values personal relationships and the protection of one's privacy, having the interviewer be someone trusted by the participants outweighed the potential disadvantage that social desirability might influence the information that the participants were willing to share. The risk of feeling coerced to participate was minimized by having another person recruit participants and obtain informed consent. The investigator concluded that the pre-existing trust allowed the participants to be more open and share their challenges, as well as their growth.

Implications for Practice

The participants had learned new behaviors, such as managing money, using a budget, going out independently, and dealing with anti-Muslim prejudices. Having left the security of their families, they reported a sense of "going alone," but acknowledged that the experience has helped them grow in life management skills. The implications of the study were for nurse educators to provide support services for international students and adapt their teaching styles to a wide range of cultures and learning styles.

Focus Groups

Focus groups were designed to obtain the participants' perceptions of a specific topic in a permissive and nonthreatening setting. One of the assumptions underlying the use of focus groups is that group dynamics can help people express and clarify their views in ways that are less likely to occur in a one-to-one interview. The group may give a sense of "safety in numbers" to those wary of researchers or those who are anxious. The recommended size of a focus group is five to eight participants. Larger focus groups are sometimes used but may be more difficult to moderate. All participants should have the opportunity to speak, which may be more difficult to achieve with a larger number. Focus groups are sometimes called group interviews (Bolderston, 2012), so the principles of interviewing such as responding in a nonjudgmental way are still applicable.

Focus groups are conducted by a moderator or facilitator, who may or may not be the researcher. Researchers may elicit the help of moderators who share common characteristics with the participants. An example would be the urban researcher who hires a health professional who grew up in a rural farming community to moderate a focus group on preventing agricultural injuries. Moderators should be thoroughly trained and understand the importance of following the procedures or script developed by the researcher (Gray, 2009).

The entire interaction is audio-recorded and, some cases, video-recorded. In addition to the recording, members of the research team may serve as observers to take notes of the proceedings. Integrating her personal experiences in conducting focus groups with the recommendations in the literature, Gray (2009) proposed that focus groups be conducted in natural settings, but noted that the researcher must plan ahead to protect the confidentiality and comfort of the participants. Confidentiality and comfort may result in richer dialogue and data.

CRITICAL APPRAISAL GUIDELINES

Focus Groups

When critically appraising studies in which data were collected using focus groups, address the following questions:
1. Were the strategies used to recruit the participants and obtain informed consent described in the research report?
2. Did the researchers describe the number, composition, length, and setting of the focus groups?
3. Did the number, composition, and length of the focus groups seem appropriate for the research question?
4. Was the setting conducive for increasing the comfort of the participants and protecting confidentiality?

RESEARCH EXAMPLE

Focus Groups

Research Study Excerpt
Researchers studying the strength of older adults had previously focused on different types of strength, such as physical or psychological. Rush, Watts, and Janke (2013) identified that no evidence existed as to whether older adults' viewed strength in a compartmentalized way. They conducted five focus groups with older adults in rural and urban settings to fulfill the purpose of their study.

"Following approval from a university behavioral research ethics board, five groups of older participants (>65 years) were purposely selected from across geographical sections in a Western Canadian province

Continued

to reflect its urban but also highly rural landscape. Sample selection sought to maximize variation in the older adult demographic, important at this exploratory stage in broadly assessing an understanding of strength.... Organized senior groups from rural and urban communities... served as the pool from which group participants were recruited.... Potential participants were invited to participate in a focus group that was scheduled in conjunction with one of the senior groups' monthly meetings and at their regular meeting location." Rush et al., 2013, pp. 11-12

"Focus groups were deemed appropriate for this exploratory study in order to obtain a breadth of perspectives related to strength. Following consent, participants completed a short demographic form.... A group facilitator used a semistructured interview guide to elicit focus group participants' perspectives.... A recorder was available to take notes and document observations of participants and their interactions. Focus groups lasted from 1 to 1½ hours and were digitally recorded." Rush et al., 2013, p. 12

Critical Appraisal

The process of recruitment was described in sufficient detail. Recruiting from pre-existing groups and meeting in the group's usual location were convenient and effective methods. However, the researchers noted that participants in seniors groups reflect the perspectives of persons who are connected to their community and may not reflect the perspectives of those who are more isolated. Groups were categorized as being rural or urban, depending on the government designation of rural and urban communities, but some participants who were identified as being urban based on group location actually considered themselves to be rural. Having a recorder to document observations of behavior and context strengthened the data collection process. Additional information about informed consent, the number who did not participate, and the effect of pre-existing relationships among the group members would have strengthened the study.

Implications for Practice

The participants in the study reported that strength was hard to describe and define. The themes were "capacity to meet variable demands," "ability to meet everyday ordinary demands," "reserve capacity to meet episodic extraordinary demands," and "resilience capacity to meet ongoing, life-changing demands" (Rush et al., 2013, p. 13). The older adults identified strategies to remain strong as giving support, receiving support, and remaining active in physical, social, and intellectual activities (p. 14).

Observation

Observation is a fundamental method of gathering data for qualitative studies, especially ethnography studies. The aim is to gather first-hand information in a naturally occurring situation. The researcher assumes the role of a learner to answer the question, "What is going on here?" The activities being observed may be automatic or routine for the participants, who may be unaware of some of their actions. The researcher looks carefully at the focus of the study, notices people and objects in the environment, and listens for what is said and unsaid. The researcher focuses on the details, including discrete events and the process of activities. Unexpected events occurring during routine activities may be significant and are carefully noted. As in any observation process, the qualitative researcher will attend to some aspects of the situation while disregarding others.

In studies that use observation, notes taken during or shortly after observations are called field notes. Waiting until the observation is over allows the researcher to focus entirely on the observational experience to avoid missing something meaningful, but may result in not all pertinent data being recorded. Another useful strategy is to videotape the events, so that careful observations and detailed notes can be taken at a later time.

CRITICAL APPRAISAL GUIDELINES

Observation

When data were collected through observation, the following questions can be asked to critically appraise the method:

1. Did the researchers describe when and where the observations occurred? Were the timing and location of the observations appropriate to address the research question? For example, if the observations occurred in a hospital, were observations conducted on all shifts and on all days of the week?
2. Did the researchers report the length of time spent observing? Was the time adequate to collect detailed and comprehensive data?
3. Did the report include information about how the data were recorded? Were field notes used?

RESEARCH EXAMPLE

Observation

Research Study Excerpt

In an ethnographic study, data about family presence during weaning from mechanical ventilation were collected by observation, interviews, and reviewing the providers' notes (Happ et al., 2007). The researchers dictated or wrote detailed notes on an observation guide developed during a previous study.

"Observations were conducted by one of the two researchers. . . . 4 to 5 days a week, including evenings and weekends, with a focus on observing weaning trials. Observations were recorded by dictated or handwritten field notes. . . . Families' talk, touch, physical stance, proximity to the patient, movement in the room, attention to electronic monitors and technologic devices were documented." Happ et al., 2007, p. 49

Family presence was the overall theme that was identified, comprised of behaviors that included touch, talk, and surveillance. Some behaviors were interpreted as being helpful to the weaning process whereas others were deemed as interfering with the process. The researchers identified the need for additional studies that could build on these findings.

Critical Appraisal

Happ and colleagues (2007) collected data over a 20-month period (201 days) from 30 patients, 41 family members, and 31 clinicians. The observations occurred when family members were present during weaning of the patient from the ventilator. The study was funded by a federal grant that supported the labor-intensive process; this allowed a comprehensive description of a complex phenomenon. The research team had conducted previous studies that allowed them to refine their methods, increasing the credibility of the study findings.

Implications for Practice

A finding in the study conducted by Happ and associates (2007) not found in previous studies was that family members can be valuable sources of clinical information about a patient's condition. Family members' ability to facilitate the weaning process and relay helpful information to the staff may be enhanced by respiratory therapists and nurses who assist family members to interpret monitors and learn comforting behaviors. Congruent with QSEN (2013) standards, the findings validated the importance of patient-centered, individualized care.

Text as a Source of Qualitative Data

In qualitative studies, text is considered a rich source of data. During a historical study, the researchers may examine texts written prior to the study, such as letters, diaries, newspaper accounts, and written descriptions of events. Other sources of pre-existing text are clinical notes in a medical record, policy manuals, and newspaper articles. Other texts may be created for the purpose of the study. For example, the researcher may ask participants to write about a particular topic. In some cases, these written narratives may be solicited by mail or e-mail rather than in person. Text provided by participants may be a component of a larger study using a variety of sources of data.

DATA MANAGEMENT

Qualitative data analysis occurs concurrently with data collection (Miles, Huberman, & Saldana, 2014), rather than sequentially, as in quantitative research. Therefore the researcher is attempting to gather, manage, and interpret a growing bulk of data simultaneously, which requires the researcher to have a plan for naming files and securely storing the data, so that specific data can be retrieved as needed.

Organizing Data Files

Keeping track of connections between various bits of data requires meticulous record keeping and may be supported by using computer-assisted qualitative data analysis software (CAQDAS) programs (Miles et al., 2014). The researchers will read, reread, and analyze the data over time to maintain a close link with—or become immersed in—the data being analyzed. The software allows the researcher to write memos about the analysis process and decisions that were reached, and it creates the audit trail of the study. The limitations on the length of manuscripts for peer-reviewed journals may prevent the researchers from reporting details of data management. However, having a general understanding of data management and analysis may provide the background needed to evaluate study proposals being considered by your facility or IRB.

Experienced researchers often create an organizational plan for the data they will collect as part of the preparation for the study. Considerations include securing computers, storage devices, and files to preserve the confidentiality of the data. Some IRBs may require that files be password-protected. Storing data files in more than one location is recommended to prevent loss of the data in case a computer crashes or a storage device becomes corrupted.

Transcribing Interviews

The most commonly used textual data in qualitative studies are transcripts of recorded interviews and focus groups. Transcription is at the heart of the qualitative research process, because a "verbatim transcript captures participants' own words, language, and expressions" and allows the researcher to "decode behavior, processes, and cultural meanings attached to people's perspectives" (Hennink & Weber, 2013, p. 700). Transcripts from such recordings can result in copious data for analysis. In a study report, researchers should describe how data were recorded during the interview, focus group, or observations and the strategies used to ensure the accuracy of the transcriptions. Typically, transcripts are prepared by typing everything in the recording word for word by the person speaking. Computer programs are now available which are voice-activated and can produce a written record of the recording. Even when computer software or a professional transcriptionist is used, the researcher will ensure accuracy by reading and correcting the transcript while listening to the recording.

DATA ANALYSIS

Data analysis is a rigorous process. Because published qualitative studies may not contain the methodology in detail, many professionals believe that qualitative research is a free-wheeling process, with little structure. Creativity and deep thought may produce innovative views to analyze the data, but the process requires discipline to develop data analysis plans consistent with the specific philosophical method of the study. For example, researchers conducting grounded theory studies use the constant comparative process by comparing concepts and themes identified through the analysis with those identified in subsequent data. In grounded theory, the analysis begins with the first participant interview, so that ideas from that participant can be integrated into questions and probes in subsequent interviews. In phenomenology, this immersion in the data is referred to as dwelling with the data. This phrase is used to indicate that the researcher spent considerable time reading and reflecting on the data.

Codes and Coding

Coding is the process of reading the data, breaking text down into subparts, and giving a label to that part of the text. These labels provide a way for the researcher to begin to identify patterns in the data, because sections of text that were coded in the same way can be compared for similarities and differences. A code is a symbol or abbreviation used to classify words or phrases in the data. Codes may be handwritten on a printed transcript. In a word-processing program or CAQDAS, you code by highlighting a section of text and making a comment in the margin or sidebar. Codes may result in themes, processes, or exemplars of the phenomenon being studied. When coding data for a phenomenological study, the researcher will first label shifts in meaning in the flow of the transcript (Liamputtong, 2009). A grounded theory researcher first labels statements using open codes to compare the data. In a qualitative study of medication adherence, participants mentioned clocks, schedules, hours, and doses that the researcher coded as "time." An exploratory-descriptive qualitative study about pain experiences of surgical patients may result in a taxonomy of types of pain, activities that resulted in pain, and types of pain relief strategies.

Themes and Interpretation

Themes emerge as codes that are combined into more abstract phrases or terms. Sometimes there are several layers of themes, with each layer further from the initial codes. Making links between these themes and the original data may become more difficult as the themes become more abstract. The rigor and clarity of the linking are of great importance, and it is the researcher who must remain rigorous in showing the links from the themes back to the original data. When you read qualitative studies that have used themes, search for evidence of links back to the original data. If you are critically appraising a qualitative study that uses themes, identify the themes and determine whether they seem sufficient and adequate for the study. During interpretation, the researcher places the findings in a larger context and may link different themes or factors in the findings to each other. The researcher is answering the question, "What do the findings mean?" Interpretation may focus on the usefulness of the findings for clinical practice or may move toward theorizing.

? CRITICAL APPRAISAL GUIDELINES

Data Analysis and Interpretation in Qualitative Studies

An important part of writing the report of a qualitative study is describing the data collection and analysis process. To appraise a qualitative study critically, you need to address the following questions:

1. Were the data analysis and interpretation processes consistent with the philosophical orientation and purpose of the study?
2. Did the researchers describe how they recorded decisions made during analysis and interpretation?
3. Did the researchers link the codes and themes used with exemplar quotations? This allows you to judge whether the codes were appropriate and adequate for the study.
4. Were the data analysis and interpretation logical and congruent with the study method?
5. Did the researchers provide adequate description of the data analysis and interpretation processes? The researcher who reports very little about the data collection and analysis process leaves the question of rigor unanswered.

RESEARCH EXAMPLE

Data Analysis and Interpretation Processes

Research Study

Häggström, Asplund, and Kristiansen (2012) thoroughly described the data analysis processes that they used in their grounded theory study of nurses facilitating patients' transitions from intensive care units. They initially collected data with focus groups and the analysis of these data resulted in 10 preliminary categories. To ensure a broad representation of nurses' experiences, they used theoretical sampling to identify additional nurses with potentially different experiences and interviewed them. The flow diagram they included in the study report indicated the different levels of codes they identified, as is appropriate for grounded theory. The flow diagram also served as documentation of the analysis and comprised part of the audit trail for the study (p. 227). The core category of "being perceptive and adjustable" was necessary to achieve the process of "balancing between patient needs and caregiver resources" (p. 229).

Critical Appraisal

Häggström and associates (2012) implemented the data analysis processes of their grounded theory study consistently with the philosophical approach of the method. They analyzed multiple sources of data (focus groups, observation, and interviews) collected in two hospitals to provide a rich picture of transitioning patients from intensive care units. In addition to the flow diagram, they provided a detailed table of when each focus group, interview, and observation occurred and how long it lasted. The report provided ample evidence that the findings emerged from the data and that the interpretation was consistent with the perspectives of the participants.

Implications for Practice

Häggström and co-workers (2012) concluded that individualized plans of care are needed because patients and their situations are unique. Discharge planning needs to begin at admission and be revised throughout the hospital stay. They also noted the challenges of meeting patient needs in organizations that are increasingly focused on efficiency, especially when resources are lacking. Their findings provide support for managers to recognize that providing patient-centered care, a QSEN (2013) expectation, requires adequate caregiver resources.

KEY CONCEPTS

- Qualitative research is a systematic approach used to elicit oral and written descriptions of life experiences from the perspective of the participants and give the experiences new meaning.
- Qualitative data are words, instead of numbers.
- Qualitative researchers set aside their own values and experiences to allow the multiple realities of the persons experiencing a phenomenon to emerge.
- Rigor in qualitative research requires critically appraising the study for congruence with the philosophical perspective; appropriateness of the collection, analysis, and interpretation of data; maintenance of an audit trail; and logic of the findings reported in the research report.
- A phenomenological researcher examines an experience and provides interpretations that enhance the meaning while staying true to the perspective of those who have lived the experience.
- Grounded theory researchers explore underlying social processes through the symbols of language, religion, relationships, and clothing and describe the deeper meaning of an event as a theoretical framework.
- Ethnographic researchers observe and interview people within a culture to understand the environment, people, power relations, and communication patterns of a work setting, community, or ethnic group.

- Exploratory-descriptive qualitative studies are conducted to provide information that will promote understanding of an experience from the perspective of the persons living the experience.
- Historical researchers explore past events by finding and examining documents from that time to gain insight into causes and factors surrounding the event.
- Data collection in qualitative studies occurs in the context of the relationship between the participant and researcher.
- Data in qualitative studies are collected through interviews, focus groups, observation, and review of documents.
- Data management, analysis, and interpretation require clear procedures to ensure methodological rigor and credibility of the findings.

REFERENCES

Ågård, A., Egerod, I., Tønnesen, E., & Lomborg, K. (2012). Struggling for independence: A grounded theory study on convalescence of ICU survivors 12 months post ICU discharge. *Intensive and Critical Care Nursing, 28,* 105–113.

Bloomberg, L., & Volpe, M. (2008). *Completing your qualitative dissertation: A roadmap from beginning to end.* Los Angeles, CA: Sage.

Bolderston, A. (2012). Conducting a research interview. *Journal of Medical Imaging and Radiation Sciences, 43* (1), 66–76.

Brown, S. J. (2014). *Evidence-based nursing: The research-practice connection* (3rd ed.). Sudbury, MA: Jones & Bartlett.

Chen, P. Y., & Chang, H. -C. (2012). The coping process of patients with cancer. *European Journal of Oncology Nursing, 16*(1), 10–16.

Connolly, C., & Gibson, M. (2011). The "White Plague" and color: Children, race, and tuberculosis in Virginia 1900–1935. *Journal of Pediatric Nursing, 26*(3), 230–238.

Converse, M. (2012). Philosophy of phenomenology: How understanding aids research. *Nurse Researcher, 20*(1), 28–32.

Creswell, J. (2013). *Qualitative inquiry and research design: Choosing among five approaches* (3rd ed.). Thousand Oaks, CA: Sage.

Dowling, M., & Cooney, A. (2012). Research approaches related to phenomenology: Negotiating a complex landscape. *Nurse Researcher, 20*(2), 21–27.

Fenwick, C., Chaboyer, W., & St. John, W. (2012). Decision-making processes for the self-management of persistent pain: A grounded theory study. *Contemporary Nurse, 42*(1), 53–66.

Flood, A. (2010). Understanding phenomenology. *Nurse Researcher, 17*(2), 2–7.

Glaser, B. G., & Strauss, A. (1967). *The discovery of grounded theory: Strategies for qualitative research.* Chicago: Aldine.

Gray, J. (2009). *Rooms, recordings, and responsibilities: The logistics of focus groups. Southern Online Journal of Nursing Research, 9*(1). Retrieved December 30, 2013 from, http://www.resourcenter.net/images/SNRS/Files/SOJNR_articles2/Vol09Num01Art05.pdf.

Grove, S. K., Burns, N., & Gray, J. R. (2013). *The practice of nursing research: Appraisal, synthesis, and generation of evidence* (7th ed.). St. Louis, MO: Elsevier Saunders.

Häggström, M., Asplund, K., & Kristiansen, L. (2012). How can nurses facilitate patient's transitions from intensive care? *Intensive and Critical Care Nursing, 28* (4), 224–233.

Happ, M. B., Swigart, V. A., Tate, J. A., Arnold, R. M., Sereika, S. M., & Hoffman, L. A. (2007). Family presence and surveillance during weaning from prolonged mechanical ventilation. *Heart & Lung, 36* (1), 47–57.

Hennink, M., & Weber, M. (2013). Quality issues of court reporters and transcriptionists for qualitative research. *Qualitative Health Research, 23*(5), 700–710.

Houghton, C., Hunter, A., & Meskell, P. (2012). Linking aims, paradigm and method in nursing research. *Nurse Researcher, 20*(2), 34–39.

Knopf, S. A. (1922). *A history of the National Tuberculosis Association.* New York: National Tuberculosis Association.

Leininger, M. M. (Ed.). (1985). *Qualitative research methods.* Orlando, FA: Grune and Stratton.

Leininger, M. M. (1988). Leininger's theory of nursing: Cultural care diversity and universality. *Nursing Science Quarterly, 1,* 152–160.

Leininger, M. M. (2002). Culture care theory: A major contribution to advance transcultural nursing knowledge and practices. *Journal of Transcultural Nursing, 13*(3), 189–192.

Letourneau, N., Young, C., Secco, L., Stewart, M., Hughes, J., & Critchley, K. (2011). Supporting mothering: Service providers' perspectives of mothers and young children affected by intimate partner violence. *Research in Nursing & Health, 34*(3), 192–203.

Liamputtong, P. (2009). *Qualitative research methods* (3rd ed.). South Melbourne, Australia: Oxford University Press.

MacGregor, C., Hamilton, A., Oishi, S., & Yano, E. (2011). Description, development, and philosophies of mental health service delivery for female veterans in the VA: A qualitative study. *Women's Health Issues, 21*(4S), S138–S144.

Mapp, T. (2008). Understanding phenomenology: The lived experience. *British Journal of Midwifery, 16*(5), 308–311.

Martsolf, D., Draucker, C., Bednarz, L., & Lea, J. (2011). Listening to the voices of important others: How adolescents make sense of troubled dating relationships. *Archives of Psychiatric Nursing, 25*(6), 430–444.

Maxwell, J. (2014). *Qualitative research design: An interactive approach* (3rd ed.). Thousand Oaks, CA: Sage.

McCready, J. (2010). Jamesian pragmatism: A framework for working toward unified diversity in nursing knowledge development. *Nursing Philosophy, 11*(3), 191–203.

McDermott-Levy, R. (2011). Going alone: The lived experience of female Arab-Muslim nursing students living and studying in the United States. *Nursing Outlook, 59*(5), 266–277.

Mead, G. H. (1934). *Mind, self and society.* Chicago: University of Chicago Press.

Miles, M., Huberman, A., & Saldana, J. (2014). *Qualitative data analysis: A methods sourcebook* (3rd ed.). Thousand Oaks, CA: Sage.

Munhall, P. L. (Ed.), (2012). *Nursing research: A qualitative perspective.* (5th ed.). Sudbury, MA: Jones & Bartlett.

Norfolk City Union of the King's Daughters Visiting Nurse Service. (1907, 1909, 1910). *Children's Hospital of the King's Daughter*s. Norfolk Virginia.

Nowak, E., & Stevens, P. (2011). Vigilance in parents' experiences of fetal and infant loss. *Journal of Obstetric, Gynecologic, and Neonate Nursing, 40*(1), 122–130.

Oliver, C. (2012). The relationship between symbolic interactionism and interpretive description. *Qualitative Health Research, 22*(3), 409–415.

Petty, N., Thomson, O., & Stew, G. (2012). Ready for a paradigm shift? Part 2: Introducing qualitative research methodologies and methods. *Manual Therapy, 17*(5), 378–384.

Ponterotto, J. (2005). Qualitative research in counseling psychology: A primer on research paradigms and philosophy of science. *Journal of Counseling Psychology, 52*(2), 126–136.

Portacolone, E. (2013). The notion of precariousness among older adults living alone in the U.S. *Journal of Aging Studies, 27*(2), 166–174.

Quality and Safety Education for Nurses (QSEN), (2013). *Pre-licensure knowledge, skills, and attitudes (KSAs).* Retrieved December 30, 2013 from, http://qsen.org/competencies/pre-licensure-ksas/.

Roberts, T. (2009). Understanding ethnography. *British Journal of Midwifery, 17*(5), 291–294.

Rogers, S. (1917). *Mortality statistics for 1915: Sixteenth annual report.* Washington, D.C.: U.S. Government Printing Office.

Roper, J. M., & Shapiro, J. (2000). *Ethnography in nursing research.* Thousand Oaks, CA: Sage.

Rush, K., Watts, W., & Janke, R. (2013). Rural and urban older adults' perspectives of strength in their daily lives. *Applied Nursing Research, 26*(1), 10–16.

Sadala, M., Stolf, N., Bocchi, E., & Bicudo, M. (2013). Caring for heart transplant recipients: The lived experience of primary caregivers. *Heart & Lung, 42*(2), 120–125.

Sandelowski, M. (2000). Whatever happened to qualitative description? *Research in Nursing & Health, 423*(5), 334–340.

Sandelowski, M. (2010). What's in a name? Qualitative description revisited. *Research in Nursing & Health, 33*(1), 77–84.

Savage, J. (2006). Ethnographic evidence: The value of applied ethnography in healthcare. *Journal of Research in Nursing, 11*(5), 383–395.

Sherwood, G., & Barnsteiner, J. (2012). *Quality and safety in nursing: A competency approach to improving outcomes.* Ames, IA: Wiley-Blackwell.

Thompson, M. E., & Keeling, A. A. (2012). Nurses' role in the prevention of infant mortality in 1884–1925: Health disparities then and now. *Journal of Pediatric Nursing, 27*(5), 471–478.

Trollvik, A., Nordbach, R., Silen, C., & Ringsberg, K. C. (2011). Children's experiences of living with asthma: Fear of exacerbations and being ostracized. *Journal of Pediatric Nursing, 26*(4), 295–303.

Walton, J., Chute, E., & Ball, L. (2011). Negotiating the role of the professional nurse: The pedagogy of simulation: A grounded theory study. *Journal of Professional Nursing, 27*(5), 299–310.

Wuerst, J. (2012). Grounded theory: The method. In P. L. Munhall (Ed.), *Nursing research: A qualitative perspective* (pp. 225–256). (5th ed.). Sudbury, MA: Jones & Bartlett.

Examining Ethics in Nursing Research

LEARNING OUTCOMES

After completing this chapter, you should be able to:

1. Identify the historical events influencing the development of ethical codes and regulations for nursing and biomedical research.

2. Describe the ethical principles that are important in conducting research on human subjects.

3. Describe the human rights that require protection in research.
4. Identify the essential elements of the informed consent process in research.
5. Describe the role of a nurse in the institutional review of research in an agency.
6. Examine the benefit-risk ratio of published studies and studies proposed for conduct in clinical agencies.
7. Describe the types of possible scientific misconduct in the conduct, reporting, and publication of healthcare research.
8. Critically appraise the protection of human rights and the informed consent and institutional review processes in published studies.
9. Critically appraise the treatment of animals reported in published studies.

KEY TERMS

Anonymity, p. 106
Assent to participate in research, p. 102
Autonomous agents, p. 101
Benefit-risk ratio, p. 119
Breach of confidentiality, p. 107
Coercion, p. 101
Confidentiality, p. 107
Consent form, p. 112
Covered entities, p. 105
Covert data collection, p. 101
Data use agreement, p. 106
Deception, p. 101
Diminished autonomy, p. 101
Discomfort and harm, p. 108

Ethical principles, p. 98
Principle of beneficence, p. 98
Principle of justice, p. 98
Principle of respect for person(s), p. 98
Fabrication in research, p. 122
Falsification of research, p. 122
Health Insurance Portability and Accountability Act (HIPAA), p. 99
Human rights, p. 100
Individually identifiable health information, p. 105
Informed consent, p. 111
Institutional review, p. 117

Complete review, p. 118
Exempt from review, p. 117
Expedited review, p. 118
Institutional review board (IRB), p. 117
Invasion of privacy, p. 105
Minimal risk, p. 118
Nontherapeutic research, p. 96
Permission to participate in research, p. 102
Plagiarism, p. 122
Privacy, p. 105
Research misconduct, p. 122
Therapeutic research, p. 96
Voluntary consent, p. 113

Ethical research is essential for generating sound empirical knowledge for evidence-based practice, but what does ethical conduct of research involve? This is a question that researchers, philosophers, lawyers, and politicians have debated for many years. The debate continues, probably because of the complexity of human rights issues, the focus of research in new and challenging arenas of technology and genetics, the complex ethical codes and regulations governing research, and the various interpretations of these codes and regulations. This chapter introduces you to the national and international codes and regulations developed to promote the ethical conduct of research.

You might think that unethical studies that violate subjects' rights are a thing of the past, but this is not the case. There are still situations in which researchers do not protect the subjects' privacy adequately or the study participants are treated unfairly or harmed during a study. Another serious ethical problem that has increased over the last 20 years is research misconduct. Research misconduct includes incidences of fabrication, falsification, or plagiarism in the process of conducting and reporting research in nursing and other healthcare disciplines (Office of Research Integrity [ORI], 2013).

You need to be able to appraise the ethical aspects of published studies and of research conducted in clinical agencies critically. Most published studies include ethical information about subject selection and treatment during data collection in the methods section of the report. Institutional review boards (IRBs) in universities and clinical agencies have been organized to examine the ethical aspects of studies before they are conducted. Nurses often are members of IRBs and participate in the review of research for conduct in clinical agencies.

To provide you with a background for examining ethical aspects of studies, this chapter describes the ethical codes and regulations that currently guide the conduct of biomedical and behavioral research. The following elements of ethical research are detailed: (1) protecting human rights; (2) understanding informed consent; (3) understanding institutional review of research; and (4) examining the balance of benefits and risks in a study. This chapter also provides critical appraisal guidelines for examining the ethical aspects of studies. The chapter concludes with a discussion of two additional important ethical issues, research misconduct and the use of animals in research.

HISTORICAL EVENTS INFLUENCING THE DEVELOPMENT OF ETHICAL CODES AND REGULATIONS

Since the 1940s, four experimental projects have been highly publicized for their unethical treatment of human subjects: the Nazi medical experiments, the Tuskegee Syphilis Study, the Willowbrook Study, and the Jewish Chronic Disease Hospital Study (Berger, 1990; Levine, 1986). Although these were biomedical studies and the primary investigators were physicians, the evidence suggests that nurses understood the nature of the research, identified potential research subjects, delivered treatments to the subjects, and served as data collectors. These unethical studies demonstrate the importance of ethical conduct for nurses while they are reviewing or participating in nursing or biomedical research (Fry, Veatch, & Taylor, 2011; Havens, 2004). These studies also influenced the formulation of ethical codes and regulations that currently direct the conduct of research.

Nazi Medical Experiments

From 1933 to 1945, the Third Reich in Europe was engaged in atrocious and unethical medical activities. The programs of the Nazi regime included sterilization, euthanasia, and medical experimentation for the purpose of producing a population of "racially pure" Germans who were destined to rule the world. The medical experiments were conducted on prisoners of war and persons considered to be racially valueless, such as Jews, who were confined in concentration camps. The experiments involved exposing subjects to high altitudes, freezing temperatures, malaria, poisons, spotted fever (typhus), or untested drugs and performing surgical procedures, usually without any form of anesthesia for the subjects. Extensive examination of the records from some of these studies indicated that they were poorly conceived and conducted. Therefore this research was not only unethical but also generated little if any useful scientific knowledge (Berger, 1990; Steinfels & Levine, 1976).

The Nazi experiments violated numerous rights of the research subjects. The selection of subjects for these studies was racially based and unfair, and the subjects had no choice—they were prisoners who were forced to participate. As a result of these experiments, subjects frequently were killed or they sustained permanent physical, mental, and social damage (Levine, 1986).

Nuremberg Code

Those involved in the Nazi experiments were brought to trial before the Nuremberg Tribunals, and their unethical research received international attention. The mistreatment of human subjects in

BOX 4-1   THE NUREMBERG CODE

The voluntary consent of the human subject is absolutely essential. . . .

The experiment should be such as to yield fruitful results for the good of society, unprocurable by other methods or means of study, and not random and unnecessary in nature.

The experiment should be so designed and based on the results of animal experimentation and a knowledge of the natural history of the disease or other problem under study that the anticipated results will justify the performance of the experiment.

The experiment should be so conducted as to avoid all unnecessary physical and mental suffering and injury.

No experiment should be conducted where there is an a priori reason to believe that death or disabling injury will occur, except, perhaps, in those experiments where the experimental physicians also serve as subjects.

The degree of risk to be taken should never exceed that determined by the humanitarian importance of the problem to be solved by the experiment.

Proper preparations should be made and adequate facilities provided to protect the experimental subject against even remote possibilities of injury, disability, or death.

The experiment should be conducted only by scientifically qualified persons. The highest degree of skill and care should be required through all stages of the experiment of those who conduct or engage in the experiment.

During the course of the experiment the human subject should be at liberty to bring the experiment to an end if he has reached the physical or mental state where continuation of the experiment seems to him to be impossible.

During the course of the experiment the scientist in charge must be prepared to terminate the experiment at any stage, if he has probable cause to believe, in the exercise of the good faith, superior skill and careful judgment required of him that a continuation of the experiment is likely to result in injury, disability, or death to the experimental subject.

From U.S. Department of Health and Human Services, Office of Human Research Protection (OHRP). 2013. *The Nuremberg Code (1949)*. Retrieved June 9, 2013 from, http://www.hhs.gov/ohrp/archive/nurcode.html.

these studies led to the development of the Nuremberg Code in 1949. Box 4-1 presents this code. The code includes guidelines that should help you evaluate the consent process, protection of subjects from harm, and balance of benefits and risks in a study (U.S. Department of Health and Human Services [U.S. DHHS], Office of Human Research Protection [OHRP], 2013).

Declaration of Helsinki

The Nuremberg Code provided the basis for the development of the Declaration of Helsinki, which was adopted in 1964 and revised most recently in 2008 by the World Medical Association (WMA, 2008). A major focus of the initial document was the differentiation of therapeutic research from nontherapeutic research. Therapeutic research provides patients with an opportunity to receive an experimental treatment that might have beneficial results. Nontherapeutic research is conducted to generate knowledge for a discipline; the results of the study might benefit future patients but probably will not benefit those acting as research participants.

The Declaration of Helsinki includes the following ethical principles: (1) the investigator should protect the life, health, privacy, and dignity of human subjects; (2) the investigator should exercise greater care to protect subjects from harm in nontherapeutic research; and (3) the investigator should conduct research only when the importance of the objective outweighs the inherent risks and burdens to the subjects. The most recent addition to the Declaration of Helsinki is that researchers must use extreme caution in studies in which participants receive a placebo or sham treatment. For example, in studies testing the effectiveness of a drug, the placebo group would receive a pill with no medication and the experimental group would receive a pill with the drug.

Researchers must provide the participants in the placebo group with access to proven diagnostic and therapeutic procedures after the study (WMA, 2008). The ethical principles of the Declaration of Helsinki are available online at http://www.wma.net/en/30publications/10policies/b3. Most institutions in which clinical research is conducted adopted the Nuremberg Code and Declaration of Helsinki; however, episodes of unethical research continued to occur in biomedical and behavioral studies.

Tuskegee Syphilis Study

In 1932 the U.S. Public Health Service initiated a study of syphilis in African American men in the small rural town of Tuskegee, Alabama (Rothman, 1982). The study, which continued for 40 years, was conducted to determine the natural course of syphilis in African American men. Many of the subjects who consented to participate in the study were not informed about the purpose and procedures of the research. Some were unaware that they were subjects in a study. By 1936 it was apparent that the men with syphilis had developed more complications than the men in the control group. Ten years later the death rate among those with syphilis was twice as high as it was for the control group. The subjects were examined periodically but were not treated for syphilis, even when penicillin was determined to be an effective treatment for the disease in the 1940s. Information about an effective treatment for syphilis was withheld from the subjects, and deliberate steps were taken to deprive them of treatment (Brandt, 1978).

Published reports of the Tuskegee Syphilis Study started appearing in 1936, and additional papers were published every 4 to 6 years. No effort was made to stop the study; in fact, in 1969 the Centers for Disease Control and Prevention (then called the Center for Disease Control) decided that the study should continue. In 1972, an account of the study in the *Washington Star* sparked public outrage; only then did the U.S. Department of Health, Education, and Welfare (DHEW) stop the study. The study was investigated and found to be ethically unjustified (Brandt, 1978).

Willowbrook Study

From the mid-1950s to the early 1970s, Dr. Saul Krugman conducted research on hepatitis at Willowbrook, an institution for the mentally retarded in Staten Island, New York (Rothman, 1982). The subjects were children who were deliberately infected with the hepatitis virus. During the 20-year study, Willowbrook closed its doors to new inmates because of overcrowded conditions. However, the research ward continued to admit new inmates, and parents had to give permission for their child to be in the study to gain admission to the institution.

From the late 1950s to the early 1970s, Krugman's research team published several articles describing the study protocol and findings. In 1966 Beecher cited the Willowbrook Study in the *New England Journal of Medicine* as an example of unethical research. The investigators defended injecting the children with the hepatitis virus because they believed that most of the children would acquire the infection on admission to the institution. They also stressed the benefits the subjects received, which were a cleaner environment, better supervision, and a higher nurse-to-patient ratio on the research ward (Rothman, 1982). Despite the controversy, this unethical study continued until the early 1970s.

Jewish Chronic Disease Hospital Study

Another highly publicized unethical study was conducted at the Jewish Chronic Disease Hospital in New York in the 1960s. The purpose of this study was to determine patients' rejection responses to live cancer cells. A suspension containing live cancer cells that had been generated from human cancer tissue was injected into 22 patients (Levine, 1986). Because researchers did not inform these patients that they were taking part in a study or that the injections they received were live cancer cells, their rights were not protected. In addition, the study was never presented for review to the research committee of the Jewish Chronic Disease Hospital, and the physicians caring for the patients were unaware that the study was being conducted. The physician directing the research was an employee of the Sloan-Kettering Institute for Cancer Research; there was no indication that this institution had conducted a review of the research project (Hershey & Miller, 1976). This unethical study was conducted without the informed consent of the subjects and without institutional review and had the potential to injure, disable, or cause the death of the human subjects. The study was stopped immediately and steps were taken to ensure proper care for the patients exposed to the cancer cells and to review all future research to be conducted by this agency.

Department of Health, Education, and Welfare, 1973: Regulations for the Protection of Human Research Subjects

The continued conduct of harmful, unethical research from the 1960s to the 1970s made additional controls necessary. In 1973 the DHEW published its first set of regulations for the protection of human research subjects. These regulations also provided protection for persons having limited capacity to consent, such as those who are ill, mentally impaired, or dying (Levine, 1986). According to the DHEW regulations, all research involving human subjects had to undergo full institutional review, which increased the protection of human subjects. However, reviewing all studies without regard for the degree of risk involved greatly increased the time for study approval and reduced the number of studies conducted.

National Commission for the Protection of Human Subjects of Biomedical and Behavioral Research

Because the DHEW regulations did not resolve the issue of protecting human subjects in research, the National Commission for the Protection of Human Subjects of Biomedical and Behavioral Research was formed in 1978. This commission was established by the National Research Act (Public Law 93-348), which was passed in 1974. The commission identified three ethical principles relevant to the conduct of research involving human subjects: respect for persons, beneficence, and justice. The principle of respect for persons indicates that people should be treated as autonomous agents, with the right to self-determination and the freedom to participate or not participate in research. Those persons with diminished autonomy, such as children, people who are terminally or mentally ill, and prisoners, are entitled to additional protection. The principle of beneficence encourages the researcher to do good and "above all, do no harm." The principle of justice states that human subjects should be treated fairly in terms of the benefits and the risks of research. Before it was dissolved in 1978, the commission developed ethical research guidelines based on these three principles and made recommendations to the U.S. DHHS in the *Belmont Report*. (Information on this report and the three ethical principles—respect for persons, beneficence, and justice—are available online at http://or.org/pdf/BelmontReport.pdf). Greaney and colleagues (2012) studied these ethical principles and provided guidelines for applying them in reviewing and conducting nursing research.

Regretfully, violations of human subjects' rights continue to occur, as evident in letters written by the Office of Human Research Protection (http://www.hhs.gov/ohrp/index.html). These violations include omitting required information from informed consent documents, failing to update the consent document when additional information was available about potential risks, and beginning data collection prior to having the study approved by the IRB. In December 2011, the Presidential Commission for the Study of Bioethics Issues released its report, *Moral Science: Protecting Participants in Human Subjects Research*, which included recommendations for enhancing the protection of human subjects.

Current Federal Regulations for the Protection of Human Subjects

In response to the recommendations presented in the Belmont Report, the U.S. DHHS developed a set of federal regulations for the protection of human research subjects in 1981, which have been revised over the years; the most current regulations were approved in 2009. The 2009 regulations are part of the *Code of Federal Regulations* (CFR), Title 45, Part 46, Protection of Human Subjects (U.S. DHHS, 2009). These regulations provide direction for the (1) protection of human subjects in research, with additional protection for pregnant women, human fetuses, neonates, children, and prisoners; (2) documentation of informed consent; and (3) implementation of the IRB process. You can access these regulations online at http://www.hhs.gov/ohrp/policy/ohrpregulations.pdf.

The DHHS Protection of Human Subjects Regulations (U.S. DHHS, 2009) and the U.S. Food and Drug Administration (FDA) govern most of the biomedical and behavioral research conducted in the United States. The FDA, within the DHHS, manages CFR Title 21—Food and Drugs, Part 50, Protection of Human Subjects (FDA, 2012a) and Part 56, Institutional Review Boards (2012b). The FDA has additional human subject protection regulations that apply to clinical investigations involving products regulated by the FDA under the federal Food, Drug, and Cosmetic Act and research that supports applications for research or marketing permits for these products. These regulations apply to studies of drugs for humans, medical devices for human use, biological products for human use, human dietary supplements, and electronic products (FDA, 2013; http://www.fda.gov). Physician and nurse researchers conducting clinical trials to generate new drugs and refine existing drug treatments must comply with these FDA regulations. Table 4-1 clarifies the focus of the regulations for the protection of human subjects of the DHHS and FDA.

The DHHS and FDA regulations provide guidelines for the protection of subjects in federally and privately funded research to ensure their privacy and the confidentiality of the information obtained through research. With the mechanisms for the electronic access and transfer of individuals' information, however, the public became concerned about the potential abuses of the health information of persons in all circumstances, including research projects. Therefore a federal regulation—the Health Insurance Portability and Accountability Act (HIPAA; Public Law 104-191)—was implemented in 2003 to protect people's private health information (U.S. DHHS, 2007a). Table 4-1 clarifies the focus of HIPAA regulations as compared with the DHHS and FDA regulations (U.S. DHHS, 2007b).

The DHHS developed regulations entitled the *Standards for Privacy of Individually Identifiable Health Information;* compliance with these regulations is known as the Privacy Rule (U.S. DHHS, 2007a). The HIPAA Privacy Rule established a category known as protected health information (PHI), which allows covered entities, such as health plans, healthcare clearinghouses, and healthcare providers that transmit health information, to use or disclose PHI to others only in certain situations. These are discussed later in this chapter.

The HIPAA Privacy Rule has an impact not only on the healthcare environment, but also on the research conducted in this environment. A person must provide his or her signed permission, or authorization, before that person's PHI can be used or disclosed for research purposes. Researchers must develop their research projects to comply with the HIPAA Privacy Rule. The DHHS has a website, *HIPAA Privacy Rule: Information for Researchers,* which addresses the impact of this rule

TABLE 4-1	CLARIFICATION OF THE FOCUS OF FEDERAL REGULATIONS AND IMPACT ON RESEARCH		
AREA OF DISTINCTION	**HIPAA PRIVACY RULE**	**U.S. DHHS PROTECTION OF HUMAN SUBJECTS REGULATIONS***	**U.S. FDA PROTECTION OF HUMAN SUBJECTS REGULATIONS†**
Overall Objective	Establish a federal floor of privacy protections for most individually identifiable health information by establishing conditions for its use and disclosure by certain healthcare providers, health plans, and healthcare clearinghouses.	To protect the rights and welfare of human subjects involved in research conducted or supported by U.S. DHHS. Not specifically a privacy regulation.	To protect the rights, safety, and welfare of subjects involved in clinical investigations regulated by the FDA. Not specifically a privacy regulation.
Applicability	Applies to HIPAA-defined covered entities, regardless of the source of funding.	Applies to human subjects' research conducted or supported by U.S. DHHS and research with private funding.	Applies to research involving products regulated by the FDA. Federal support is not necessary for FDA regulations to be applicable. When research subject to FDA jurisdiction is federally funded, both the DHHS Protection of Human Subjects Regulations and FDA Protection of Human Subjects Regulations apply.

*Title 45, CFR Part 46.
†Title 21 CFR, Parts 50 and 56.
From U.S. Department of Health and Human Services (U.S. DHHS). (2007b). *How do other privacy protections interact with the privacy rule?* Retrieved May 29, 2013, from *http://privacyruleandresearch.nih.gov/pr_05.asp.*

on the informed consent and IRB processes in research and answers common questions about HIPAA (http://privacyruleandresearch.nih.gov; U.S. DHHS, 2007a). The HIPAA Privacy Rule has had a negative effect on researchers' abilities to conduct studies; the Institute of Medicine and other professional organizations are encouraging lessening the impact or removing research from the HIPAA regulation (Infectious Diseases Society of America, 2009).

PROTECTING HUMAN RIGHTS

What are human rights? How are these rights protected during research? Human rights are claims and demands that have been justified in the eyes of an individual or by the consensus of a group of people. Nurses who critically appraise published studies, review research for conduct in their agencies, or assist with data collection for a study have an ethical responsibility to determine whether the rights of the research participants are protected. The human rights that require protection in research are the rights to (1) self-determination, (2) privacy, (3) anonymity and confidentiality, (4) fair selection and treatment, and (5) protection from discomfort and harm (American Nurses

Association [ANA], 2001; American Psychological Association [APA], 2010; Fawcett & Garity, 2009; Fowler, 2010; Fry et al., 2011). The ANA Code of Ethics for Nurses (2001) provides nurses with guidelines for ethical conduct in nursing practice and research. This code focuses on protecting the rights of patients and research participants. Fowler (2010) provides a detailed interpretation and application of the statements in this code.

Right to Self-Determination

The right to self-determination is based on the ethical principle of respect for persons, and it indicates that humans are capable of controlling their own destiny. People should be treated as autonomous agents who have the freedom to conduct their lives as they choose, without external controls. Researchers treat subjects as autonomous agents in a study when they (1) inform them about the study, (2) allow them to choose whether or not to participate, and (3) allow them to withdraw from the study at any time, without penalty (ANA, 2001; Banner & Zimmer, 2012; Greaney et al., 2012).

Violation of the Right to Self-Determination

A subject's right to self-determination can be violated through the use of coercion, covert data collection, and deception. Coercion occurs when one person intentionally presents an overt threat of harm or an excessive reward to another to obtain compliance. Some subjects are coerced (forced) to participate in research because they fear harm or discomfort if they do not participate. For example, some patients believe that their medical and nursing care will be negatively affected if they do not agree to be research participants. Others are coerced to participate in studies because they believe that they cannot refuse the excessive rewards offered, such as large sums of money, special privileges, or jobs (U.S. DHHS, 2009; Emanuel, 2004; Fry et al., 2011).

With covert data collection, subjects are unaware that research data are being collected (Reynolds, 1979). For example, in the Jewish Chronic Disease Hospital Study, most of the patients and their physicians were unaware of the study. The subjects were informed that they were receiving an injection of cells, but the word *cancer* was omitted (Beecher, 1966).

The use of deception, the actual misinforming of subjects for research purposes, can also violate a subject's right to self-determination (Kelman, 1967). A classic example of deception is seen in the Milgram study (1963), in which the subjects thought they were administering electric shocks to another person, but the person was really a professional actor who pretended to feel the shocks. If deception is used in a study, the research report should indicate how the subjects were deceived, provide a rationale for the use of deception, and discuss when the subjects were informed of the actual research activities and the findings (U.S. DHHS, 2009).

Persons with Diminished Autonomy

Persons have diminished autonomy when they are vulnerable and less advantaged because of legal or mental incompetence, terminal illness, or confinement to an institution (U.S. DHHS, 2009; FDA, 2012a). They require additional protection of their right to self-determination because of their decreased ability or inability to give informed consent. In addition, they are vulnerable to coercion and deception. The research report should include justification for the use of these subjects, and the need for justification increases as the subjects' risks and vulnerability increase.

Study participants with legal and mental diminished autonomy. Minors (neonates and children), pregnant women and fetuses, mentally impaired persons, and unconscious patients are legally and/or mentally unable to give informed consent. These individuals have diminished

De-Identifying Protected Health Information under the Privacy Rule

Covered entities, such as healthcare providers and agencies, can allow researchers access to health information if the information has been de-identified. De-identifying health data involves removing the elements that could identify a specific person or that person's relatives, employer, or household members. You need to be aware of these elements to ensure that a patient's PHI is kept confidential in the healthcare agencies in which you work or are a student. The elements that require de-identifying are (U.S. DHHS, 2007a):

- Names
- All geographic subdivisions smaller than a state, including street address, city, county, precinct, ZIP code, and their equivalent geographic codes, except for the initial three digits of a ZIP code
- All elements of dates (except year) for dates directly related to an individual, including birth date, admission date, discharge date, date of death, and all ages over 89 years and all elements of dates (including year) indicative of such age, except that such ages and elements may be aggregated into a single category of age 90 years or older
- Telephone numbers
- Facsimile numbers
- Electronic mail (e-mail) addresses
- Social Security numbers
- Medical record numbers
- Health plan beneficiary numbers
- Account numbers
- Certificate and/or license numbers
- Vehicle identifiers and serial numbers, including license plate numbers
- Device identifiers and serial numbers
- Web universal resource locators (URLs)
- Internet protocol (IP) address numbers
- Biometric identifiers, including fingerprints and voiceprints
- Full-face photographic images and any comparable images
- Any other unique identifying number, characteristic, or code, unless otherwise permitted by the Privacy Rule for re-identification

A person's health information also can be de-identified using statistical methods. However, the covered entity and researcher must ensure that the individual subject cannot be identified, or that there is a very small risk that the subject could be identified from the information collected. The statistical method used for de-identification of the health data must be documented, and the study must certify that the elements for identification have been removed or revised to prevent identification of a specific person. This certification information must be kept for a period of 6 years by the researcher.

Limited Data Set and Data Use Agreement

Covered entities—healthcare provider, health plan, and healthcare clearinghouse—may use and disclose a limited data set to a researcher for a study without an individual subject's authorization or IRB waiver. However, a limited data set is considered PHI, and the covered entity and researcher need to have a data use agreement. The data use agreement limits how the data set may be used and how it will be protected.

Right to Anonymity and Confidentiality

On the basis of the right to privacy, the research subject has the right to anonymity and the right to assume that the data collected will be kept confidential. Complete anonymity exists when the .

subject's identity cannot be linked, even by the researcher, with his or her individual responses (Grove, Burns, & Gray, 2013). In most studies, researchers know the identity of their subjects, and they promise the subjects that their identity will be kept anonymously from others and that the research data will be kept confidential. **Confidentiality** is the researcher's safe management of information or data shared by a subject to ensure that the data are kept private from others. The researcher must refrain from sharing this information without the authorization of the subject. Confidentiality is grounded in the following premises (ANA, 2001; Fowler, 2010):

1. Individuals can share personal information to the extent that they wish and are entitled to have secrets.
2. One can choose with whom to share personal information.
3. Those accepting information in confidence have an obligation to maintain confidentiality.
4. Professionals, such as researchers and nurses, have a duty to maintain confidentiality that goes beyond ordinary loyalty.

A breach of confidentiality can occur when a researcher, by accident or direct action, allows an unauthorized person to gain access to the raw data of a study. Confidentiality also can be breached in reporting or publishing a study if a participant's identity is accidentally revealed, violating his or her right to anonymity. Breach of confidentiality is of special concern in qualitative studies that have few study participants and involve the reporting of long quotes made by those participants. In addition, qualitative researchers and participants often have relationships in which detailed stories of the participants' lives are shared, requiring careful management of study data to ensure confidentiality (Eide & Kahn, 2008; Munhall, 2012a). Breaches of confidentiality that can be especially harmful to participants include those regarding religious preferences, sexual practices, income, racial prejudices, drug use, child abuse, and personal attributes, such as intelligence, honesty, and courage. Research reports need to be examined closely for evidence that the participants' confidentiality was maintained during data collection, analysis, and reporting (Munhall, 2012a; Sandelowski, 1994). In addition, the research findings in a published study should be reported so that a participant or group of participants cannot be identified by their responses.

Right to Fair Selection and Treatment

The right to fair selection and treatment is based on the ethical principle of justice. According to this principle, people must be treated fairly and receive what they are owed or is comparable to other persons in the same situation. The research report needs to indicate that the selection of subjects and their treatment during the study were fair.

Fair Selection and Treatment of Subjects

Injustices in subject selection have resulted from social, cultural, racial, and sexual biases in society. For many years, research was conducted on categories of people who were thought to be especially suitable as research subjects, such as those living in poverty, charity patients, prisoners, slaves, peasants, dying persons, and others who were considered undesirable (Reynolds, 1979). Researchers often treated these subjects carelessly and had little regard for the harm and discomfort they experienced. The Nazi medical experiments, Tuskegee Syphilis Study, Willowbrook Study, and Jewish Chronic Disease Hospital Study all exemplify unfair subject selection (Levine, 1986).

Another concern with subject selection is that some researchers select subjects because they like them and want them to receive the specific benefits of a study. Other researchers have been swayed by power or money to make certain patients subjects so that these patients can receive potentially beneficial treatments. Random selection of subjects can eliminate some of the researchers' biases that may influence subject selection and strengthens the design of the study (see Chapter 9).

Each study must include a specific researcher-subject agreement or consent form regarding the researcher's role and subject's participation in a study (U.S. DHHS, 2009; FDA, 2012a). While conducting the study, the researcher must treat subjects fairly and respect that agreement. For example, the activities or procedures that subjects are to perform should not be changed without the subjects' and IRB's consent. The benefits promised to the subjects should be provided. Also, subjects who participate in studies should receive equal benefits regardless of age, race, or socioeconomic level.

The research report needs to indicate that the selection and treatment of the subjects were fair. Subjects must have been selected for reasons directly related to the problem being studied and not for their easy availability, compromised position, manipulability, or friendship with the researcher (Greaney et al., 2012; National Commission for the Protection of Human Subjects of Biomedical and Behavioral Research, 1978). In addition, the procedures section of the research report must indicate fair and equal treatment of the subjects during data collection (Fawcett & Garity, 2009).

Right to Protection from Discomfort and Harm

The right to protection from discomfort and harm in a study is based on the ethical principle of beneficence, which states that one should do good and, above all, do no harm. According to this principle, members of society must take an active role in preventing discomfort and harm and promoting good in the world around them (ANA, 2001, APA, 2010). In research, discomfort and harm can be physical, emotional, social, or economic or any combination of these four (Weijer, 2000). Reynolds (1972) identified five categories of studies based on levels of discomfort and harm—no anticipated effects, temporary discomfort, unusual levels of temporary discomfort, risk of permanent damage, and certainty of permanent damage.

No Anticipated Effects

No positive or negative effects are expected for the subjects in some studies. For example, studies that involve reviewing patients' records, students' files, pathology reports, or other documents have no anticipated effects on the research subjects. These studies involve no direct interaction between the researchers and subjects. However, there is still a potential risk of invading a subject's privacy. A subject's IIHI must be protected during data collection and analysis and in publication of the final report for the study to be compliant with the HIPAA regulations (U.S. DHHS, 2007a, 2009).

Temporary Discomfort

Studies that cause temporary discomfort are described as minimal-risk studies, in which the discomfort is similar to what the subject would encounter in his or her daily life and is temporary, ending with termination of the experiment (U.S. DHHS, 2009). Many nursing studies require the completion of questionnaires or participation in interviews, which usually involve minimal risk or are a mere inconvenience for the subjects. The physical discomfort may include fatigue, headache, or muscle tension. The emotional and social risks may include anxiety or embarrassment associated with answering certain questions. The economic risks may include the time commitment for the study or travel costs to the study site.

Most clinical nursing studies examining the effect of a treatment involve minimal risk. For example, a study may involve examining the effects of exercise on the blood glucose levels of diabetic subjects. For the study, the subjects are asked to test their blood glucose level one extra time per day. Discomfort occurs when the blood is obtained, and there is a potential risk of physical changes that may occur with exercise. The subjects may also feel anxiety and fear associated with the additional blood testing, and the testing may be an added expense. The diabetic subjects in this study will encounter similar discomforts in their daily lives, however, and the discomfort will cease with the termination of the study.

Unusual Levels of Temporary Discomfort

In studies that involve unusual levels of temporary discomfort, subjects frequently have discomfort during the study and after they have completed it. For example, subjects may have prolonged muscle weakness, joint pain, and dizziness after participating in a study that required them to be confined to bed for 7 days to determine the effects of immobility. Studies that require subjects to experience failure, extreme fear, or threats to their identity or to act in unnatural ways involve unusual levels of temporary discomfort. In some qualitative studies, researchers ask participants questions that open old wounds or involve reliving a traumatic event (Eide & Kahn, 2008; Fawcett & Garity, 2009). For example, asking participants to describe their sexual assault experience could precipitate feelings of extreme anger, fear, or sadness or any combination of these emotions. In such studies, the IRB protocol is required to include information on the resources to which researchers can refer subjects who have difficulties. Investigators need to indicate in the research report that they were vigilant in assessing the participants' discomfort and referred them as necessary for appropriate professional intervention.

Risk of Permanent Damage

In some studies, the possibility exists for subjects to sustain permanent damage; this is more common in biomedical research than in nursing research. For example, new drugs and surgical procedures being tested in medical studies have the potential to cause subjects permanent physical damage. Some topics investigated by nurses have the potential to cause permanent damage to subjects, emotionally and socially. Studies examining sensitive information, such as sexual behavior, child abuse, HIV-AIDS status, or drug use, can be very risky for subjects. These studies have the potential to cause permanent damage to a subject's personality or reputation. There also are potential economic risks, such as those resulting from a decrease in job performance or loss of employment.

Certainty of Permanent Damage

In some research, such as the Nazi medical experiments and the Tuskegee Syphilis Study, the subjects have a certainty of experiencing permanent damage. Conducting research that has a certainty of causing permanent damage to study subjects is highly questionable, regardless of the benefits that will be gained. Frequently, the benefits gained from such a study are experienced not by the research participants, but by others in society. Studies causing permanent damage to subjects violate the fifth principle of the Nuremberg Code and probably should not be conducted (see Box 4-1).

Critical Appraisal Guidelines to Examine Protection of Human Rights in Studies

The human rights that require protection in research include the rights to (1) self-determination, (2) privacy, (3) confidentiality, (4) fair selection and treatment, and (5) protection from discomfort and harm. The guidelines that follow will assist you in critically appraising a study to ensure the protection of human rights.

? CRITICAL APPRAISAL GUIDELINES

Protection of Human Rights

When critically appraising studies, evaluate whether the participants' human rights are protected by asking questions such as the following:

1. Did the study participants or subjects have diminished autonomy because of legal or mental incompetence, terminal illness, or confinement to an institution? If they did, were special precautions taken in obtaining consent from these participants and their parents or guardians (U.S. DHHS, 2009)?
2. Were the participants' right to privacy protected and confidentiality of research data maintained during data collection, analysis, and reporting?
3. Was the individually identifiable health information protected in compliance with the HIPAA Privacy Rule (U.S. DHHS, 2007a)?
4. Were the participants selected in a fair way for the study?
5. Were the participants treated in a fair way during the conduct of the study?
6. Were the participants protected from discomfort or harm (U.S. DHHS, 2009; FDA, 2012a)?

⚐ RESEARCH EXAMPLE

Ethical Conduct of Research with Children and Adolescents

Research Study Excerpt

Cerdan, Alpert, Moonie, Cyrkiel, and Rue (2012) conducted a correlational study to examine the relationships of children and adolescents' asthma severity and sociodemographic factors with parents' quality of life (QOL). The ethical aspects of the study are described in the following excerpt; the human rights protected are identified in brackets.

Research Design and Methodology

"This correlational study utilized a convenience sample of parents of children and adolescents, aged 7 to 17 years, with medical diagnoses of mild intermittent to severe persistent asthma. This study was reviewed and approved by the institutional review board [IRB] at the University of Nevada, Las Vegas [IRB approval].... Parents surveyed were legal guardians of the asthmatic children.... The clinic was chosen by the investigators because the clinic had patients with a greater variety of asthma severity (mild, moderate, or severe) and sociodemographic factors (e.g., health insurance coverage, parental age and ethnicity, and other variables) [right to fair selection]....

One of the researchers reviewed the charts of all scheduled patients to verify asthma diagnosis and age. Those deemed to be eligible to participate were approached in the waiting room by the researcher as patients and parents came in for their scheduled appointments. All potential participants were told that the researcher was not an employee of the clinic. They were also told that their participation was voluntary and declining participation would not jeopardize their relationships with their doctor or office staff [right to self-determination and protection from discomfort or harm]. Those who agreed to participate completed the informed consent and their children offered assent [right to self-determination and informed consent]....

Prior to completing the three questionnaires, the researcher gave parents explicit instructions on how to answer the items for each questionnaire, including the option not to answer questions that made them feel uncomfortable [right to fair treatment].... To maintain participant confidentiality, participant questionnaires were assigned numbers, and participant names or any other identifying information such as address, telephone number, or birth date were not recorded. The parents returned the questionnaires to the researcher in unmarked manila envelope to further ensure confidentiality" [right to anonymity, confidentiality, and privacy; compliance with HIPAA]. Cerdan et al., 2012, pp.132-133

Critical Appraisal

Cerdan and associates (2012) clearly described their sampling process, which indicated a fair selection of study participants who reflected diversity in asthma severity, parental and child age and ethnicity, and insurance status. The researchers also recognized that these children and adolescents have diminished autonomy because they are younger than the adult age of 18 years. The study was explained to the children and adolescents and their parents (legal guardian), and assent was obtained from the children and adolescents and consent from the parents to participate in the study. The study participants were identified with numbers, and all other identifying information was not recorded to ensure confidentiality and privacy of information according to HIPAA U.S. DHHS 2009 regulations. The children, adolescents, and their parents' rights to self-determination, privacy, confidentiality, fair selection and treatment, and protection from discomfort and harm were protected by the informed consent process and the ethical conduct of this study, according to federal regulations (U.S. DHHS, 2007a, 2009).

Implications for Practice

The study findings of Cerdan and co-workers (2012) were consistent with previous research, which indicated that a number of factors, such as asthma severity and sociodemographic factors, influenced the parents' QOL. Programs are needed to take into consideration the parents and their experiences when their children have asthma. Nurses working with families of asthmatic children need to educate children and parents aggressively and vigilantly monitor their health status to improve their health outcomes. Quality and Safety Education for Nurses (QSEN) implications are focused on the competencies of providing evidence-based, safe, and patient- and family-centered care (QSEN, 2013; Sherwood & Barnsteiner, 2012).

UNDERSTANDING INFORMED CONSENT

What is informed consent? How is informed consent obtained from research subjects and documented in the research report? *Informing* is the transmission of essential ideas and content from the investigator to the prospective subject. *Consent* is the prospective subject's agreement to participate in a study as a subject. Every prospective subject, to the degree that he or she is capable, should have the opportunity to choose whether to participate in research (U.S. DHHS, 2009; FDA, 2012a). Informed consent includes four elements: (1) disclosure of essential study information to the study participant; (2) comprehension of this information by the participant; (3) competence of the participant to give consent; and (4) voluntary consent of the participant to take part in the study.

Essential Information for Consent

Informed consent requires the researcher to disclose specific information to all prospective subjects. The following information is essential for obtaining informed consent from research subjects (U.S. DHHS, 2009; FDA, 2012a):

1. *Introduction of research activities.* The initial information presented to prospective subjects clearly indicates that a study is to be conducted and that they are being asked to participate as subjects.
2. *Statement of the research purpose.* The researcher states the immediate purpose of the research and any long-range goals related to the study.
3. *Selection of research subjects.* The researcher explains to prospective subjects why they were selected to participate in the study.
4. *Explanation of procedures.* Prospective subjects receive a complete description of the procedures to be followed and any procedures that are experimental in the study are identified

5. *Description of risks and discomforts.* Prospective subjects are informed of any reasonably foreseeable risks or discomforts (physical, emotional, social, and economic) that might result from the study.
6. *Description of benefits.* The investigator describes any benefits to the subjects or to other people or future patients that may reasonably be expected from the research, including any financial advantages or other rewards for participating in the study.
7. *Disclosure of alternatives.* The investigator discloses the appropriate alternative procedures or courses of treatment, if any, that might be advantageous to the subjects (U.S. DHHS, 2009; FDA, 2012a). For example, the researchers in the Tuskegee Syphilis Study should have informed the subjects with syphilis that penicillin was an effective treatment for the disease.
8. *Assurance of anonymity and confidentiality.* Prospective subjects should know the extent to which their responses and records will be kept confidential. Subjects are promised that their identity will remain anonymous in presentations and publication of the study.
9. *Offering to answer questions.* The researcher offers to answer any questions that the prospective subjects may have.
10. *Voluntary participation.* The consent form includes a statement that participation is voluntary and that refusal to participate will involve no penalty or loss of benefits to which the subject is otherwise entitled.
11. *Option to withdraw.* Subjects are informed that they may discontinue participation (withdraw from a study) at any time, without penalty or loss of benefits.
12. *Consent to incomplete disclosure.* In some studies, subjects are not completely informed of the study purpose because that knowledge would alter their actions. However, prospective subjects must be told when certain information is being withheld deliberately.

A consent form is a written document that includes the elements of informed consent required by U.S. DHHS (2009) and FDA (2012a) regulations. In addition, a consent form may include other information required by the institution in which the study is to be conducted or by the agency funding the study. An example of a consent form is presented in Figure 4-1. The boldface terms indicate the essential consent information.

Comprehension of Consent Information

Informed consent implies not only that the researcher has imparted information to the subjects, but also that the prospective subjects have comprehended that information. The researcher must take the time to teach the subjects about the study. The amount of information to be taught depends on the subjects' knowledge of research and the specific research topic. Researchers need to discuss the benefits and risks of a study in detail, with examples that the potential subjects or participants can understand. Nurses often serve as patient advocates in clinical agencies and need to assess whether patients involved in research understand the purpose and potential risks and benefits of their participation in a study (ANA, 2001; Banner & Zimmer, 2012; Fry et al., 2011).

Competence to Give Consent

nomous persons, who are capable of understanding the benefits and risks of a proposed study,
ompetent to give consent. Persons with diminished autonomy because of legal or mental
mpetence or confinement to an institution frequently are not legally competent to consent
rticipate in research (see earlier, "Right to Self-Determination"). In the research report, investors need to indicate the competence of the subjects and the process that was used for obtaining med consent (Banner & Zimmer 2012; U.S. DHHS, 2009; FDA, 2012a).

Study title: The Needs of Family Members of Critically Ill Adults
Investigator: Linda L. Norris, R.N.

Ms. Norris is a registered nurse studying the emotional and social needs of family members of patients in the Intensive Care Units **(research purpose)**. Although the study will not benefit you directly, it will provide information that might enable nurses to identify family members' needs and to assist family members with those needs **(potential benefits)**.

The study and its procedures have been approved by the appropriate people and review boards at The University of Texas at Arlington and X hospital **(IRB approval)**. The study procedures might cause fatigue for you or your family **(potential risks)**. The procedures include: (1) responding to a questionnaire about the needs of family members of critically ill patients and (2) completing a demographic data sheet **(explanation of procedures)**. Participation in this study will take approximately 20 minutes **(time commitment)**. You are free to ask any questions about the study or about being a subject and you may call Ms. Norris at (999) 999-9999 (work) or (999) 999-9999 (disposable cell phone) if you have further questions **(offer to answer questions)**.

Your participation in this study is voluntary; you are under no obligation to participate **(alternative option and voluntary consent)**. You have the right to withdraw at any time and the care of your family member and your relationship with the healthcare team will not be affected **(option to withdraw)**.

The study data will be coded so they will not be linked to your name. Your identity will not be revealed while the study is being conducted or when the study is reported or published. All study data will be collected by Ms. Norris, stored in a secure place, and not shared with any other person without your permission **(assurance of anonymity and confidentiality)**.

I have read this consent form and voluntarily consent to participate in this study.

(If Appropriate)

_____   _____
Subject's Signature   Date   Legal Representative   Date

I have explained this study to the above subject and have sought his/her understanding for informed consent.

_____
Investigator's Signature   Date

FIG 4-1 Sample Consent Form. Words in parentheses and boldface identify common essential consent information and would not appear in an actual consent form.

Voluntary Consent

Voluntary consent means that the prospective subject has decided to take part in a study of his or her own volition, without coercion or any undue influence (U.S. DHHS, 2009). Researchers obtain voluntary consent after the prospective subject receives the essential information about the study and has demonstrated comprehension of this information. All these elements of informed consent need to be documented in a consent form and discussed in the research report.

Documentation of Informed Consent

The documentation of informed consent depends on (1) the level of risk involved in the study and (2) the discretion of the researcher and those reviewing the study for institutional approval. Most studies require a written consent form that the subject signs, although in some studies, the requirement for written consent is waived. Nurses may be asked to identify subjects for studies, obtain consent forms for studies, collect study data, or participate in an IRB to review the ethics of a study. As a result, you need to be aware of the process for documenting informed consent in research.

Written Signed Consent Waived

The requirements for written signed consent may be waived in research that "presents no more than minimal risk of harm to subjects and involves no procedures for which written consent is normally required outside of the research context" (U.S. DHHS, 2009, 45 CFR, Section 46.117c). For example, researchers using questionnaires to collect relatively harmless data do not require a signed consent form from the subjects. Therefore, the subjects' completion of the questionnaire online or through the mail may serve as consent. The top of the questionnaire might contain a statement such as, "Your completion of this questionnaire indicates your consent to participate in this study."

Written signed consent also is waived in a situation in which "the only record linking the subject and the research would be the consent document and the principal risk would be potential harm resulting from a breach of confidentiality. Each subject will be asked whether he or she wants documentation linking them with the research, and the subject's wishes will govern" (U.S. DHHS, 2009, 45 CFR, Section 46.117c). In this situation, subjects are given the option to sign or not sign a consent form that links them to the research. The four elements of consent—disclosure, comprehension, competency, and voluntariness—are essential in all studies, whether written signed consent is waived or required.

Written Short Form Consent Documents

The short form consent document includes the following statement: "The elements of informed consent required by Section 46.116 (see earlier, "Essential Information for Consent") have been presented orally to the subject or the subject's legally authorized representative" (U.S. DHHS, 2009, 45 CFR, Section 46.117a). The researcher must develop a written summary of what is to be said to the subject in the oral presentation, and an IRB must approve the summary. When the researcher makes the oral presentation to the subject or to the subject's representative, a witness is required. The subject or representative must sign the short form consent document. "The witness shall sign both the short form and a copy of the summary, and the person actually obtaining consent shall sign a copy of the summary" (U.S. DHHS, 2009, 45 CFR, Section 46.117a). Copies of the summary and short form are given to the subject and witness, and the researcher retains the original documents. The researcher must keep these documents for 3 years. The short form written consent documents typically are used in studies that present minimal or moderate risk to the subjects.

Formal Written Consent Document

The formal written consent document includes the elements of informed consent required by U.S. DHHS (2009) and FDA (2012a) regulations (see earlier, "Essential Information for Consent"). The consent form can be read by the subject or read to the subject by the researcher; however, it is also prudent to explain the study to the subject. The form is signed by the subject and witnessed by the investigator or research assistant collecting the data (see example consent form in Figure 4-1). This type of consent can be used for any type of study, from minimal risk to high risk. All persons signing the consent form—including the subject, researcher, and any witnesses—must receive a copy of it. The original consent form is kept by the researcher for a period of 3 years.

Studies that involve subjects with diminished autonomy require a written signed consent form. If these prospective subjects have some comprehension of the study and agree to participate as subjects, they must sign the consent form. However, the subject's legally authorized representative must sign the form. The representative indicates his or her relationship with the subject under the signature (see Figure 4-1). Sometimes nurses are asked to sign a consent form as a witness for a

biomedical study. They must know the study purpose and procedures and the subject's comprehension of the study before signing the form. To ensure the consistent implementation of the
consent process, nurses and others involved in the consent process are educated about the study
and consent process. Larson, Cohn, Meyer, and Boden-Albala (2009) identified problems with
the lack of standardization of the informed consent process in health-related studies that leads
to disparities in those participating in studies. Certain individuals elect not to participate in
research because of the way the study is presented to them during the consent process. Larson
and co-workers (2009, p. 95) recommended a formal educational program for researchers and
those involved in the consent process "to reduce disparities in research participation by improving
communication between research staff and potential participants."

Health Insurance Portability and Accountability Act Privacy Rule: Authorization for Research Uses and Disclosure

The HIPAA Privacy Rule provides people, as research subjects, with the right to authorize covered
entities (healthcare provider, health plan, and healthcare clearinghouse) to use or disclose their
PHI for research purposes (U.S. DHHS, 2007a). HIPAA regulates this authorization in addition
to the informed consent process regulated by the U.S. DHHS (2009) and FDA (2012a). The authorization focuses on the privacy risks and states how, why, and to whom the PHI will be shared.
The authorization core elements and a sample authorization form can be found online at
http://privacyruleandresearch.nih.gov/authorization.asp (U.S. DHHS, 2007a). The authorization
information can be included as part of the consent form or as a separate form.

Critical Appraisal Guidelines to Examine Informed Consent in Studies

All studies require obtaining informed consent from the study participants or subjects. The consent process must meet the U.S. DHHS (2009), FDA (2012a), and HIPAA (U.S. DHHS, 2007a)
regulations for the conduct of ethical research with human subjects. Research reports often discuss
the consent process and identify some of the essential consent information that was provided to the
potential subjects. Some mention of the consent process for that study is required, but the depth of
the discussion will vary according to the research purpose and types of participants or subjects
included in the study. The consent process is usually presented in the methods section under a
discussion of study procedures or data collection process. The following critical appraisal guidelines will assist you in examining the consent process of a published study or for a study to be
conducted in your clinical agency.

---

⑦ CRITICAL APPRAISAL GUIDELINES

Examining Informed Consent Process

Consider the following questions when critically appraising the consent process of a study (Banner & Zimmer,
2012; U.S. DHHS, 2009; FDA, 2012a; Simpson, 2010):
1. Was informed consent obtained from the subjects or participants?
2. Was the essential information for consent provided and comprehended by the subjects?
3. Were the subjects competent to give consent? If the subjects were not competent to give consent, who
   acted as their legally authorized representatives?
4. Did it seem that the subjects participated voluntarily in the study?

RESEARCH EXAMPLE

Informed Consent

Research Study Excerpt

Franklin and Harrell (2013) conducted a study to examine the influence of rheumatoid arthritis (RA)–related fatigue on the psychological outcomes of depressive symptoms, perceived health impairment, and satisfaction with abilities in adults with RA. The following excerpt documents the process for obtaining informed consent from the participants in this study.

Methods

Participants

"The sample for this study was recruited from the general community, including local senior centers, independent and assisted living facilities, community organizations, and retirement communities in East Central Florida. . . . Eligibilty criteria included . . . willingness to participate, including signing the informed consent form, with acknowledgment that the participant understood the information presented within the consent form. Participants did not receive compensation for their participation. . . ."

Procedure

"The study and all procedures were approved by the university's human subject institutional review board. Questionnaires and consent forms were provided to community agencies. The agencies distributed the instruments to their members or residents who expressed a willingness to complete the questionnaires. Informed consent was obtained in the presence of agency personnel who had been briefed on the study so they could address participant questions. In addition, participants were provided with a phone number to contact researchers with any questions. Completed questionnaires and consent forms were returned to the researchers via mail, using a provided self-addressed, stamped envelope. Names appeared only on the signature line of the consent forms, which were separated from the completed questionnaires and maintained separately to insure anonymity of participants." Franklin & Harrell, 2013, pp. 204-205

Critical Appraisal

Franklin and Harrell (2013) identified the essential elements of the informed consent process in their research report. They indicated that the study participants were provided information about the study and their signing of the consent form indicated that they understood the information presented. The consent process was voluntary because only those individuals willing to participate were asked to sign a consent form and complete the study questionnaire. The study participants were given the right to ask questions and their information was kept confidential. The consent process would have been strengthened by a discussion of the benefits and risks of the study and compliance with HIPAA regulations.

Implications for Practice

Franklin and Harrell (2013) found that RA-related fatigue had a clinically and statistically significant impact on psychological well-being (depressive symptoms, perceived health impairment, and satisfaction with ability) of older adults. Because the sample was comprised of older adults (age range, 55 to 89 years; mean age, 66.7 years), the findings cannot be generalized to other adults with RA. The researchers recommended future research using a larger sample to include males and younger patients to determine the influence of age and gender on the relationship of fatigue with psychological well-being.

UNDERSTANDING INSTITUTIONAL REVIEW

In institutional review, a study is examined for ethical concerns by a committee knowledgeable about research and clinical practice. The first federal policy statement on protection of human subjects by institutional review was issued by the Public Health Service (PHS) in 1966. The statement required that research involving human subjects must be reviewed by a committee of peers or associates to confirm that (1) the rights and welfare of the persons involved were protected, (2) the appropriate methods were used to secure informed consent, and (3) the potential benefits of the investigation were greater than the risks (Levine, 1986).

In 1974, DHEW passed the National Research Act, which required that all research involving human subjects undergo institutional review. The DHHS reviewed and revised these guidelines several times, with the last revision in 2009 (45 CFR, Sections 46.107-46.115). The FDA (2012b, 21 CFR, Part 56) also has very similar guidelines for institutional review of research. The regulations describe the membership, functions, and operations of the body responsible for institutional review. An institutional review board (IRB) is a committee that reviews research to ensure that the investigator is conducting the research ethically. Universities, hospitals, corporations, and many managed care centers have IRBs to promote the conduct of ethical research and protect the rights of prospective subjects at their institutions (Fry et al., 2011; Munhall, 2012b).

Each IRB has at least five members of varying backgrounds (cultural, economic, educational, gender, racial) to promote complete, scholarly, and fair review of research commonly conducted in an institution. If an institution regularly reviews studies with vulnerable subjects, such as children, neonates, pregnant women, prisoners, and the mentally disabled, the IRB must include one or more members with knowledge about and experience in working with these subjects. The members must have sufficient experience and expertise to review a variety of studies, including quantitative, qualitative, and outcomes research studies (Grove et al., 2013; Munhall, 2012b). The IRB members must not have a conflicting interest related to a study conducted in an institution. Any member having a conflict of interest with a research project being reviewed must excuse himself or herself from the review process for that study, except to provide information requested by the IRB. The IRB also must include one member whose primary concern is nonscientific, such as an ethicist, lawyer, or minister. At least one of the IRB members must be someone who is not affiliated with the institution (U.S. DHHS, 2009; FDA, 2012b). IRBs in hospitals often are composed of physicians, nurses, lawyers, scientists, clergy, and community laypersons.

The FDA (2012b) regulations were revised to require all IRBs to register through a system maintained by the DHHS. The registration information includes contact information for IRB members (e.g., addresses, telephone numbers, and e-mail), the number of active protocols involving FDA-regulated products reviewed during the preceding 12 months, and a description of the types of FDA-regulated products involved in the protocols reviewed (FDA, 2012b). The IRB registration requirement was implemented to make it easier for the FDA to inspect IRBs and communicate information to them. IRB registration must be renewed every 3 years and can be done online at http://ohrp.cit.nih.gov/efile.

Levels of Reviews Conducted by Institutional Review Boards

The functions and operations of an IRB involve the review of research at three different levels: (1) exempt from review, (2) expedited review, and (3) complete review. The IRB chairperson and/or committee, not the researcher, decide the level of the review required for each study. Studies usually are exempt from review if they pose no apparent risks for the research subjects. A common type of exempt study is when de-identified data from patient charts are analyzed. Nursing studies that carry no foreseeable risks for subjects often are considered exempt from review by the IRB committee.

Studies that carry some risks, which are viewed as minimal, qualify for an expedited review. Minimal risk means that "the probability and magnitude of harm or discomfort anticipated in the research are not greater in and of themselves than those ordinarily encountered in daily life or during the performance of routine physical or psychological examinations or tests" (U.S. DHHS, 2009, 45 CFR, Section 46.102i). Expedited review procedures also can be used to review minor changes in previously approved research. Under expedited review procedures, the review may be carried out by the IRB chairperson or one or more experienced reviewers designated by the chairperson from among members of the IRB. In reviewing the research, the reviewers may exercise all the authority of the IRB, except disapproval of the research. A research activity may be disapproved only after a complete review of the IRB (U.S. DHHS, 2009; FDA, 2012b). Descriptive studies, in which subjects are asked to respond to questionnaires, commonly need only expedited review.

A study that carries greater than minimal risks must receive a complete review by an IRB. To obtain IRB approval, researchers must ensure that (1) risks to subjects are minimized, (2) risks to subjects are reasonable in relation to anticipated benefits, (3) selection of subjects is equitable, (4) informed consent will be sought from each prospective subject or the subject's legally authorized representative, (5) informed consent will be appropriately documented, (6) the research plan makes adequate provision for monitoring data collection for subject's safety, and (7) adequate provisions are made to protect the privacy of subjects and maintain the confidentiality of data (U.S. DHHS, 2009; FDA, 2012b).

Most studies indicate that IRB approval was obtained, but do not indicate whether the study was exempt from review, expedited review, or complete review. If a researcher is affiliated with a university, the study needs to be approved by the IRB of that university before seeking IRB approval from the clinical agency in which the study is to be conducted. In the study conducted by Cerdan and colleagues (2012, p. 132; see earlier), the researchers obtained "IRB approval at the University of Nevada, Las Vegas. . . . The participants were chosen from a pediatric pulmonology outpatient clinic located in Las Vegas, Nevada." The researchers did not identify the IRB approval from the clinic, but it might have been part of the university medical center.

If a study is conducted in more than one clinical agency, researchers must obtain IRB approval from all clinical sites in which the study is to be conducted. A research report needs to identify the IRBs that reviewed and approved a study for implementation clearly. For example, Elshatarat, Stotts, Engler, and Froelicher (2013) conducted a descriptive study of the knowledge and beliefs about smoking and goals of smoking cessation in men hospitalized with cardiovascular disease. "The Committee on Human Research at the University of California, San Francisco approved this study as did the Directors of Nursing and the Chief Medical Officers of the two hospitals. All subjects provided written informed consent" (p. 127). These researchers documented IRB approval of the university and administrative approval of the two hospitals in which the study was conducted.

Influence of Health Insurance Portability and Accountability Act Privacy Rule on Institutional Review Boards

Under the HIPAA Privacy Rule, an IRB or institutional established privacy board can act on requests for a waiver or an alteration of the authorization requirement for a research project. If an IRB and privacy board both exist in an agency, the approval of only one board is required;

it will probably be the IRB for research projects. Researchers can choose to obtain a signed authorization form from potential subjects or can ask for a waiver or alteration of the authorization requirement. An altered authorization requirement is when an IRB approves a request that some, but not all, of the required 18 elements be removed from health information to be used in research. The researcher can also request a partial or complete waiver of the authorization requirement from the IRB. The partial waiver involves the researcher's obtaining PHI to contact and recruit potential subjects for a study. An IRB can give a researcher a complete waiver of authorization in studies in which the requirement for a written or signed consent form was waived (U.S. DHHS, 2007a). The HIPAA regulations related to IRBs can be found online at http://privacyruleandresearch.nih.gov/irbandprivacyrule.asp. The HIPAA Privacy Rule does not change the IRB membership and functions that are designated under the U.S. DHHS (2009) and FDA (2012b) IRB regulations.

EXAMINING THE BENEFIT-RISK RATIO OF A STUDY

Nurses who serve on an IRB for their agency, serve as patient advocates when research is conducted in their agency, or are asked to collect data for a study should examine the balance of benefits and risks in studies. To determine this balance, or benefit-risk ratio, the benefits and risks associated with the sampling method, consent process, procedures, and potential outcomes of the study are assessed (Figure 4-2). Informed consent must be obtained from subjects, and

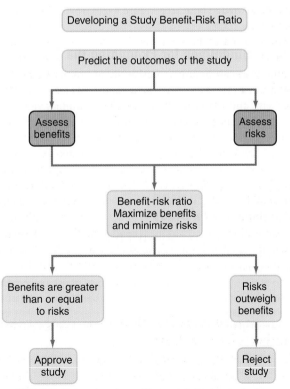

FIG 4-2 Balancing benefits and risks for a study.

selection and treatment of subjects during the study must be fair. An important outcome of research is the development and refinement of knowledge. The type of knowledge that might be obtained from the study and who will be influenced by the knowledge also need to be identified.

The type of research conducted—therapeutic or nontherapeutic—affects the potential benefits for subjects. In therapeutic research, subjects might benefit from the study procedures in areas such as skin care, range of motion, touch, and other nursing interventions. The benefits might include improved physical condition, which could facilitate emotional and social benefits. Some researchers have noted that participation in qualitative research has encouraged subjects to process and disclose thoughts regarding life-altering events, and that these actions have been beneficial to the subjects' health and well-being (Eide & Kahn, 2008, Munhall, 2012a). Nontherapeutic nursing research does not benefit subjects directly, but is important because it generates and refines nursing knowledge for future patients, the nursing profession, and society. Most subjects involved in a study do benefit by having an increased understanding of the research process and knowing the findings from a particular study.

Examining the benefit-risk ratio also involves assessing the type, degree, and number of risks that subjects might encounter while participating in a study. The risks involved depend on the purpose of the study and procedures used to conduct the study. Risks can be physical, emotional, social, or economic and can range from no anticipated risk or mere inconvenience to certain risk of permanent damage (see earlier, "Right to Protection from Discomfort and Harm"; Fry et al., 2011; Reynolds, 1972). If the risks outweigh the benefits, the study probably is unethical and should not be conducted. If the benefits outweigh the risks, the study probably is ethical and has the potential to add to nursing's knowledge base (see Figure 4-2; Grove et al., 2013).

Critical Appraisal Guidelines for Examining the Ethical Aspects of Studies

The following guidelines can be used to critically appraise the ethical aspects of a study. These guidelines include (1) examination of the benefit-risk ratio of the study, (2) IRB approval, (3) informed consent, and (4) protection of subjects' human rights. This information needs to be included in published studies.

? CRITICAL APPRAISAL GUIDELINES

Examining the Ethical Aspects of a Study

When conducting a study, researchers must meet the U.S. DHHS (2009), FDA (2012a, 2012b), and HIPAA (U.S. DHHS, 2007a) regulations for the conduct of ethical research with human subjects. Consider the following questions when critically appraising the ethical aspects of a study:

1. Was the benefit-risk ratio of the study acceptable? Was the level of risk reasonable for the study and did the benefits outweigh the risks? (Use Figure 4-2 to examine the benefit-risk ratio of the study.)
2. Was the study approved by the appropriate IRB(s)?
3. Was informed consent obtained from the subjects? (Refer to the previous guidelines for examining the consent process in studies.)
4. Were the rights of the subjects protected during the study? (Refer to the previous guidelines for examining the protection of subjects' rights in research.)

RESEARCH EXAMPLE

Determining the Ethics of a Study

Research Study Excerpt

Rew, Horner, and Fouladi (2010) conducted a study of school-age children's health behaviors to determine if they were precursors of adolescents' health-risk behaviors. The sample included Hispanic and non-Hispanic children and their parents. The ethical aspects of the study are described in the following quote.

Setting and Sample

"The study took place in a rural setting in central Texas, a state with a rapidly expanding population of Hispanics, primarily of Mexican descent. The nonprobability sample was composed of 1,934 children in grades 4 ($n=781$), 5 ($n=621$), and 6 ($n=532$) who were enrolled in three rural school districts in central Texas and one of their parents." Rew et al., 2010, p. 158

Data Collection Procedure

"After study approval was obtained from the university's institutional review board [IRB] and each of the school administrators, a packet was mailed to parents of all the children in grades 4 through 6 in three rural school districts. The packets included a cover letter from the child's school, an explanatory letter from the researchers, and consent forms. All materials were written in English and Spanish, with forward and backward translations by independent speakers, and were reviewed by bilingual members of the community for translation clarity and accuracy before mailing. Informational meetings were held at the schools after parent-teacher meetings. At those school meetings, the study was explained to the children, questions were answered, and signed permissions were obtained from parents. Data were later collected during school hours using audio (optional), computer-assisted, self-interviewing (A-CASI) technology using laptop computers after the children who agreed to participate provided written assent. . . .

The children were oriented to the A-CASI format and were directed to select either the English or Spanish language versions to complete. For children who had difficulty with reading, audio support was engaged on the laptop computer and the children listened with an earpiece as the items were read to them in their preferred language. . . . As each child completed the questionnaires, the research assistants saved the data record to a secure Web site." Rew et al., 2010, p. 160

Critical Appraisal

Rew and associates (2010) presented the essential information about the protection of the participants' rights, informed consent process, and IRB approval in their research report. They provided a detailed description of the protection of the children and their parents' rights. The study was described in informational meetings held at the school in a language of choice, with an offer to answer questions. The parents agreed to their child's participation in the study through signed permission forms. The children gave written assent to participate in the study. IRB approvals of the university and school administrators were obtained, and the storage of study data in a secure location protected the privacy of the participants. All these activities promoted the ethical conduct of this study, according to the U.S. DHHS (2009) regulations. The benefit-risk ratio of this study was acceptable because the risk level of completing an online survey was minimal and the benefits of understanding adolescents' health-promoting and health-risk behaviors provide a basis for developing school wellness programs.

Implications for Practice

Rew and co-workers (2010) found that girls have more health-focused behaviors than boys, and the health behaviors decreased from grades 4 to 6. In addition, the school environment was found to be an important place for promoting healthy behaviors. The researchers encouraged school nurses, administrators, teachers, and parents to develop wellness policies and programs within the schools to increase the students' health-promoting behaviors and decrease their health-risk behaviors. Consistent with QSEN (2013) competencies, the findings could be integrated with other research evidence and used in practice, with the goal of providing evidence-based nursing care (Brown, 2014).

UNDERSTANDING RESEARCH MISCONDUCT

The goal of research is to generate sound scientific knowledge, which is possible only through the honest conduct, reporting, and publication of studies. However, since the 1980s, a number of fraudulent studies have been conducted and published in prestigious scientific journals. An example of research misconduct is the work of Marc Hauser, a former professor at Harvard University. He was found to have committed eight incidences of research misconduct in his studies of the development of human and monkey cognition (Office of Research Integrity, 2012b). He was cited for miscoding data, fabricating data, and misrepresenting study methods. Another example of research misconduct was evident in the publications of Dr. Robert Slutsky, a heart specialist at the University of California, San Diego, School of Medicine, whose study results raised questions of data fabrication (Friedman, 1990). In 6 years, Slutsky published 161 articles, and at one time, he was completing an article every 10 days. Of these articles, 18 were found to be fraudulent and have retraction notations, and 60 articles were judged to be questionable.

In response to the increasing incidences of scientific misconduct, the federal government developed the Office of Research Integrity (ORI) in 1989 within the U.S. DHHS. The ORI was to supervise the implementation of the rules and regulations related to research misconduct and to manage any investigations of misconduct. The most current regulations implemented by the ORI (2005) are CFR 42, Parts 50 and 93, Policies of General Applicability, discussed in the following section.

Role of the Office of Research Integrity in Promoting the Conduct of Ethical Research

The ORI was responsible for defining important terms used in the identification and management of research misconduct. Research misconduct is defined as "the fabrication, falsification, or plagiarism in processing, performing, or reviewing research, or in reporting research results. It does not include honest error or differences in opinion" (ORI, 2005, 42 CFR, Section 93.103). Fabrication in research is the making up of results and recording or reporting them. Falsification of research is manipulating research materials, equipment, or processes or changing or omitting data or results such that the research is not accurately represented in the research record. Fabrication and falsification of research data are two of the most common acts of research misconduct managed by ORI (2013) over the last 5 years. Plagiarism is the appropriation of another person's ideas, processes, results, or words without giving appropriate credit, including those obtained through confidential review of others' research proposals and manuscripts.

Currently, ORI promotes the integrity of biomedical and behavioral research in approximately 4000 institutions worldwide (ORI, 2012a). ORI applies federal policies and regulations to protect the integrity of the PHS's extramural and intramural research programs. The extramural program provides funding to research institutions, and the intramural program provides funding for research conducted within the federal government.

The ORI classifies research misconduct as (1) an act that involves a significant departure from the acceptable practice of the scientific community for maintaining the integrity of the research record, (2) an act that was committed intentionally, and (3) an allegation that can be proved by a preponderance of evidence. ORI has a section on their website (http://ori.U.S.DHHS.gov/case_summary) entitled "Handling Misconduct," which includes a summary of the allegations and investigations managed by its office from 1994 to present (ORI, 2013). The most common sites for the investigations were medical schools (68%), hospitals (11%), and research institutes (10%). The individuals charged with misconduct were primarily men with a doctorate or medical degree and were mostly associate professors, professors, and postdoctoral fellows.

Research misconduct has also been reported in the nursing profession (Habermann, Broome, Pryor, & Ziner, 2010; Rankin & Esteves, 1997). A specific example of a nurse found guilty of research misconduct was Scott Weber, who was found to have plagiarized significant portions of published articles, including using prior studies' data in graphs in his publications (ORI, 2011). He also changed the years of some cited articles in his reference lists to avoid detection of plagiarism. Habermann and colleagues (2010) conducted a study of research coordinators' experiences with scientific misconduct and research integrity and found that research coordinators often learned of the misconduct firsthand, and the principal investigator was usually identified as the responsible party. They identified five major categories of misconduct: "protocol violations, consent violations, fabrication, falsification, and financial conflict of interest" (Habermann et al., 2010, p. 51). They indicated that the definition of research misconduct might need to be expanded beyond fabrication, falsification, and plagiarism.

When research misconduct was documented, the actions taken against the researchers or agencies included debarment from receiving federal funding for periods ranging from 18 months to 8 years, prohibition from PHS advisory services, and other actions requiring supervised research, certification of data, certification of sources, and correction or retraction of articles (ORI, 2013). More information on the handling of research misconduct can be found on the ORI website (http://ori.U.S.DHHS.gov/handling-misconduct).

EXAMINING THE USE OF ANIMALS IN RESEARCH

The use of animals as research participants is a controversial issue of growing interest to nurse researchers. A small but increasing number of nurse scientists are conducting physiological studies that require the use of animals. For decades, animals have been used in the conduct of biomedical and biobehavioral research and have significantly contributed to our understanding of disease processes. Animals will also play an important role in genetics research. Renn and Dorsey (2011) have provided some important information to assist researchers in determining when and how animals might best be used to generate research knowledge. Selected animal rights groups, however, are very opposed to research using animals. Many scientists, especially physicians, believe that the current animal rights' movement could threaten the future of healthcare research. The goal of these groups is to raise the consciousness of researchers and society to ensure that animals are used wisely and treated humanely in the conduct of research. However, some of these animal rights groups have tried to frighten the public with somewhat distorted stories about the inhumane treatment of animals in research. Some activist leaders have made broad comparisons between human life and animal life. For example, a major animal rights group, People for the Ethical Treatment of Animals (PETA), has a website that posts videos and blogs about the unethical treatment of animals in research (http://www.peta.org/tv/videos/investigations-animal-experimentation). Some of these activists have now progressed to violence, using physical attacks, including real bombs, arson, and vandalism. Even more damage is being done to research through lawsuits that have blocked the conduct of research and the development of new research centers. Health science centers now spend millions of dollars annually for security, public education, and other efforts to defend research conducted with animals.

Because more nurses are conducting research with animals, the ethics of these studies need to be critically appraised. An important question to address is: What mechanisms ensured that the animals were treated humanely in the conduct of the study? Animals are just one of a variety of types of subjects used in research; others include humans, plants, and computer data sets. If possible, most researchers use nonanimal subjects, because they are generally less expensive (Latham, 2012). In low-risk studies, as are most nursing studies, humans are often used as subjects.

Some studies, however, require the use of animals to answer the research question. Approximately 17 to 22 million animals are used in research each year, and 90% of them are rodents, with the combined percentage of dogs and cats being only 1% to 2% (Goodwin & Morrison, 2000; Renn & Dorsey, 2011). Studies using animals comprise about one eighth of published studies (Osborne, Payne, & Newman, 2009). Because animals are deemed valuable subjects for selected research projects, the question concerning their humane treatment must be addressed. Recent studies have indicated that animals experience a wider variety of harm, including fear and pain, than was previously thought (Ferdowsian, 2011).

Currently at least five separate types of regulations exist to protect research animals from mistreatment. The federal government, state governments, independent accreditation organizations, professional societies, and individual institutions work to ensure that research animals are used only when necessary and only under humane conditions. At the federal level, animal research is conducted according to the guidelines of the PHS Policy on Humane Care and Use of Laboratory Animals, which was adopted in 1986 and reprinted essentially unchanged in 1996. The most current addition to this federal policy is the revised guidelines for euthanasia of animals. These policies are managed by the Office of Laboratory Animal Welfare (OLAW, 2013), and are available on their website at http://grants.nih.gov/grants/olaw/olaw.htm.

The Humane Care and Use of Laboratory Animals Regulations define animal as any live, vertebrate animal used or intended for use in research, research training, experimentation, or biological testing or for related purposes. Any institution proposing research involving animals must have a written animal welfare assurance statement acceptable to the PHS that documents compliance with PHS policy. Every assurance statement is evaluated by the National Institutes of Health's Office for Protection from Research Risks (OPRR) to determine the adequacy of the institution's proposed program for the care and use of animals in activities conducted or supported by the PHS (OLAW, 2011). Researchers using animals are required to develop an animal use protocol that describes the following elements: (1) research project; (2) rationale for animal use and consideration of alternatives; (3) justification for the choice of species and numbers of animals; (4) research procedures involving animals; (5) procedures to minimize pain and distress; (6) animal living conditions and veterinary care; (7) names and qualifications of personnel who will perform work with animals; (8) method of euthanasia; and (9) endpoint criteria. The OLAW (2011) website includes guidelines for the care and use of animals in research (http://grants.nih.gov/grants/policy/air/researchers_institutions.htm).

Institutions' assurance statements about compliance with PHS policy have promoted the humane care and treatment of animals in research. In addition, more than 700 institutions conducting health-related research have sought accreditation by the American Association for Accreditation of Laboratory Animal Care (AAALAC), which was developed to ensure the humane treatment of animals in research (OLAW, 2011). In conducting research, each investigator must carefully select the type of participant needed; if animals are used in a study, they require humane treatment. Osborne and associates (2009) conducted a study to determine journals' editorial policies regarding animal research. They found that journals need clear policies on the essential information to be included in a research report to reflect the fair treatment of animals in studies. In critically appraising studies, you need to ensure that animals were the appropriate subjects for a study and that they were treated humanely during the conduct of the study (OLAW, 2011, 2013).

Sharma, Ryals, Gajewski, and Wright (2010) noted that the molecular basis for the positive effects of exercise on chronic pain was poorly understood. Therefore they conducted an experimental study of the effects of aerobic exercise on analgesia and neurotrophin-3 (NT-3) synthesis in female mice. They noted that "all experiments were approved by the Institutional Animal Care and Use Committee of the University of Kansas Medical Center and adhered to the university's animal care guidelines" (Sharma et al., 2010, p. 715). Following these guidelines provided for the humane treatment of the animals in this study. The researchers found that moderate-intensity aerobic exercise reduced cutaneous and deep tissue pain and stimulated NT-3 synthesis in skeletal muscle, providing a possible molecular basis for the effects of exercise training on muscle pain. However, these results are limited to animals; further research is needed to determine the effects of exercise on humans with chronic pain.

KEY CONCEPTS

- Four experimental projects have been highly publicized for their unethical treatment of human subjects: (1) the Nazi medical experiments; (2) the Tuskegee Syphilis Study; (3) the Willowbrook Study; and (4) the Jewish Chronic Disease Hospital Study.
- Two historical documents, the Nuremberg Code and Declaration of Helsinki, have had a strong impact on the conduct of research.
- U.S. DHHS (2009) and FDA (2012a, b) regulations have been implemented to promote ethical conduct in research, including (1) general requirements for informed consent and (2) guidelines for IRB review of research.
- The HIPAA Privacy Rule (2007a) was enacted to protect the privacy of people's health information.
- The human rights that require protection in research are the right to (1) self-determination, (2) privacy, (3) anonymity and confidentiality, (4) fair selection and treatment, and (5) protection from discomfort and harm.
- Informed consent involves (1) transmission of essential study information to the potential subject, (2) comprehension of that information by the potential subject, (3) competence of the potential subject to give consent, and (4) voluntary consent by the potential subject to participate in the study.
- An institutional review board consists of a committee of peers who examine studies for ethical concerns with three levels of review—exempt, expedited, and complete.
- To balance the benefits and risks of a study, the type, degree, and number of risks are examined, and the potential benefits are identified. The benefits should overshadow the risks.
- Research misconduct is a serious ethical problem concerned with the conducting, reporting, and publication of fraudulent research.
- Animals are important for the conduct of certain studies, and they must be treated humanely during the study.

REFERENCES

American Nurses Association, (2001). *Code of ethics for nurses with interpretive statements.* Washington, DC: Author.

American Psychological Association, (2010). *Ethical principles of psychologists and code of conduct.* Retrieved June 9, 2013 from, http://www.apa.org/ethics/code/index.aspx.

Banner, C., & Zimmer, L. (2012). Informed consent in research: An overview for nurses. *Canadian Journal of Cardiovascular Nursing, 22*(1), 26–30.

Beebe, L. H., & Smith, K. (2010). Informed consent to research in persons with schizophrenia spectrum disorders. *Nursing Ethics, 17*(4), 425–434.

Beecher, H. K. (1966). Ethics and clinical research. *New England Journal of Medicine, 274*(24), 1354–1360.

Berger, R. L. (1990). Nazi science: The Dachau hypothermia experiments. *New England Journal of Medicine, 322*(20), 1435–1440.

Brandt, A. M. (1978). Racism and research: The case of the Tuskegee syphilis study. *Hastings Center Report, 8*(6), 21–29.

Broome, M. E. (1999). Consent (assent) for research with pediatric patients. *Seminars in Oncology Nursing, 15*(2), 96–103.

Brown, S. J. (2014). *Evidence-based nursing: The research-practice connection* (3rd ed.). Sudbury, MA: Jones & Bartlett.

Cerdan, N. S., Alpert, P. T., Moonie, S., Cyrkiel, D., & Rue, S. (2012). Asthma severity in children and the quality of life of their parents. *Applied Nursing Research, 25*(3), 131–137.

Eide, P., & Kahn, D. (2008). Ethical issues in the qualitative researcher-participant relationship. *Nursing Ethics, 15*(2), 199–207.

Elshatarat, R. A., Stotts, N. A., Engler, M., & Froelicher, E. S. (2013). Knowledge and beliefs about smoking and goals for smoking cessation in hospitalized men with cardiovascular disease. *Heart & Lung, 42*(2), 126–132.

Emanuel, E. J. (2004). Ending concerns about undue inducement. *The Journal of Law, Medicine & Ethics: A Journal of the American Society of Law, Medicine & Ethics, 32*(1), 100–105.

Fawcett, J., & Garity, J. (2009). *Evaluating research for evidence-based nursing practice.* Philadelphia: F. A. Davis.

Ferdowsian, H. (2011). Human and animal research guidelines: Aligning ethical constructs with new scientific developments. *Bioethics, 25*(8), 472–478.

Fowler, M. D. M. (2010). *Guide to the code of ethics for nursing: Interpretation and application.* Silver Spring, MD: American Nurses Association.

Franklin, A. L., & Harrell, T. H. (2013). Impact of fatigue on psychological outcomes in adults living with rheumatoid arthritis. *Nursing Research, 62*(3), 203–209.

Friedman, P. J. (1990). Correcting the literature following fraudulent publication. *Journal of the American Medical Association, 263*(10), 1416–1419.

Fry, S. T., Veatch, R. M., & Taylor, C. (2011). *Case studies in nursing ethics* (4th ed.). Sudbury, MA: Jones & Bartlett Learning.

Goodwin, F. K., & Morrison, A. R. (2000). Science and self-doubt. *Reason, 32*(5), 22–28.

Greaney, A., Sheehy, A., Heffernan, C., Murphy, J., Mhaolrunaigh, S. N., Heffernan, E., et al. (2012). Research ethics application: A guide for the novice nurse researcher. *British Journal of Nursing, 21*(1), 38–43.

Grove, S. K., Burns, N., & Gray, J. R. (2013). *The practice of nursing research: Appraisal, synthesis, and generation of evidence* (7th ed.). Philadelphia: Elsevier Saunders.

Habermann, B., Broome, M., Pryor, E. R., & Ziner, K. W. (2010). Research coordinators' experiences with scientific misconduct and research integrity. *Nursing Research, 59*(1), 51–57.

Hadley, E. K., Smith, C. A., Gallo, A. M., Angst, D. B., & Knafl, K. A. (2007). Parents' perspectives on having their children interviewed for research. *Research in Nursing & Health, 31*(1), 4–11.

Havens, G. A. (2004). Ethical implications for the professional nurse of research involving human subjects. *Journal of Vascular Nursing, 22*(1), 19–23.

Hershey, N., & Miller, R. D. (1976). *Human experimentation and the law.* Rockville, MD: Aspen.

Infectious Diseases Society of America, (2009). Grinding to a halt: The effects of the increasing regulatory burden on research and quality improvement efforts. *Clinical Infectious Diseases, 49*(3), 328–335.

Kelman, H. C. (1967). Human use of human subjects: The problem of deception in social psychological experiments. *Psychological Bulletin, 67*(1), 1–11.

Larson, E. L., Cohn, E. G., Meyer, D. D., & Boden-Albala, B. (2009). Consent administrator training to reduce disparities in research participation. *Journal of Nursing Scholarship, 41*(1), 95–103.

Latham, S. (2012). U. S. law and animal experimentation. *Hastings Center Reports, 42*, S35–S39.

Levine, R. J. (1986). *Ethics and regulation of clinical research* (2nd ed.). Baltimore: Urban & Schwarzenberg.

Milgram, S. (1963). Behavioral study of obedience. *Journal of Abnormal and Social Psychology, 67*(4), 371–378.

Munhall, P. L. (2012a). Ethical considerations in qualitative research. In P. L. Munhall (Ed.), *Nursing research: A qualitative perspective* (pp. 491–502). (5th ed.). Sudbury, MA: Jones & Bartlett Learning.

Munhall, P. L. (2012b). Institutional review of qualitative research proposals: A task of no small consequence. In P. L. Munhall (Ed.), *Nursing research: A qualitative perspective* (pp. 503–515). (5th ed.). Sudbury, MA: Jones & Bartlett Learning.

National Commission for the Protection of Human Subjects of Biomedical and Behavioral Research,

(1978). *Belmont report: Ethical principles and guidelines for research involving human subjects.* DHEW Publication No. (05) 78-0012. Washington, DC: U.S. Government Printing Office.

Office of Laboratory Animal Welfare (OLAW), (2011). *For researchers and institutions: Good animal care and good science go hand-in-hand.* Retrieved June 9, 2013 from, http://grants.nih.gov/grants/policy/air/researchers_institutions.htm.

Office of Laboratory Animal Welfare (OLAW), (2013). *OLAW policies and laws.* Retrieved June 9, 2013 from, http://grants.nih.gov/grants/olaw/olaw.htm.

Office of Research Integrity (ORI), (2005). Public health service policies on research misconduct. *Code of Federal Regulations,* Title 42, Parts 50 and 93, Policies of General Applicability. Retrieved June 9, 2013 from, http://ori.U.S.DHHS.gov/documents/FR_Doc_05-9643.shtml.

Office of Research Integrity (ORI), (2011). *Case summary: Weber, Scott.* Retrieved June 8, 2013 from, http://ori.hhs.gov/content/case-summary-weber-scott.

Office of Research Integrity (ORI), (2012a). *About ORI.* Retrieved June 9, 2013 from, http://ori.U.S.DHHS.gov/about-ori.

Office of Research Integrity (ORI), (2012b). *Case summary: Hauser, Marc.* Retrieved June 8, 2013 from, http://ori.hhs.gov/content/case-summary-hauser-marc.

Office of Research Integrity (ORI), (2013). *Handling misconduct—Case summaries.* Office of Research Integrity. Retrieved May 29, 2013 from, *http://ori.U.S.DHHS.gov/misconduct/cases/.*

Olsen, D. P. (2003). Methods: HIPAA privacy regulations and nursing research. *Nursing Research, 52*(5), 344–348.

Osborne, N. J., Payne, D., & Newman, M. L. (2009). Journal editorial policies, animal welfare, and the 3Rs. *The American Journal of Bioethics, 9*(12), 55–59.

Quality and Safety Education for Nurses (QSEN), (2013). *Pre-licensure knowledge, skills, and attitudes (KSAs).* Retrieved February 11, 2013 from, http://qsen.org/competencies/pre-licensure-ksas/.

Rankin, M., & Esteves, M. D. (1997). Perceptions of scientific misconduct in nursing. *Nursing Research, 46*(5), 270–276.

Renn, C. L., & Dorsey, S. G. (2011). From mouse to man: The efficacy of animal models of human disease in genetic and genomic research. *Annual Review of Nursing Research, 29,* 99–112.

Rew, L., Horner, S. D., & Fouladi, R. T. (2010). Factors associated with health behaviors in middle childhood. *Journal of Pediatric Nursing, 25*(3), 157–166.

Reynolds, P. D. (1972). On the protection of human subjects and social science. *International Social Science Journal, 24*(4), 693–719.

Reynolds, P. D. (1979). *Ethical dilemmas and social science research.* San Francisco: Jossey-Bass.

Rosato, J. (2000). The ethics of clinical trials: A child's view. *The Journal of Law, Medicine & Ethics: A Journal of the American Society of Law, Medicine & Ethics, 28*(4), 362–378.

Rotenberg, M. A., & Rudnick, A. (2011). Reporting of ethics procedures in psychiatric rehabilitation peer-reviewed empirical research publications in the last decade. *American Journal of Psychiatric Rehabilitation, 14*(2), 97–108.

Rothman, D. J. (1982). Were Tuskegee and Willowbrook "studies in nature?" *Hastings Center Report, 12*(2), 5–7.

Sandelowski, M. (1994). Focus on qualitative methods: The use of quotes in qualitative research. *Research in Nursing & Health, 17*(6), 479–482.

Savage, E., & McCarron, S. (2009). Research access to adolescents and young adults. *Applied Nursing Research, 22*(1), 63–67.

Sharma, N. K., Ryals, J. M., Gajewski, B. J., & Wright, D. E. (2010). Aerobic exercise alters analgesia and neurotropin-3 synthesis in an animal model of chronic widespread pain. *Physical Therapy, 90*(5), 714–725.

Sherwood, G., & Barnsteiner, J. (2012). *Quality and safety in nursing: A competency approach to improving outcomes.* Ames, IA: Wiley-Blackwell.

Simpson, C. (2010). Decision-making capacity and informed consent to participate in research by cognitively impaired individuals. *Applied Nursing Research, 23*(4), 221–226.

Steinfels, P., & Levine, C. (1976). Biomedical ethics and the shadow of Nazism. *Hastings Center Report, 6*(4), 1–20.

Stone, P. W. (2003). Ask an expert: HIPAA in 2003 and its meaning for nurse researchers. *Applied Nursing Research, 16*(4), 291–293.

Thompson, P. J. (1987). Protection of the rights of children as subjects for research. *Journal of Pediatric Nursing, 2* (6), 392–399.

U.S. Department of Health and Human Services (U.S. DHHS), (1981). Final regulations amending basic HHS policy for the protection of human research subjects. *Code of Federal Regulations,* Title 45, Part 46.

U.S. Department of Health and Human Services (U.S. DHHS), (2007a). *HIPAA privacy rule: Information for researchers.* Retrieved May 29, 2013 from, http://privacyruleandresearch.nih.gov/.

U.S. Department of Health and Human Services (U.S. DHHS), (2007b). *How do other privacy protections interact with the privacy rule?.* Retrieved May 29, 2013 from, http://privacyruleandresearch.nih.gov/pr_05.asp.

U.S. Department of Health and Human Services (U.S. DHHS), (2009). Protection of human subjects. *Code of Federal Regulations,*Title 45, Part 46. Retrieved May 30, 2013 from, http://www.hhs.gov/ohrp/policy/ohrpregulations.pdf.

U.S. Department of Health and Human Services (U.S. DHHS), Office of Human Research Protection (OHRP), (2013). *The Nuremberg Code (1949).* Retrieved June 9, 2013 from, http://www.hhs.gov/ohrp/archive/nurcode.html.

U.S. Food and Drug Administration (FDA), (2003). *Pediatric Research Equity Act.* Retrieved May 31, 2013, from, http://frwebgate.access.gpo.gov/cgi-bin/getdoc.cgi?dbname=108_cong_public_laws&docid=f:publ155.108.

U.S. Food and Drug Administration (FDA), (2012a). Protection of human subjects (informed consent).

*Code of Federal Regulations,*Title 21, Part 50. Retrieved May 15, 2013 from, http://www.accessdata.fda.gov/scripts/cdrh/cfdocs/cfcfr/CFRsearch.cfm?CFRPart=50.

U.S. Food and Drug Administration (FDA), (2012b). Institutional review boards. *Code of Federal Regulations,* Title 21, Part 56. Retrieved May 29, 2013 from, http://www.accessdata.fda.gov/scripts/cdrh/cfdocs/cfcfr/CFRsearch.cfm?CFRPart=56.

U.S. Food and Drug Administration (FDA), (2013). *Protecting and promoting your health.* Retrieved May 29, 2013 from, http://www.fda.gov.

Weijer, C. (2000). The ethical analysis of risk. *The Journal of Law, Medicine & Ethics: A Journal of the American Society of Law, Medicine & Ethics, 28*(4), 344–361.

World Medical Association, (2008). *Regulations and ethical guidelines. World Medical Association Declaration of Helsinki.* Retrieved June 9, 2013 from, http://www.wma.net/en/30publications/10policies/b3/17c.pdf.

Research Problems, Purposes, and Hypotheses

LEARNING OUTCOMES

After completing this chapter, you should be able to:

1. Identify research topics, problems, and purposes
   in published quantitative, qualitative, and
   outcomes studies.
2. Critically appraise the research problems and
   purposes in studies.
3. Critically appraise the feasibility of a
   study problem and purpose by examining
   the researcher's expertise, money commitment,
   availability of subjects, facilities, and equipment,
   and the study's ethical considerations.

4. Differentiate among the types of hypotheses
   (simple versus complex, nondirectional
   versus directional, associative versus causal,
   and statistical versus research) in published
   studies.
5. Critically appraise the quality of
   objectives, questions, and hypotheses presented
   in studies.
6. Differentiate the types of variables in
   studies.

7. Critically appraise the conceptual and operational definitions of variables in published studies.

8. Critically appraise the demographic variables measured and the sample characteristics described in studies.

KEY TERMS

Associative hypothesis, p. 149
Background for a problem, p. 131
Causal hypothesis, p. 149
Complex hypothesis, p. 150
Conceptual definition, p. 155
Confounding variables, p. 155
Demographic variables, p. 157
Dependent (outcome) variable, p. 153
Directional hypothesis, p. 150
Environmental variables, p. 154
Extraneous variables, p. 154

Feasibility of a study, p. 143
Hypothesis, p. 149
Independent (treatment or intervention) variable, p. 153
Nondirectional hypothesis, p. 150
Null hypothesis (H_0), p. 151
Operational definition, p. 155
Problem statement, p. 131
Research concepts, p. 156
Research hypothesis, p. 151
Research objective or aim, p. 145

Research problem, p. 131
Research purpose, p. 131
Research question, p. 147
Research topic, p. 130
Research variables, p. 154
Sample characteristics, p. 157
Significance of a research problem, p. 131
Simple hypothesis, p. 150
Statistical hypothesis, p. 151
Testable hypothesis, p. 152
Variables, p. 153

We are constantly asking questions to gain a better understanding of ourselves and the world around us. This human ability to wonder and ask creative questions is the first step in the research process. By asking questions, clinical nurses and nurse researchers are able to identify significant research topics and problems to direct the generation of research evidence for use in practice. A research topic is a concept or broad issue that is important to nursing, such as acute pain, chronic pain management, coping with illness, or health promotion. Each topic contains numerous research problems that might be investigated through quantitative, qualitative, and outcomes studies. For example, chronic pain management is a research topic that includes research problems such as "What is it like to live with chronic pain?" and "What strategies are useful in coping with chronic pain?" Qualitative studies have been conducted to investigate these problems or areas of concern in nursing (Munhall, 2012). Quantitative studies have been conducted to address problems such as "What is the most accurate way to assess chronic pain?" and "What interventions are effective in managing chronic pain?" Outcomes research methodologies have been used to examine patient outcomes and the cost-effectiveness of care provided in chronic pain management centers (Doran, 2011).

The problem provides the basis for developing the research purpose. The purpose is the goal or focus of a study that guides the development of the objectives, questions, or hypotheses in quantitative and outcomes studies. The objectives, questions, or hypotheses bridge the gap between the more abstractly stated problem and purpose and the detailed design for conducting the study. Objectives, questions, and hypotheses include the variables, relationships among the variables, and often the population to be studied. In qualitative research, the purpose and broadly stated research questions guide the study of selected research concepts.

This chapter includes content that will assist you in identifying problems and purposes in a variety of quantitative, qualitative, and outcomes studies. Objectives, questions, and hypotheses are discussed, and the different types of study variables are introduced. Also presented are guidelines that will assist you in critically appraising the problems, purposes, objectives, questions, hypotheses, and variables or concepts in published quantitative, qualitative, and outcomes studies.

WHAT ARE RESEARCH PROBLEMS AND PURPOSES?

A research problem is an area of concern in which there is a gap in the knowledge needed for nursing practice. Research is required to generate essential knowledge to address the practice concern, with the ultimate goal of providing evidence-based nursing care (Brown, 2014; Craig & Smyth, 2012). In a study, the research problem (1) indicates the significance of the problem, (2) provides a background for the problem, and (3) includes a problem statement. The significance of a research problem indicates the importance of the problem to nursing and health care and to the health of individuals, families, and communities. The background for a problem briefly identifies what we know about the problem area, and the problem statement identifies the specific gap in the knowledge needed for practice. Not all published studies include a clearly expressed problem, but the problem usually can be identified in the first page of the report.

The research purpose is a clear, concise statement of the specific goal or focus of a study. In quantitative and outcomes studies, the goal of a study might be to identify, describe, or examine relationships in a situation, examine the effectiveness of an intervention, or determine outcomes of health care. In qualitative studies, the purpose might be to explore perceptions of a phenomenon, describe elements of a culture, develop a theory of a health situation or issue, or describe historical trends and patterns. The purpose includes the variables or concepts, the population, and often the setting for the study. A clearly stated research purpose can capture the essence of a study in a single sentence and is essential for directing the remaining steps of the research process.

The research problem and purpose from the study of Piamjariyakul, Smith, Russell, Werkowitch, and Elyachar (2013) of the effectiveness of a telephone coaching program on heart failure home management by family caregivers are presented as an example. This example is critically appraised using the following guidelines.

? CRITICAL APPRAISAL GUIDELINES

Problems and Purposes in Studies

1. Is the problem clearly and concisely expressed early in the study?
2. Does the problem include the significance, background, and problem statement?
3. Does the purpose clearly express the goal or focus of the study?
4. Is the purpose focused on the study problem statement?
5. Are the study variables and population identified in the purpose?

⚡ RESEARCH EXAMPLE

Problem and Purpose of a Quantitative Study

Research Study Excerpt
Problem Significance
"Results of meta-analyses and American Heart Association (AHA) guidelines emphasize the critical importance of family caregivers' involvement in home management of heart failure (HF). Family caregivers perform daily HF home management and provide essential support for patients in recognizing worsening symptoms (i.e., edema, shortness of breath; Riegel et al., 2009)." Piamjariyakul et al., 2013, p. 32

Continued

RESEARCH EXAMPLE—cont'd

Problem Background

"Results of several studies have shown that HF rehospitalization is frequently precipitated by excess dietary sodium, inappropriate changes or reductions in taking prescribed medications, and respiratory infections, most of which family caregivers could help prevent if they were educated to be alert for these problems. . . . One intervention program found that a family partnership program on HF home care was helpful in adherence to diet with significant reductions in patients' urine sodium (Dunbar et al., 2005)." Piamjariyakul et al., 2013, p. 32

Problem Statement

"Yet, the few available studies on providing instruction for family caregivers are limited in content and lack guidance for implementing HF self-management strategies at home. . . . Also, in developing interventions that involve family caregivers, researchers need to measure caregiver outcomes (i.e., burden) to ensure that interventions do improve patient outcomes but do not have untoward negative impacts on the caregivers." Piamjariyakul et al., 2013, pp. 32-33

Research Purpose

"The purpose of this study was to determine the feasibility and evaluate the helpfulness and costs of a coaching program for family caregiver HF home care management." Piamjariyakul et al., 2013, p. 33

Critical Appraisal

Research Problem

Piamjariyakul and colleagues (2013) presented a clear, concise research problem that had the relevant areas of (1) significance, (2) background, and (3) problem statement. HF is a significant, costly chronic illness to manage, and family caregivers are essential to the management process. A concise background of the problem was provided by discussing studies of the effects of caregivers on the outcomes of patients with HF. The discussion of the problem concluded with a concise problem statement that indicated the gap in the knowledge needed for practice and provided a basis for the study conducted by these researchers. Each problem provides the basis for generating a variety of research purposes and, in this study, the knowledge gap regarding the effectiveness of interventions on HF home management by family caregivers provides clear direction for the formulation of the research purpose.

Research Purpose

In a published study, the purpose frequently is reflected in the title of the study, stated in the study abstract, and restated after the literature review. Piamjariyakul and associates (2013) included the purpose of their study in all three places. The focus of this study was to examine the effectiveness of a telephone coaching program on HF home management (independent variable) on caregiving burden, confidence in providing HF care, preparedness, satisfaction, and program cost (dependent variables) for family caregivers (population). The purpose indicated the type of study conducted (quasi-experimental) and clearly identified the independent variable (telephone coaching program), population (patients with HF and their families), and setting (home). However, the dependent variables are not clearly identified in the study purpose but were discussed in the methods section of the study. The study purpose would have been strengthened by the inclusion of the dependent variables measured in this study.

Implications for Practice

The findings from the study by Piamjariyakul and co-workers (2013, p. 38) indicated that "The telephone coaching program was shown to reduce the caregiving burden and improve caregiver confidence and preparedness in HF home care management. . . . The cost for the program is considerably less than the cost for home healthcare providers ($120-160 per each visit), a single emergency department visit, or one inpatient hospitalization for HF due to poor HF home management." This study has potential for use in practice to improve the quality of care provided to patients and families; however, the researchers did recognize the need for additional testing of the coaching program with a larger sample to determine its effectiveness. This type of study supports the Quality and Safety Education for Nurses (QSEN, 2013; Sherwood & Barnsteiner, 2012) prelicensure competency to ensure safe, quality, and cost- effective health care that actively involves patients and families in this care process.

IDENTIFYING THE PROBLEM AND PURPOSE IN QUANTITATIVE, QUALITATIVE, AND OUTCOMES STUDIES

Quantitative, qualitative, and outcomes research approaches enable nurses to investigate a variety of research problems and purposes. Examples of research topics, problems, and purposes for different types of quantitative, qualitative, and outcomes studies are presented in this section.

Problems and Purposes in Types of Quantitative Studies

Example research topics, problems, and purposes for the different types of quantitative research (descriptive, correlational, quasi-experimental, and experimental) are presented in Table 5-1. If little is known about a topic, researchers usually start with descriptive and correlational studies and progress to quasi-experimental and experimental studies as knowledge expands in an area. An examination of the problems and purposes in Table 5-1 will reveal the differences and similarities among the types of quantitative research. The research purpose usually reflects the type of study that was conducted (Grove, Burns, & Gray, 2013). The purpose of descriptive research is to identify and describe concepts or variables, identify possible relationships among variables, and delineate differences between or among existing groups, such as males and females or different ethnic groups.

TABLE 5-1   QUANTITATIVE RESEARCH
Topics, Problems, and Purposes

TYPE OF RESEARCH	RESEARCH TOPIC	RESEARCH PROBLEM AND PURPOSE
Descriptive research	Hand hygiene (HH), HH opportunities, HH adherence, infection control, pediatric extended care facilities (ECFs), clinical and nonclinical caregivers	*Title of study:* "Hand hygiene opportunities in pediatric extended care facilities" (Buet et al., 2013, p. 72). *Problem:* "The population in pediatric ECFs [extended care facilities] is increasingly complex, and such children are at high risk of healthcare-associated infections (HAIs), which are associated with increased morbidity, mortality, resources use, and cost (Burns et al., 2010) [problem significance]. . . . The Centers for Disease Control and Prevention (CDC) . . . and the World Health Organization (WHO, 2009) have published evidence-based guidelines confirming the causal relationship between poor infection control practices, particularly hand hygiene (HH), and increased risk of HAIs [problem background]. However, most of the HH research has been focused in adult long term care facilities and acute care settings and findings from such studies are unlikely to be applicable to HH in pediatric ECFs given the different care patterns, including the relative distribution of different devices" [problem statement] (Buet et al., 2013, pp. 72-73). *Purpose:* "The purpose of this observational study was to assess the frequency and type of HH opportunities initiated by clinical (e.g., physicians and nurses) and non-clinical (e.g., parents and teachers) care givers, as well as evaluate HH adherence using the WHO's '5 Moments for HH' observation tool" (Buet et al., 2013, p. 73).

Continued

The purpose of correlational research is to examine the type (positive or negative) and strength of relationships among variables. In their correlational study, Bindler, Bindler, and Daratha (2013) examined the prediction of insulin resistance (IR) in adolescents using anthropometric measurements (height, weight, body mass index [BMI], and waist circumference), systolic and diastolic blood pressure, laboratory values [lipid and triglyceride levels], and the inflammatory marker of high-sensitivity, C-reactive protein (see Table 5-1). The researchers found that waist circumference and triglycerides were the strongest predictors of IR in adolescents. The findings from this study stressed the importance of nurses measuring waist circumference, height, and weight; calculating BMI; and examining lipid levels to identify youths at risk for IR.

Quasi-experimental studies are conducted to determine the effect of a treatment or independent variable on designated dependent or outcome variables (Shadish, Cook, & Campbell, 2002). Nyamathi and colleagues (2009) conducted a quasi-experimental study to examine the effectiveness of a nurse case-managed intervention on hepatitis A and B vaccine completion among homeless adults. The research topics, problem, and purpose for this study are presented in Table 5-1. The findings from this study "revealed that a culturally sensitive comprehensive program, which included nurse case management plus targeted hepatitis education, incentives, and client tracking, performed significantly better than did a usual care program" (Nyamathi et al., 2009, p. 21). Thus the researchers recommended that public health program planners and funders use this type of program to promote increased completion of hepatitis A and B vaccinations for high-risk groups.

Experimental studies are conducted in highly controlled settings, using a highly structured design to determine the effect of one or more independent variables on one or more dependent variables (Grove et al., 2013). Sharma, Ryals, Gajewski, and Wright (2010) conducted an experimental study to determine the effects of an aerobic exercise program on pain like behaviors and neurotrophin-3 synthesis in mice with chronic widespread pain (see Table 5-1). These researchers found that moderate-intensity aerobic exercise had the effect of deep tissue mechanical hyperalgesia on chronic pain in mice. This finding provides a possible molecular basis for aerobic exercise training in reducing muscular pain in fibromyalgia patients.

Problems and Purposes in Types of Qualitative Studies

The problems formulated for qualitative research identify areas of concern that require investigation to gain new insights, expand understanding, and improve comprehension of the whole (Munhall, 2012). The purpose of a qualitative study indicates the focus of the study, which may be a concept such as pain, an event such as loss of a child, or a facet of a culture such as the healing practices of a specific Native American tribe. In addition, the purpose often indicates the qualitative approach used to conduct the study. The basic assumptions for this approach are discussed in the research report (Creswell, 2014). Examples of research topics, problems, and purposes for the types of qualitative research—phenomenological, grounded theory, ethnographic, exploratory-descriptive, and historical—commonly found in nursing are presented in Table 5-2.

Phenomenological research is conducted to promote a deeper understanding of complex human experiences as they have been lived by the study participants (Munhall, 2012). Trollvik, Nordbach, Silen, and Ringsberg (2011) conducted a phenomenological study to describe children's experiences of living with asthma. The research topics, problem, and purpose for this study are presented in Table 5-2. Findings from this study described two themes with five subthemes (identified in parentheses): fear of exacerbation (body sensations, frightening experiences, and loss of control) and fear of being ostracized (experiences of being excluded and dilemma of keeping the asthma secret or being open about it). The findings from this study emphasize that asthma management is not only a major issue for the children involved but also for their parents,

TABLE 5-3 O...
Topics, Problem...

TYPE OF RESEARCH	RE...
Outcomes research	Work... saf... Proce... nur... wo... nee... Outc... eve... sat...

TABLE 5-2 QUALITATIVE RESEARCH
Topics, Problems, and Purposes

TYPE OF RESEARCH	RESEARCH TOPIC	RESEARCH PROBLEM AND PURPOSE
Phenomenological research	Lived experience of children, asthma, health promotion, child health, chronic illness, fears of exacerbations, fears of being ostracized	*Title of study:* "Children's experiences of living with asthma: Fear of exacerbations and being ostracized" (Trollvik et al., 2011, p. 295). *Problem:* "Asthma is the most common childhood disease and long-term medical condition affecting children (Masoli et al., 2004). The prevalence of asthma is increasing, and atopic diseases are considered to be a worldwide health problem and an agent of morbidity in children significance]. . . . Studies show that children with asthma have more emotional/behavioral problems than healthy children. . . It has also been found that asthma control in children is poor and that healthcare professionals (HCPs) and children focus on different aspects of having asthma (Price et al., 2002) [problem background]. . . . Few studies have considered very young children's, 7-10 years old, perspectives; this study might contribute to new insights into their lifeworld experiences" [problem statement] (Trollvik et al., 2011, pp. 295-296). *Purpose:* "The aim of this study was to explore and describe children's everyday experiences of living with asthma to tailor an Asthma Education Program based on their perspectives. . . . In this study, a phenomenological and hermaneutical approach was used to gain an understanding of the children's lifeworld" (Trollvik et al., 2011, p. 296).
Grounded theory research	Foster care, pregnancy prevention, prevention of sexually transmitted infections, patient-provider relationship	*Title of study:* "Where do youth in foster care receive information about preventing unplanned pregnancy and sexually transmitted infections [STIs]" (Hudson, 2012, p. 443). *Problem:* "Within the United States, approximately 460,000 children live in foster care, and adolescents comprise half of this population. . . . Children enter the foster care system as a result of sexual abuse, physical abuse, or physical neglect and abandonment (Child Welfare League of America, 2007) [problem significance]. . . . With limited access to health promotion information and education about high-risk sexual behavior, it is not surprising that these young people have a high incidence of unplanned pregnancy and STIs compared with youth not in foster care [problem background]. Little research exists on the extent to which foster youth receive information about sexual activity from healthcare providers" [problem statement] (Hudson, 2012, p. 443-444). *Purpose:* A grounded theory study was conducted to "describe how and where foster youth receive reproductive health and risk reduction information to prevent pregnancy and sexually transmitted infections. Participants also were asked to describe their relationship with their primary healthcare provider while they were in foster care" (Hudson, 2012, p. 443).

Continued

quality of n...
and mortal...
(EBP) so th...
Overholt, 2...
interventio...
and co-wor...
failure (HF...
developed...
Interventio...
ment of EF...
Sherwood &...

Builds or

A significar...
introductio...
current stu...
in the area...

for and document the significance of the study's purpose. The study by Piamjariyakul and colleagues (2013; see earlier) indicated what was known about the effectiveness of management in the home of HF patients' outcomes. What was not known was the effectiveness of a telephone coaching intervention on caregivers' confidence and skill in managing HF patients in the home and their caregiving burden. This gap in the research knowledge base provides the basis for developing a study to examine the effectiveness of an intervention in improving HF patients' and caregivers' outcomes.

Promotes Theory Testing or Development

Significant problems and purposes in quantitative studies are supported by theory, and often the focus of these studies is theory testing (Chinn & Kramer, 2011). The focus of qualitative studies is often on developing theory (Munhall, 2012). A detailed discussion of the different types of theory tested and/or developed through research is presented in Chapter 7.

Addresses Nursing Research Priorities

Over the last 40 years, expert researchers, professional organizations, and funding agencies have identified research priorities to encourage studies in the most important areas for nursing. The research priorities for clinical practice were initially identified in a study by Lindeman (1975). Those original research priorities included nursing interventions related to stress, care of the aged, pain management, and patient education, which continue to be priorities for nursing research today.

Many professional nursing organizations use websites to communicate their current research priorities. For example, the current research priorities of the American Association of Critical-Care Nurses (AACN, 2013) are identified on the website as:

(1) effective and appropriate use of technology to achieve optimal patient assessment, management, and/or outcomes; (2) creation of a healing, humane environment; (3) processes and systems that foster the optimal contribution of critical care nurses; (4) effective approaches to symptom management; and (5) prevention and management of complications.

AACN, 2013; http://www.aacn.org/wd/practice/content/research/
research-priority-areas.pcms?menu=practice

AACN (2013) has also identified future research needs under the following topics: medication management, hemodynamic monitoring, creating healing environments, palliative care and end-of-life issues, mechanical ventilation, monitoring neuroscience patients, and noninvasive monitoring. You can review these research priorities by going to the AACN website (http://www.aacn.org) and searching for the research priority areas.

A significant funding agency for nursing research is the National Institute of Nursing Research (NINR). A major initiative of the NINR is the development of a national nursing research agenda that involves identifying nursing research priorities, outlining a plan for implementing priority studies, and obtaining resources to support these priority projects.

To advance the science of health, NINR will invest in research to:
- *Enhance health promotion and disease prevention.*
- *Improve quality of life by managing symptoms of acute and chronic illness.*
- *Improve palliative and end-of-life care.*
- *Enhance innovation in science and practice.*
- *Develop the next generation of nurse scientists.*

NINR, 2011; http://www.ninr.nih.gov/AboutNINR/NINRMissionandStrategicPlan

Another federal agency with emphasis on funding healthcare research is the Agency for Healthcare Research and Quality (AHRQ). The mission for AHRQ is "to improve the quality, safety, efficiency, and effectiveness of health care for all Americans" (AHRQ, 2013). The research priorities and funded projects are presented on the AHRQ website (http://www.ahrq.gov/legacy/fund/ragendix. htm). These are important areas for nursing and the focus of the QSEN (2013) competencies for undergraduate nursing students, which include the areas of patient-centered care, teamwork and collaboration, EBP, quality improvement, safety, and informatics. The research generated through AHRQ will provide sound evidence for providing quality and safe care in nursing.

World Health Organization (WHO) is encouraging the identification of priorities for a common nursing research agenda among countries. A quality healthcare delivery system and improved patient and family health have become global goals. By 2020, the world's population is expected to increase by 94%, with the older adult population increasing by almost 240%. Seven of every 10 deaths are expected to be caused by noncommunicable diseases, such as chronic conditions (heart disease, cancer, depression) and injuries (unintentional and intentional). The priority areas for research identified by WHO are to:

(1) improve the health of the world's most marginalized populations; (2) study new diseases that threaten public health around the world; (3) conduct comparative analyses of supply and demand of the health workforce of different countries; (4) analyze the feasibility, effectiveness, and quality of education and practice of nurses; (5) conduct research on healthcare delivery modes; and (6) examine the outcomes for healthcare agencies, providers, and patients around the world.

WHO, 2013; http://www.who.int/entity/en.

The *Healthy People 2020* website identifies and prioritizes the health topics and objectives of all age groups over the next decade (U.S. Department of Health and Human Services [U.S. DHHS], 2013). These health topics and objectives direct future research in the areas of health promotion, illness prevention, illness management, and rehabilitation and can be accessed online (http://www. healthypeople.gov/2020/topicsobjectives2020/default.aspx).

In summary, expert nurse researchers, professional nursing organizations, and national and international agencies and organizations have identified research priorities to direct the future conduct of healthcare research to improve the outcomes for patients and families, nurses, and healthcare systems. When conducting a critical appraisal of a study, you need to examine the study's contribution to nursing practice and determine whether the study's problem and purpose are based on previous research, theory, and current research priorities. These four elements help determine a study's significance in developing and refining knowledge to build an EBP for nursing (Brown, 2014).

EXAMINING THE FEASIBILITY OF A PROBLEM AND PURPOSE

A critical appraisal of research begins by determining the feasibility of the problem and purpose of the study. The feasibility of a study is determined by examining the researchers' expertise; money commitment; availability of subjects, facilities, and equipment; and the study's ethical considerations (Rogers, 1987). The feasibility of Piamjariyakul and associates' (2013) study of the effectiveness of a telephone coaching program on heart failure (HF) home management by family caregivers was critically appraised and presented as an example as follows. You can review the problem and purpose for this study presented at the beginning of this chapter. The critical appraisal involves addressing the following questions about a study's feasibility.

Researcher Expertise

The research problem and purpose studied need to be within the area of expertise of the researchers. Research reports usually identify the education of the researchers and their current positions, which indicate their expertise to conduct a study. Also, examine the reference list to determine whether the researchers have conducted additional studies in this area. If you need more information, you can search the Internet for the researchers' accomplishments and involvement in research (Grove et al., 2013).

Piamjariyakul is a PhD-prepared nurse employed by the School of Nursing at the University of Kansas Medical Center. The reference list includes additional publications by this author in the area of HF patient management in the home by family caregivers. Thus Piamjariyakul has the research, education, and academic position that support her expertise to conduct this study. Smith is also PhD-prepared and is on the faculty at the School of Nursing and Department of Preventive Medicine and Public Health at the University of Kansas Medical Center. She is an author of previous publications with Piamjariyakul. Russell, Werkowitch, and Elyachar demonstrate clinical expertise with certifications in their clinical areas and are employed by the University of Kansas Medical Center. Piamjariyakul and her co-authors demonstrate strong research, educational, and clinical expertise for conducting this study.

Money Commitment

The problem and purpose studied are influenced by the amount of money available to the researchers. The cost of a research project can range from a few dollars for a student's small study to hundreds of thousands and even millions of dollars for complex projects. Critically appraising a study involves examining the financial resources available to the researchers in conducting their study. Sources of funding for a study usually are identified in the article.

Studies might be funded by grants from national institutions, professional organizations, or private foundations. The researchers may have received financial assistance from companies that provided necessary equipment or support from the agency where they work. Receiving funding for a study indicates that it was reviewed by peers who chose to support the research financially. Piamjariyakul and co-workers' (2013) study was supported by an award from the American Association of Heart Failure Nurses (AAHFN), a Bernard Saperstein Caregiver Grant, and partially by the National Heart, Lung, and Blood Institute (NHLBI). This study had strong financial support from a variety of national funding sources.

Availability of Subjects, Facilities, and Equipment

Researchers need to have adequate sample size, facilities, and equipment to implement their study. Most published studies indicate the sample size and setting(s) in the methods section of the research report. Often, nursing studies are conducted in natural or partially controlled settings, such as a home, hospital unit, or clinic. Many of these facilities are easy to access, and the hospitals and clinics provide access to large numbers of patients. Piamjariyakul and colleagues (2013, p. 33) conducted a pilot study with a sample of 12 caregivers who "were recruited from a group of HF patients receiving care at a large Midwestern University Medical Center." They recognized the small sample size as a study limitation but the findings were significant, in that the telephone coaching program reduced the caregivers' burden. Thus the researchers recommended that the intervention be tested with a larger sample to determine its efficacy.

A review of the methods section of the research article will determine if adequate and accurate equipment was available. Nursing studies frequently require a limited amount of equipment, such as a tape or video recorder for interviews, or physiological instruments, such as an electrocardiograph or thermometer. Piamjariyakul and associates (2013) gave each family caregiver program materials from American Heart Association handouts and the caregivers' guidebook, *The Comfort of Home*™ *for Chronic Heart Failure: A Guide for Caregivers*. The handouts and book were used during the telephone coaching sessions provided by five nurse interventionists, who had received training to ensure the fidelity of the intervention implementation.

Ethical Considerations

The purpose selected for investigation must be ethical, which means that the subjects' rights and the rights of others in the setting are protected (Grove et al., 2013). An ethical study confers more benefits than risks in its conduct and will generate useful knowledge for practice (see Chapter 4). Piamjariyakul and co-workers (2013) provided a detailed discussion of the ethical aspects of their study in the following:

> "The procedures for the study were approved by the university medical center Institutional Review Board (IRB). All individually identifiable information collected during the study was handled confidentially in accordance with university IRB policies and in compliance with HIPAA [Health Insurance Portability and Accountability Act] regulations. Consent was obtained from caregivers and nurse interventionists as well as the patients for medical record review of demographic data." Piamjariyakul et al., 2013, p. 34

EXAMINING RESEARCH OBJECTIVES, QUESTIONS, AND HYPOTHESES IN RESEARCH REPORTS

Research objectives, questions, and hypotheses evolve from the problem, purpose, literature review, and study framework, and direct the remaining steps of the research process. In a published study, the objectives, questions, or hypotheses usually are presented after the literature review section and right before the methods section. The content in this section is provided to assist you in identifying and critically appraising the objectives, questions, and hypotheses in published studies.

Research Objectives or Aims

A research objective or aim is a clear, concise, declarative statement expressed in the present tense. The objectives are sometimes referred to as aims and are generally used in descriptive and correlational quantitative studies. For clarity, an objective or aim usually focuses on one or two variables and indicates whether they are to be identified or described. Sometimes the purpose of objectives is to identify relationships among variables or determine differences between two or more existing groups regarding selected variables.

Qualitative research is most appropriate when the focus of the study is to obtain a personal perspective of a situation, experience, or event (Hale, Treharne, & Kitas, 2007). The research objectives or aims formulated for quantitative and qualitative studies have some similarities because they focus on exploration, description, and determination of relationships. However, the objectives directing qualitative studies are commonly broader in focus and include concepts that are more complex and abstract than those of quantitative studies. The aims or objectives in qualitative studies focus on obtaining a holistic, comprehensive understanding of the area of study (Creswell, 2014; Munhall, 2012).

Tenfelde, Finnegan, Miller, and Hill (2012) used aims to direct their study of the risk of breastfeeding cessation among low-income women, infants, and children. This correlational study demonstrated the logical flow from research problem and purpose to research aims used to guide this study. The questions in the following box were used to conduct a critical appraisal of this study.

? CRITICAL APPRAISAL GUIDELINES

Research Objectives and Questions

1. Are the objectives (aims) or questions clearly and concisely expressed in the study?
2. Are the study aims or questions based on the study purpose?
3. Do the aims or questions appear to direct the study methodology and interpretation of results?

RESEARCH EXAMPLE

Problem, Purpose, and Aims

Research Study Excerpt

Research Problem

"A major goal of the Special Supplemental Nutrition Program for Women, Infants, and Children (WIC) is to improve the nutritional status of infants. . . . On the basis of the scientific evidence supporting breastfeeding and the use of mother's milk, mothers who received WIC services are encouraged to breastfeed their infants, unless medically contraindicated (Gartner et al., 2005). In a national sample of WIC recipients, only 26% breastfed until 6 months and 12% breastfed until 12 months. . . . These breastfeeding duration rates fall well below the *Healthy People 2020* benchmarks of 61% at 6 months and 34% at 12 months postpartum (U.S. DHHS, 2010) [problem significance].

Breastfeeding protects infants and mothers against a broad spectrum of adverse health outcomes, including gastrointestinal infections, ear infections, diabetes, and obesity (Gartner et al., 2005). . . . Mothers who breastfeed for longer periods are less likely to retain pregnancy weight gain [problem background]. . . . Although predictors of early breastfeeding cessation among low-income women have been identified in previous studies, studies focusing solely on WIC participants were limited. Moreover, in no studies were statistical methods used that enabled identification of the timing of breastfeeding cessation in relation to specific maternal background and intrapersonal variables" [problem statement] (Tenfelde et al., 2012, pp. 86-87).

Research Purpose

"The purpose of this study was to identify the maternal background and intrapersonal predictors associated with the timing of breastfeeding cessation in WIC participants over the course of 12-month postpartum period" (Tenfelde et al., 2012, p. 87).

Research Objectives

"Study aims were to determine (a) the risk of breastfeeding cessation over time and (b) how the risk of breastfeeding cessation varied in relation to maternal background and intrapersonal variables" (Tenfelde et al., 2012, p. 87).

Critical Appraisal

Tenfelde and colleagues (2012) identified a significant problem of the low breastfeeding rates and early cessation of breastfeeding among WIC participants. Their breastfeeding rates for 6 and 12 months were significantly lower than the *Healthy People 2020* benchmarks. The problem background clearly identified the contributions of breastfeeding to the health of infants and mothers. The problem statement indicated what was not known and provided a basis for the purpose and aims of this study. The purpose clearly indicated the focus of the study was to identify maternal background and intrapersonal predictors related to breastfeeding cessation in a population of WIC participants. The study aims built on the problem and purpose and provide more clarity regarding the focus of the study. The first study aim focused on describing risk of breastfeeding cessation over time and the second aim focused on relationships of maternal background and intrapersonal variables to risk of breastfeeding cessation. This study identified a significant problem and a feasible purpose for research. In addition, the study aims provided clear direction for the conduct of the study and the interpretation of the study results.

Implications for Practice

In the following study excerpt, Tenfelde and associates (2012) identified key findings and made recommendations for practice and research.

"Similar to national findings, the WIC participants in this study did not reach the *Healthy People 2020* goals for breastfeeding duration. Women who had consistently high monthly risks of breastfeeding cessation were younger, were not of Mexican descent, had no previous breastfeeding experience, and had no breastfeeding support systems. . . . Clinicians and researchers can use the findings from this study to develop interventions that are targeted to periods of greatest risk of premature breastfeeding cessation to prolong breastfeeding duration in this vulnerable population" (Tenfelde et al., 2012, p. 93).

Research Questions

A **research question** is a clear, concise interrogative statement that is worded in the present tense, includes one or more variables, and is expressed to guide the implementation of studies. The foci of research questions in quantitative studies are description of variable(s), examination of relationships among variables, use of independent variables to predict dependent variable, and determination of differences between two or more groups regarding selected variable(s). These research questions are usually narrowly focused and inclusive of the study variables and population. It is really a matter of choice whether researchers identify objectives or questions in their study but, more often, questions are stated to guide studies. Piamjariyakul and co-workers (2013) conducted a pilot study to examine the feasibility of a telephone coaching program on HF home management for family caregivers. The problem and purpose for this study were noted earlier. They identified research questions to direct the implementation of their study. The critical appraisal guidelines for examining research objectives or questions in a study were applied to this example.

RESEARCH EXAMPLE

Questions from a Quantitative Study

Research Study Excerpt
Research Questions

"The research questions were:
1. Did the family caregivers completing the program and nurse interventionists implementing the coaching program evaluate the program as helpful for HF home management?
2. Were there improvements in outcomes data for caregivers' level of HF caregiving burden, confidence, and preparedness in providing HF home care?
3. What were the costs of the program materials and delivery?" Piamjariyakul et al., 2013, p. 33.

Continued

RESEARCH EXAMPLE—cont'd

Critical Appraisal

Piamjariyakul and colleagues (2013) clearly stated their problem and purpose, as indicated earlier, and the research questions build on these and clarified the foci of this study. The first question focuses on description of the quality of the telephone coaching program from the perspectives of the family caregivers and the nurses. The second question focuses on differences in outcomes before and after the implementation of the telephone coaching program for the caregivers. The third question focuses on a description of the costs related to the program. These questions are addressed by the study methodology and were used to organize the study results.

Implications for Practice

The implications for practice for the Piamjariyakul and associates' (2013) study were discussed earlier.

The research questions directing qualitative studies are often limited in number, broadly focused, and inclusive of variables or concepts that are more complex and abstract than those of quantitative studies. Marshall and Rossman (2011) indicated that the questions developed to direct qualitative research might be theoretical, which can be studied with different populations or in a variety of sites, or the questions could be focused on a particular population or setting. The specific study questions formulated are very important for the selection of the qualitative research method to be used to conduct the study (Hale et al., 2007). Thompson and Keeling (2012) conducted a historical study to examine the PHNs' role in the prevention of infant mortality from 1884 to 1925. Table 5-2 includes the problem and purpose for this study; the questions used to guide this study are presented in the following study excerpt.

RESEARCH EXAMPLE

Questions from a Qualitative Study

Research Questions

"1. What was the state of the art of medicine and nursing regarding childhood malnutrition in the late 19th and early 20th century?

2. How did ethnicity and class influence the care given and what were the socioeconomic and political issues of that time?" Thompson, & Keeling, 2012, p. 472.

Critical Appraisal

Thompson and Keeling (2012) identified a significant problem of infant mortality and conducted a historical study to examine the role of early PHNs on improving understanding of childhood health issues today. The problem statement indicated what was not known and provided the basis for the research purpose (see Table 5-2). The research questions provided clear direction for the conduct of this qualitative study. Question 1 focused on a description of nursing and medical practice regarding childhood malnutrition from 1884 to 1925. Question 2 focused on a description of socioeconomic and political issues of that time. These questions directed the study and the interpretation of the results.

Implications for Practice

Thompson and Keeling (2012, p. 477) identified the following implications for practice:

"Nurses made a significant impact on infant mortality a century ago, and today, we can learn from their example to do the same for child health issues such as childhood obesity. Nurses and nurse practitioners, particularly, are an integral part of this fight against obesity in targeting at risk children from disadvantaged backgrounds who might not otherwise receive optimal care."

Hypotheses

A hypothesis is a formal statement of the expected relationship(s) between two or more variables in a specified population. The hypothesis translates the research problem and purpose into a clear explanation or prediction of the expected results or outcomes of selected quantitative and outcome studies. A clearly stated hypothesis includes the variables to be manipulated or measured, identifies the population to be examined, and indicates the proposed outcomes for the study. Hypotheses also influence the study design, sampling method, data collection and analysis process, and interpretation of findings (Fawcett & Garity, 2009). Quasi-experimental and experimental quantitative studies are conducted to test the effectiveness of a treatment or intervention; these types of studies should include hypotheses to predict the study outcomes. In this section, types of hypotheses are described and the elements of a testable hypothesis are discussed so that you can critically appraise hypotheses in published studies.

Types of Hypotheses

Different types of relationships and numbers of variables are identified in hypotheses. A study might have one, four, or more hypotheses, depending on its complexity. The type of hypothesis developed is based on the purpose of the study. Hypotheses can be described using four categories: (1) associative versus causal; (2) simple versus complex; (3) nondirectional versus directional; and (4) statistical versus research.

Associative versus causal hypotheses. The relationships identified in hypotheses are associative or causal. An associative hypothesis proposes relationships among variables that occur or exist together in the real world, so that when one variable changes, the other changes (Reynolds, 2007). Associative hypotheses identify relationships among variables in a study but do not indicate that one variable causes an effect on another variable. Ausserhofer, Schubert, Desmedt, Belgen, De Geest, and Schwendimann (2013) used an associative hypothesis to direct their outcomes study (the problem and purpose for this study are presented in Table 5-3 for your review). They hypothesized that "higher levels of PSC [patient safety climate] would be associated with less frequent nurse-reported adverse events (medication errors, patient falls, pressure ulcers, and healthcare-associated infections) and higher patient satisfaction" (Ausserhofer et al., 2013, p. 242). This associative hypothesis identified the expected negative relationship between PSC and nurse-reported adverse events (as PSC increased, adverse events were less frequent) and the positive relationship between PSC and patient satisfaction (as PSC increased, patient satisfaction was higher). These relationships are diagrammed below:

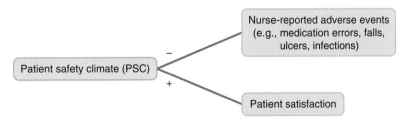

A causal hypothesis proposes a cause and effect interaction between two or more variables, referred to as independent and dependent variables. The independent variable (treatment or experimental variable) is manipulated by the researcher to cause an effect on the dependent or outcome variable. The researcher then measures the dependent variable to examine the effect created by the independent variable (Fawcett & Garity, 2009). A format for stating a causal hypothesis is the following: the subjects in the experimental group, who are exposed to the independent variable (treatment), demonstrate greater change, as measured by the dependent variable, than the subjects in the comparison group who receive standard care. Bernard and colleagues (2013) conducted a quasi-experimental study to examine the effect of a counseling and exercise intervention on smoking reduction in patients with schizophrenia. They hypothesized that "the participants would decrease tobacco consumption at the end of the intervention compared to baseline" (Bernard et al., 2013, p. 24). The counseling and exercise intervention (independent variable) was proposed to cause a decrease in tobacco consumption (dependent variable) in patients with schizophrenia. This causal hypothesis might be diagrammed as follows, with an arrow ($\rightarrow$) to indicate cause and effect versus association:

Counseling and exercise intervention $\longrightarrow$ Decreased tobacco consumption

Simple versus complex hypotheses. A simple hypothesis states the relationship (associative or causal) between two variables. Bernard and co-workers' (2013) study included a simple causal hypothesis, with one independent variable and one dependent variable. A complex hypothesis states the relationships (associative or causal) among three or more variables. Ausserhofer and colleagues' (2013) study included a complex associative hypothesis that examined the relationships between PSC and nurse-reported adverse events (e.g., medication errors, patient falls, pressure ulcers, healthcare-associated infections) and between PSC and patient satisfaction. These researchers examined associations or relationships among six variables (PSC, four specific adverse events or outcomes, and patient satisfaction).

Nondirectional versus directional hypotheses. A nondirectional hypothesis states that a relationship exists but does not predict the nature (positive or negative) of the relationship. If the direction of the relationship being studied is not clear in clinical practice or in the theoretical or empirical literature, the researcher has no clear indication of the nature of the relationship. Under these circumstances, nondirectional hypotheses are developed, such as "hours playing video games is related to body mass index in school-age children." This is an example of a simple (two variables), associative, and nondirectional hypothesis.

A directional hypothesis states the nature (positive or negative) of the interaction between two or more variables. The use of terms such as positive, negative, less, more, increase, decrease, greater, higher, or lower in a hypothesis indicates the direction of the relationship. Directional hypotheses are developed from theoretical statements (propositions), findings of previous studies, and clinical experience. As the knowledge on which a study is based increases, researchers are able to make a prediction about the direction of a relationship between the variables being studied. For example, Ausserhofer and associates (2013, p. 242) stated a directional hypothesis: "that *higher* levels of PSC would be associated with *less frequent* nurse-reported adverse events (medication errors, patient falls, pressure ulcers, and healthcare-associated infections) and *higher* patient satisfaction." The italicized words indicate the nature of the relationships in this complex, associative, directional hypothesis. The diagram of this hypothesis (see earlier) indicates that the relationship of PSC and adverse events is negative and the relationship of PSC and patient satisfaction is positive.

A causal hypothesis predicts the effect of an independent variable on a dependent variable, specifying the direction of the relationship. The independent variable increases or decreases each dependent variable. Thus all causal hypotheses are directional. Bernard and co-workers (2013) conducted a quasi-experimental study to test a simple, causal, directional hypothesis to guide their study. They predicted that a counseling and exercise intervention would decrease tobacco consumption in patients with schizophrenia. The results of this study were statistically significant, and this hypothesis was supported at the end of the intervention and at 6 weeks postintervention.

Statistical versus research hypotheses. The statistical hypothesis, also referred to as a null hypothesis (H_0), is used for statistical testing and for interpreting statistical outcomes. Even if the null hypothesis is not stated, it is implied, because it is the converse of the research hypothesis (Kerlinger & Lee, 2000). Some researchers state the null hypothesis because it is more easily interpreted on the basis of the results of statistical analyses. The null hypothesis is also used when the researcher believes that there is no relationship between two variables and when theoretical or empirical information is inadequate to state a research hypothesis. A statistical or null hypothesis can be simple or complex and associative or causal. Schultz, Drew, and Hewitt (2002) conducted a quasi-experimental study to determine the effectiveness of heparinized and normal saline flushes in maintaining the patency of 24-gauge (G) intermittent peripheral intravenous (IV) catheters in neonates in intensive care. "The hypothesis stated that there would be no significant difference in the duration of patency of a 24-G IV lock in a neonatal patient when flushed with 0.5 mL [millimeters] of heparinized saline (2 U/mL), our standard practice, compared with 0.5 mL of 0.9% normal saline" (Schultz et al., 2002, p. 30). This is a simple null hypothesis with one independent variable (0.9% normal saline flush) and one dependent variable (patency of 24-G IV catheter). The comparison group received standard care of a heparinized saline flush, and the population was neonates in an intensive care setting. The findings of the study did not support the null hypothesis because the catheters flushed with heparinized saline were patent significantly longer than the catheters flushed with normal saline. Thus the researchers recommended continuing the use of heparinized saline as the standard for flushing 24-G catheters in infants, which is the current practice.

A research hypothesis is the alternative hypothesis (H_1 or H_A) to the null or statistical hypothesis and states that a relationship exists between two or more variables. All the hypotheses stated earlier in this chapter have been research hypotheses. Research hypotheses can be simple or complex, nondirectional or directional, and associative or causal.

? CRITICAL APPRAISAL GUIDELINES

Hypotheses in Studies

1. Are the hypotheses formally stated in the study? If the study is quasi-experimental or experimental, hypotheses are needed to direct the study.
2. Do the hypotheses clearly identify the relationships among the variables of the study?
3. Are the hypotheses associative or causal, simple or complex, directional or nondirectional, and research or null (statistical)?
4. If hypotheses are included in a study, are they used to organize research results and interpret study findings?

⚡ RESEARCH EXAMPLE

Hypothesis

Research Study

Polman, de Castro, and van Aken (2007) conducted a study of the effects of playing versus watching violent video games on children's aggressive behavior. These researchers developed the following complex causal hypothesis to direct the conduct of their study:

"It was hypothesized that playing a violent video game will lead to higher levels of aggression than watching a violent video game or playing a non-violent game." (Polman et al., 2007, p. 257)

Continued

RESEARCH EXAMPLE—cont'd

Critical Appraisal

Polman and colleagues (2007) conducted a quasi-experimental study to examine the effects of three independent variables or interventions (playing violent video game, watching a violent video game, and playing a nonviolent game) on the dependent variable level of aggression. It is important that a hypothesis was developed to direct this type of study. The hypothesis clearly identifies the independent and dependent variables but not the population, which included children (boys and girls) in this study. The study included three groups, and each group included both boys and girls who were exposed to one of the interventions or independent variables. The causal relationships examined in this study are presented in the following diagrams.

Group 1 **Playing a violent video game → Level of aggression**

Group 2 **Watching a violent video game → Level of aggression**

Group 3 **Playing a nonviolent game → Level of aggression**

Implications for Practice

This hypothesis was supported by the study findings for boys but not for girls. Polman and associates (2007) found that boys who played violent video games were more aggressive than if they watched violent video games. However, there was no relationship between game conditions and aggressive behavior in girls. The researchers recommended additional studies with larger samples to investigate not only whether violent video games lead to aggression, but why. They also recommended that parents and caregivers pay special attention to the regulation of violent video game play by boys.

Testable Hypothesis

The value of a hypothesis ultimately is derived from whether it is testable in the real world. A testable hypothesis is one that clearly predicts the relationships among variables and contains variables that are measurable or able to be manipulated in a study. The independent variable must be clearly defined, often by a protocol, so that it can be implemented precisely and consistently as an intervention in a study. The dependent variable must be clearly defined to indicate how it will be precisely and accurately measured.

A testable hypothesis also needs to predict a relationship that can be "supported" or "not supported," as indicated by the data collected and analyzed. If the hypothesis states an associative relationship, correlational analyses are conducted on the data to determine the existence, type, and strength of the relationship between the variables studied. The hypothesis that states a causal link between the independent and dependent variables is evaluated using statistics that examine differences between the experimental and comparison or control groups, such as the t-test or ANOVA (see Chapter 11). It is the statistical or null hypothesis (stated or implied) that is tested to determine whether the independent variable produced a significant effect on the dependent variable.

Hypotheses are clearer without specifying the presence or absence of a "significant difference," because determination of the level of significance is only a statistical technique applied to sample data. In addition, hypotheses should not identify methodological points, such as techniques of sampling, measurement, and data analysis (Kerlinger & Lee, 2000). Therefore, such phrases as "measured by," "in a random sample of," and "using ANOVA" (analysis of variance) are inappropriate because they limit the hypothesis to the measurement methods, sample, or analysis techniques identified for one study. In addition, hypotheses need to reflect the variables and population outlined in the research purpose.

In summary, the research objectives, questions, and hypotheses must be clearly focused and concisely expressed in studies. Both objectives and questions are used in qualitative studies and descriptive and correlational quantitative studies, but questions are more common. Some correlational studies focus on predicting relationships and may include hypotheses. Quasi-experimental and experimental studies should be directed by hypotheses.

UNDERSTANDING STUDY VARIABLES AND RESEARCH CONCEPTS

The research purpose and objectives, questions, and hypotheses include the variables or concepts to be examined in a study. Variables are qualities, properties, or characteristics of persons, things, or situations that change or vary. Variables should be concisely defined to promote their measurement or manipulation within quantitative or outcomes studies (Chinn & Kramer, 2011). Research concepts are usually studied in qualitative research and are at higher levels of abstraction than variables. In this section, different types of variables are described, and conceptual and operational definitions of variables are discussed. The research concepts investigated in qualitative research are also discussed.

Types of Variables in Quantitative Research

Variables are classified into a variety of types to explain their use in research. Some variables are manipulated; others are controlled. Some variables are identified but not measured; others are measured with refined measurement devices. The types of variables presented in this section include independent, dependent, research, and extraneous variables (Fawcett & Garity, 2009; Reynolds, 2007).

Independent and Dependent Variables

The relationship between independent and dependent variables is the basis for formulating hypotheses for correlational, quasi-experimental, and experimental studies. An independent variable is an intervention that is manipulated or varied by the researcher to create an effect on the dependent variable. The independent variable is also called an intervention, treatment, or experimental variable. A dependent variable is the outcome that the researcher wants to predict or explain. Changes in the dependent variable are presumed to be caused by the independent variable. In the quasi-experimental study by Piamjariyakul and associates (2013; see earlier), the independent variable telephone coaching program was implemented to determine its effects on the dependent variables of caregiving burden and caregiver confidence, preparedness, and satisfaction. In the study by Bernard and co-workers (2013), the independent variable of a counseling and exercise intervention was implemented to determine its effect on tobacco consumption (dependent variable) in patients with schizophrenia.

In predictive correlational studies, the variables measured to predict a single dependent variable are also called independent variables (Grove et al., 2013). For example, Bindler and colleagues (2013) conducted a predictive correlational study to predict IR (insulin resistance) in young adolescents (see Table 5-1 for the problem and purpose of this study). The independent variables of height, weight, BMI, waist circumference, systolic and diastolic blood pressures, lipid values, triglycerides, and high-sensitivity C-reactive protein levels were measured and used to predict the dependent variable of IR.

Research Variables

Descriptive and correlational quantitative studies involve the investigation of research variables. Research variables are the qualities, properties, or characteristics identified in the research purpose and objectives or questions that are observed or measured in a study. Research variables are used when the intent of the study is to observe or measure variables as they exist in a natural setting without the implementation of a treatment. Thus no independent variables are manipulated and no cause and effect relationships are examined. Buet and associates (2013) described the research variables of HH (hand hygiene) opportunities and HH adherence for clinical caregivers (e.g., nurses, physicians) and nonclinical caregivers (e.g., parents, teachers) in pediatric extended-care facilities (see Table 5-1).

Extraneous Variables

Extraneous variables exist in all studies and can affect the measurement of study variables and the relationships among these variables. Extraneous variables are of primary concern in quantitative studies because they can interfere with obtaining a clear understanding of the relational or causal dynamics within these studies. These variables are classified as recognized or unrecognized and controlled or uncontrolled. Some extraneous variables are not recognized until the study is in progress or has been completed, but their presence influences the study outcome.

Researchers attempt to recognize and control as many extraneous variables as possible in quasi-experimental and experimental studies, and specific designs, intervention protocols, and sample criteria have been developed to control the influence of extraneous variables that might influence the outcomes of studies. Piamjariyakul and co-workers (2013) developed a detailed protocol for the implementation of their telephone coaching program to family caregivers of HF patients. This protocol was based on evidence-based national clinical guidelines for the management of HF patients and was included in the journal article. Five nurse interventionists were trained to implement this intervention consistently during the study. The sample criteria were strong in that only primary caregivers for HF patients who assisted them daily were included in the study, and caregivers of HF patients with Alzheimer's disease were excluded because of their different needs. The study would have been stronger if the sample size had been larger ($n = 12$) and the study design had included two groups—a comparison group in addition to the experimental group (see Chapter 8).

The extraneous variables that are not recognized until the study is in process, or are recognized before the study is initiated but cannot be controlled, are referred to as confounding variables. Sometimes extraneous variables can be measured during the study and controlled statistically during analysis. However, extraneous variables that cannot be controlled or measured are a design weakness and can hinder the interpretation of findings (see Chapter 8). As control in correlational, quasi-experimental, and experimental studies decreases, the potential influence of confounding variables increases.

Environmental variables are a type of extraneous variable that compose the setting in which the study is conducted. Examples of these variables include climate, family, healthcare system, and governmental organizations. If a researcher is studying humans in an uncontrolled or natural setting, it is impossible and undesirable to control all the extraneous variables. In qualitative and some quantitative studies (descriptive and correlational), little or no attempt is made to control extraneous variables. The intent is to study subjects in their natural environment, without controlling or altering that setting or situation (Fawcett & Garity, 2009; Munhall, 2012). The environmental variables in quasi-experimental and experimental research can be controlled by using a laboratory setting or a specially constructed research unit in a hospital. Environmental control is an extremely important part of conducting an experimental study. For example, Sharma and co-workers (2010) conducted an experimental study using mice in a laboratory setting (see Table 5-1). The laboratory controlled for many of the environmental variables, so they did not have an impact on the study outcomes.

Conceptual and Operational Definitions of Variables in Quantitative Research

A variable is operationalized in a study by the development of conceptual and operational definitions. A conceptual definition provides the theoretical meaning of a variable (Chinn & Kramer, 2011) and is often derived from a theorist's definition of a related concept. In a published study, the framework includes concepts and their definitions, and the variables are selected to represent these concepts. The variables are conceptually defined, indicating the link with the concepts in the framework. An operational definition is derived from a set of procedures or progressive acts that a researcher performs to receive sensory impressions (e.g., sound, visual, or tactile impressions) that indicate the existence or degree of existence of a variable (Reynolds, 2007). Operational definitions need to be independent of time and setting so that variables can be investigated at different times and in different settings using the same operational definitions. An operational definition is developed so that a variable can be measured or manipulated in a concrete situation; the knowledge gained from studying the variable will increase the understanding of the theoretical concept that this variable represents.

Two variables are operationalized as an example from Piamjariyakul and colleagues' (2013) study of the effect of a telephone coaching program on HF home management for family caregivers. The conceptual and operational definitions for the independent variable telephone coaching program and one of the dependent variables, caregiving burden, are presented in the following research example. The guidelines identified in the following box were used to critically appraise the variables and their definitions in this study.

🔍 CRITICAL APPRAISAL GUIDELINES

Study Variables

1. Are the variables clearly identified in the study purpose and/or research objectives, questions, or hypotheses?
2. What types of variables are examined in the study? Are independent and dependent variables or research variables examined in the study?
3. If a quasi-experimental or experimental study is conducted, are the extraneous variables identified and controlled?
4. Are the variables conceptually defined?
5. Are the variables operationally defined?

🔧 RESEARCH EXAMPLE

Conceptual and Operational Definitions of Variables

Independent Variable: Telephone Coaching Program
Conceptual Definition
The telephone coaching program was developed based on the study framework of coaching by healthcare professionals. The program included evidence-based coaching strategies designed to improve intermediate and long-term caregivers' outcomes (Piamjariyakul et al., 2013).

Continued

⚡ RESEARCH EXAMPLE—cont'd

Operational Definition
The telephone coaching program was an intervention implemented by five nurse interventionists to family caregivers using a detailed protocol, which included specific educational objectives and selected coaching activities based on the evidence-based national clinical guidelines for management of HF patients (see protocol in Piamjariyakul et al., 2013, p. 35; this article can be accessed from the Elsevier website for this text).

Dependent Variable: Caregiving Burden
Conceptual Definition
Caregiving burden is a long-term outcome thought to be improved by the implementation of evidence-based coaching strategies by health professionals (Piamjariyakul et al., 2013).

Operational Definition
"Caregiving burden of HF homecare management was measured using a 17-item five-point Likert-type scale, with higher scores indicating more burden or difficulty in providing HF home caregiving." Piamjariyakul et al., 2013, p. 34
This scale was modified based on the original Oberst Caregiving Burden Scale.

Critical Appraisal
The variables in this study were clearly identified and defined. The independent and dependent variables were identified in the research questions (see earlier). The conceptual definitions for the telephone coaching program and caregiving burden were based on the study framework (see the model and description in Piamjariyakul et al., 2013, p. 33). The operational definitions for the variables were found in the methods section of the research report. These definitions were strong and provided clear direction for the implementation of the intervention and measurement of the dependent variable in the study.

Implications for Practice
Findings from this study were discussed earlier in this chapter when the problem and purpose of this study were presented as examples.

Research Concepts Investigated in Qualitative Research

The variables in quasi-experimental and experimental research are narrow and specific in focus and can be quantified (converted to numbers) or manipulated using specified steps that are often developed into a protocol. In addition, the variables are objectively defined to decrease researcher bias, as indicated in the previous section. Qualitative research is more abstract, subjective, and holistic than quantitative research and involves the investigation of research concepts versus research variables. Research concepts include the ideas, experiences, situations, or events that are investigated in qualitative research. For example, Trollvik and associates (2011, p. 295) conducted a qualitative study to explore the phenomenon of "children's experiences of living with asthma." The problem and purpose for this phenomenological study are presented in Table 5-2. The research concept explored was "experiences of living with asthma" as perceived by children. In many qualitative studies, the focus of the study is to define or describe the concept(s) being studied (Munhall, 2012). In this study, the research concept of living with asthma was defined as including two themes—fear of exacerbations and fear of being ostracized. The fear of exacerbations included the subthemes of bodily sensations, frightening experiences, and loss of control. The fear of being ostracized included the subthemes of experiences of being excluded and the dilemma of keeping the asthma secret or being open about it. More details on the research concepts studied in qualitative research are found in Chapter 3.

Demographic Variables

Demographic variables are attributes of subjects that are collected to describe the sample. The demographic variables are identified by the researcher when a proposal is developed for conducting a study. Some common demographic variables are age, education, gender, ethnic origin (race), marital status, income, job classification, and medical diagnosis. Once data are collected from the study subjects on these demographic variables and analyzed, the results are called sample characteristics used to describe the sample. A study's sample characteristics can be presented in table format and/or narrative. Piamjariyakul and co-workers (2013), in a study discussed earlier, presented most of their sample characteristics in a table and discussed others in the narrative of their article. Table 5-4 identifies the sample characteristics for the family caregivers and patients with HF. The demographic variables described for the family caregivers and patients with HF included age, gender, employment, education, and race. These are common demographic variables examined to describe study samples and are the basis for comparison with samples from other studies. Two other demographic variables were described in Table 5-4, caregivers' relationship to the patient with HF and the patient's EF (ejection fraction). In the narrative of the article, 10 of the 12 "caregivers reported having one or more chronic health problems (osteoarthritis, hypertension, asthma, myocardial infarction, and diabetes mellitus). . . . One caregiver did not have health insurance

TABLE 5-4	SAMPLE CHARACTERISTICS OF HF PATIENTS AND THEIR CAREGIVERS ENROLLED IN THIS PILOT STUDY ($n=12$)		
CAREGIVER CHARACTERISTICS	**PERCENTAGE/MEAN (SD) N (%)**	**PATIENT CHARACTERISTICS**	**PERCENTAGE/MEAN (SD) N (%)**
Caregiver Age (years)	62.6 (13.7); range=38-81	**Patient Age (years)**	61.6 (12.8); range=43-79
Caregiver Gender		**Patient Gender**	
Female	9 (75)	Female	4 (33.3)
Male	3 (25)	Male	8 (66.7)
Employment		**Employment**	
Full or part time	3 (25)	Full or part time	1 (8.3)
Retired	7 (58.3)	Retired	6 (50)
Retired/disabled	2 (16.7)	Retired/disabled	4 (33.3)
		Missing (did not answer)	1 (8.3)
Education		**Education**	
High school	1 (8.3)	High school or lower	5 (41.7)
Technical/some college	7 (58.3)	Technical/some college	6 (50)
College or more	4 (33.3)	College or more	1 (8.3)
Race		**Race**	
White	8 (66.7)	Caucasian	6 (50)
African American	4 (33.3)	African American	5 (41.7)
Relationship		Other	1 (8.3)
Spouse	8 (66.7)		
Adult child	1 (8.3)	**EF**	
Mother	1 (8.3)	≤40%	9 (75)
Other	2 (16.7)	>40%	3 (25)

EF, Ejection fraction; *HF,* heart failure; *n,* sample size; *N,* frequency; *SD,* standard deviation.
From Piamjariyakul, U., Smith, C. E., Russell, C., Werkowitch, M., & Elyachar, A. (2013). The feasibility of a telephone coaching program on heart failure home management for family caregivers. *Heart & Lung, 42*(1), 37.

coverage" (Piamjariyakul et al., 2013, p. 36). The demographic variables of chronic illnesses and insurance coverage were also described for the caregivers. The researchers provided a quality description of their sample characteristics in their study.

KEY CONCEPTS

- The research problem is an area of concern in which there is a gap in the knowledge base needed for nursing practice. The problem includes significance, background, and problem statement.
- The research purpose is a concise, clear statement of the specific goal or focus of the study.
- A significant problem and purpose influence nursing practice, build on previous research, promote theory development, and/or address current concerns or priorities in nursing.
- Study feasibility is evaluated by examining the researchers' expertise, money commitments, availability of subjects, facilities, and equipment, and the study's ethical considerations.
- Research objectives, questions, or hypotheses are formulated to bridge the gap between the more abstractly stated research problem and purpose and the detailed quantitative design and data analysis.
- A qualitative study often includes problem, purpose, and research questions or aims to direct the study.
- A hypothesis is the formal statement of the expected relationship(s) between two or more variables in a specified population in a quantitative or outcomes study.
- Hypotheses can be described using four categories: (1) associative versus causal; (2) simple versus complex; (3) nondirectional versus directional; and (4) statistical versus research.
- Variables are qualities, properties, or characteristics of persons, things, or situations that change or vary.
- An independent variable is an intervention or treatment that is manipulated or varied by the researcher to create an effect on the dependent variable.
- A dependent variable is the outcome that the researcher wants to predict or explain.
- In predictive correlational studies, independent variables are measured to predict a dependent variable.
- Research variables are the qualities, properties, or characteristics that are observed or measured in descriptive and correlational studies.
- A variable is operationalized in a study by developing conceptual and operational definitions.
- A conceptual definition provides the theoretical meaning of a variable and is derived from a theorist's definition of a related concept.
- Operational definitions indicate how a treatment or independent variable will be implemented and how the dependent or outcome variable will be measured.
- Research concepts include the ideas, experiences, situations, or events that are investigated in qualitative research.
- Research concepts are defined and described during the conduct of qualitative studies.
- Demographic variables are collected and analyzed to determine sample characteristics for describing the study subjects or participants.

REFERENCES

Agency for Healthcare Research and Quality (AHRQ), (2013). *AHRQ research funding priorities.* Retrieved July 2, 2013 from, http://www.ahrq.gov/legacy/fund/ragendix.htm.

American Association of Critical-Care Nurses (AACN), (2013). *AACN's research priority areas.* Retrieved July 2, 2013 from, http://www.aacn.org, and search for Research Priorities.

Ausserhofer, D., Schubert, M., Desmedt, M., Belgen, M. A., De Geest, S., & Schwendimann, R. (2013). The association of patient safety climate and nurse-related organizational factors with selected patient outcomes: A cross-sectional survey. *International Journal of Nursing Studies, 50*(2), 240–252.

Bernard, P. P. N., Esseul, E. C., Raymond, L., Dandonneau, L., Xambo, J., Carayol, M. S., et al. (2013). Counseling and exercise intervention for smoking reduction in patients with schizophrenia: Feasibility study. *Archives of Psychiatric Nursing, 27*(1), 23–31.

Bindler, R. J., Bindler, R. C., & Daratha, K. B. (2013). Biological correlates and predictors of insulin resistance among early adolescents. *Journal of Pediatric Nursing, 28*(1), 20–27.

Brown, S. J. (2014). *Evidence-based nursing: The research-practice connection* (3rd ed.). Sudbury, MA: Jones & Bartlett.

Buet, A., Cohen, B., Marine, M., Scully, F., Alper, P., Simpser, E., et al. (2013). Hand hygiene opportunities in pediatric extended care facilities. *Journal of Pediatric Nursing, 28*(1), 72–76.

Burns, K. H., Casey, P. H., Lyle, R. E., Bird, T. M., Fussell, J. J. , & Robbins, J. M. (2010). Increasing prevalence of medically complex children in U.S. hospitals. *Pediatrics, 126*(4), 638–646.

Centers for Disease Control and Prevention (CDC), (2006). A comprehensive immunization strategy to eliminate transmission of hepatitis B virus infection in the United States. *Morbidity and Mortality Weekly Report, 55*(RR-16), 1–25.

Centers for Disease Control and Prevention (CDC), (2008). Surveillance for acute viral hepatitis—United States, 2006. *Morbidity and Mortality Weekly Report, 57* (SS02), 1–24.

Child Welfare League of America, (2007). *Quick facts about foster care.* Retrieved March 14, 2013 from, http://cwla.org/programs/fostercare/factsheet.htm.

Chinn, P. L., & Kramer, M. K. (2011). *Integrated theory and knowledge development in nursing* (8th ed.). St. Louis: Elsevier Mosby.

Craig, J., & Smyth, R. (2012). *The evidence-based practice manual for nurses* (3rd ed.). Edinburgh: Churchill Livingstone Elsevier.

Creswell, J. W. (2014). *Research design: Qualitative, quantitative, and mixed methods approaches* (4th ed.). Thousand Oaks, CA: Sage.

Doran, D. M. (2011). *Nursing outcomes: The state of the science* (2nd ed.). Canada: Jones & Bartlett Learning.

Dunbar, S. B., Clark, P. C., Deaton, C., Smith, A. L., De, A. K., & O'Brien, M. C. (2005). Family education and support interventions in heart failure: A pilot study. *Nursing Research, 54*(2), 158–166.

Fawcett, J., & Garity, J. (2009). *Evaluating research for evidence-based nursing practice.* Philadelphia: F. A. Davis.

Gartner, L. M., Morton, J., Lawrence, R. A., Naylor, A. J., O'Hare, D., Schanler, R. J., et al. American Academy of Pediatrics Section on Breastfeeding. (2005). Breastfeeding and the use of human milk. *Pediatrics, 115*(2), 496–506.

Grove, S. K., Burns, N., & Gray, J. R. (2013). *The practice of nursing research: Appraisal, synthesis, and generation of evidence* (7th ed.). St. Louis: Elsevier Saunders.

Hale, E. D., Treharne, G. J., & Kitas, G. D. (2007). Qualitative methodologies I: Asking research questions with reflexive insight. *Musculoskeletal Care, 5*(3), 139–147.

Happ, M. B., Swigart, V. A., Tate, J. A., Arnold, R. M., Sereika, S. M., & Hoffman, L. A. (2007). Family presence and surveillance during weaning from prolonged mechanical ventilation. *Heart & Lung, 36* (1), 47–57.

Hudson, A. L. (2012). Where do youth in foster care receive information about preventing unplanned pregnancy and sexually transmitted infections? *Journal of Pediatric Nursing, 27*(5), 443–450.

Institute of Medicine, (2004). *Patient safety: Achieving a new standard for care.* Washington, DC: National Academies Press.

Kerlinger, F. N., & Lee, H. B. (2000). *Foundations of behavioral research* (4th ed.). Fort Worth, TX: Harcourt College.

Letourneau, N., Young, C., Secco, L., Stewart, M., Hughes, J., & Critchley, K. (2011). Supporting mothering: Service providers' perspectives of mothers and young children affected by intimate partner violence. *Research in Nursing & Health, 34*(3), 192–203.

Li, C., Ford, E. S., Huang, T. T., Sun, S. S., & Goodman, E. (2009). Patterns of change in cardiometabolic risk factors associated with the metabolic syndrome among children and adolescents: The Fels Longitudinal Study. *Journal of Pediatrics, 155*(S5), e9–e16.

Lindeman, C. A. (1975). Delphi survey of priorities in clinical nursing research. *Nursing Research, 24*(6), 434–441.

Litrownik, A. J., Newton, R., Hunter, W. M., English, D., & Everson, M. D. (2003). Exposure to family violence in young at-risk children: A longitudinal look at the effects of victimization and witnessed physical and psychological aggression. *Journal of Family Violence, 18*(1), 59–73.

Lundy, K. S. (2012). Historical research. In P. L. Munhall (Ed.), *Nursing research: A qualitative perspective* (pp. 381–397) (5th ed.). Sudbury, MA: Jones & Bartlett Learning.

Marshall, C., & Rossman, G. B. (2011). *Designing qualitative research* (5th ed.). Los Angeles: Sage.

Masoli, M., Fabian, D., Holt, S., & Beasley, R. Global Initiative for Asthma (GINA) Program. (2004). The global burden of asthma: Executive summary of the GINA Dissemination Committee Report. *Allergy, 59* (5), 469–478.

Melnyk, B. M., & Fineout-Overholt, E. (2011). *Evidence-based practice in nursing & healthcare: A guide to best practice* (2nd ed.). Philadelphia: Lippincott, Williams & Wilkins.

Munhall, P. L. (2012). *Nursing research: A qualitative perspective* (5th ed.). Sudbury, MA: Jones & Bartlett Learning.

National Institute of Nursing Research (NINR), (2011). *Mission and strategic plan.* Retrieved March 16, 2013 from, http://www.ninr.nih.gov/aboutninr/ninr-mission-and-strategic-plan.

Nyamathi, A., Liu, Y., Marfisee, M., Shoptaw, S., Gregerson, P., Saab, S., et al. (2009). Effects of a nurse-managed program on hepatitis A and B vaccine completion among homeless adults. *Nursing Research, 58*(1), 13–22.

Piamjariyakul, U., Smith, C. E., Russell, C., Werkowitch, M., & Elyachar, A. (2013). The feasibility of a telephone coaching program on heart failure home management for family caregivers. *Heart & Lung, 42* (1), 32–39.

Polman, H., de Castro, B. O., & van Aken, M. A. (2007). *Experimental study of the differential effects of playing versus watching violent video games on children's aggressive behavior. Aggressive Behavior, 34,* 256–264. Retrieved March 12, 2009 from, www.interscience.wiley.com.

Price, D., Ryan, D., Pearce, L., Bawden, R., Freeman, D., Thomas, M., et al. (2002). The burden of pediatric asthma is higher than health professionals think: Results from the Asthma In Real Life (AIR) study. *Primary Care Respiratory Journal, 11*(1), 30–33.

Quality and Safety Education for Nurses (QSEN), (2013). *Pre-licensure knowledge, skills, and attitudes (KSAs).* Retrieved July 2, 2013 from, http://qsen.org/competencies/pre-licensure-ksas.

Reutter, L., & Kushner, K. E. (2010). Healthy equity through action on the social determinants of health: Taking up the challenge in nursing. *Nursing Inquiry, 17* (3), 269–280.

Reynolds, P. D. (2007). *A primer in theory construction.* Boston: Allyn & Bacon Classics.

Riegel, B., Moser, D. K., Anker, S. D., Appel, L. J., Dunbar, S. B., Grady, K. L., et al. (2009). State of the science: Promoting self-care in persons with heart failure: A scientific statement from the American Heart Association. *Circulation, 120*(12), 1141–1163.

Rogers, B. (1987). Research corner: Is the research project feasible? *American Association of Occupational Health Nurses Journal, 35*(7), 327–328.

Rohrbeck, J., Jordan, K., & Croft, P. (2007). The frequency and characteristics of chronic widespread pain in general practice: A case-control study. *British Journal of General Practice, 57*(535), 109–115.

Schultz, A. A., Drew, D., & Hewitt, H. (2002). Comparison of normal saline and heparinized saline for patency of IV locks in neonates. *Applied Nursing Research, 15*(1), 28–34.

Shadish, W. R., Cook, T. D., & Campbell, D. T. (2002). *Experimental and quasi-experimental designs for generalized causal inference.* Chicago: Rand McNally.

Sharma, N. K., Ryals, J. M., Gajewski, B. J., & Wright, D. E. (2010). Aerobic exercise alters analgesia and neurotrophin-3 synthesis in an animal model of chronic widespread pain. *Physical Therapy, 90*(5), 714–725.

Sherwood, G., & Barnsteiner, J. (2012). *Quality and safety in nursing: A competency approach to improving outcomes.* Ames, IA: Wiley-Blackwell.

Tenfelde, S. M., Finnegan, L., Miller, A. M., & Hill, P. D. (2012). Risk of breastfeeding cessation among low-income women, infants, and children. *Nursing Research, 61*(2), 86–95.

Thompson, M. E., & Keeling, A. A. (2012). Nurses' role in the prevention of infant mortality in 1884–1925: Health disparities then and now. *Journal of Pediatric Nursing, 27*(5), 471–478.

Trollvik, A., Nordbach, R., Silen, C., & Ringsberg, K. C. (2011). Children's experiences of living with asthma: Fear of exacerbations and being ostracized. *Journal of Pediatric Nursing, 26*(4), 295–303.

U.S. Department of Health and Human Services (U.S. DHHS). (2010). *Healthy People 2020.* Retrieved July 2, 2013 from, http://www.healthypeople.gov/hp2020.

U.S. Department of Health and Human Services (U.S. DHHS). (2013). *Healthy People 2020: Topics and objectives.* Retrieved July 2, 2013 from, http://healthypeople.gov/2020/topicsobjectives2020.

Wasley, A., Miller, J. T., & Finelli, L. (2007). Surveillance for acute viral hepatitis—United States, 2005. *Morbidity and Mortality Weekly Report. CDC Surveillance Summaries, 56*(3), 1–24.

Whiteside, A., Hansen, S., & Chaudhuri, A. (2004). Exercise lowers pain threshold in chronic fatigue syndrome. *Pain, 109*(3), 497–499.

Wolf, Z. R. (2012). Ethnography: The method. In P. L. Munhall (Ed.), *Nursing research: A qualitative perspective* (pp. 285–338) (5th ed.). Sudbury, MA: Jones & Bartlett Learning.

World Health Organization (WHO). (2009). *Guidelines for hand hygiene in health care.* Retrieved July 2, 2013 from, http://who.int/gpsc/5may/tools/9789241597906/en.

World Health Organization (WHO). (2011). *Obesity and overweight.* Retrieved July 2, 2013 from, http://www.who.int/mediacentre/factsheets/fs311/en.

World Health Organization (WHO). (2013). *Programmes and projects.* Retrieved March 17, 2013 from, http://www.who.int/entity/en.

Wuest, J. (2012). Grounded theory: The method. In P. L. Munhall (Ed.), *Nursing research: A qualitative perspective* (pp. 225–256) (5th ed.). Sudbury, MA: Jones & Bartlett Learning.

CHAPTER

6

Understanding and Critically Appraising the Literature Review

LEARNING OUTCOMES

After completing this chapter, you should be able to:

1. Discuss the purposes of the literature review in quantitative and qualitative research.
2. Identify the sources included in a literature review.
3. Differentiate a primary source from a secondary source.
4. Critically appraise the literature review section of a published study.

5. Conduct a computerized search of the literature.
6. Read and critically appraise literature to develop a synthesis of the literature.
7. Write a literature review to promote the use of evidence-based knowledge in nursing practice.

KEY TERMS

Article, p. 166
Bibliographic database, p. 177
Citation, p. 165
Clinical journals, p. 166
Comprehending a source, p. 180
Conclusion, p. 184

Conference proceedings, p. 166
Current sources, p. 167
Data-based literature, p. 167
Digital object identifiers
   (DOI), p. 184
Dissertation, p. 166

Empirical literature, p. 167
Encyclopedia, p. 166
Keywords, p. 178
Landmark studies, p. 167
Literature, p. 165
Monograph, p. 166

A high-quality review of literature contains the current theoretical and scientific knowledge about a specific topic. The review identifies what is known and unknown about the topic. Nurses in clinical practice review the literature to synthesize the available evidence to find a solution to a problem in practice or because they want to remain current in their practice. As they read studies, they must critically appraise the literature review, as well as the other components of the study. Critically appraising a review of the literature begins with understanding the purpose of the literature review in quantitative and qualitative studies and the relative quality of the different types of references that are cited. The critical appraisal guidelines for literature reviews listed in this chapter can be applied to both quantitative and qualitative studies. In addition, examples are provided of critical appraisals of the literature reviews in a quantitative study and another in a qualitative study.

You may be required to review the literature as part of a course assignment or project in the clinical setting, especially projects in Magnet hospitals. Nurses in Magnet hospitals must implement evidence-based practice, identify problems, and assist with data collection for research studies (American Nurses Credentialing Center [ANCC], 2013). Reviewing the literature is a first step in implementing evidence-based practice and identifying problems. (Chapter 13 identifies the research responsibilities of nurses in Magnet facilities.)

A review of literature is the process of finding relevant research reports, critically appraising the studies, and synthesizing the study results. The written description of the literature that results from the process is also called a review of the literature. As a foundation for this process, this chapter includes information on how to find references, select those that are relevant, organize what you find, and write a logical summary of the findings.

PURPOSE OF THE LITERATURE REVIEW

Literature reviews in published research reports provide the background for the problem studied. Such reviews include (1) describing the current knowledge of a practice problem, (2) identifying the gaps in this knowledge base, and (3) explaining how the study being reported contributed to building knowledge in this area. The scope of a literature review must be broad enough to allow the reader to become familiar with the research problem and narrow enough to include only the most relevant sources.

Purpose of the Literature Review in Quantitative Research

The review of literature in quantitative research is conducted to direct the planning and execution of a study. The major literature review is performed at the beginning of the research process (before the study is conducted). A limited review is conducted after the study is completed to identify studies published since the original literature review, especially if it has been 1 year or longer since the study began. Additional articles may be retrieved to find information relevant to interpreting the findings. The results of both reviews are included in the research report. The purpose of the literature review is similar for the different types of quantitative studies—descriptive, correlational, quasi-experimental, and experimental.

Quantitative research reports may include citations to relevant sources in all sections of the report. The researchers include sources in the introduction section to summarize the background and significance of the research problem. Citations about the number of patients affected, cost of treatment, and consequences in terms of human suffering and physical health may be included. The review of literature section may not be labeled but be integrated into the introduction. The review includes theoretical and research references that document current knowledge about the problem studied.

A quantitative study develops its framework section (not always so labeled) from the theoretical literature and sometimes from research reports, depending on the focus of the study. The methods section of the research report describes the design, sample and the process for obtaining the sample, measurement methods, treatment, and data collection process. References may be cited in various parts of the methods section as support for the appropriateness of the methods used in the study. The results section includes the results of the statistical analyses, but also includes sources to validate the analytical techniques that were used to answer the research questions. Sources might also be included to compare the analysis of the data in the present study with the results of previous studies. The discussion section of the research report provides the comparison of the findings to other studies' findings, if not already included in the results section. The discussion section also incorporates conclusions that are a synthesis of the findings from previous research and those from the present study.

Purpose of the Literature Review in Qualitative Research

In qualitative research reports, the introduction will be similar to the same section in the quantitative study report because the researchers document the background and significance of the research problem. Researchers often include citations to support the need to study the selected topic (Creswell, 2013). However, additional review of the literature may not be cited for two reasons. One reason is that qualitative studies are often conducted on topics about which we know very little, so little literature is available to review. The other reason is that some qualitative researchers deliberately do not review the literature deeply prior to conducting the study because they do not want their expectations about the topic to bias their data collection, data analysis, and findings (Munhall, 2012). This is consistent with the expectation that qualitative researchers remain open to the perspectives of the participants. In the methods, results, and discussion sections, qualitative researchers will incorporate literature to support the use of specific methods and place the findings in the context of what is already known.

The purpose, extent, and timing of the literature review vary across the different qualitative approaches (Grove, Burns, & Gray, 2013). Phenomenologists are among those who are likely to delay literature review until after data collection and initial analysis have been completed (Munhall, 2012). These researchers will review the literature in the later stages of the analysis and as they interpret the findings in the larger context of theoretical and empirical knowledge. Grounded theory researchers include a minimal review of relevant studies at the beginning of the research process. This review is merely a means of making the researcher aware of what studies have been conducted and that a research problem exists (Corbin & Strauss, 2008), but the information from these studies is not used to direct data collection or theory development for the current study (Walls, Pahoo, & Fleming, 2010). The researcher uses the literature primarily to explain, support, and extend the theory generated in the study (Wuerst, 2012).

The review of literature in ethnographic research is similar to that in quantitative research. In early ethnographies of unexplored groups of people in distant locations, culture-specific literature was not available to review prior to data collection. Theoretical and philosophical literature, however, was and continues to be used to provide a framework or perspective through which researchers approach data collection. The research problem for an ethnography is based on a review of the literature that identifies how little is known about the culture of interest (Wolf, 2012). The review also informs the research process by providing a general understanding of the cultural characteristics to be examined. For example, the literature review for an ethnography of nursing in Uganda would reveal that the healthcare system has referral hospitals, district hospitals, and health centers. With this information, the researcher might decide to develop a data collection plan to observe nurses in each setting, or the researcher might decide to narrow the ethnography to health centers. Another example would be the ethnographer studying health behaviors of Burmese refugees in a specific neighborhood. From the literature, the researcher learned that older community members are highly respected and, as a result, the researcher would seek support of older refugees to facilitate access to others in the community. Ethnographers return to the literature during analysis and interpretation of the data to expand the readers' understanding of the culture.

Researchers using the exploratory-descriptive qualitative and historical approaches may be conducting the study because they have reviewed the literature and found that little knowledge is available. Exploratory-descriptive qualitative researchers want to understand a situation or practice problem better so solutions can be identified (Grove et al., 2013). Historical researchers conduct an initial review of current literature and identify an event or time in history about which little is known and that has possible implications for nursing and health care today. Publications contemporary to the event or time are the sources of data. The researchers develop an inventory of sources, locate these sources, and examine them (Lundy, 2012). Because historical research requires an extensive review of literature that is sometimes difficult to locate, the researcher can spend months and even years locating and examining sources. Chapter 3 contains additional information about literature reviews in qualitative studies.

SOURCES INCLUDED IN A LITERATURE REVIEW

The literature is all written sources relevant to the topic you have selected, including articles published in periodicals or journals, Internet publications, monographs, encyclopedias, conference papers, theses, dissertations, clinical journals, textbooks, and other books. Websites and reports developed by government agencies and professional organizations are also included. Each source reviewed by the author and used to write the review is cited. A citation is the act of quoting a source, paraphrasing content from a source, using it as an example, or presenting it as support for a position taken. Each citation should have a corresponding reference in the reference list. The reference is documentation of the origin of the cited quote or paraphrased idea and provides enough information for the reader to locate the original material. This information is typically the original author's name, year, and title of publication and, when necessary, periodical or monograph title, volume, pages, and other location information as required by standard style writing manuals. The style developed by the American Psychological Association (APA, 2010) is commonly used in nursing education programs and journals. More information about APA style is provided later in this chapter.

Types of Publications

An article is a paper about a specific topic and may be published together with other articles on similar themes in journals (periodicals), encyclopedias, or edited books. As part of an edited book, articles may be called chapters. A periodical such as a journal is published over time and is numbered sequentially for the years published. This sequential numbering is seen in the year, volume, issue, and page numbering of a journal. A monograph, such as a book on a specific subject, a record of conference proceedings, or a pamphlet, usually is a one-time publication. Periodicals and monographs are available in a variety of media, including online and print. An encyclopedia is an authoritative compilation of information on alphabetized topics that may provide background information and lead to other sources, but is rarely cited in academic papers and publications. Some online encyclopedias are electronic publications that have undergone the same level of review as published encyclopedias. Other online encyclopedias, such as Wikipedia, are in an open, editable format and, as a result, the credibility of the information is variable. Using Wikipedia as a professional source is controversial (Luyt, Ally, Low, & Ismail, 2010; Younger, 2010). When you are writing a review of the literature, Wikipedia may provide ideas for other sources that you may want to find but check with your faculty about whether Wikipedia or any other encyclopedia may be cited for course assignments.

Major professional organizations may publish papers selected by a review process that were presented at their conference, called conference proceedings. These publications may be in print or online. Conference proceedings may include the findings of pilot studies and preliminary findings of ongoing studies. A thesis is a report of a research project completed by a postgraduate student as part of the requirements for a master's degree. A dissertation is a report of an extensive, sometimes original, research project that is completed as the final requirement for a doctoral degree. Theses and dissertations can be cited in a literature review. In some cases, an article may be published based on the student's thesis or dissertation. Clinical journals are periodicals that include research reports and non-research articles about practice problems and professional issues. You are familiar with textbooks as a source of information for academic courses. Other books on theories, methods, and events may also be cited in a literature review. To evaluate the quality of a book, consider the qualifications of the author related to the topic, and review the evidence that the author provides to support the book's premises and conclusions. With textbooks and other books, chapters in an edited book might have been written by different people, which are cited differently than the book as a whole. This is important to note when checking citations and writing your own literature reviews.

Electronic access to articles and books has increased dramatically, making many types of published literature more widely available. In addition, websites are an easily accessible source of information. Not all websites are valid and appropriate, however, for citation in a literature review. The website of a company that sells diuretic medications may not be an appropriate source for hypertension statistics. In contrast, websites prepared and sponsored by government agencies and professional organizations are considered appropriate references to cite.

Content of Publications

References cited in literature reviews contain two main types of content, (1) theoretical and (2) empirical. Theoretical literature includes concept analyses, models, theories, and conceptual frameworks that support a selected research problem and purpose. Theoretical sources can be found in books, periodicals, and monographs. Nursing theorists have written books to describe the development and content of their theories. Other books contain summaries of several theories. In a published study, theoretical and conceptual sources are described and summarized to reflect the current understanding of the research problem and provide a basis for the study framework.

Empirical literature in this context refers to knowledge derived from research. In other words, the knowledge is based on data from research (data-based). Data-based literature consists of reports of research and includes published studies, usually in journals, on the Internet, or books, and unpublished studies, such as master theses and doctoral dissertations.

Quality of Sources

Most references cited in quality literature reviews are primary sources that are peer-reviewed. A primary source is written by the person who originated or is responsible for generating the ideas published. A research report written by the researchers who conducted the study is a primary source. A theorist's development of a theory or other conceptual content is a primary source. A secondary source summarizes or quotes content from primary sources. Authors of secondary sources paraphrase the works of researchers and theorists and present their interpretation of what was written by the primary author. As a result, information in secondary sources may be misinterpretations of the primary authors' thoughts. Secondary sources are used only if primary sources cannot be located, or the secondary source provides creative ideas or a unique organization of information not found in a primary source. Peer-reviewed means that the author of the research report, clinical description, or theoretical explanation has submitted a manuscript to a journal editor, who identified scholars familiar with the topic to review the manuscript. These scholars provide input to the editor about whether the manuscript in its current form is accurate, meets standards for quality, and is appropriate for the journal. A peer-reviewed paper has undergone significant scrutiny and is considered trustworthy.

Quality literature reviews include relevant and current sources. Relevant studies are those with a direct bearing on the problem of concern. Current sources are those published within 5 years before publication of the manuscript. Sources cited should be comprehensive as well as current. Some problems have been studied for decades, and the literature review often includes seminal and landmark studies that were conducted years ago. Seminal studies are the first studies on a particular topic that signaled the beginning of a new way of thinking on the topic and sometimes are referred to as classical studies. Landmark studies are significant research projects that have generated knowledge that influences a discipline and sometimes society as a whole. Such studies frequently are replicated or serve as the basis for the generation of additional studies. Some authors may describe a landmark study as being a groundbreaking study. Citing a few older studies significant to the development of knowledge on the topic being reviewed is appropriate. Most publications cited, however, should be current. Replication studies are reproductions or repetitions of a study that researchers conduct to determine whether the findings of the original study could be found consistently in different settings and with different subjects. Replication studies are important to build the evidence for practice. A replication study that supports the findings of the original study increases the credibility of the findings and strengthens the evidence for practice. A replication that does not support the original study findings raises questions about the credibility of the findings.

Syntheses of research studies, another type of data-based literature, may be cited in literature reviews. A research synthesis may be a systematic review of the literature, meta-analysis of quantitative studies, meta-synthesis of qualitative studies, or a mixed-method systematic review. These publications are valued for their rigor and contributions to evidence-based practice (see Chapters 1 and 13).

CRITICALLY APPRAISING LITERATURE REVIEWS

Appraising the literature review of a published study involves examining the quality of the content and sources presented. A correctly prepared literature review includes what is known and not known about the study problem and identifies the focus of the present study. As a result, the review provides a basis for the study purpose and may be organized according to the variables (quantitative) or concepts (qualitative) in the purpose statement. The sources cited must be relevant and current for the problem and purpose of the study. The reviewer must locate and review the sources or respective abstracts to determine whether these sources are relevant. To judge whether all the relevant sources are cited, the reviewer must search the literature to determine the relevant sources. This is very time-consuming and usually is not done for appraisal of an article. However, you can review the reference list and determine the focus of the sources, the number of data-based and theoretical sources cited, and where and when the sources were published. Sources should be current, up to the date the paper was accepted for publication. Most articles indicate when they were accepted for publication on the first page of the study.

Although the purpose of the literature review for a quantitative study is different from the purpose of the literature review for a qualitative study, the guidelines for critically appraising the literature review of quantitative and qualitative studies are the same. However, because the purposes of literature reviews are different, the type of sources and the extent of the literature cited may vary.

⚡ CRITICAL APPRAISAL GUIDELINES

Literature Reviews

1. Inclusion of relevant literature
   - Did the researchers describe previous studies and relevant theories?
   - What other types of literature were cited?
2. Currency of sources
   - Are the references current (number and percentage of sources in the last 10 years and in the last 5 years)?
   - Are landmark, seminal, and/or replication studies included?
3. Breadth of the review
   - Identify the disciplines of the authors of studies cited in this paper and the journals in which they published their studies.
   - Does it appear that the author searched databases outside of the Cumulative Index of Nursing and Allied Health Literature (CINAHL) for relevant studies?
4. Synthesis of strengths and weaknesses of available evidence
   - Are the studies critically appraised and synthesized (Fawcett & Garity, 2009; Grove et al., 2013; Hart, 2009)?
   - Is a clear, concise summary presented of the current empirical and theoretical knowledge in the area of the study, including identifying what is known and not known (O'Mathuna, Fineout-Overholt, & Jonston, 2011)?
   - Is the literature review organized to demonstrate the progressive development of evidence from previous research?
   - Does the literature review summary provide direction for the formation of the research purpose?

Critical Appraisal of a Literature Review in a Quantitative Study

The anxiety related to having a surgical or diagnostic procedure can have adverse effects. Brand, Munroe, and Gavin (2013, p. 708) conducted a quasi-experimental study to "determine the effects of hand massage on patient anxiety in the ambulatory surgical setting." The section entitled "Literature Review" (pp. 709-710) is included as an example and is critically appraised. In addition to the references included in the review of the literature, these authors cited references throughout the research report. The reference list, previously formatted in the style of medical literature, is included in APA format in this chapter. All the cited references are considered in the critical appraisal.

RESEARCH EXAMPLE

Literature Review

"Anxiety is considered a normal part of the preoperative experience (Bailey, 2010). Because it is common, however, does not mean it should be ignored. Part of the nurse's role in the perioperative setting is to manage patient anxiety to support positive surgical outcomes and satisfaction with the surgical experience. The shift from inpatient hospital stays for surgery to same-day surgery has been monumental; most patients undergoing surgeries that once required an overnight hospital stay now go home within hours of surgery (Mitchell, 2003). Unfortunately, nurses and physicians have a fraction of the time they once had to achieve all of the postoperative goals and outcomes, including, but not limited to, pain management and postoperative education (Mitchell, 2003).

Grieve (2002) described causes of anxiety in the preoperative patient. . . . Yellen and Davis (2001) reviewed the effects of anxiety and found that it can be detrimental to physical and emotional recovery, and that anxiety can contribute to poor outcomes and longer hospitalizations. These researchers also learned that when patients felt valued and attained a high level of comfort, these beliefs were strong predictors of patient satisfaction.

Anxiety triggers the stress response, stimulating the release of epinephrine and norepinephrine, which raises blood pressure and increases heart rate, cardiac output, and blood glucose levels (Forshee, Clayton, & McCance, 2010). Poorly managed anxiety can be life-threatening in patients diagnosed with hypertension and coronary artery disease, increasing the chances for myocardial infarction or potential stroke (Forshee, Clayton, & McCance, 2010). Anxiety can also have a major effect on psychological symptoms and can inhibit learning, concentration, and routine tasks (Gilmartin & Wright, 2008; Vaughn, Wichowski, & Bosworth, 2007). . . . Armed with this knowledge, nurses in the perioperative setting should be concerned about how anxiety can affect the outcomes for all surgical patients.

There is a link between preoperative anxiety and postoperative pain. In their systematic review of predictors for postoperative pain, Ip et al. (2009) found that anxiety ranked as the highest predictor. . . . According to Lin and Wang (2005), unrelieved postoperative pain has a negative effect on patients and delays postoperative recovery. In their literature review, Vaughn et al. (2007) found studies that correlated anxiety and pain, and concluded that 'preoperative planning for patients with high levels of anxiety should be implemented to obtain optimal postoperative pain control' (p. 601).

In her review of studies for strategies to decrease patient anxiety, Bailey (2010) found that perioperative education and music therapy were successful. McRee et al. (2003) researched the use of music and massage as forms of improving postoperative outcomes. . . . The findings provided evidence that patients who received preoperative music or music with massage had reduced anxiety, stress, and pain (McRee et al., 2003).

In their review, Cooke et al. (2005) identified 12 studies that focused on the effect of music on anxiety in patients waiting for surgery or other procedures in the ambulatory setting. . . . The studies of the effects of music interventions in relation to anxiety and pain reduction have similar findings (Nilsson, 2008; Yung, Chui-Kam, French, & Chan, 2002). . . . The types of music that are relaxing to patients may need to be individualized, however, thus posing challenges to implementing this intervention.

Braden et al. (2009) studied the use of oil lavandin, which has relaxant and sedative effects, as a means to reduce preoperative anxiety in surgical patients. . . . Similar to music, olfactory and topical application of oil lavandin has a low risk of adverse effects and is a cost-effective intervention that has proven successful in lowering patient anxiety on OR transfer (Braden et al., 2009). However, the use of essential oils may pose

Continued

RESEARCH EXAMPLE—cont'd

challenges with infection control standards, which often specify the brand name (i.e., source) of lotion products that can be used in the healthcare facility.

Kim et al. (2001) researched the effects of preoperative hand massage on patient anxiety before and during cataract surgery.... The researchers concluded that hand massage decreased the psychological and physiological anxiety levels in patients having cataract surgery under local anesthesia (Kim et al., 2001).

Of all the alternative methods used to alleviate anxiety in preoperative patients, we identified hand massage as a strategy that was consistent with the time constraints in the perioperative setting. Massage can be readily learned by nursing personnel, surgical patients' hands are easily accessible, and massage can be accomplished in 10 minutes. We were curious to see whether hand massage would improve patient outcomes and overall patient satisfaction. Results of previous research have shown that significant psychological and physiological changes take place after a hand massage (Kim et al., 2001). Hand massage is also a high-touch nursing care procedure that supports the concept of patients feeling valued and feeling the highest level of comfort during a time of stress and uncertainty."

References

Bailey, L. (2010). Strategies for decreasing patient anxiety in the perioperative setting. *AORN Journal, 92*(4), 445–457.

Braden, R., Reichow, S., & Halm, M. A. (2009). The use of the essential oil lavandin to reduce preoperative anxiety in surgical patients. *Journal of Perianesthesia Nursing, 24*(6), 348–355.

Chlan, L. L. (2004). Relationship between two anxiety instruments in patients receiving mechanical ventilatory support. *Journal of Advanced Nursing, 48*(5), 493–499.

Cline, M. E., Herman, J., Shaw, E. R., & Morton, R. D. (1992). Standardization of the visual analog scale. *Nursing Research, 41*(6), 378–380.

Cooke, M., Chaboyer, W., Schluter, P., & Hiratos, M. (2005). The effect of music on preoperative anxiety in day surgery. *Journal of Advanced Nursing, 52*(1), 47–54.

Creating the patient experience. (2011). DeKalb, IL: Kish Health System.

D'Arcy, Y. (2011). Controlling pain. New thinking about fibromyalgia pain. *Nursing, 41*(2), 63–64.

Forshee, B. A., Clayton, M. F., & McCance, K. L. (2010). Stress and disease. In K. L. McCance, S. E. Huether, V. L. Brashers & N. S. Rote (Eds.), *Pathophysiology: The biologic basis for disease in adults and children* (6th ed., pp. 336–358). St. Louis, MO: Mosby.

Gilmartin, J., & Wright, K. (2008). Day surgery: Patients felt abandoned during the preoperative wait. *Journal of Clinical Nursing, 17*(18), 2418–2425.

Grieve, R. J. (2002). Day surgery preoperative anxiety reduction and coping strategies. *British Journal of Nursing, 11*(10), 670–678.

Ip, H. Y., Abrishami, A., Peng, P. W., Wong, J., & Chung, F. (2009). Predictors of postoperative pain and analgesic consumption. *Anesthesiology, 111*(3), 657–677.

Kim, M. S., Cho, K. S., Woo, H. M., & Kim, J. H. (2001). Effects of hand massage on anxiety in cataract surgery using local anesthesia. *Journal of Cataract and Refractive Surgery, 27*(6), 884–890.

Leach, M., Zernike, W., & Tanner, S. (2000). How anxious are surgical patients? *ACORN Journal, 13*(1), 30–31, 34–35.

Lin, L. Y., & Wang, R. H. (2005). Abdominal surgery, pain and anxiety: Preoperative nursing intervention. *Journal of Advanced Nursing, 51*(3), 252–260.

McRee, L. D., Noble, S., & Pasvogel, A. (2003). Using massage and music therapy to improve postoperative outcomes. *AORN Journal, 78*(3), 433–447.

Mitchell, M. (2003). Patient anxiety and modern elective surgery: A literature review. *Journal of Clinical Nursing, 1*(6), 806–815.

Nilsson, U. (2008). The anxiety- and pain-reducing effects of music interventions: A systematic review. *AORN Journal, 87*(4), 780–807.

Oshodi, T. O. (2007). The impact of preoperative education on postoperative pain. *British Journal of Nursing*, *16*(3), 790–797.

Quattrin, R., Zanini, A., & Buchini, S., et al. (2006). Use of reflexology foot massage to reduce anxiety in hospitalized cancer patients in chemotherapy treatment: Methodology and outcomes. *Journal of Nursing Management*, *14*(2), 96–105.

Salmore, R. G., & Nelson, J. P. (2000). The effect of preprocedure teaching, relaxation instruction and music on anxiety as measured by blood pressures in an outpatient gastrointestinal endoscopy laboratory. *Gastroenterology Nursing*, *23*(3), 102–110.

Statistical package for the social sciences. Version 18.0. (2008). Chicago, IL: SPSS, Inc.

Vaughn, F., Wichowski, H., & Bosworth, G. (2007). Does preoperative anxiety level predict postoperative pain? *AORN Journal*, *85*(3), 589–604.

Wang, S. M., Caldwell-Andrews, A., & Kain, Z. N. (2003). The use of complementary and alternative medicines by surgical patients: A follow-up survey study. *Anesthesia and Analgesia*, *97*(4), 1010–1015.

Wagner, D., Byrne, M., & Kolcaba, K. (2003). Effects of comfort warming on perioperative patients. *AORN Journal*, *84*(3), 427–448.

Watson, J. (2008). *Nursing. The philosophy and science of caring* (revised ed.). Boulder, CO: University Press of Colorado.

Williams, V. S., Morlock, R. J., & Feltner, D. (2010). Psychometric evaluation of a visual analog scale for the assessment of anxiety. *Health and Quality of Life Outcomes*, *8*, 57. Available from http://www.hqlo.com/content/8/1/57.

Yellen, E., & Davis, G. (2001). Patient satisfaction in ambulatory surgery. *AORN Journal*, *74*(4), 483–498.

Yung, P. M., Chui-Kam, S., French, P., & Chan, T. (2002). A controlled trial of music and pre-operative anxiety in Chinese men undergoing transurethral resection of the prostate. *Journal of Advanced Nursing*, *39*(4), 352–359.

Critical Appraisal

1. Inclusion of Relevant Literature

Brand and colleagues (2013) cited 28 references in their research report, including 15 research or data-based papers. Three of these were reviews synthesizing findings of several studies on the topic. Watson's theory of caring (2008) was the only theoretical source cited, but Brand and associates did reference Forshee and co-workers (2010), a chapter in a pathophysiological book. Pathophysiological principles can be considered scientific theory. In the literature review section, Brand and colleagues described four studies in detail because these studies were the most pertinent to the research problem. They also cited the statistical software that was used, two clinical summaries of anxiety-minimizing nursing interventions, and three journal articles to support the reliability, validity, and scoring of the visual analog (also spelled analogue) scale used to measure anxiety.

2. Currency of Sources

Twenty (71%) of the references were published in the past 10 years (in or since 2003) and 10 (36%) were published in the past 5 years (in or since 2008). Brand and associates (2013) cited Cline and co-workers (1992) to support how to use the visual analog scale. Cline and colleagues (1992) is a landmark article and the authority on scoring visual analog scales. The only concern is that four of the articles cited as research findings were older than 10 years. A search of CINAHL revealed four articles published since 2009 about hand massage and stress that were not included in the reference list, but none specifically addressed hand massage and anxiety.

3. Breadth of the Review

The journals cited were primarily nursing journals (20 of 24 journal citations), and most authors were nurses. The nursing journal citations were split evenly between journals published in the United States and journals published in Britain. Three of the non-nursing journals were medical and one was a journal with a focus on health quality of life outcomes. The researchers searched databases other than CINAHL, because not all the cited publications are included in CINAHL. A search of four other health-related databases only revealed one additional article with possible relevance for the study.

Continued

RESEARCH EXAMPLE—cont'd

4. Synthesis of Strengths and Weaknesses of Available Evidence

In the review, Brand and associates (2013) indicated the studies that included random assignment to groups were an indication of more rigorous study designs. As noted, they cited three research reviews and indicated the number of studies in each review. They focused their discussion of the studies, however, on the applicability and feasibility of using the interventions, rather than on the strength of the studies.

The review was organized with the first paragraph describing the changes that have occurred in health care that made this an important study to conduct. Subsequent paragraphs reviewed the literature related to causes and effects of anxiety, the negative consequences of anxiety, and the connection between preoperative anxiety and postoperative pain. The last half of the review consisted of the research on the effects of anxiety-reducing interventions. Brand and co-workers (2013) concluded the review by providing their rationale for using hand massage as an intervention for preoperative and preprocedure anxiety. They did note that previous studies had indicated that "significant psychological and physiological changes take place after hand massage" (p. 710). The review provided a logical argument supporting the selection of the intervention for the study and the purpose of the study. The logical argument is a strength of the review, which was longer than is often allowed in a journal. The review could have been strengthened by Brand and colleagues (2013) by providing critical appraisal information about the cited studies and identifying the type of research syntheses included, such as a systematic review or meta-analysis (see Chapters 1 and 13).

Summary of the Study and Its Findings

Brand and associates (2013) developed a hand massage procedure and a script for obtaining informed consent. Nurses were trained to do hand massage following the procedure. Of the 101 recruited subjects, 15 (14%) did not complete the post-test measurement, resulting in a sample of 86 subjects with complete data. The change in the pretest and post-test anxiety level of subjects in the intervention group ($n=45$) was statistically significant. The change in pretest and post-test anxiety of subjects in the control group ($n=41$) was not statistically significant. Pretest anxiety levels of the two groups were statistically equivalent. However, the difference in post-test anxiety levels of the intervention group and control group was statistically significant, indicating that hand massage reduced anxiety. An unexpected observation was that the insertion of the preoperative intravenous access was easier to complete in the intervention group, explained as being a result of the hand massage warming the hands and causing vasodilation. Brand and co-workers (2013) recommended future multisite studies with larger and more culturally and gender diverse samples.

Implications for Practice

One relatively small study is not adequate evidence to support a recommendation for using hand massage to lower anxiety in all preoperative patients. Hand massage, however, has few contraindications and is a low-cost, easily implemented intervention within the scope of nurses. Individual nurses might choose to learn hand massage techniques and use the intervention in practice to reduce the anxiety of preoperative patients. Consistent with Quality and Safety Education for Nurses (QSEN) competencies, using hand massage to reduce anxiety in preoperative patients is an example of providing patient-centered care and contributing to safety by reducing the likelihood of anxiety-related complications in cardiac patients undergoing day surgery (QSEN, 2013).

Critical Appraisal of a Literature Review in a Qualitative Study

In Chapter 3, a qualitative study conducted by Trollvik, Nordbach, Silen, and Ringsberg (2011) was used as an example of phenomenology. The research report of their study of children's perceptions of living with asthma does not have a section titled "Literature Review." Trollvik and colleagues (2011) cited references primarily in the background and discussion sections. The background section and reference list are included here as an example of critical appraisal of the literature review in a qualitative study (pp. 295-296, 303). The discussion section was not included because the focus of this chapter is on the literature review.

⚡ RESEARCH EXAMPLE

Example Literature Review (2011)

Background

"Asthma is the most common childhood disease and long-term medical condition affecting children (Masoli, Fabian, Holt, Beasley, & Global Initiative for Asthma [GINA] Program, 2004). The prevalence of asthma is increasing, and atopic diseases are considered to be a worldwide health problem and an agent of morbidity in children (Masoli et al., 2004). A Norwegian cohort study among 10-year-old children concluded that lifetime prevalence of asthma was 20.2%, current asthma was 11.1%, and doctor diagnosis of asthma was 16.1%, the highest number ever reported in Scandinavia; boys are more affected than girls (Carlsen et al., 2006). A Nordic study of children aged 2-17 years found that asthma, allergies, and eczema were the most commonly reported long-term illnesses (Berntsson, 2000). Many children and their families are thus affected by asthma directly or indirectly. Rydström, Englund, and Sandman (1999) found that children with asthma show signs of uncertainty, guilt, and fear and sometimes they felt like participants, other times like outsiders, in everyday life. Studies show that children with asthma have more emotional/behavioral problems than healthy children (Reichenberg & Broberg, 2004). Chiang, Huang, and Fu (2006) observed that children with asthma, especially girls, participate less in physical activity. It has also been found that asthma control in children is poor and that health care professionals (HCPs) and children focus on different aspects of having asthma (Price et al., 2002); HCPs focus on symptoms, whereas children focus on activity limitations. Guyatt, Juniper, Griffith, Feeny, and Ferrie (1997) stated that children as young as 7 years are able to accurately report changes in symptoms for periods as long as 1 month. These studies, however, are mainly from a caregiver's perspective than from the perspective of the child's own experience. Few studies have considered very young children's, 7-10 years old, perspectives; this study might contribute to new insights into their lifeworld experiences. The aim of the study was to explore and describe children's everyday experiences of living with asthma to tailor an Asthma Education Program based on their perspectives."

References

"Antonovsky, A. (1996). The salutogenic model as a theory to guide health promotion. *Health Promotion International, 11*, 11 – 18. http://dx.doi.org/10.1093/heapro/11.1.7.

Berntsson, L. (2000). *Health and well-being of children in the five Nordic countries in 1984 and 1996.* (Doctoral thesis). Gothenburg, Sweden: Nordic School of Public Health.

Canham, D. L., Bauer, L., Concepcion, M., Luong, J., Peters, J., & Wilde, C. (2007). An audit of medication administration: A glimpse into school health offices. *Journal of School Nursing, 23*, 21 – 27. http://dx.doi.org/10.1177/10598405070230010401.

Carlsen, K., Haland, G., Devulapalli, C., Munthe-Kaas, M., Pettersen, M., Granum, B., et al. (2006). Asthma in every fifth child in Oslo, Norway: A 10-year follow up of a birth cohort study. *Allergy: European Journal of Allergy & Clinical Immunology, 61*, 454 – 460. http://dx.doi.org/10.1111/j.1398- 9995.2005.00938.

Chiang, L. C., Huang, J. L., & Fu, L. S. (2006). Physical activity and physical self-concept: Comparison between children with and without asthma. *Journal of Advanced Nursing, 54*, 653 – 662. http://dx.doi.org/ 10.1111/ j.1365-2648.2006.03873.

Christensen, P., & James, A. (2008). *Research with children. Perspectives and practices* (2nd ed.). London: Routledge.

Dahlberg, K. M. E., & Dahlberg, H. K. (2004). Description vs. interpretation—A new understanding of an old dilemma in human research. *Nursing Philosophy, 5*, 268 – 273. http://dx.doi.org/10.1111/j.1466-769X. 2004.00180.

Darbyshire, P., MacDougall, C., & Schiller, W. (2005). Multiple methods in qualitative research with children: More insight or just more? *Qualitative Research, 5*, 417. http://dx.doi.org/10.1177/ 1468794105056921.

Continued

RESEARCH EXAMPLE—cont'd

Driessnack, M. (2005). Children's drawings as facilitators of communication: A meta-analysis. *Journal of Pediatric Nursing, 20,* 415–423. http://dx.doi.org/10.1016/j.pedn.2005.03.011.

Guyatt, G. H., Juniper, E. F., Griffith, L. E., Feeny, D. H., & Ferrie, P. J. (1997). Children and adult perceptions of childhood asthma. *Pediatrics, 99,* 165–168. http://dx.doi.org/10.1542/peds.99.2.165.

Hummelvoll, J. K., & Barbosa da Silva, A. (1998). The use of the qualitative research interview to uncover the essence of community psychiatric nursing. *Journal of Holistic Nursing, 16,* 453–477. http://dx.doi.org/10.1177/089801019801600406.

Kirk, S. (2007). Methodological and ethical issues in conducting qualitative research with children and young people: A literature review. *International Journal of Nursing Studies, 44,* 1250–1260. http://dx.doi.org/10.1016/j.ijnurstu.2006.08.015.

Kvale, S. (1997). *Interviews. An introduction to qualitative research interviewing.* London: Sage Publications.

Masoli, M., Fabian, D., Holt, S., Beasley, R., & Global Initiative for Asthma (GINA) Program. (2004). The global burden of asthma: Executive summary of the GINA Dissemination Committee Report. *Allergy, 59,* 469–478. http://dx.doi.org/10.1111/j.1398-9995.2004.00526.

McCann, D., McWhirter, J., Coleman, H., Devall, I., Calvert, M., Weare, K., et al. (2002). The prevalence and management of asthma in primary-aged schoolchildren in the south of England. *Health Education Research, 17*(2), 181–194.

Merleau-Ponty, M. (2004). *Phenomenology of perception.* London: Routledge.

Patton, M. Q. (2002). *Qualitative research and evaluation methods* (3rd ed.). Thousand Oaks, CA: Sage Publications.

Price, D., Ryan, D., Pearce, L., Bawden, R., Freeman, D., Thomas, M., et al. (2002). The burden of paediatric asthma is higher than health professionals think: Results from the Asthma In Real Life (AIR) study. *Primary Care Respiratory Journal, 11*(2), 30–33.

Reichenberg, K., & Broberg, A. (2004). Emotional and behavioural problems in Swedish 7- to 9-year olds with asthma. *Chronic Respiratory Disease, 1,* 183–189. http://dx.doi.org/10.1191/1479972304cd041oa.

Rootman, I., Goodstadt, M., Hyndman, B., McQueen, D., Potvin, L., & Springett, J. (2001). *Evaluation in health promotion: Principles and perspectives.* Copenhagen: WHO Regional Office Europe.

Rydström, I., Englund, A. C., & Sandman, P. O. (1999). Being a child with asthma. *Pediatric Nursing, 25*(6), 589–90, 593–596.

Sällfors, C., Hallberg, L., & Fasth, A. (2001). Coping with chronic pain: In-depth interviews with children suffering from juvenile chronic arthritis. *Scandinavian Journal of Disability Research, 3,* 3–20. http://dx.doi.org/10.1080/15017410109510765.

The Act of 2 July 1999 No. 63 relating to Patients' Rights (the Patients' Rights Act). (1999). *Norwegian government.* Retrieved March 16, 2010 from http://www.ub.uio.no/ujur/ulovdata/lov-19990702-063-eng.pdf.

Trollvik, A., & Severinsson, E. (2005). Influence of an Asthma Education Program on parents with children suffering from asthma. *Nursing & Health Sciences, 7,* 157–163. http://dx.doi.org/10.1111/j.1442-2018.2005.00235.

UNICEF. (2008). *Convention on the rights of the child.* Retrieved May 20, 2010 from http://www2.ohchr.org/english/law/pdf/crc.pdf.

Woodgate, R. (2009). The experience of dyspnea in school-age children with asthma. *American Journal of Maternal/Child Nursing, 34,* 154–161. http://dx.doi.org/10.1097/01.NMC.0000351702.58632.9e.

Williams, C. (2000). Doing health, doing gender: Teenagers, diabetes and asthma. *Social Science & Medicine, 50,* 387–396. http://dx.doi.org/10.1016/S0277- 9536(99)00340-8." Trollvik et al., 2011, p. 303

Critical Appraisal

1. Inclusion of Relevant Literature

Of the 27 references cited by Trollvik and associates (2011) in their research report, 15 (55%) were citations of studies or database sources. Most of the total references (70%) were journal articles. One theoretical source (Antonovky, 1996), the oldest reference, was cited in the discussion as an explanation of one of the findings. A theoretical framework was not identified, as is often the case with phenomenological studies (Munhall, 2012). Trollvik and co-workers (2011) described the philosophical orientation and qualitative approach of phenomenology in the methods section. Four books and one statistical analysis software were cited in the methods section. A government website and a website of an international organization were cited as well.

2. Currency of Sources

Eight citations were publications older than 10 years. The remainder (70%) were cited in the 10 years prior to the article's publication (in or since 2001), but only seven publications (26%) were cited in the 5 years prior to the publication (in or since 2006). Because qualitative researchers often study topics that have been rarely researched, it is not uncommon for the literature they cite to be older. As noted earlier, Antonovsky (1996) was the oldest reference cited. Inclusion of this older article is appropriate because his theory was a landmark publication and was one of the first theories to describe health as more than the absence of disease.

3. Breadth of the Review

The authors and journals cited were from multiple disciplines, with nursing journals cited seven times and medical journals cited eight times. The researchers had searched databases outside of nursing to find these references. The multidisciplinary nature of the journals cited are an indication that other health professionals and scientists from other disciplines authored the cited publications.

4. Synthesis of Strengths and Weaknesses of Available Evidence

Although Trollvik and colleagues (2011) included little detail about the strengths and weaknesses of the cited studies, they did acknowledge, as a major threat to the validity of previous studies, that the studies had been conducted on the perspective of parents, rather than the children living with asthma. Selected studies were reviewed prior to the discussion of the method, with additional references cited in the discussion of the findings. Trollvik and associates (2011) clearly described the need for the study in terms of disease prevalence. The last few sentences of the background section identified the research problem as the logical conclusion of the review. The research problem was directly linked to the purpose of the study and the potential contribution of the study's findings.

Summary of the Study and Its Findings

In interviews, 15 children were asked to describe their experiences with asthma in daily life. The interviewers also asked the children to describe their feelings and body sensations of asthma and how they communicated with teachers and peers about having asthma. Of these children, 14 drew a picture about living daily with asthma as another source of data. Trollvik and co-workers (2011, p. 297) found two major themes, "fear of exacerbation and fear of being ostracized." See Chapter 3 for more information about the study.

Implications for Practice

Trollvik and colleagues (2011, p. 302) identified that "using drawing . . . is a good tool for initiating a dialogue and gaining access to children's inner thoughts." They also emphasized the need to develop asthma patient education in collaboration with children with asthma to ensure that the education meets their needs. Including patients in the developing of teaching materials is an example of incorporating the QSEN competency of patient-centered care into practice (QSEN, 2013).

REVIEW

Searching professional electronic databases has many advantages, but one challenge is that you will have to select relevant sources from a much larger number of articles. You can narrow the number of articles and retrieve fewer but relevant articles by using keywords to search. Keywords are terms that serve as labels for publications on a topic. For example, a quasi-experimental study of providing text message reminders to patients living with heart failure who are taking five or more medications might be found by searching for keywords, such as electronic communication, instant messaging, medication adherence, patient teaching, quasi-experimental designs, and heart failure. When you find one article on your topic, look under the abstract to determine whether the search terms are listed. Using search terms or keywords to search is a skill you can teach yourself, but also remember that a librarian is an information specialist. Consulting a librarian may save you time and make searching more effective.

Conducting the Literature Review

Search the selected databases. The actual search of the databases may be the easiest step of the process. One method of decreasing the time to search is to search multiple databases simultaneously, an approach that is possible when several databases are available within a search engine, such as Elton B. Stephens Company host (EBSCOhost). To avoid duplicating your work, keep a list of searches that you have completed. This is especially important if you have limited time and will be searching in several short sessions, instead of one long one.

Use a table or other method to document the results of your search. A very simple way to document your search is to use a table, such as that shown in Table 6-2. On the table, you will record the search terms, time frame you used, and the results. With most electronic databases, you can sign up for an account and keep your search history. Reference management software, such as RefWorks (http://www.refworks.com) and EndNotes (http://www.endnote.com), can make tracking the references you have obtained through your searches considerably easier. You can use reference management software to conduct searches and store the information on all search fields for each reference obtained in a search. Within the software, you can store articles in folders with other similar articles. For example, you may have a folder for theory sources, another for methodological sources, and a third for relevant research topics. As you read the articles, you can also insert comments into the reference file about each one. By exporting search results from the bibliographic database to your reference management software, all the needed citation information and abstract are readily available to you electronically when you write the literature review.

Refine your Search. As seen in Table 6-2, a search may identify thousands of references, many more than you can read and include in any literature review. Open a few articles that were identified and see what key terms were used. Reconsider the topic and determine how you can narrow

TABLE 6-2 RECORD OF SIMPLE LITERATURE SEARCH FOR PATIENT SAFETY				
DATABASE SEARCHED	DATE OF SEARCH	SEARCH TERMS	YEARS	NO. OF SOURCES FOUND
CINAHL Complete	8/10/2013	Patient safety	2003-2013	28,842
Academic Search Complete	8/10/2013	Patient safety	2003-2013	17,745
Health Source: Nursing/Academic Edition	8/10/2013	Patient safety	2003-2013	7,392

TABLE 6-3   RESULTS OF REFINED SEARCHES FOR PATIENT SAFETY SOURCES

DATABASE SEARCHED	DATE OF SEARCH	SEARCH TERMS AND STRATEGY	YEARS	NO. OF SOURCES FOUND
CINAHL Complete	8/10/2013	• Patient safety	2008-2013	18,788
CINAHL Complete	8/10/2013	• Patient safety *and* nurses	2008-2013	2,917
CINAHL Complete	8/10/2013	• Patient safety *and* nurses • Abstracts only	2008-2013	846
CINAHL Complete	8/10/2013	• Patient safety *and* nurses • Abstracts only • Limited to full text available	2008-2013	336
CINAHL Complete	8/10/2013	• Patient safety *and* nurses *and* older adults • Abstracts only • Limited to full text available	2008-2013	2
CINAHL Complete	8/10/2013	• Patient safety *and* nurses *and* older adults • Limited to full text available	2008-2013	8
CINAHL Complete	8/10/2013	• Patient safety *and* older adults • Limited to full text available	2008-2013	36

your search. One strategy is to decrease the range of years you are searching. Some electronic databases allow you to limit the search to certain types of articles, such as scholarly, peer-reviewed articles. Combining terms or searching for the terms only in the abstracts will decrease the number of articles identified. For undergraduate course assignments, it may be appropriate to limit the search to only full-text articles. The recommendation would be, however, that graduate students avoid limiting searches to full-text articles because doing so might result in missing sources that are needed. Table 6-3 provides the results of patient safety searches in CINAHL using different strategies, including an example of narrowing a search tightly and ending up with few results. When that occurs, you can retry the search with one or more search terms and limitations removed.

Review the abstracts to identify relevant studies. The abstract provides pertinent information about the article. You can easily determine if the article is a research report, description of a clinical problem, or theoretical article, such as a concept analysis. You will identify the articles that seem to be the most relevant to your topic and the purpose of the review. If looking for evidence on which to base clinical practice, you can identify the research reports and select those conducted in settings similar to yours. If writing a literature review for a course assignment, you will review the abstracts to identify different types of information. For example, you may need information on mortality and morbidity, as well as descriptions of available treatments. Mark the abstracts of the relevant studies or save in an electronic folder.

Obtain full-text copies of relevant articles. Using the abstracts of relevant articles, you will retrieve and save the electronic files of full-text articles on your computer to review more thoroughly. You may want to rename the electronic file using a file name that includes the first author's last name and the year or a file name with a descriptive phrase. For articles not available as full-text online, you will search your library's holdings to determine if the journal is available to you in print form. If your library does not have the journal, you may be able to obtain the article through interlibrary loan. Check with your library's website or a librarian to learn the process for using the interlibrary loan system. If you prefer reading print materials to electronic materials, you may choose to print the articles. It is important to obtain the full-text of the article because the abstract does not include the detail needed for a literature review.

Ensure that information needed to cite the source is recorded. As you retrieve and save the articles, note if the article includes all the information needed for the citation. The bibliographic information on a source should be recorded in a systematic manner, according to the format that you will use in the reference list. The purpose for carefully citing sources is that readers can retrieve the reference for themselves, confirm your interpretation of the findings, and gather additional information on the topic. You will need the authors' names, year, article title, journal name, journal volume and issue, and page numbers. If a book chapter has been photocopied or retrieved electronically, ensure that the publisher's name, location, and year of publication are recorded. Notice specifically whether the chapter is in an edited book and if the chapter has an author other than the editor. If you are using an electronic personal bibliographic software such as RefWorks, the software records the citation information for you.

Processing the Literature

Processing the literature is among the more difficult phases of the literature review. This section includes reading the articles and appraising, analyzing, and synthesizing the literature.

Read the articles. As you look at the stack of printed articles or scan the electronic copies of several articles, you may be asking yourself, "Am I expected to read every word of the available sources?" The answer is no. Reading every word of every source would result in you being well read and knowledgeable, but with no time left to prepare the course assignment or paper. With the availability of full-text online articles, you can easily forget the focus of the review. Becoming a skilled reviewer of the literature involves finding a balance and learning to identify the most pertinent and relevant sources. On the other hand, you cannot critically appraise and synthesize what you have not read. Skim over information provided by the author that is not relevant to your task. Learn what is normally included in different sections of an article so you can read the sections pertinent to your task more carefully. Chapter 2 provides you with ideas on how to read the literature.

Comprehending and critically appraising sources leads to an understanding of the current state of knowledge related to a research problem. Although you may skim or only read selected sections of some references that you find, you will want to read the articles most relevant to your topic word for word and probably more than once. Comprehending a source begins by reading and focusing on understanding the main points of the article or other sources. Highlight the content you consider important or make notes in the margins. Record your notes on photocopies or electronic files of articles. The type of information you highlight or note in the margins of a source depends on the type of study or source. With theory articles, you might make note of concepts, definitions, and relationships among the concepts. For a research article, the research problem, purpose, framework, major variables, study design, sample size, measurement methods, data collection, analytical techniques, results, and findings are usually highlighted. You may wish to record quotations (including page numbers) that might be used in a review of a literature section. The decision to paraphrase these quotes can be made later. Also make notes about what you think about the article, such as how this content fits with other information that you have read.

Appraise, analyze, and synthesize the literature. Analysis is required to determine the value of a reference as you make the decision about what information to include in the review. First, you need to appraise the individual studies critically. The process of appraising individual studies is discussed in Chapter 12. To appraise the article critically, you will identify relevant content in the articles and make value judgments about their validity or credibility. However, the critical appraisal of individual studies is only the first step in developing an adequate review of the literature. Any written literature review that simply appraises individual studies paragraph by paragraph is inadequate. A literature review that is a series of paragraphs, in which each paragraph is a description of a single study, with no link to other studies being reviewed, does not provide evidence of adequate analysis of the literature. Refer to the paragraph on preoperative anxiety and postoperative pain in Trollvik and colleagues' (2011) example presented earlier in the chapter. In this paragraph, the researchers described and compared the findings of three studies on the topic, an example of summarizing and synthesizing.

Analysis requires manipulation of what you are finding, literally making it your own (Garrard, 2011). Pinch (1995, 2001) was the first nurse to publish a strategy to synthesize research findings using a literature summary table. More recently, Kable, Pich, and Maslin-Prothero (2012) presented a table to organize studies that are reviewed for possible inclusion into a proposal (Table 6-4). Other examples of literature summary tables are provided in Tables 6-5 and 6-6 to demonstrate how the column headers might vary, depending on the type of research. Table 6-5 contains information from the Brand and associates' (2013) article as an example of using the table. The content in Table 6-6 is from Trollvik and co-workers (2011). If using reference management software, it may allow you to generate summary tables from information you record about each study. Another way to manipulate the information you have retrieved and transform it into knowledge is known as *mapping* (Hart, 2009). Your nursing faculty may have taught you how to map conceptually what you are studying to make connections between facts and principles (Vacek, 2009). The same strategy applied to a literature review is to classify the sources and arrange them into a graphic or diagrammatic format that requires you to become familiar with key concepts (Hart, 2009). The map may connect studies with similar methodologies or key ideas.

As you continue to analyze the literature you have found, you will make comparisons among the studies. This analysis allows you to appraise the existing body of knowledge critically in relation to the research problem. You may want to record theories that have been used, methods that have been used to study the problem, and any flaws with these theories and methods. You will begin to work toward summarizing what you have found by describing what is known and what is not known about the problem. The information gathered by using the table formats shown in Tables 6-5 and 6-6 or displayed in a conceptual map can be useful in making these comparisons. Pay special attention to conflicting findings, because they may provide clues for gaps in knowledge that represent researchable problems.

TABLE 6-4 **EXAMPLE OF LITERATURE SUMMARY TABLE FOR STUDIES**				
AUTHOR (YEAR), AND COUNTRY	**STUDY DESIGN**	**SAMPLE SIZE AND SITE**	**COMMENTS AND KEY FINDINGS**	**QUALITY APPRAISAL: INCLUDE, EXCLUDE**

Adapted from Kabe, A., Pich, J. & Maslin-Prothero, S. (2012). A structured approach to documenting a search strategy for publication: A 12-step guideline for authors. *Nurse Education Today, 32*(8), 882.

TABLE 6-5 LITERATURE SUMMARY TABLE FOR QUANTITATIVE STUDIES

AUTHOR, YEAR	PURPOSE	FRAMEWORK	SAMPLE	MEASURES	TREATMENT	RESULTS	FINDINGS
Brand et al., 2013	"Determine the effects of hand massage on patient anxiety in the ambulatory surgery setting" (p. 708).	Watson's human caring theory	86 patients	Demographic data; VAS for anxiety	Hand massage	Intervention group had significantly lower anxiety ($t = 4.85$; $p = .000$).	"Pre-operative hand massage has a significant effect on patient-reported anxiety" (p. 715).

TABLE 6-6 LITERATURE SUMMARY TABLE FOR QUALITATIVE STUDIES

AUTHOR AND YEAR	PURPOSE	QUALITATIVE APPROACH	SAMPLE	DATA COLLECTION	KEY FINDINGS	COMMENTS
Trollvik et al. (2011)	"Explore children's experiences of asthma to tailor a learning program based on their perspectives" (p. 295).	Phenomenology	14 children with asthma, 9 boys and 6 girls	Interviews. Drawing by the child of a situation described in the interview	Fear of exacerbation (subthemes of bodily sensations, frightening experiences, loss of control) Fear of being ostracized (subthemes of being excluded, dilemma about keeping asthma a secret)	Supports need for including children in developing of patient education

The sources to be included in your research proposal can be organized by the section in which you plan to cite them. For example, sources that provide background and significance for the study are included in the introduction. You may decide to include theoretical sources to describe the framework for the study. Methodologically strong studies may be cited to support the development of the research design, guide the selection of data collection, whether by survey or interview, and plans for data analysis.

The synthesis of sources involves thinking deeply about what you have found and identifying the main themes of information that you want to present. Through synthesis, you will cluster and describe connections among what you have found (Hart, 2009). From the clusters of connections, you can begin to draw some conclusions about what is known and make additional connections to the topic being studied. Note these sentences from the review of the literature in the Brand and colleagues' (2013) article: "Anxiety can also have a major effect on psychological symptoms and can inhibit learning, concentration, and routine tasks (Gilmartin & Wright, 2008; Vaughn, Wichowski, & Bosworth, 2007). Keeping anxiety to a minimum is important because, if patients are anxious, then they may not be able to retain important home care instructions" (Brand et al., 2013, p. 709). Brand and associates (2013) synthesized information from two articles to make a conclusion and link the information to the significance of studying anxiety in this population.

One strategy for synthesizing is to review the tables or mind maps that you have developed and make a list of findings that are similar and those that are different. For example, you have read five intervention studies of end-of-life care in children with leukemia. As you review your notes, you notice that four studies were conducted in home settings with samples of children from ages 7 to 10 years and had similar statistically significant results when using a parent-administered intervention. The remaining study, with nonsignificant results, also used a parent-administered intervention, but was set in an inpatient hospice unit and had a sample of younger children. The main ideas that you identify may be that the effectiveness of parent-administered interventions may vary, depending on the setting and age of the child. Another strategy for synthesis is to talk about the articles you have reviewed with another student, nurse, or friend. Verbalizing the characteristics of the studies and explaining them to another person can cause you to think differently about the studies than you do when you are reading your notes. Your enhanced thinking may result in the identification of main ideas or conclusions of the review.

Writing the Review of the Literature

Talking about the main ideas of the review can prepare you for the final steps of writing the literature review. Step 11 is organizing your information by developing an outline prior to writing the major sections of the review. The final steps are creating the reference list and checking the review and reference list for correctness.

Develop an outline to organize the information from the review. Before beginning to write your review, develop an outline based on your synthesis of what you have read using the sections of the review as major headings in the outline. Depending on the purpose of the written literature review, you will determine what the major sections of the paper will be. Frequently, a comprehensive literature review has four major sections: (1) introduction; (2) discussion of theoretical literature; (3) discussion of empirical literature; and (4) summary. The introduction and summary are standard sections, but the discussion of sources should be organized by the main ideas that you have identified or the concepts of the theoretical framework you will use in the study. Under the major headings of the outline, make notes about which sources you want to mention in the different sections of the paper. The introduction will include the focus or purpose of the review and present the organizational structure of the review. In this section, you should make clear what you will and will not be covering.

The discussion section may be divided into theoretical and empirical subsections or divided by the themes of the review findings. A theoretical literature section might include concept analyses, models, theories, or conceptual frameworks relevant to the topic. The empirical section, if it is a separate section, will include the research findings of the articles reviewed. In addition to the synthesis, you want to incorporate the strengths and weaknesses of the overall body of knowledge, rather than a detailed presentation and critical appraisal of each study. In the summary section of the outline, make notes of your conclusions. A conclusion is a statement about the state of knowledge in relation to the topic area.

Write each section of the review. Start each paragraph with a theme sentence that describes the main idea of the paragraph. Present the relevant studies in each paragraph that support the main idea stated in the theme sentence. End each paragraph with a concluding sentence that transitions to the next claim. Each paragraph can be compared to a train with an engine (theme sentence), freight cars connected to each other (sentences with evidence), and a caboose (summary sentence linking to next paragraph).

Avoid using direct quotes from an author. Your analysis and synthesis of the sources will allow you to paraphrase the authors' ideas. Paraphrasing involves expressing the ideas clearly and in your own words. The meanings of these sources are then connected to the proposed study. If the written review is not clear or cohesive, you may need to look at your notes and sources again to ensure that you have synthesized the literature adequately. The defects of a study or body of knowledge need to be described, but maintain a respectful tone and avoid being highly critical of other researchers' work.

As you near the end of the review, write the summary as a concise presentation of the current knowledge base for the research problem. The findings from the studies will have been logically presented in the previous sections so that the reader can see how the body of knowledge in the research area evolved. You will make conclusions about the gaps in the knowledge base. You may also conclude with the potential contribution of the proposed study to the body of knowledge.

Create the reference list. Many journals and academic institutions use the format developed by the APA (2010). The sixth edition of the *APA Publication Manual* (2010) provides revised guidelines for citing electronic sources and direct quotations from electronic sources and for creating the reference list. The APA standard for direct quotations from a print source is to cite the page of the source on which the quotation appears. The reference lists in this text are presented in APA format, with the exception that we have not included digital object identifiers (DOIs). Digital object identifiers (DOIs) have become standard for the International Standards Organization (http://www.doi.org), but have not yet received universal support. The use of DOIs seems to be gaining in credibility because the DOI "provides a means of persistent identification for managing information on digital networks" (APA, 2010, p. 188). CrossRef is a registration agency for DOIs so that citations can be linked across databases and disciplines (http://www.crossref.org).

The sources included in the list of the references are only those that were cited in the paper. Each citation on an APA-style reference list is formatted as a paragraph with a hanging indent, meaning that the first line is on the left margin and subsequent lines are indented (see citation examples below). If you do not know how to format a paragraph this way, search the Help tool in your word processing program to find the correct command to use. The inclusion of an article published in a print journal in a reference list includes the journal number, volume, and issue. For most journals, the numbering of the volumes of the journal represents all the articles published during a specific year. APA (2010) has requirements for formatting each component of the entry in the reference list for a journal article. Table 6-7 presents the components of common references with the correct formatting.

TABLE 6-7	AMERICAN PSYCHOLOGICAL ASSOCIATION FORMATTING OF CITATIONS		
REFERENCE COMPONENT	**TYPE OF FONT**	**CAPITALIZATION**	**EXAMPLE**
Article title	Regular font	• First word of title and subtitle • Proper nouns	Nursing students' fears of failing NCLEX Grounded theory methods: Similarities and differences.
Journal title	Italicized font	• All key words	*Journal of Clinical Information Systems Health Promotion Journal*
Book title	Italicized font	• First word of title and subtitle • Proper nouns	*Qualitative methods: Grounded theory expanded.* *Human resources for health in Uganda.*

An entry on a reference list for a book is listed by the author and includes the publisher and its location. The University Press, located in Boulder, Colorado, published a revised edition of Dr. Watson's philosophy of nursing in 2008. The entry on the reference list would be as follows:

Watson, J. (2008). *Nursing. The philosophy and science of caring* (Revised ed.). Boulder, CO: University Press of Colorado.

Some chapters are compiled by editors, with each chapter having its own author(s). The chapter by Wolf on ethnography is in a qualitative research book edited by Munhall (2012). The chapter title is formatted like an article title and the page numbers of the chapter are included:

Wolf, M. (2012). Ethnography: The method. In P. L. Munhall (Ed.), *Nursing research: A qualitative perspective* (5th ed.) (pp. 285-338). Sudbury, MA: Jones & Bartlett.

When you retrieve an electronic source in *p*ortable *d*ocument *f*ormat (pdf), you cite the source in the same way as if you had made a copy of the print version of the article. When you retrieve an electronic source in html (*h*yper*t*ext *m*arkup *l*anguage) format, you will not have page numbers for the citation. Providing the URL (*u*niform *r*esource *l*ocator) that you used to retrieve the article is not helpful because it is unique to the path you used to find the article and reflects your search engines and bibliographic databases. The updated APA standard is to provide the URL for the home page of the journal from which the reader can navigate and find the source.

Check the review and the reference list. You may complete the first draft of your review of the literature and feel a sense of accomplishment. Before you leave the review behind, a few tasks remain that will ensure the quality of your written review. Begin by rereading the review. It is best to delay this step for a day or at least a few hours to allow you to take a fresh look at the final written product. One way to identify awkward sentences or disjointed paragraphs is to read the review aloud. Ask a fellow student or trusted colleague to read the review and provide constructive feedback.

A critical final step is to compare the sources cited in the paper to the reference list. Be sure that the authors' names and year of publication match. If you are missing sources on the reference list, add them. If you have sources on the reference list that you did not cite, you can remove them. Downloading citations from a database directly into a reference management system and using the system's manuscript formatting functions reduce some errors but do not eliminate all of them. You want your references to be accurate as a reflection of your attention to detail and quality of your work.

KEY CONCEPTS

- The review of literature in a research report is a summary of current knowledge about a particular practice problem and includes what is known and not known about this problem.
- The literature is reviewed to complete an assignment for a course and summarize knowledge for use in practice.
- Reviews of the literature can be critically appraised for their relevance, comprehensiveness, and inclusion of current studies.
- A checklist for reviewing the literature includes preparing, conducting the search, processing the information, and writing the review.
- Electronic databases to be searched are selected based on the types of sources that they include and the fit of those sources to the purpose of the literature review being conducted.
- The size and efficiency of electronic databases allows for the identification of a large number of sources quickly.
- Keywords and search terms will allow you to find more relevant references when you search databases.
- Consult a librarian to help you identify relevant references.
- Reference management software should be used to track the references obtained through the searches.
- The articles to be included in a review can be further limited by reviewing the abstracts.
- A literature summary table or conceptual map can be used to help you process the information in numerous studies and identify the main ideas.
- The literature review usually begins with an introduction, includes database sources, and concludes with a summary of current knowledge.
- Well-written literature reviews are syntheses of what is known and not known.
- Careful checking of the review for grammatical correctness and logical flow are essential to producing a quality product.
- The reference list must be accurate and complete to allow readers to retrieve the cited sources.

REFERENCES

American Nurses Credentialing Center, (2013). *Magnet: Program overview.* Silver Springs, MD: Author, a subsidiary of American Nurses Association. Retrieved July 17, 2013 from, *http://www.nursecredentialing.org/ Magnet/ProgramOverview.*

American Psychological Association (APA), (2010). *Publication manual of the American Psychological Association* (6th ed.). Washington, DC: Author.

Brand, L., Munroe, D., & Gavin, J. (2013). The effect of hand massage on preoperative anxiety in ambulatory surgery patients. *AORN Journal, 97*(6), 708–716.

Corbin, J., & Strauss, A. (2008). *Basics of qualitative research* (3rd ed.). Thousand Oaks, CA: Sage.

Creswell, J. (2013). *Qualitative inquiry & research design: Choosing among five approaches* (3rd ed.). Thousand Oaks, CA: Sage.

Fawcett, J., & Garity, J. (2009). *Evaluating research for evidence-based nursing practice.* Philadelphia: F. A. Davis.

Garrard, J. (2011). *Health sciences literature review made easy: The matrix method* (3rd ed.). Sudbury, MA: Jones & Bartlett.

Grove, S. K., Burns, N., & Gray, J. (2013). *The practice of nursing research: Conduct, critique, and utilization* (7th ed.). St. Louis: Elsevier Saunders.

Hart, C. (2009). *Doing a literature review: Releasing the social science imagination.* Thousand Oaks, CA: Sage.

Kable, A., Pich, J., & Maslin-Prothero, S. (2012). A structured approach to documenting a search strategy for publication: A 12-step guideline for authors. *Nurse Education Today, 32*(8), 878–886.

Lundy, K. (2012). Historical research. In P. L. Munhall (Ed.), *Nursing research: A qualitative perspective* (pp. 381–399). (5th ed.). Sudbury, MA: Jones & Bartlett.

Luyt, B., Ally, Y., Low, N., & Ismail, N. (2010). Librarian perception of Wikipedia: Threats or opportunities for librarianship? *Libri, 60*(1), 57–64.

Munhall, P. L. (2012). *Nursing research: A qualitative perspective* (5th ed.). Sudbury, MA: Jones & Bartlett.

O'Mathuna, D. P., Fineout-Overholt, E., & Jonston, L. (2011). Critically appraising quantitative evidence for clinical decision making. In B. M. Melnyk & E. Fineout-Overholt (Eds.), *Evidence-based practice in nursing & healthcare: A guide to best practice* (pp. 81–134). (2nd ed.). Philadelphia: Lippincott Williams & Wilkins.

Pinch, W. J. (1995). Synthesis: Implementing a complex process. *Nurse Educator, 20*(1), 34–40.

Pinch, W. J. (2001). Improving patient care through use of research. *Orthopaedic Nursing, 20*(4), 75–81.

Quality and Safety Education for Nurses (QSEN), (2013). *Pre-licensure knowledge, skills, and attitudes (KSAs).* Retrieved August 10, 2013 from, http://qsen.org/competencies/pre-licensure-ksas/.

Trollvik, A., Nordbach, R., Silen, C., & Ringsberg, K. C. (2011). Children's experiences of living with asthma: Fear of exacerbations and being ostracized. *Journal of Pediatric Nursing, 26*(4), 295–303.

Vacek, J. E. (2009). Using a conceptual approach with a concept map of psychosis as an exemplar to promote critical thinking. *Journal of Nursing Education, 48*(1), 49–53.

Walls, P., Pahoo, K., & Fleming, P. (2010). The role and place of knowledge and literature in grounded theory. *Nurse Researcher, 17*(4), 8–17.

Watson, J. (2008). *Nursing. The philosophy and science of caring* (Revised ed.). Boulder, CO: University Press of Colorado.

Wolf, M. (2012). Ethnography: The method. In P. L. Munhall (Ed.), *Nursing research: A qualitative perspective* (pp. 285–338). (5th ed). Sudbury, MA: Jones & Bartlett.

Wuerst, J. (2012). Grounded theory: The method. In P. L. Munhall (Ed.), *Nursing research: A qualitative perspective* (pp. 225–256). (5th ed.). Sudbury, MA: Jones & Bartlett.

Younger, P. (2010). Using wikis as an online health information resource. *Nursing Standard, 24*(36), 49–56.

Understanding Theory and Research Frameworks

CHAPTER OVERVIEW

LEARNING OUTCOMES

After completing this chapter, you should be able to:

1. Define theory and the elements of theory (concepts, relational statements, and propositions).
2. Distinguish between the levels of theoretical thinking.
3. Describe the use of middle range theories as frameworks for studies.
4. Describe the purpose of a study framework.
5. Identify study frameworks developed from nursing theories.
6. Critically appraise the frameworks in published studies.

KEY TERMS

Abstract, p. 190
Assumptions, p. 191
Concepts, p. 190
Conceptual definition, p. 192
Conceptual models, p. 194
Concrete, p. 190
Constructs, p. 191
Framework, p. 198
Grand nursing theories, p. 194

Implicit framework, p. 198
Maps or models, p. 198
Middle range theories, p. 195
Phenomenon (phenomena), p. 190
Philosophies, p. 191
Practice theories, p. 197
Propositions, p. 193
Relational statement, p. 193

Scientific theory, p. 198
Specific proposition, p. 193
Statements, p. 190
Substantive theories, p. 196
Tentative theory, p. 198
Theory, p. 190
Variables, p. 191

Theories are the ideas and knowledge of science. In a psychology course, you may have studied theories of the mind, defense mechanisms, and cognitive development that provide explanations of thinking and behavior. In nursing, we also have theories that provide explanations, but our theories explain human responses to illness and other phenomena important to clinical practice. For example, nursing has a theory of using music and movement to improve health outcomes (Murrock & Higgins, 2009). A theory of adaptation to chronic pain (Dunn, 2004, 2005) has also been developed, as well as a theory of unpleasant symptoms (Lenz, Pugh, Milligan, Gift, & Suppe, 1997). With the increased focus on quality and safety (Sherwood & Barnsteiner, 2012), a theory has been developed to describe a culture of safety in a hospital (Groves, Meisenbach, & Scott-Cawiezell, 2011). Theories guide nurses in clinical practice and in conducting research.

As a researcher develops a plan for conducting a quantitative study, the theory on which the study is based is expressed as the framework for the study. A study framework is a brief explanation of a theory or those portions of a theory that are to be tested in a study. The major ideas of the study, called concepts, are included in the framework. The framework with the concepts and their connections to each other may be described in words or in a diagram. When the study is conducted, the researcher can then answer the question, "Was this theory correct in its description of reality?" Thus a study tests the accuracy of theoretical ideas proposed in the theory. In explaining the study findings, the researcher will interpret those findings in relation to the theory (Grove, Burns, & Gray, 2013).

Qualitative studies may be based on a theory or may be designed to create a theory. Because the assumptions and underlying philosophy of qualitative research (see Chapter 3) are not the same as quantitative research, the focus of this chapter is on theory as related to quantitative studies. To assist you in learning about theories and their use in research, the elements of theory are described, types of theories are identified, and how theories provide frameworks for studies are discussed. You may notice that references in this chapter are older, because we cited primary sources for the theories, many of which were developed 10 or more years ago. You are also provided with guidelines for critically appraising study frameworks, and these guidelines are applied to a variety of frameworks from published studies.

WHAT IS A THEORY?

Scientific professions, such as nursing, use theories to organize their body of knowledge and establish what is known about a phenomenon. Formally, a theory is defined as a set of concepts and statements that present a view of a phenomenon. Concepts are terms that abstractly describe and name an object, idea, experience, or phenomenon, thus providing it with a separate identity or meaning. Concepts are defined in a particular way to present the ideas relevant to a theory. For example Dunn (2004, 2005) developed definitions for the concepts of adaptation and chronic pain in her theory. The statements in a theory describe how the concepts are connected to each other. A phenomenon (the plural form is phenomena) is the appearance, objects, and aspects of reality as we experience them (Rodgers, 2005). You may understand the phenomenon of taking an examination in a course or the phenomenon of receiving news of your acceptance into nursing school. As nurses, we intervene in the phenomena of pain, fear, and uncertainty of our patients.

Theories are abstract, rather than concrete. When you hear the term *social support,* you have an idea about what the phrase means and how you have observed or experienced social support in different situations. The concept of social support is abstract, which means that the concept is the expression of an idea, apart from any specific instance. An abstract idea focuses on a general view of a phenomenon. Concrete refers to realities or actual instances—it focuses on the particular, rather than on the general. For example, a concrete instance of social support might be a time when a friend listened to your frustrations about a difficult clinical situation.

At the abstract level, you may also encounter a philosophy. Philosophies are rational intellectual explorations of truths or principles of being, knowledge, or conduct. Philosophies describe viewpoints on what reality is, how knowledge is developed, and which ethical values and principles should guide our practice. Other abstract components of philosophies and theories are assumptions, which are statements that are taken for granted or considered true, even though they have not been scientifically tested. For example, a fairly common assumption made by nurses is that "People want to assume control of their own health problems." Your clinical experiences may give you reason to accept or doubt the truth of assumptions. Nonetheless, theorists begin with some assumptions, explicit or implicit.

UNDERSTANDING THE ELEMENTS OF THEORY

To understand theories, you need to be familiar with their components–concepts and relational statements. Concepts are the building blocks and relational statements indicate how the concepts are connected.

Concepts

The phenomenon termed social support introduced earlier is a concept. A concept is the basic element of a theory. Each concept in a theory needs to be defined by the theorist. The definition of a concept might be detailed and complete, or it might be vague and incomplete and require further development (Chinn & Kramer, 2011). Theories with clearly identified and defined concepts provide a stronger basis for a study framework.

Two terms closely related to concept are construct and variable. In more abstract theories, concepts have very general meanings and are sometimes referred to as constructs. A construct is a broader category or idea that may encompass several concepts. For example, a construct for the concept of social support might be resources. Another concept that is a resource might be household income. At a more concrete level, terms are referred to as variables and are narrow in their definition. Thus a variable is more specific than a concept. The word variable implies that the term is defined so that it is measurable and suggests that numerical values of the term are able to vary (are variable) from one instance to another. The levels of abstraction of constructs, concepts, and variables are illustrated with an example in Figure 7-1.

A variable related to social support might be emotional support. The researchers might define emotional support as a study subject's rating of the extent of emotional encouragement or affirmation that he or she receives during a stressful time. The measurement of the variable is a specific method for assigning numerical values to varying amounts of emotional social support. Subjects would respond to questions on a survey or questionnaire about emotional support and their individual answers would be reported as scores. For example, the Functional Social Support Questionnaire has a three-item subscale that measures perceived emotional support (Broadhead, Gehlbach, de Gruy, & Kaplan, 1988; Mas-Expósito, Amador-Campos, Gómez-Benito, & Lalucat-Jo, 2011). One of the items was "People care what happens to me," and the others addressed whether the respondent felt loved and received praise for doing a good job (Broadhead et al., 1988, p. 722). If the Functional Social Support Questionnaire was used by researchers in a study, the subjects' answers to the three items would be added together as the total score. The subjects' total scores on the three questions would be the measurement of the variable of perceived emotional support. (Chapter 10 provides a detailed discussion of measurement methods.)

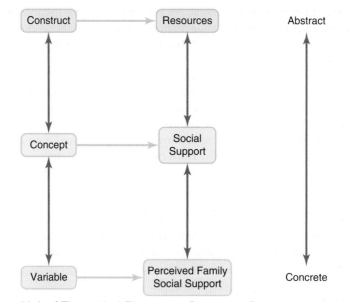

FIG 7-1 Link of Theoretical Elements—Construct, Concept, and Variable.

Defining concepts allows consistency in the way the term is used. Concepts from theories have conceptual definitions that are developed by the theorist and differ from the dictionary definition of a word. A conceptual definition is more comprehensive than a denotative (or dictionary) definition and includes associated meanings that the word may have. A conceptual definition is referred to as connotative, because the term brings to mind memories, moods, or images, subtly or indirectly. For example, a conceptual definition of home might include feelings of security, love, and comfort, which often are associated with a home, whereas the dictionary definition is narrower and more specific—home is a dwelling in which a group of people who may or may not be related live. Some of the words or terms that are used frequently in nursing language have not been clearly defined. Terms used in theory or research need connotative meanings based on professional literature. Connotative definitions are clear statements of the concepts' meaning in the particular theory or study.

The conceptual definition that a researcher identifies or develops for a concept comes from a theory and provides a basis for the operational definition. Remember that in quantitative studies, each variable is ideally associated with a concept, conceptual definition, and operational definition. The operational definition is how the concept can be manipulated, such as an intervention or independent variable, or measured, such as a dependent or outcome variable (see Chapter 5). Conceptual definitions may be explicit or implicit. It is important that you identify the researcher's conceptual definitions of study variables when you critically appraise a study. Nichols, Rice, and Howell (2011) conducted a study with 73 overweight children who were 9 to 11 years old to examine the relationships among anger, stress, and blood pressure. Although the researchers did not identify the conceptual definitions in the report of the study, the definitions can be extracted from the study's framework. The implicit conceptual definition and operational definition for one concept in the study, trait anger, are presented in Table 7-1. Conceptual and operational definitions of variables are described in detail in Chapter 5.

TABLE 7-1	CONCEPTUAL AND OPERATIONAL DEFINITIONS FOR TRAIT ANGER IN THE STUDY OF OVERWEIGHT CHILDREN		
CONCEPT	VARIABLE	CONCEPTUAL DEFINITION	OPERATIONAL DEFINITION
Anger	Trait anger	Enduring personality characteristic reflected in the fury, rage, and displeasure experienced over time (Nichols, Rice, & Howell, 2011)	Trait anger subscale of the Jacobs Pediatric Trait Anger Scale (PPS-2; Jacobs & Blumer, 1984; Nichols et al., 2011, p. 449)

Adapted from Jacobs, G. & Blumer, C. (1984). *The Pediatric Anger Scale.* Vermillion, SD: University of South Dakota, Department of Psychology; and from Nichols, Rice, & Howell, 2011.

Relational Statements

A relational statement clarifies the type of relationship that exists between or among concepts. For example, in the study just mentioned, Nichols and colleagues (2011) proposed that high levels of trait anger were related to high blood pressure in overweight children. They also proposed that high blood pressure was influenced by patterns of anger expression and stress. In regard to the effects of stress on blood pressure, they provided more detail about how stress affected blood pressure by describing the relationships among the corticotropin-releasing factor, stress response, rate and stroke volume of the heart, cardiac output, and constriction of the blood vessels that result in changes in blood pressure. The statements of the physiological processes explaining the connections between stress and blood pressure were also relational statements. Figure 7-2 is the diagram that the researchers provided to display the relationships of their framework.

The relational statements are what are tested through research. The researcher obtains data for the variables that represent the concepts in the study's framework and analyzes the data for possible significant relationships among the variables using specific statistical tests. Testing a theory involves determining the truth of each relational statement in the theory. As more researchers provide evidence about the relationships among concepts, the accuracy or inaccuracy of the relational statements is determined. Many studies are required to validate all the relational statements in a theory.

In theories, propositions (relational statements) can be expressed at various levels of abstraction. Theories that are more abstract (grand nursing theories) contain relational statements that are called general propositions (Grove et al., 2013). Stating a relationship in a more narrow way makes the statement more concrete and testable and results in a specific proposition. Specific propositions in less abstract frameworks (middle range theories) may lead to hypotheses. Hypotheses are developed based on propositions from a grand or middle range theory that comprise the

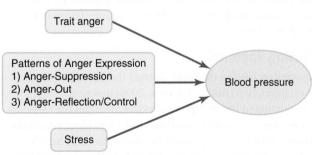

FIG 7-2 Framework of Trait Anger, Patterns of Anger Expression, Stress, and Blood Pressure. (From Nichols, K. H., Rice, M., & Howell, C. [2011]. Anger, stress, and blood pressure in overweight children. *Journal of Pediatric Nursing, 26*[5], 448.)

TABLE 7-2   **EXAMPLES OF LOGICAL LINKS* IN A STUDY OF TRAIT ANGER, PATTERNS OF ANGER EXPRESSION, STRESS, AND BLOOD PRESSURE IN OVERWEIGHT CHILDREN**

GENERAL PROPOSITION	SPECIFIC PROPOSITION	HYPOTHESIS
Enduring personality traits are associated with physiological responses to the environment.	Trait anger is associated with blood pressure.	Among overweight children, high levels of trait anger are associated with high systolic and diastolic blood pressures.
Patterns of emotional responses are associated with physiological responses to the environment.	Patterns of anger expression are associated with blood pressure.	Among overweight children, anger expressed outwardly is associated with high systolic and diastolic blood pressures.
Emotional stress is associated with physiological responses to the environment.	Stressful events are associated with blood pressure.	Among overweight children, high levels of perceived daily stress are associated with high systolic and diastolic blood pressures.

*Between relational statements from abstract to concrete.
From Nichols, K. H., Rice, M., & Howell, C. (2011). Anger, stress, and blood pressure in overweight children. *Journal of Pediatric Nursing, 26*(5), 446-455.

study's framework. Hypotheses, written at a lower level of abstraction, are developed to be tested in a study. Statements at varying levels of abstraction that express relationships between or among the same conceptual ideas can be arranged in hierarchical form, from general to specific. Table 7-2 provides three examples of relationships between two concepts that are written as general propositions, specific propositions, and hypotheses. The first general proposition includes the constructs of enduring personality traits and physiological responses and could be applied to enduring personality traits, such as determination or self-confidence. In this case, the specific proposition indicates that the enduring personality trait is trait anger and the physiological response is blood pressure. The hypothesis proposes a specific relationship between trait anger and blood pressure that was tested in the study (Nichols et al., 2011).

LEVELS OF THEORETICAL THINKING

Theories can be abstract and broad, or they can be more concrete and specific. Between abstract and concrete, there are several levels of theoretical thinking. Understanding the degree of abstraction or level of theoretical thinking will help you to determine whether a theory is applicable to your research problem.

Grand Nursing Theories

Early nurse scholars labeled the most abstract theories as conceptual models or conceptual frameworks. For example, Roy (Roy & Andrews, 2008) described adaptation as the primary phenomenon of interest to nursing in her model. This model identifies the elements considered essential to adaptation and describes how the elements interact to produce adaptation and thus health. In contrast, Orem (Orem & Taylor, 2011) presents her descriptions of health phenomena in terms of self-care, self-care deficits, and nursing systems. Both these theories have been called conceptual models.

What can be confusing is that other scholars do not label Roy's and Orem's writings as conceptual models, but classify them as grand nursing theories (Peterson & Bredow, 2009). Because of

TABLE 7-3	SELECTED GRAND NURSING THEORIES	
NAME	AUTHOR (YEAR)	BRIEF DESCRIPTION
Adaptation Model	Roy & Andrews (2008)	In response to focal, contextual, and residual stimuli, people adapt by using a variety of processes and systems, some of which are automatic and some of which are learned. The overall goal is to return to homeostasis and promote growth.
Self-Care Deficit Theory of Nursing	Orem (2001)	Individuals' ability to care for themselves is affected by developmental stage, presence of disease, and available resources and may result in a self-care deficit. The goal of nursing is to provide care in proportion to the person's self-care capacity.
Systems Model	Neuman & Fawcett (2002)	Stressors can pose a threat to the core processes of the individual. The core is protected by concentric circles of resistance and defense.
Theory of Caring	Watson (1985)	Human caring is a central process of life that influences health. A nurse may create caring moments with a patient by being an authentic human and acknowledging the uniqueness of the patient.

this lack of agreement, we will use the term *grand nursing theories* in this book to describe the nursing theories that are more abstract. We will reserve the term *model* to refer to a diagram that graphically presents the concepts and relationships of a framework being used to guide a study. Table 7-3 lists several well-known grand nursing theories, with a brief explanation.

Building a body of knowledge related to a particular grand nursing theory requires an organized program of research and a group of scholars. The Roy Adaptation Model (RAM) has been used as the basis for studies for over 25 years. The Roy Adaptation Association is a group of researchers who "analyze, critique, and synthesize all published studies in English based on the RAM" (Roy, 2011, p. 312). The Society of Rogerian Scholars continues to conduct studies and develop knowledge related to Martha Rogers' Science of Unitary Human Beings (http://www.societyofrogerianscholars.org/index.html). The International Orem Society publishes a journal, *Self-Care, Dependent-Care, & Nursing*, to disseminate research and clinical applications of Dorothea Orem's theory of self-care. These are examples of researchers who maintain a network to communicate with each other and other nurses about their work with a specific theoretical approach.

Middle Range and Practice Theories

Middle range theories are less abstract and narrower in scope than grand nursing theories. These types of theories specify factors such as a patient's health condition, family situation, and nursing actions and focus on answering particular practice questions (Alligood & Tomey, 2010). Middle range theories are more closely linked to clinical practice and research than grand nursing theories and therefore have a greater appeal to nurse clinicians and researchers. They may emerge from a grounded theory study, be deduced from a grand nursing theory, or created through a synthesis of theories on a particular topic. Middle range theories also can be used as the framework for a study, thus contributing to the validation of the middle range theory (Peterson & Bredow, 2009). Table 7-4 lists some of the middle range theories currently being used as frameworks in nursing studies. These published middle range theories have clearly identified concepts, definitions of concepts, and

TABLE 7-4   MIDDLE RANGE THEORIES

THEORY	RELEVANT THEORETICAL SOURCES
Acute pain	Good, 1998; Good & Moore, 1996
Acute pain management	Huth & Moore, 1998
Adaptation to chronic pain	Dunn, 2004, 2005
Adapting to diabetes mellitus	Whittemore & Roy, 2002
Adolescent vulnerability to risk behaviors	Cazzell, 2008
Caregiver stress	Tsai, 2003
Caring	Swanson, 1991
Chronic pain	Tsai, Tak, Moore, & Palencia, 2003
Chronic sorrow	Eakes, Burke, & Hainsworth, 1998
Client Expression Model	Holland, Gray, & Pierce, 2011
Crisis emergencies for individuals with severe, persistent mental illnesses	Brennaman (2012)
Comfort	Kolcaba, 1994
Culturing brokering	Jezewski, 1995
Health promotion	Pender, Murdaugh, & Parsons, 2006
Home care	Smith, Pace, Kochinda, Kleinbeck, Koehler, & Popkess-Vawter, 2002
Nursing intellectual capital	Covell, 2008
Peaceful end of life	Ruland & Moore, 1998
Postpartum weight management	Ryan, Weiss, Traxel, & Brondino, 2011
Resilience	Polk, 1997
Self-care management for vulnerable populations	Dorsey & Murdaugh, 2003
Uncertainty in illness	Mishel, 1988, 1990
Unpleasant symptoms	Lenz, Pugh, Milligan, Gift, & Suppe, 1997
Urine control theory	Jirovec, Jenkins, Isenberg, & Baiardi, 1999

relational statements and are referred to as substantive theories. These theories are labeled as substantive because they are closer to the substance of clinical practice. For example, clinical practice involves nursing actions to help the patient be comfortable. Kolcaba and Kolcaba (1991) analyzed the concept of comfort. They defined comfort as the state of relief, ease, and transcendence that is experienced in the physical, psychospiritual, environmental, and social contexts of a person. From that concept analysis, a middle range theory of comfort was developed that is applicable to practice and research. "According to the theory, enhanced comfort strengthens recipients....to engage in activities necessary to achieving health and remaining healthy" (Kolcaba & DiMarco, 2005, p.189).

The theory of comfort has three major constructs (Kolcaba, 1994, 2001) in addition to comfort. Comfort is "a dynamic state, subject to positive or negative change very quickly" (Kolcaba & Wilson, 2002). Comfort encompasses relief, ease, and transcendence. Relief is experienced when pain, nausea, anxiety, or other unsettling experiences are mitigated. Ease occurs when the person is not having a stressful or painful experience. Transcendence occurs when a person rises above his or her difficulties or learns to live in a less than desirable situation. When these three components are present, the person is stronger and able to initiate health-seeking behaviors. Health-seeking behaviors may be internal behaviors such as healing or external behaviors such as exercising. A peaceful death is seen as a normal, health-seeking behavior for persons in the later stages of life. The relationship of nursing interventions to patient comfort is often altered by intervening variables, such as the number of nurses available to provide care to hospitalized patients. Note in Figure 7-3, in the

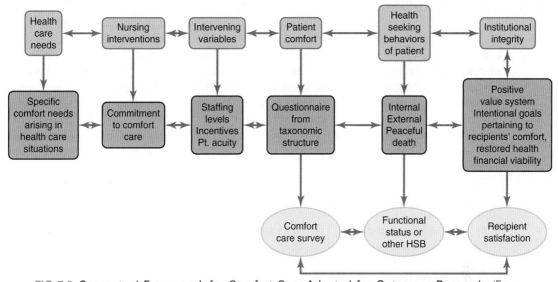

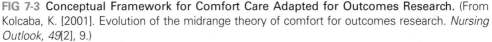

FIG 7-3 Conceptual Framework for Comfort Care Adapted for Outcomes Research. (From Kolcaba, K. [2001]. Evolution of the midrange theory of comfort for outcomes research. *Nursing Outlook, 49*[2], 9.)

top row of the model, that the arrows between the concepts indicate two-way relationships. Patient comfort is near the middle of the top row and can lead to health-seeking behaviors (HSB). The institution can influence health-seeking behaviors and health-seeking behaviors can influence the integrity of the institutional (two-way arrow). The second row of Figure 7-3 has less abstract concepts that can be manipulated, observed, or measured in a specific study or practice setting. Comfort care theory has also been applied in a similar way to perianesthesia nursing (Kolcaba & Wilson, 2002) and pediatric nursing (Kolcaba & DiMarco, 2005).

Practice theories are a type of middle range theories that are more specific. They are designed to propose specific approaches to particular nursing practice situations. Some scholars call them situation-specific theories. Brennaman (2012) proposed a situation-specific theory by applying the middle range theory of crisis for individuals with severe, persistent mental illnesses (ISPMIs; Ball, Links, Strike, & Boydell, 2005) to care provided in emergency departments. From the perspective of the individual with SPMI, Ball and associates (2005) described a crisis as feeling overwhelmed or out of control. In the midst of the crisis, the individual decides whether to manage alone or seek care. Brennaman extended the middle range theory by identifying that a subset of crises was mental health emergencies that posed a risk of imminent suicide or harm to others. When ISPMIs seek help in a crisis, the health provider in the emergency department must first assess the extent of potential risk and determine whether a mental health emergency exists. In the presence of a mental health emergency, the provider must immediately intervene to prevent harm. In situations in which the crisis has not progressed to an emergency, the provider can refer the person to a mental health specialist. The ideal outcome is a resolution to the crisis. As seen in this example, applying a middle range theory to a specific situation identifies appropriate nursing actions. For this reason, practice theories are sometimes referred to as prescriptive theories. Evidence-based practice guidelines are a good source for practice and prescriptive theories (see Chapter 13).

Study Frameworks

A framework is an abstract, logical structure of meaning, such as a portion of a theory, which guides the development of the study and enables the researcher to link the findings to nursing's body of knowledge. Every quantitative study has an implicit or explicit framework. This is true whether the study has a physiological, psychological, social, or cultural focus. A clearly expressed framework is one indication of a well-developed quantitative study. Perhaps the researcher expects one variable to cause a change in another variable, such as the independent variable of an aerobic exercise program affecting the dependent variable of weight loss. In a well-developed quantitative study, the researcher explains abstractly in the framework why one variable is expected to influence the other. The idea is expressed concretely as a hypothesis to be tested through the study methodology.

One strategy for expressing a theory or framework is a diagram with the concepts and relationships graphically displayed. These diagrams are sometimes called maps or models (Grove et al., 2013). For clarity, we are using the term *research framework* to refer to the concepts and relationships being addressed in a study. The researcher develops or applies the framework to explain the concepts contributing to or partially causing an outcome. The researcher cites articles and books in support of the explanation. The model is the diagram used to display the concepts and relationships that allows the reader to grasp of the "wholeness" of a phenomenon.

A model includes all the major concepts in a research framework. Arrows between the concepts indicate the proposed linkages between them. Each linkage shown by an arrow is a graphic illustration of a relational statement (proposition) of the theory. Nichols and co-workers (2011) included a diagram of their conceptual framework (see Figure 7-2). In the diagram, the arrows between trait anger, patterns of anger expression, stress, and blood pressure represent the potential relationships among these concepts.

Unfortunately, in some quantitative studies, the ideas that compose the framework remain nebulous and are vaguely expressed. Although the researcher believes that the variables being studied are related in some fashion, this notion is expressed only in concrete terms. The researcher may make little attempt to explain why the variables are thought to be related. However, the rudiment of a framework is the expectation (perhaps not directly expressed) that one or more variables are linked to other variables. Sometimes basic ideas for the framework are expressed in the introduction or literature review, in which linkages among variables found in previous studies are discussed, but then the researcher stops, without fully developing the ideas as a framework. These are referred to as implicit frameworks. In most cases, a careful reader can extract an implicit framework from the text of the research report. When researchers do not clearly describe the framework, you may want to draw a model based on the information provided. Having a model helps you visualize the framework and how the variables are linked. Implicit frameworks provide limited guidance for the development and conduct of a study and limit the contribution of study findings to nursing knowledge.

Research frameworks can come from grand nursing theories, middle range theories from nursing and other professions, syntheses of concepts and relationships from more than one theory, or syntheses of research findings. In some quantitative studies, the framework that is newly proposed can be called tentative theory. Syntheses of concepts and relationships from more than one theory or syntheses of research findings are also examples of tentative theories that are usually developed for a particular study.

Frameworks for physiological studies are usually derived from physiology, genetics, pathophysiology, and physics. This type of theory is called scientific theory. Scientific theory has extensive evidence to support its claims. Valid and reliable methods exist for measuring each concept and relational statement in scientific theories. Because the knowledge in these areas has been well tested through research, the theoretical relationships are often referred to as laws and principles. In addition, propositions can be developed and tested using these laws and principles and then applied to nursing problems. However, scientific theories remain open to possible contrary evidence that would require their revision. For example, prior to this century, scientists believed that they knew the functions and interactions of various genes. The knowledge gained through the Human Genome Project (http://www.genome.gov/10001772) has required that scientists revise some of their theories.

⟨?⟩ CRITICAL APPRAISAL GUIDELINES

Framework of a Study

The quality of a framework in a quantitative study needs to be critically appraised to determine its usefulness for directing the study and interpreting the study findings. The following questions were developed to assist you in evaluating the quality of a study's framework:

1. Is the study framework explicitly expressed in the study?
2. What is the name of the theory and theorist used for the framework?
3. What are the concepts in the framework?
4. Is each study variable or concept conceptually defined in the study?
5. Are the operational definitions of the variables consistent with their associated conceptual definitions?
6. Do the researchers clearly identify the relationship statement(s) or proposition(s) from the framework being examined by the study design?
7. Are the study findings linked back to the framework?

Critically appraising a framework of a quantitative study requires that you go beyond the framework itself to examine its linkages to other components of the study, such as measurement of the variables and implementation of an intervention, if applicable. Begin by identifying the concepts and conceptual definitions from the written text in the introduction, literature review, or discussion of the framework. Then you must judge the adequacy of the linkages of concepts to variables, measurement of research or dependent variables, and implementation of independent variables. You also need to determine if the study findings have been linked back to the study framework. Researchers usually link the findings back to the framework and other literature in the discussion section of the research report.

EXAMPLES OF CRITICAL APPRAISAL

In this section, critical appraisal guidelines are applied to frameworks that were derived from a grand nursing theory, middle range theory, tentative theory, and/or scientific theory.

Framework from a Grand Nursing Theory

One of the challenges with grand nursing theories is their abstractness and difficulty in measuring their concepts. Some researchers have deduced middle range theories from grand nursing theories and used middle range theories to guide their studies. Other researchers have used a grand nursing theory as an overall framework but have not directly linked the variables to the theory constructs. Other researchers, such as Tao, Ellenbecker, Chen, Zhan, and Dalton (2012), have identified a proposition from a grand nursing theory and tested hypotheses derived from the proposition.

RESEARCH EXAMPLE

Self-Care Deficits

Research Study

The Centers for Medicare and Medicaid services (CMS) will no longer pay for the care of Medicare patients who have been hospitalized for acute myocardial infarction, heart failure, and pneumonia and are admitted again within 30 days of being discharged (CMS, 2013). This makes Tao and colleagues' study highly relevant. The researchers (Tao et al., 2012) used Orem's theory of self-care deficits to "examine the relationship of social environmental factors to home healthcare patients' rehospitalizations" (p. 346) and stated that their second purpose was to "test a hypothesis from Orem's theory" (p. 350). Using a retrospective correlational study, the researchers obtained data without names and other identifying information from a standardized database, the Outcome and Assessment Information Set (OASIS). These patients were 65 to 99 years of age and received home health care after being hospitalized. The researchers proposed that some of the patients had been readmitted to the hospital because of self-care deficits.

Orem proposed that a self-care deficit occurs when people need more care than they can provide for themselves. Self-care deficit is the difference between a person's health-related needs and his or her ability to meet these needs. She also proposed that people have a certain amount of ability and motivation to provide care for themselves and labeled the concept *self-care agency* (Orem & Taylor, 2011). Therapeutic self-care demand occurs when the person must take additional actions because of being acutely or chronically ill. The framework of the study included two propositions from Orem's theory:

"Orem's conceptual model proposes that basic conditional factors (BCFs) and power components (PCs) affect a patient's self-care agency. Therapeutic self-care demand (TSCD) and self-care agency are interrelated and, when known, can predict a patient's self-care deficit or ability. . . .Figure 7-4 presents the conceptual framework that guides this study. The difference between the clinical status score and the functional ability score (therapeutic self-care demand minus self-care agency) relates to rehospitalization (self-care deficit). The patient's functional ability (self-care agency), in turn, is influenced by the patient's cognitive functioning and the BCFs of age, gender, risk characteristics, and social environmental factors. The influences of the social environmental factors are poorly understood and are the focus of this study." (Tao et al., 2012, pp. 347-348)

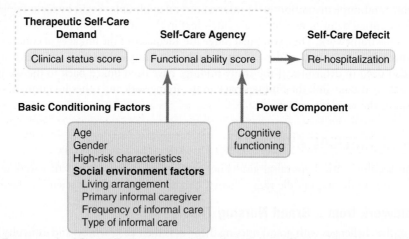

FIG 7-4 **Framework of Social Environmental Factors Affecting Rehospitalization of Medicare Patients.** (From Tao, H., Ellenbecker, C., Chen, J., Zhan, L., & Dalton, J. [2012]. The influence of social environmental factors on hospitalization among patients receiving home health care services. *Advances in Nursing Science, 35*[4], 346-358.)

In Figure 7-4, the basic conditional factors are displayed in a box and are listed as age, gender, high risk characteristics, and societal environmental factors. The social environmental factors specifically being studied are listed; these include living arrangement, primary informal caregiver, frequency of informal care, and type of informal care. The arrow from the BCFs box to the functional ability score in the box above represents the relationship from the theory that BCFs affect self-care agency. Cognitive function was identified as an aspect of the power component, another concept that affects self-care agency. Therapeutic self-care demand and self-care agency are within a box made of dotted lines to indicate that they are associated with each other. The researchers provided a table of concepts, variables, and scoring for each variable. We have summarized the connections among the concepts and variables in Table 7-5.

TABLE 7-5	CONSTRUCTS, CONCEPTS, VARIABLES, AND DATA RELATED TO OREM'S SELF-CARE DEFICIT THEORY*	
CONSTRUCT	**CONCEPT**	**VARIABLE**
Therapeutic self-care demand	Health status	Clinical status score = case mix measure of diagnoses, therapies, presence of pain, pressure ulcers, incontinence, and behavior problems
Self-care agency	Functional ability	Functional ability score = case mix measure of activities of daily living such as ability to dress, bath, toilet, and ambulate
Power component	Cognitive functioning	Cognitive function score = score on the Cognitive Function Scale
Basic conditioning factors	Risk characteristics Personal characteristics Informal caregiving	Total risk factors = heavy smoking, obesity, alcohol dependency, and drug dependency Age, gender, living arrangements Presence of informal caregiver, frequency of caregiving, type of primary informal care
Self-deficit	Rehospitalization Number of days	Readmission within 60 days Days between discharge and rehospitalization

*As used by Tao and colleagues in their study of Medicare patients receiving home healthcare: Tao H., Ellenbecker, C., Chen, J., Zhan, L., & Dalton, J. (2012). The influence of social environmental factors on hospitalization among patients receiving home health care services. *Advances in Nursing Science, 35*(4), 346-358.

In the OASIS data set for one home health agency, 1268 patients were identified as being eligible to be included in the study. The analysis revealed support for the first hypothesis. Patients who were men, had other assistance at home, lived alone, or received frequent care had high functional ability. Patients who were obese and older patients were most likely to be rehospitalized. Also, "higher levels of cognitive functioning were related to higher levels of functional ability" (p. 352). Tao and colleagues (2012) also learned that the greater the difference between clinical status and functional status, the more likely it was that the patient had been rehospitalized.

"This study supported that social environmental factors contributed to rehospitalization (self-care deficit) through functional ability (self-care agency) by altering the balance between the self-care demand and self-care agency." (Tao et al., 2012, p. 354)

Clinical Appraisal
Tao and associates (2012) made strong connections between the theory and the study. First, they clearly identified the name of the theory and theorists. They explicitly identified the theory's concepts to be studied and defined them (see Table 7-5). The operational definitions were consistent with the conceptual definitions of the variables. The propositions were identified, along with the hypotheses. In the discussion section of the report, the researchers indicated how the findings were consistent with the framework.

"Specifically, the study determined that increasing age, obesity, lower levels of cognitive functioning, and receiving less care from [an] informal caregiver are related to lower functional ability and may increase the possibility of rehospitalization." (Tao et al., 2012, p. 354)

Continued

⚡ **RESEARCH EXAMPLE—cont'd**

Implications for Practice

The researchers began the report by noting the need to inform policy makers about the factors contributing to rehospitalization and to educate home health nurses about the importance of social environmental factors. At the end of the report, they returned to the implications for policy and practice.

> "The results of this study have implications for home health care reimbursement policy strategies for reducing unnecessary hospitalizations and improving the quality of home health care. Findings may help home healthcare nurses recognize those patients who are in need of certain services that may reduce rehospitalization, such as those that lack the support of the patient's family or assistance from paid informal caregivers...When health problems arise, those with adequate social environmental support are more likely to seek medical care before the problems become more serious. The importance of social environmental support and its ability to motivate patients to increased levels of functioning has the potential to reduce rates of rehospitalizations." (Tao et al., 2012, pp. 355-356)

Before these findings are broadly applied, however, the study needs to be replicated with a nationally representative sample because this sample was from a single home healthcare agency.

Framework Based on Middle Range Theory

Many frameworks for nursing studies are based on middle range theories. These studies test the validity of the middle range theory and examine the parameters within which the middle range theory can be applied. Some nursing researchers have used middle range theories developed by non-nurses. Other researchers have used middle range theories that they or other nurses have developed to explain nursing phenomena. In either case, middle range theories should be tested before being applied to nursing practice.

⚡ **RESEARCH EXAMPLE**

Framework based on Middle Range Theory

Research Study

Park, Stotts, Douglas, Donesky-Cuenco, and Carrieri-Kohlman (2012) adapted the middle range theory of unpleasant symptoms (Lenz et al., 1997) for their study of symptoms related to asthma and chronic obstructive pulmonary disease. Their sample was 86 Korean immigrants in outpatient settings. From the theory, they used the theorists' influencing factors and multiple symptoms and linked them to functional performance to create the framework for the study (see Figure 7-5, in this example). Functional performance is the outcome concept and is shown on the right side of the model. Multiple symptoms are connected to functional performance by a one-way arrow, indicating the direction of influence. In other words, the experience of multiple symptoms affects functional performance. On the left side of the model, influencing factors has been divided into smaller components. Physiological factors are identified as age, gender, disease group, duration of the disease, comorbidities, and dyspnea. Each of the influencing factor boxes has the variables that will be used to measure that concept. There may be additional relationships among these concepts but those displayed are the relationships being analyzed in the study.

Consistent with the main premise of the theory of unpleasant symptoms, Park and colleagues (2012, p. 227) assessed symptom clusters of the subjects because "multiple symptoms are experienced simultaneously" and increase exponentially in their effect as the number of symptoms increases. For example, the experience of having nausea and dyspnea at the same time is more than adding together the experiences of having each alone. The combination of experiencing nausea and dyspnea at the same time makes the situation more distressing. The researchers also analyzed the relationships among symptoms and functional performance. Table 7-6 presents the concepts of the middle range theory with the operational definitions.

Park and colleagues (2012, p. 233) described the subjects' symptoms by severity, frequency, persistence, distress, and burden and found three clusters (groups) of symptoms that when they occurred together, affected

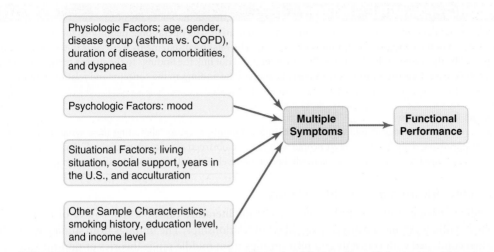

FIG 7-5 Framework of Symptoms in Chronic Obstructive Pulmonary Disease and Asthma Patients. (Adapted from Park, S. K., Stotts, N., Douglas, M., Donesky-Cuenco, D., & Carrieri-Kohlman, V. [2012]. Symptoms and functional performance in Korean immigrants with asthma or chronic obstructive pulmonary disease. *Heart & Lung, 41*[3], 226-237.)

TABLE 7-6	CONCEPTUAL AND OPERATIONAL DEFINITIONS FOR THE STUDY OF SYMPTOMS AND FUNCTIONAL PERFORMANCE*	
CONCEPT	**CONCEPTUAL DEFINITION**	**OPERATIONAL DEFINITION**
Symptoms	"Multidimensional experience that incorporates intensity, timing, distress, and quality" (p. 227)	"The Memorial Symptom Assessment Scale (MSAS) is a self-report questionnaire designed to measure the multidimensional experience of symptoms" (p. 228).
Influencing factors	"Physiological (pathological problems), psychological (mood), and situational (social support)" (p. 227)	"The Profile of Moods States—Short Form (POMS-SF) was used to measure the moods of the participants" (p. 229). Other tools measured the other influencing factors.
Consequences of symptoms	Experiencing a symptom affects one's performance.	"The Functional Performance Inventory-Short Form (FPI-SF) was used to elicit participants' descriptions of their functional performance" (p. 229).

*In Korean immigrants with asthma or chronic obstructive pulmonary disease.
From Park, S. K., Stotts, N., Douglas, M., Donesky-Cuenco, D., & Carrieri-Kohlman, V. (2012). Symptoms and functional performance in Korean immigrants with asthma or chronic obstructive pulmonary disease. *Heart & Lung, 41*(3), 226-237.

functional status. One cluster was comprised of "age, level of education, working status, level of acculturation, and mean severity score of 7 symptoms" and explained a significant amount of the variance in functional status. Another factor was a set of emotional responses, such as feeling sad or nervous, and physiological responses, such as dyspnea. The third cluster had only two elimination-related symptoms—constipation and urinary problems. The second and third groups (clusters) of characteristics and symptoms also were found to affect functional status.

Critical Appraisal
The researchers provided a model of the study's framework (see Figure 7-5) and provided the names of the theorists for the middle range theory from which it was adapted (Lenz et al. 1997). The concepts in the framework were

Continued

RESEARCH EXAMPLE—cont'd

identified in the model (see Figure 7-5) and defined in the narrative. The operational definitions for the concepts were consistent with the conceptual definitions (Table 7-6). The relational statements were clear in the model and were supported by the study results. However, the researchers did not link the findings to the study's framework. The researchers could have done this by discussing the application of the findings to the concepts and relationships of the framework.

Implications for Practice

The researchers indicated nurses should evaluate coexisting symptoms, because "alleviating these symptoms may be important in improving daily functioning in people with chronic obstructive pulmonary disease" (Park et al., 2012, p. 235). They recognized that more research is needed prior to developing interventions to alleviate symptoms.

Framework from a Tentative Theory

Findings from completed studies reported in the literature can be a rich source of frameworks when synthesized into a coherent, logical set of relationships. The findings from studies, especially when combined with concepts and relationships from middle range theories or non-nursing theories, can be synthesized into a tentative theory that provides a framework for a particular study. The study by Nichols and associates (2011) that was used as an example earlier in the chapter will be described in more detail here and its framework critically appraised.

RESEARCH EXAMPLE

Framework from a Tentative Theory

Research Study

Nichols and co-workers (2011, p. 447) conducted a study to describe "levels of trait anger, patterns of anger expression, and stress in overweight and obese 9- to 11-year-old children." They also compared the influences of these concepts on the blood pressure of the children. Following the review of literature, the researchers explicitly stated their framework, as follows:

> "Anger, a feeling varying in intensity from mild displeasure to fury or rage (Spielberger, Reheiser, & Sydeman, 1995), can be examined both as the level of trait anger and as the patterns used to express that anger [see Figure 7-2 earlier in the chapter]. Trait anger is more stable and reflects the extent of the experience of angry feelings over time (Spielberger et al., 1995). Equally important is the pattern used to express anger, such as anger-in (holding in anger or denying angry feelings), anger-out (expressing anger openly), or anger reflection-control (using a cognitive, problem-solving approach to dealing with anger; (Jacobs, Phelps, & Rhors, 1989; Siegman & Smith, 1994) . . . In addition to anger, stress can have an impact on the physiological functioning of children through activation of the hypothalamic-pituitary-adrenocortical (HPA) system (McEwen, 2007; Ryan-Wenger, et al., 2000) and of the sympathetic nervous system (Institute of Medicine, 2001; McEwen, 2007). . . . The body responds by (a) increasing the rate and stroke volume of the heart contraction and thereby increasing cardiac output and (b) constricting vessels in the blood reservoirs and thus increasing BP (McEwen, 2007; Severtsen & Copstead, 2000)." (Nichols et al., 2011, pp. 448-449)

Critical Appraisal

Nichols and colleagues (2011) clearly described their framework by providing a description and a model of the concepts and relationships (see Figure 7-3). The theory was a synthesis of evidence from published studies, so there was no theorist identified. The concepts in the model were defined conceptually and operationally. For example, trait anger was conceptually defined as the "extent of the experience of angry feelings over time (Spielberger et al., 1995)" (Nichols et al., 2011, p. 448). Nichols and associates provided an operational definition of trait anger that was "measured by the 10-item trait anger subscale of the Jacobs Pediatric Trait Anger Scale" (PPS-2; Jacobs & Blumer, 1984, p. 449). The operational definition of each concept was consistent with its conceptual definition. Gender, an important factor in two of the research questions, was not included in the model and was not defined. The relational statements were embedded in the review of literature and conceptual framework sections but were not stated as propositions and no hypotheses were developed for testing in this study. The model did graphically present the relationships. The study would have been stronger if the propositions expressed in the model were linked to hypotheses that might have been tested in the study. This would have provided clearer links of the concepts and relationships in the model and the variables expressed in the hypotheses. Nichols and co-workers (2011, p.453) linked the findings back to the framework in the discussion section.

"The conceptual framework as depicted was partially supported by the findings. A significant amount of the variance in SBP [systolic blood pressure] in the group as a whole was accounted for by trait anger, patterns of anger expression, and stress. Trait anger was an independent predictor of SBP. However, this set of variables did not explain a significant amount of the variance in DBP [diastolic blood pressure]."

Implications for Practice

Nichols and colleagues (2011, pp. 453-454) stated the study implications for practice in their conclusions and indicated that the relationships among these concepts in overweight children warrants additional research.

"...it is important for healthcare providers to assess BP and to consider treatments for such elevations. Because overweight and obese children are particularly vulnerable to elevations in BP (McNiece et al., 2007), assessment of BP and weight in school-aged children is critical... healthcare providers may also need to assess trait anger, patterns of anger expression, and stress."

Framework for Physiological Study

Developing a physiological framework to express the logic on which the study is based clearly is helpful to the researcher and readers of the published study. The critical appraisal of a physiological framework is no different from that of other frameworks. However, concepts and conceptual definitions in physiological frameworks may be less abstract than concepts and conceptual definitions in psychosocial studies. Concepts in physiological studies might be such terms as *cardiac output, dyspnea, wound healing, blood pressure, tissue hypoxia, metabolism,* and *functional status.* For example, in mechanically ventilated patients, nurse researchers have described the risk of bacteremia (concept) after oral care (Jones, Munro, Grap, Kitten, & Edmond, 2010). Among cardiac patients, they have studied the effects of beta blockers on fatigue (concept) in chronic heart failure (Tang, Yu, & Yeh, 2010) and compared the inflammatory biomarkers (concept) of persons with coronary artery disease to those without coronary artery disease (Jha, Divya, Prasad, & Mittal, 2010).

Another example is a study conducted by Corbett, Daniel, Drayton, Field, Steinhardt, and Garrett (2010) to describe the effects of dietary supplements on anesthesia. In this study, the researchers wanted to determine the effects of specific physiological processes and therefore needed high levels of control in the study. To accomplish this without harming human subjects, an animal study was designed using the scientific theory.

◢ RESEARCH EXAMPLE

Study Framework from Scientific Theories of Inflammation and Dietary Supplements

Research Study

Increasing numbers of people are using herbal and dietary supplements. As certified registered nurse anesthetists, Corbett and associates (2010) were concerned about the risks of dietary supplements having negative interactions with anesthesia. They were also interested in the potential positive effects of dietary supplements on inflammation. They identified ellagic acid that can be extracted from pomegranate juice as the specific substance that they wanted to test.

Continued

RESEARCH EXAMPLE—cont'd

"The primary objective of this study was to investigate the anti-inflammatory effects of ellagic acid compared with known selective and non-selective COX [cyclooxygenase] inhibitors in male Sprague-Dawley rats as measured by paw volume assessment. The secondary objective investigated [about] whether there is an interaction between ellagic acid and the anesthesia adjunct ketorolac or the COX-2 inhibitor meloxicam." (Corbett et al., 2010, p. 216)

The researchers provided a model with the physiological pathways that resulted in inflammation of the rat paw or homeostasis after an injection of a noxious substance (see Figure 7-6). In the model, tissue injury affects the phospholipids, which release arachidonic acid. They proposed that ellagic acid interfered with the release of cyclooxygenase-2 (COX-2), which causes inflammation. The experiment was conducted using six groups that received different combinations of ellagic acid, ketorolac, meloxicam, and the solution used to inject the substances into the rats. At 4 and 8 hours after injection of the noxious substance, edema was reduced in the paws into which ellagic acid was also injected.

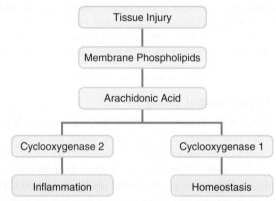

FIG 7-6 Framework of Ellagic Acid and Anti-Inflammation Effects. (From Corbett, S., Daniel, J., Drayton, R., Field, M., Steinhardt, R., & Garrett, N. [2010]. Evaluation of the anti-inflammatory effects of ellagic acid. *Journal of PeriAnesthesia, 25*[4], 216.)

Critical Appraisal

Corbett and co-workers (2010) developed the study framework from scientific theories of inflammation and dietary supplements. They provided a model, which would have been clearer had it included ellagic acid as a concept. COX-1 and COX-2 were defined in the caption for the figure, but are not clearly described in the text of the paper. The extent of inflammation was operationalized as paw edema, with a detailed procedure for obtaining the measurement. The relationships among the concepts were displayed in the model as nondirection connections between the concepts and were not stated as propositions. The study findings were not linked back to the framework. The findings were congruent with the findings of other studies and supported the framework in that ellagic acid decreased inflammation (edema). Although not directly tested, ellagic acid appears to decrease the effects of COX-2, which in turn decreases inflammation.

Implications for Practice

Corbett and colleagues (2010, p. 219) stated the following implications for practice:

"Clearly, the rise in the use of dietary supplements, specifically ellagic acid, poses both potential risks and benefits during the perianesthesia period and should be carefully evaluated and considered by the anesthesia provider during patient assessment."

Additional laboratory and animal studies are needed to confirm the findings and determine the mechanisms whereby ellagic acid interferes with inflammation. Another approach would be to conduct a retrospective study of surgery patients to describe their responses to anesthesia in relation to their use of dietary supplements.

KEY CONCEPTS

- Theory is essential to research because it is the initial inspiration for developing a study and links the study findings back to the knowledge of the discipline.
- A theory is an integrated set of concepts, definitions, and statements that presents a view of a phenomenon.
- The elements of theories are concepts and relational statements.
- Conceptual models or grand nursing theories are very abstract and broadly explain phenomena of interest.
- Middle range and tentative theories are less abstract and narrower in scope than conceptual models.
- Every study has a framework, although some frameworks are poorly expressed or are implicit.
- A framework is an abstract, logical structure of meaning, such as a portion of a theory, that guides the development of the study, is tested in the study, and enables the researcher to link the findings to nursing's body of knowledge.
- To be used appropriately, the study framework must include the concepts and their definitions. The relational statements or propositions being examined need to be clear and represented by a model or map.
- Frameworks for studies may come from grand nursing theories, middle range theories, research findings, non-nursing theories, tentative theories, and scientific theories.
- Scientific theories are derived from physiology, genetics, pathophysiology, and physics and are supported by extensive evidence.
- Critically appraising a framework requires the identification and evaluation of the concepts, their definitions, and the statements linking the concepts. Then the study findings are examined in the context of the framework to determine the usefulness of the framework in describing reality.

REFERENCES

Alligood, M. R., & Tomey, A. M. (2010). *Nursing theorists and their work* (7th ed.). Maryland Heights, MO: Mosby Elsevier.

Ball, J. S., Links, P. S., Strike, C., & Boydell, K. M. (2005). It's overwhelming...everything seems to be too much: A theory of crisis for individuals with severe persistent mental illness. *Psychiatric Rehabilitation Journal, 29*(1), 10–17.

Brennaman, L. (2012). Crisis emergencies for individuals with severe, persistent mental illnesses: A situation-specific theory. *Archives of Psychiatric Nursing, 26*(4), 251–260.

Broadhead, W. E., Gehlbach, S. H., de Gruy, F., & Kaplan, B. H. (1988). The Duke-UNC Functional Social Support Questionnaire: Measurement of social support in family medicine patients. *Medical Care, 26*(7), 709–723.

Cazzell, M. (2008). Linking theory, evidence, and practice in assessment of adolescent inhalant use. *Journal of Addictions Nursing, 19*(1), 17–25.

Centers for Medicare and Medicaid Services, (2013). *Readmission reduction program*. Retrieved July 1, 2013 from, http://www.cms.gov/Medicare/Medicare-Fee-for-Service-Payment/AcuteInpatientPPS/Readmissions-Reduction-Program.html.

Chinn, P. L., & Kramer, M. K. (2011). *Integrated theory and knowledge development in nursing* (8th ed.). St. Louis: Elsevier Mosby.

Corbett, S., Daniel, J., Drayton, R., Field, M., Steinhardt, R., & Garrett, N. (2010). Evaluation of the anti-inflammatory effects of ellagic acid. *Journal of PeriAnesthesia Nursing, 25*(4), 214–220.

Covell, C. L. (2008). The middle-range theory of nursing intellectual capital. *Journal of Advanced Nursing, 63*(1), 94–103.

Dorsey, C. J., & Murdaugh, C. L. (2003). The theory of self-care management for vulnerable populations. *Journal of Theory Construction & Testing, 7*(2), 43–49.

Dunn, K. S. (2004). Toward a middle-range theory of adaptation to chronic pain. *Nursing Science Quarterly, 17*(1), 78–84.

Dunn, K. S. (2005). Testing a middle-range theoretical model of adaptation to chronic pain. *Nursing Science Quarterly, 18*(2), 146–156.

Eakes, G. G., Burke, M. L., & Hainsworth, M. A. (1998). Middle-range theory of chronic sorrow. *Journal of Nursing Scholarship, 30*(2), 179–184.

Good, M. A. (1998). A middle range theory of acute pain management: Use in research. *Nursing Outlook, 46*(3), 120–124.

Good, M., & Moore, S. M. (1996). Clinical practice guidelines as a new source of middle range theory: Focus on acute pain. *Nursing Outlook, 44*(2), 74–79.

Grove, S. K., Burns, N., & Gray, J. R. (2013). *The practice of nursing research: Appraisal, synthesis, and generation of evidence* (7th ed.). St. Louis: Elsevier Saunders.

Groves, P., Meisenbach, R., & Scott-Cawiezell, J. (2011). Keeping patients safe in healthcare organizations: A structuration theory of safety culture. *Journal of Advanced Nursing, 67*(8), 1846–1855.

Holland, B., Gray, J., & Pierce, T. (2011). The client experience model: Synthesis and application to African Americans with multiple sclerosis. *Journal of Theory Construction & Testing, 15*(2), 36–40.

Huth, M. M., & Moore, S. M. (1998). Prescriptive theory of acute pain management in infants and children. *Journal of the Society of Pediatric Nurses, 3*(1), 23–32.

Institute of Medicine, (2001). *Health and behavior: The interplay of biological, behavioral, and societal influences.* Washington, DC: National Academy of Science.

Jacobs, G., & Blumer, C. (1984). *The Pediatric Anger Scale.* Vermillion, SD: University of South Dakota, Department of Psychology.

Jacobs, G., Phelps, M., & Rhors, B. (1989). Assessment of anger in children: The Pediatric Anger Expression Scale. *Personality and Individual Differences, 10*(1), 59–65.

Jezewski, M. A. (1995). Evolution of a grounded theory: Conflict resolution through culture brokering. *Advances in Nursing Science, 17*(3), 14–30.

Jha, H., Divya, A., Prasad, J., & Mittal, A. (2010). Plasma circulatory markers in male and female patients with coronary artery disease. *Heart & Lung, 39*(4), 296–303.

Jirovec, M. M., Jenkins, J., Isenberg, M., & Baiardi, J. (1999). Urine control theory derived from Roy's conceptual framework. *Nursing Science Quarterly, 12*(3), 251–255.

Jones, D., Munro, C., Grap, M. J., Kitten, T., & Edmond, M. (2010). Oral care and bacteremia risk in mechanically ventilated adults. *Heart & Lung, 39*(6S), S57–S65.

Kolcaba, K. (1994). A theory of comfort for nursing. *Journal of Advanced Nursing, 19*(6), 1178–1184.

Kolcaba, K. (2001). Evolution of the mid range theory of comfort for outcomes research. *Nursing Outlook, 49*(2), 86–92.

Kolcaba, K., & DiMarco, M. (2005). Comfort theory and its application to pediatric nursing. *Pediatric Nursing, 31*(3), 187–194.

Kolcaba, K., & Kolcaba, R. (1991). An analysis of the concept of comfort. *Journal of Advanced Nursing, 16* (11), 1301–1310.

Kolcaba, K., & Wilson, L. (2002). Comfort care: A framework for perianesthesia nursing. *Journal of PeriAnesthesia Nursing, 17*(2), 102–114.

Lenz, E. R., Pugh, L. C., Milligan, R., Gift, A., & Suppe, F. (1997). The middle range theory of unpleasant symptoms: An update. *Advances in Nursing Science, 19* (3), 14–27.

Mas-Expósito, L., Amador-Campos, J., Gómez-Benito, J., & Lalucat-Jo, L. Research Group on Severe Mental Disorder. (2011). The World Health Organization Quality of Life Scale Brief Version: A validation study in patients with schizophrenia. *Quality of Life Research, 20* (7), 1079–1089.

McEwen, B. (2007). Physiology and neurobiology of stress and adaptation. *Physiological Reviews, 87*(3), 873–904.

McNiece, K., Poffenbarger, T., Turner, J., Franco, F., Sorof, J., & Portman, R. (2007). Prevalence of hypertensions and pre-hypertension among adolescents. *Journal of Pediatrics, 150*(6), 640–644.

Mishel, M. H. (1988). Uncertainty in illness. *Journal of Nursing Scholarship, 20*(4), 225–232.

Mishel, M. H. (1990). Reconceptualization of the uncertainty in illness theory. *Journal of Nursing Scholarship, 22*(3), 256–262.

Murrock, C., & Higgins, P. (2009). The theory of music, mood, and movement to improve health outcomes. *Journal of Advanced Nursing, 65*(10), 2249–2257.

Neuman, B., & Fawcett, J. (2002). *The Neuman systems model* (4th ed.). Upper Saddle River, NJ: Prentice-Hall.

Nichols, K. H., Rice, M., & Howell, C. (2011). Anger, stress, and blood pressure in overweight children. *Journal of Pediatric Nursing, 26*(5), 446–455.

Orem, D. E. (2001). *Nursing: Concepts of practice* (6th ed.). St. Louis: Mosby.

Orem, D. E., & Taylor, S. G. (2011). Reflections on nursing practice science: The nature, the structure, and the

KEY TERMS

A research design is a blueprint for conducting a study. Over the years, several quantitative designs have been developed for conducting descriptive, correlational, quasi-experimental, and experimental studies. Descriptive and correlational designs are focused on describing and examining relationships of variables in natural settings. Quasi-experimental and experimental designs were developed to examine causality, or the cause and effect relationships between interventions and outcomes. The designs focused on causality were developed to maximize control over factors that could interfere with or threaten the validity of the study design. The strengths of the design validity increase the probability that the study findings are an accurate reflection of reality. Well-designed studies, especially those focused on testing the effects of nursing interventions, are essential for generating sound research evidence for practice (Brown, 2014; Craig & Smyth, 2012).

Being able to identify the study design and evaluate design flaws that might threaten the validity of the findings is an important part of critically appraising studies. Therefore this chapter introduces you to the different types of quantitative study designs and provides an algorithm for determining whether a study design is descriptive, correlational, quasi-experimental, or experimental. Algorithms are also provided so that you can identify specific types of designs in published studies. A background is provided for understanding causality in research by defining the concepts of multicausality, probability, bias, control, and manipulation. The different types of validity—statistical conclusion validity, internal validity, construct validity, and external validity—are described. Guidelines are provided for critically appraising descriptive, correlational, quasi-experimental, and experimental designs in published studies. In addition, a flow diagram is provided to examine the quality of randomized controlled trials conducted in nursing. The chapter concludes with an introduction to mixed-method approaches, which include elements of quantitative designs and qualitative procedures in a study.

IDENTIFYING DESIGNS USED IN NURSING STUDIES

A variety of study designs are used in nursing research; the four most commonly used types are descriptive, correlational, quasi-experimental, and experimental. These designs are categorized in different ways in textbooks (Fawcett & Garity, 2009; Hoe & Hoare, 2012; Kerlinger & Lee, 2000). Sometimes, descriptive and correlational designs are referred to as nonexperimental designs because the focus is on examining variables as they naturally occur in environments and not on the implementation of a treatment by the researcher. Some of these nonexperimental designs include a time element. Designs with a cross-sectional element involve data collection at one point in time. Cross-sectional design involves examining a group of subjects simultaneously in various stages of development, levels of education, severity of illness, or stages of recovery to describe changes in a phenomenon across stages. The assumption is that the stages are part of a process that will progress over time. Selecting subjects at various points in the process provides important information about the totality of the process, even though the same subjects are not monitored throughout the entire process (Grove, Burns, & Gray, 2013). Longitudinal design involves collecting data from the same subjects at different points in time and might also be referred to as repeated measures. Repeated measures might be included in descriptive, correlational, quasi-experimental, or experimental study designs.

Quasi-experimental and experimental studies are designed to examine causality or the cause and effect relationship between a researcher-implemented treatment and selected study outcome. The designs for these studies are sometime referred to as experimental because the focus is on examining the differences in dependent variables thought to be caused by independent variables or treatments. For example, the researcher-implemented treatment might be a home monitoring program for patients initially diagnosed with hypertension, and the dependent or outcome variable could be blood pressure measured at 1 week, 1 month, and 6 months. This chapter introduces you to selected experimental designs and provides examples of these designs from published nursing studies. Details on other study designs can be found in a variety of methodology sources (Campbell & Stanley, 1963; Creswell, 2014; Grove et al., 2013; Kerlinger & Lee, 2000; Shadish, Cook, & Campbell, 2002).

The algorithm shown in Figure 8-1 may be used to determine the type of design (descriptive, correlational, quasi-experimental, and experimental) used in a published study. This algorithm includes a series of yes or no responses to specific questions about the design. The algorithm starts with the question, "Is there a treatment?" The answer leads to the next question, with the four types of designs being identified in the algorithm. Sometimes, researchers combine elements of different designs to accomplish their study purpose. For example, researchers might conduct a cross-sectional, descriptive, correlational study to examine the relationship of body mass index (BMI) to blood lipid levels in early adolescence (ages 13 to 16 years) and late adolescence (ages 17 to 19 years). It is important that researchers clearly identify the specific design they are using in their research report.

DESCRIPTIVE DESIGNS

Descriptive studies are designed to gain more information about characteristics in a particular field of study. The purpose of these studies is to provide a picture of a situation as it naturally happens. A descriptive design may be used to develop theories, identify problems with current practice,

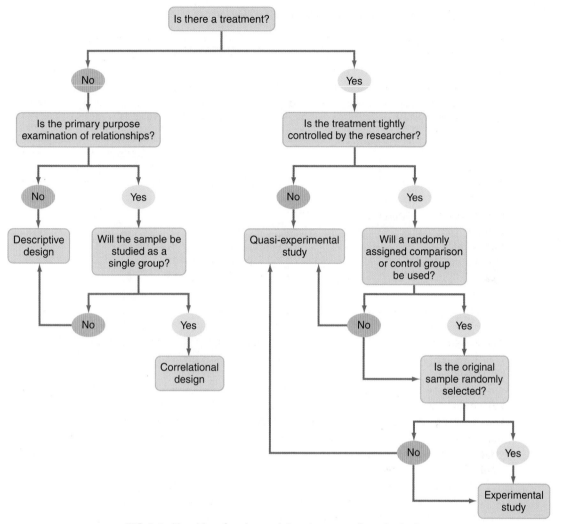

FIG 8-1 Algorithm for determining the type of study design.

make judgments about practice, or identify trends of illnesses, illness prevention, and health promotion in selected groups. No manipulation of variables is involved in a descriptive design. Protection against bias in a descriptive design is achieved through (1) conceptual and operational definitions of variables, (2) sample selection and size, (3) valid and reliable instruments, and (4) data collection procedures that might partially control the environment. Descriptive studies differ in level of complexity. Some contain only two variables; others may include multiple variables that are studied over time. You can use the algorithm shown in Figure 8-2 to determine the type of descriptive design used in a published study. Typical descriptive and comparative descriptive designs are discussed in this chapter. Grove and colleagues (2013) have provided details about additional descriptive designs.

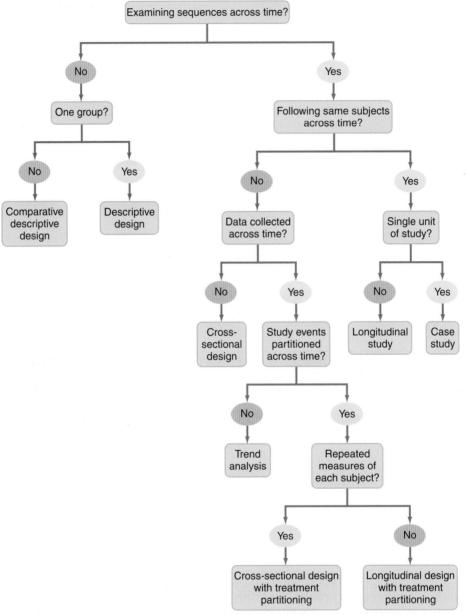

FIG 8-2 Algorithm for determining the type of descriptive design.

Typical Descriptive Design

A **typical descriptive design** is used to examine variables in a single sample (Figure 8-3). This descriptive design includes identifying the variables within a phenomenon of interest, measuring these variables, and describing them. The description of the variables leads to an interpretation of the theoretical meaning of the findings and the development of possible relationships or hypotheses that might guide future correlational or quasi-experimental studies.

CLARIFICATION ⟶ MEASUREMENT ⟶ DESCRIPTION ⟶ INTERPRETATION

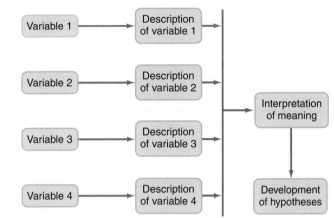

FIG 8-3 Typical descriptive design.

⚡ CRITICAL APPRAISAL GUIDELINES

Descriptive and Correlational Designs

When critically appraising the designs of descriptive and correlational studies, you need to address the following questions:

1. Is the study design descriptive or correlational? Review the algorithm in Figure 8-1 to determine the type of study design.
2. If the study design is descriptive, use the algorithm in Figure 8-2 to identify the specific type of descriptive design implemented in the study.
3. If the study design is correlational, use the algorithm in Figure 8-5 to identify the specific type of correlational design implemented in the study.
4. Does the study design address the study purpose and/or objectives or questions?
5. Was the sample appropriate for the study?
6. Were the study variables measured with quality measurement methods?

🔍 RESEARCH EXAMPLE

Typical Descriptive Design

Research Study Excerpt

Maloni, Przeworski, and Damato (2013) studied women with postpartum depression (PPD) after pregnancy complications for the purpose of describing their barriers to treatment for PPD, use of online resources for assistance with PPD, and preference for Internet treatment for PPD. This study included a typical descriptive design; key aspects of this study's design are presented in the following excerpt.

"Methods

An exploratory descriptive survey design was used to obtain a convenience sample of women who self-report feelings of PPD across the past week [sample size $n=53$]. Inclusion criteria were women between

Continued

---

⑤ RESEARCH EXAMPLE—cont'd

2 weeks and 6 months postpartum who had been hospitalized for pregnancy complications. Women were excluded if they had a score of <6 on the Edinburgh Postnatal Depression Scale (EPDS). . . . EPDS is a widely used screening instrument to detect postpartum depression. . . .

In addition, a series of 26 descriptive questions assessed women's barriers to PPD treatment, whether they sought information about depression after birth from any sources and their information seeking about PPD from the Internet, how often they sought the information, and whether the information was helpful. Questions were developed from review of the literature. . . . Content validity was established by a panel of four experts. . . . The survey was posted using a university-protected website using standardized software for surveys." (Maloni et al., 2013, pp. 91-92)

Critical Appraisal

Maloni and associates (2013) clearly identified their study design as descriptive and indicated that the data were collected using an online survey. This type of design was appropriate to address the study purpose. The sample section was strengthened by using the EPDS to identify women with PPD and using the sample criteria to ensure that the women had been hospitalized for pregnancy complications. However, the sample size of 53 was small for a descriptive study. The 26-item questionnaire had content validity and was consistently implemented online using standard survey software. This typical descriptive design was implemented in a way to provide quality study findings.

Implications for Practice

Maloni and co-workers (2013) noted that of the 53 women who were surveyed because they reported PPD, 70% had major depression. The common barriers that prevented them from getting treatment included time and the stigma of PPD diagnosis. Over 90% of the women did use the Internet as a resource to learn about coping with PPD and expressed an interest in a web-based PPD treatment.

Comparative Descriptive Design

A comparative descriptive design is used to describe variables and examine differences in variables in two or more groups that occur naturally in a setting. A comparative descriptive design compares descriptive data obtained from different groups, which might have been formed using gender, age, educational level, medical diagnosis, or severity of illness. Figure 8-4 provides a diagram of this design's structure.

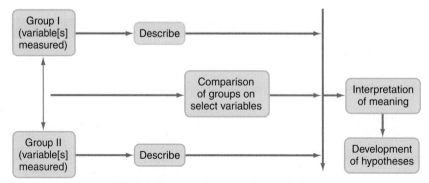

FIG 8-4 Comparative descriptive design.

RESEARCH EXAMPLE

Comparative Descriptive Design

Research Study Excerpt

Buet and colleagues (2013) conducted a comparative descriptive study to describe and determine differences in the hand hygiene (HH) opportunities and adherence of clinical (e.g., nurses and physicians) and nonclinical (e.g., teachers and parents) caregivers for patients in pediatric extended-care facilities (ECFs). The following study excerpt includes key elements of this comparative descriptive design:

> "Eight children across four pediatric ECFs were observed for a cumulative 128 hours, and all caregiver HH opportunities were characterized by the World Health Organization [WHO] '5 Moments for HH.'... A convenience sample of two children from each site (*n*=8) was observed. ... Four observers participated in two hours of didactic training and two hours of monitored practice observations at one of the four study sites to ensure consistent documentation and interpretation of observations. Observers learned how to accurately record HH opportunities and HH adherence using the WHO '5 Moments of HH' data acquisition tool, discussed below. Throughout the study, regular debriefings were also held to review and discuss data recording....The World Health Organization (WHO, 2009) '5 Moments for HH' define points of contact when healthcare workers should perform HH: 'before touching a patient, before clean/aseptic procedures, after body fluid exposure/risk, after touching a patient, and after touching patient surroundings. ... During approximately 128 hours of observation, 865 HH opportunities were observed." (Buet et al., 2013, pp. 72-73)

Critical Appraisal

Buet and associates (2013) clearly described the aspects of their study design but did not identify the specific type of design used in their study. The design was comparative descriptive because the HH opportunities and adherence for clinical and nonclinical caregivers were described and compared. The study included 128 hours of observation (16 hours per child) of 865 HH opportunities in four different ECF settings. Thus the sampling process was strong and seemed focused on accomplishing the study purpose. The data collectors were well trained and monitored to ensure consistent observation and recording of data. HH was measured using an observational tool based on international standards (WHO, 2009) for HH.

Implications for Practice

Buet and co-workers (2013) found that the HH of the clinical caregivers was significantly higher than the nonclinical caregivers. However, the overall HH adherence for the clinical caregivers was only 43%. The low HH adherence suggested increased potential for transmission of infections among children in ECFs. Additional HH education is needed for clinical and nonclinical caregivers of these children to prevent future adverse events. Quality and Safety Education for Nurses (QSEN, 2013) implications from this study encourage nurses to follow evidence-based practice (EBP) guidelines in adhering to HH measures to ensure safe care of their patients and reduce their risk of potentially life-threatening infections (Sherwood & Barnsteiner, 2012).

CORRELATIONAL DESIGNS

The purpose of a correlational design is to examine relationships between or among two or more variables in a single group in a study. This examination can occur at any of several levels—descriptive correlational, in which the researcher can seek to describe a relationship, predictive correlational, in which the researcher can predict relationships among variables, or the model testing design, in which all the relationships proposed by a theory are tested simultaneously.

In correlational designs, a large range in the variable scores is necessary to determine the existence of a relationship. Therefore the sample should reflect the full range of scores possible on the variables being measured. Some subjects should have very high scores and others very low scores, and the scores of the rest should be distributed throughout the possible range. Because of the need for a wide variation on scores, correlational studies generally require large sample sizes. Subjects are not divided into groups, because group differences are not examined. To determine the type of correlational design used in a published study, use the algorithm shown in Figure 8-5. More details on correlational designs referred to in this algorithm are available from other sources (Grove et al., 2013; Kerlinger & Lee, 2000).

Descriptive Correlational Design

The purpose of a descriptive correlational design is to describe variables and examine relationships among these variables. Using this design facilitates the identification of many interrelationships in a situation (Figure 8-6). The study may examine variables in a situation that has already occurred or is currently occurring. Researchers make no attempt to control or manipulate the situation. As with descriptive studies, variables must be clearly identified and defined conceptually and operationally (see Chapter 5).

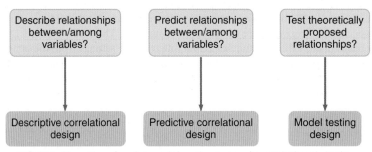

FIG 8-5 Algorithm for determining the type of correlational design.

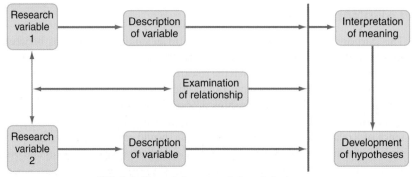

FIG 8-6 Descriptive correlational design.

Descriptive Correlational Design

Research Study Excerpt

Burns, Murrock, and Graor (2012) conducted a correlational study to examine the relationship between BMI and injury severity in adolescent males attending a National Boy Scout Jamboree. The key elements of this descriptive correlational design are presented in the following study excerpt.

"Design

This study used a descriptive, correlational design to examine the relationship between obesity and injury severity.... The convenience sample consisted of the 611 adolescent males, aged 11-17 years, who received medical attention for an injury at one of eight participating medical facilities. Exclusion criteria were adolescent males presenting with medical complaints unrelated to an injury (e.g., sore throat, dehydration, insect bite) and those who were classified as 'special needs' participants because of the disability affecting their mobility or requiring the use of an assistive device.... There were 20 medical facilities located throughout the 2010 National Boy Scout Jamboree. Each facility was equipped to manage both medical complaints and injuries...." (Burns et al., 2012, pp. 509–510)

"Measures

Past medical history, weight (in pounds) and height (in inches) were obtained from the HMR [health and medical record]. BMI [body mass index] and gender-specific BMI percentage were calculated electronically using online calculators from the Centers for Disease Control and Prevention and height and weight data. The BMI value was plotted on the CDC's gender-specific BMI-for-age growth chart to obtain a percentile ranking (BMI-P).... BMI-P defines four weight status categories: less than 5% is considered underweight, 5% to less than 85% is categorized healthy weight, 85% to less than 95% is the overweight category, and 95% or greater is categorized as obese. Age was measured in years and was self-reported.

Severity of injury was measured using the ESI [Emergency Severity Index] Version 4. This five-level triage rating scale was developed by the Agency for Healthcare Research and Quality and provides rapid, reproducible, clinically relevant stratification of patients into levels based on acuity and resource needs.... Training sessions were held for each medical facility to educate staff on the project, process, data collection techniques, and injury severity scoring methods.... All BMI and BMI-P values were recalculated to verify accuracy. To assess interrater reliability for injury severity scoring, ESI scores reported were compared with the primary researcher's scores. When discrepancies were found, the primary researcher reviewed the treatment record to determine the most accurate score." (Burns et al., 2012, p. 510)

Critical Appraisal
Descriptive Correlational Design

Burns and colleagues (2012) clearly identified their study design in their research report. The sampling method was a nonrandom sample of convenience that is commonly used in descriptive and correlational studies. Nonrandom sampling methods decrease the sample's representativeness of the population; however, the sample size was large and included 20 medical facilities at a national event. The exclusion sampling criteria ensured that the subjects selected were most appropriate to address the study purpose. The adolescents' height and weight were obtained from their medical records but the researchers did not indicate if these were reported or measured by the healthcare professionals. Self-reported height and weight for subjects could decrease the accuracy of the BMI and BMI-P calculated in a study. The BMI-P and severity injury scores were obtained using reliable and valid measurement methods, and the data from the medical facilities were checked for accuracy. The design of this study seemed strong and the knowledge generated provides a basis for future research.

Implications for Practice

Burns and associates (2012) found a significant relationship between BMI-P and injury severity. They noted that overweight/obese adolescents may have increased risks of serious injuries. Additional research is needed to examine the relationship of BMI to injury risk and to identify ways to prevent injuries in these adolescents. The findings from this study also emphasize the importance of healthy weight in adolescents to prevent health problems. QSEN (2013) implications are that evidence-based knowledge about the relationship between obesity and severity of injury provides nurses and students with information for educating adolescents to promote their health.

Predictive Correlational Design

The purpose of a **predictive correlational design** is to predict the value of one variable based on the values obtained for another variable or variables. Prediction is one approach to examining causal relationships between variables. Because causal phenomena are being examined, the terms dependent and independent are used to describe the variables. The variable to be predicted is classified as the dependent variable, and all other variables are independent or predictor variables. A predictive correlational design study attempts to predict the level of a dependent variable from the measured values of the independent variables. For example, the dependent variable of medication adherence could be predicted using the independent variables of age, number of medications, and medication knowledge of patients with congestive heart failure. The independent variables that are most effective in prediction are highly correlated with the dependent variable but are not highly correlated with other independent variables used in the study. The predictive correlational design structure is presented in Figure 8-7. Predictive correlational designs require the development of a theory-based mathematical hypothesis proposing variables expected to predict the dependent variable effectively. Researchers then use regression analysis to test the hypothesis (see Chapter 11).

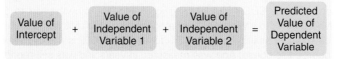

FIG 8-7 Predictive correlational design.

🖾 RESEARCH EXAMPLE

Predictive Correlational Design

Research Study Excerpt
Coyle (2012) used a predictive correlational design to determine if depressive symptoms were predictive of self-care behaviors in adults who had suffered a myocardial infarction (MI). The following study excerpt presents key elements of this design.

"Design, Setting, and Sample
    A descriptive correlational design examined the relationship between the independent variable of depressive symptoms [agitation and loss of energy] and the dependent variable of self-care. Data were collected from 62 patients in one hospital, who were recovering from an MI in the metropolitan Washington, areaA...." (Coyle, 2012, p. 128)

Measures
"Beck Depression Inventory II
    Depressive symptoms were measured using the BDI-II [Beck Depression Inventory II], a well-validated, 21-item scale designed to measure self-reported depressive symptomatology.... Internal-consistency estimates coefficient alpha of the total scores were .92 for psychiatric outpatients and .93 for college students. Construct validity was .93 (p < .001) when correlated with the BDI-I. In this study, the BDI-II Cronbach's alpha was .68 at baseline." (Coyle, 2012, p. 128)

"Health Behavior Scale
    Self-care behaviors after an MI were measured by the Health Behavior Scale (HBS), developed specifically for measuring the extent to which persons with cardiac disease perform prescribed self-care behaviors.... This

self-report, a 20-item instrument, assesses the degree to which patients perform five types of prescribed self-care (following diet, limiting smoking, performing activities, taking medications, and changing responses to stressful situations).... Cronbach's alphas for different self-care behaviors ranged from .82 to .95. In this study, reliability was measured by Cronbach's alpha and was .62 at 2 weeks and .71 at 30 days....Prior to hospital discharge, the Medical and Demographic Characteristics Questionnaire and BDI-II were administered by the researcher.... At 2 weeks and at 30 days after hospital discharge, participants were contacted by telephone to determine responses to the HBS." (Coyle, 2012, pp. 128-129)

Critical Appraisal

Coyle (2012) might have identified her study design more clearly as predictive correlational but did clearly identify the dependent variable as self-care and the independent variables as depressive symptoms. The design also included the longitudinal measurement of self-care with the HBS at 2 weeks and 30 days. The design was appropriate to accomplish the study purpose. The sample of 62 subjects was adequate because the study findings indicated significant results. The BDI-II has documented reliability (Cronbach's alphas > 0.7) and validity from previous studies, but the reliability of .68 was low in this study. Reliability indicates how consistently the scale measured depression and, in this study, it had 68% consistency and 32% error ($1.00 - .68 = .32 \times 100\% = 32\%$; see Chapter 10). HBS had strong reliability in previous studies but the validity of the scale was not addressed. The reliability of HBS was limited at 2 weeks (62% reliable and 38% error) but acceptable at 30 days (71% reliable and 29% error). This study has a strong design with more strengths than weaknesses, and the findings are probably an accurate reflection of reality. The study needs to be replicated with stronger measurement methods and a larger sample.

Implications for Practice

Coyle (2012) found that depressive symptoms of agitation and loss of energy were significantly predictive of self-care performance in patients with an MI at 30 days post–hospital discharge. Coyle recommended screening post-MI patients for depressive symptoms so that their symptoms might be managed before they were discharged. Further research is recommended to examine depression and self-care behaviors after hospital discharge to identify and treat potential problems.

Model Testing Design

Some studies are designed specifically to test the accuracy of a hypothesized causal model (see Chapter 7 for content on middle range theory). The model testing design requires that all concepts relevant to the model be measured and the relationships among these concepts examined. A large heterogeneous sample is required. Correlational analyses are conducted to determine the relationships among the model concepts, and the results are presented in the framework model for the study. This type of design is very complex; this text provides only an introduction to a model testing design implemented by Battistelli, Portoghese, Galletta, and Pohl (2013).

◢ RESEARCH EXAMPLE

Model Testing Design

Research Study

Battistelli and co-workers (2013) developed and tested a theoretical model to examine turnover intentions of nurses working in hospitals. The concepts of work-family conflict, job satisfaction, community embeddedness, and organizational affective commitment were identified as predictive of nurse turnover intention. The researchers collected data on these concepts using a sample of 440 nurses from a public hospital. The analysis of study data identified significant relationships ($p < 0.05$) among all concepts in the model. The results of this study are presented in Figure 8-8 and indicate the importance of these concepts in predicting nurse turnover intention.

Continued

RESEARCH EXAMPLE—cont'd

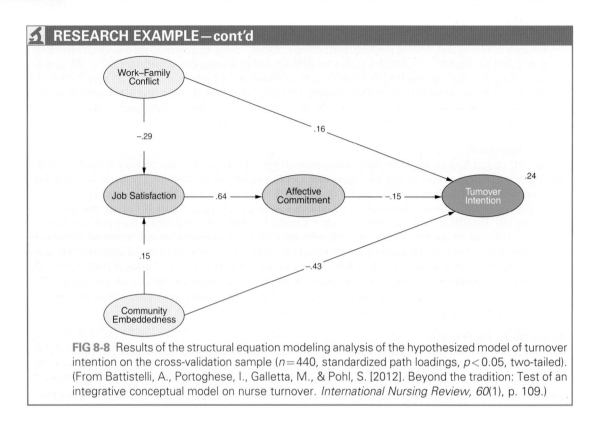

FIG 8-8 Results of the structural equation modeling analysis of the hypothesized model of turnover intention on the cross-validation sample ($n=440$, standardized path loadings, $p<0.05$, two-tailed). (From Battistelli, A., Portoghese, I., Galletta, M., & Pohl, S. [2012]. Beyond the tradition: Test of an integrative conceptual model on nurse turnover. *International Nursing Review, 60*(1), p. 109.)

UNDERSTANDING CONCEPTS IMPORTANT TO CAUSALITY IN DESIGNS

Quasi-experimental and experimental designs were developed to examine causality or the effect of an intervention on selected outcomes. **Causality** basically says that things have causes, and causes lead to effects. In a critical appraisal, you need to determine whether the purpose of the study is to examine causality, examine relationships among variables (correlational designs), or describe variables (descriptive designs). You may be able to determine whether the purpose of a study is to examine causality by reading the purpose statement and propositions within the framework (see Chapter 7). For example, the purpose of a causal study may be to examine the effect of a specific, preoperative, early ambulation educational program on length of hospital stay. The proposition may state that preoperative teaching results in shorter hospitalizations. However, the preoperative early ambulation educational program is not the only factor affecting length of hospital stay. Other important factors include the diagnosis, type of surgery, patient's age, physical condition of the patient prior to surgery, and complications that occurred after surgery. Researchers usually design quasi-experimental and experimental studies to examine causality or the effect of an intervention (independent variable) on a selected outcome (dependent variable), using a design that controls extraneous variables. Critically appraising studies designed to examine causality requires an understanding of such concepts as multicausality, probability, bias, control, and manipulation.

Multicausality

Very few phenomena in nursing can be clearly linked to a single cause and a single effect. A number of interrelating variables can be involved in producing a particular effect. Therefore studies developed from a multicausal perspective will include more variables than those using a strict causal orientation. The presence of multiple causes for an effect is referred to as multicausality. For example, patient diagnosis, age, presurgical condition, and complications after surgery will be involved in causing the length of hospital stay. Because of the complexity of causal relationships, a theory is unlikely to identify every element involved in causing a particular outcome. However, the greater the proportion of causal factors that can be identified and examined or controlled in a single study, the clearer the understanding will be of the overall phenomenon. This greater understanding is expected to increase the ability to predict and control the effects of study interventions.

Probability

Probability addresses relative rather than absolute causality. A cause may not produce a specific effect each time that a particular cause occurs, and researchers recognize that a particular cause *probably* will result in a specific effect. Using a probability orientation, researchers design studies to examine the probability that a given effect will occur under a defined set of circumstances. The circumstances may be variations in multiple variables. For example, while assessing the effect of multiple variables on length of hospital stay, researchers may choose to examine the probability of a given length of hospital stay under a variety of specific sets of circumstances. One specific set of circumstances may be that the patients in the study received the preoperative early ambulation educational program, underwent a specific type of surgery, had a particular level of health before surgery, and experienced no complications after surgery. Sampling criteria could be developed to control most of these factors. The probability of a given length of hospital stay could be expected to vary as the set of circumstances are varied or controlled in the design of the study.

Bias

The term bias means a slant or deviation from the true or expected. Bias in a study distorts the findings from what the results would have been without the bias. Because studies are conducted to determine the real and the true, researchers place great value on identifying and removing sources of bias in their study or controlling their effects on the study findings. Quasi-experimental and experimental designs were developed to reduce the possibility and effects of bias. Any component of a study that deviates or causes a deviation from a true measurement of the study variables contributes to distorted findings. Many factors related to research can be biased; these include attitudes or motivations of the researcher (conscious or unconscious), components of the environment in which the study is conducted, selection of the individual subjects, composition of the sample, groups formed, measurement methods, data collection process, data, and statistical analyses. For example, some of the subjects for the study might be taken from a unit of the hospital in which the patients are participating in another study involving high-quality nursing care or one nurse, selecting patients for the study, might assign the patients who are most interested in the study to the experimental group. Each of these situations introduces bias to the study.

   An important focus in critically appraising a study is to identify possible sources of bias. This requires careful examination of the methods section in the research report, including strategies for obtaining subjects, implementing a study treatment, and performing measurements. However, not all biases can be identified from the published report of a study. The article may not provide sufficient detail about the methods of the study to detect some of the biases.

Control

One method of reducing bias is to increase the amount of control in the design of a study. Control means having the power to direct or manipulate factors to achieve a desired outcome. For example, in a study of preoperative early ambulation educational program, subjects may be randomly selected and then randomly assigned to the experimental group or control group. The researcher may control the duration of the educational program or intervention, content taught, method of teaching, and teacher. The time that the teaching occurred in relation to surgery also may be controlled, as well as the environment in which it occurred. Measurement of the length of hospital stay may be controlled by ensuring that the number of days, hours, and minutes of the hospital stay is calculated exactly the same way for each subject. Limiting the characteristics of subjects, such as diagnosis, age, type of surgery, and incidence of complications, is also a form of control. The greater the researcher's control over the study situation, the more credible (or valid) the study findings.

Manipulation

Manipulation is a form of control generally used in quasi-experimental and experimental studies. Controlling the treatment or intervention is the most commonly used manipulation in these studies. In descriptive and correlational studies, little or no effort is made to manipulate factors in the circumstances of the study. Instead, the purpose is to examine the situation as it exists in a natural environment or setting. However, when quasi-experimental and experimental designs are implemented, researchers must manipulate the intervention under study. Researchers need to develop quality interventions that are implemented in consistent ways by trained individuals. This controlled manipulation of a study's intervention decreases the potential for bias and increases the validity of the study findings. Examining the quality of interventions in studies is discussed in more detail later in this chapter.

EXAMINING THE VALIDITY OF STUDIES

Determining the validity of a study's design and its findings is essential to the critical appraisal process. Study validity is a measure of the truth or accuracy of the findings obtained from a study. The validity of a study's design is central to obtaining quality results and findings from a study. Critical appraisal of studies requires that you think through the threats to validity or the possible problems in a study's design. You need to make judgments about how serious are these threats and how they might affect the quality of the study's findings. Strengths and threats to a study's validity provide a major basis for making decisions about which findings are accurate and might be ready for use in practice (Brown, 2014). Shadish and associates (2002) have described four types of validity—statistical conclusion validity, internal validity, construct validity, and external validity. Table 8-1 describes these four types of validity and summarizes the threats common to each. Understanding these types of validity and their possible threats are important in critically appraising quasi-experimental and experimental studies.

Statistical Conclusion Validity

The first step in inferring cause is to determine whether the independent and dependent variables are related. You can determine this relationship through statistical analysis. Statistical conclusion validity is concerned with whether the conclusions about relationships or differences drawn from statistical analysis are an accurate reflection of the real world. The second step is to identify

TABLE 8-1   TYPES OF VALIDITY CRITICALLY APPRAISED IN STUDIES

TYPES OF VALIDITY	DESCRIPTION	THREATS TO VALIDITY
Statistical conclusion validity	Validity is concerned with whether the conclusions about relationships or differences drawn from statistical analysis are an accurate reflection of the real world.	**Low statistical power**: Concluding that there are no differences between samples when one exists (type II error), which is usually caused by small sample size. **Unreliable measurement methods**: Scales or physiological measures used in a study are not consistently measuring study variables. **Unreliable intervention implementation**: The intervention in a study is not consistently implemented because of lack of study protocol or training of individuals implementing the intervention. **Extraneous variances in study setting**: Extraneous variables in the study setting influence the scores on the dependent variables, making it difficult to detect group differences.
Internal validity	Validity is focused on determining if study findings are accurate or are the result of extraneous variables.	**Subject selection and assignment to group concerns**: The subjects are selected by nonrandom sampling methods and are not randomly assigned to groups. **Subject attrition**: The percentage of subjects withdrawing from the study is high or more than 25%. **History**: An event not related to the planned study occurs during the study and could have an impact on the findings. **Maturation**: Changes in subjects, such as growing wiser, more experienced, or tired, which might affect study results.
Construct validity	Validity is concerned with the fit between the conceptual and operational definitions of variables and that the instrument measures what it is supposed to in the study.	**Inadequate definitions of constructs**: Constructs examined in a study lack adequate conceptual or operational definitions, so the measurement method is not accurately capturing what it is supposed to in a study. **Mono-operation bias**: Only one measurement method is used to measure the study variable. **Experimenter expectancies (Rosenthal effect)**: Researchers' expectations or bias might influence study outcomes, which could be controlled by blinding researchers and data collectors to the group receiving the study intervention.
External validity	Validity is concerned with the extent to which study findings can be generalized beyond the sample used in the study.	**Interaction of selection and treatment**: The subjects participating in the study might be different than those who decline participation. If the refusal to participate is high, this might alter the effects of the study intervention. **Interaction of setting and treatment**: Bias exists in study settings and organizations that might influence implementation of a study intervention. For example, some settings are more supportive and assist with a study, and others are less supportive and might encourage patients not to participate in a study. **Interaction of history and treatment**: An event, such as closing a hospital unit, changing leadership, or high nursing staff attrition, might affect the implementation of the intervention and measurement of study outcomes, which would decrease generalization of findings.

differences between groups. There are reasons why false conclusions can be drawn about the presence or absence of a relationship or difference. The reasons for the false conclusions are called threats to statistical conclusion validity (see Table 8-1). This text discusses some of the more common threats to statistical conclusion validity that you might identify in studies, such as low statistical power, unreliable measurement methods, unreliable intervention implementation, and extraneous variances in study setting. Shadish et al. –([2002)- provide a more detailed discussion of statistical conclusion validity.

Low Statistical Power

Low statistical power increases the probability of concluding that there is no significant difference between samples when actually there is a difference (type II error). A type II error is most likely to occur when the sample size is small or when the power of the statistical test to determine differences is low (Cohen, 1988). You need to ensure that the study has adequate sample size and power to detect relationships and differences. The concepts of sample size, statistical power, and type II error are discussed in detail in Chapters 9 and 11.

Reliability or Precision of Measurement Methods

The technique of measuring variables must be reliable to reveal true differences. A measure is reliable if it gives the same result each time the same situation or factor is measured. If a scale used to measure depression is reliable, it should give similar scores when depression is repeatedly measured over a short time period (Waltz, Strickland, & Lenz, 2010). Physiological measures that consistently measure physiological variables are considered precise. For example, a thermometer would be precise if it showed the same reading when tested repeatedly on the same patient within a limited time (see Chapter 10). You need to examine the measurement methods in a study and determine if they are reliable.

Reliability of Intervention Implementation

Intervention reliability ensures that the research treatment or intervention is standardized and applied consistently each time it is implemented in a study. In some studies, the consistent implementation of the treatment is referred to as intervention fidelity (see later). If the method of administering a research intervention varies from one person to another, the chance of detecting a true difference decreases. The inconsistent or unreliable implementation of a study intervention creates a threat to statistical conclusion validity.

Extraneous Variances in the Study Setting

Extraneous variables in complex settings (e.g., clinical units) can influence scores on the dependent variable. These variables increase the difficulty of detecting differences between the experimental and control groups. Consider the activities that occur on a nursing unit. The numbers and variety of staff, patients, health crises, and work patterns merge into a complex arena for the implementation of a study. Any of the dynamics of the unit can influence manipulation of the independent variable or measurement of the dependent variable. You might review the methods section of the study and determine how extraneous variables were controlled in the study setting.

Internal Validity

Internal validity is the extent to which the effects detected in the study are a true reflection of reality rather than the result of extraneous variables. Although internal validity should be a concern in all studies, it is usually addressed in relation to studies examining causality than in other studies. When examining causality, the researcher must determine whether the dependent variables may have been influenced by a third, often unmeasured, variable (an extraneous variable). The possibility of an alternative explanation of cause is sometimes referred to as a rival hypothesis (Shadish et al., 2002). Any study can contain threats to internal design validity, and these validity threats can lead to false-positive or false-negative conclusions (see Table 8-1). The researcher must ask, "Is there another reasonable (valid) explanation (rival hypothesis) for the finding other than the one I have proposed?" Some of the common threats to internal validity, such as subject selection and assignment to groups, subject attrition, history, and maturation, are discussed in this section.

Subject Selection and Assignment to Groups

Selection addresses the process whereby subjects are chosen to take part in a study and how subjects are grouped within a study. A selection threat is more likely to occur in studies in which randomization is not possible (Grove et al., 2013; Shadish et al., 2002). In some studies, people selected for the study may differ in some important way from people not selected for the study. In other studies, the threat is a result of the differences in subjects selected for study groups. For example, people assigned to the control group could be different in some important way from people assigned to the experimental group. This difference in selection could cause the two groups to react differently to the treatment or intervention; in this case, the intervention would not have caused the differences in group outcomes. Random selection of subjects in nursing studies is often not possible, and the number of subjects available for studies is limited. The random assignment of subjects to groups decreases the possibility of subject selection being a threat to internal validity.

Subject Attrition

Subject attrition involves participants dropping out of a study before it is completed. Subject attrition becomes a threat when (1) those who drop out of a study are a different type of person from those who remain in the study or (2) there is a difference between the types of people who drop out of the experimental group and the people who drop out of the control or comparison group (see Chapter 9).

History

History is an event that is not related to the planned study but that occurs during the time of the study. History could influence a subject's response to the treatment and alter the outcome of the study. For example, if you are studying the effect of an emotional support intervention on subjects' completion of their cardiac rehabilitation program, and several nurses quit their job at the center during your study, this historical event would create a threat to the study's internal design validity.

Maturation

In research, maturation is defined as growing older, wiser, stronger, hungrier, more tired, or more experienced during the study. Such unplanned and unrecognized changes are a threat to the study's internal validity and can influence the findings of the study.

Construct Validity

Construct validity examines the fit between the conceptual and operational definitions of variables. Theoretical constructs or concepts are defined within the study framework (conceptual definitions). These conceptual definitions provide the basis for the operational definitions of the variables. Operational definitions (methods of measurement) must validly reflect the theoretical constructs. (Theoretical constructs were discussed in Chapter 7; conceptual and; operational definitions of variables and concepts are discussed in Chapter 5.) The process of developing construct validity for an instrument often requires years of scientific work, and researchers need to discuss the construct validity of the instruments that they used in their study (Shadish et al., 2002; Waltz et al., 2010). (Instrument construct validity is discussed in Chapter 10.) The threats to construct validity are related to previous instrument development and to the development of measurement techniques as part of the methodology of a particular study. Threats to construct validity are described here and summarized in Table 8-1.

Inadequate Definitions of Constructs

Measurement of a construct stems logically from a concept analysis of the construct by the theorist who developed the construct or by the researcher. The conceptual definition should emerge from the concept analysis, and the method of measurement (operational definition) should clearly reflect both. A deficiency in the conceptual or operational definition leads to low construct validity (see Chapter 5).

Mono-operation Bias

Mono-operation bias occurs when only one method of measurement is used to assess a construct. When only one method of measurement is used, fewer dimensions of the construct are measured. Construct validity greatly improves if the researcher uses more than one instrument (Waltz et al., 2010). For example, if pain were a dependent variable, more than one measure of pain could be used, such as a pain rating scale, verbal reports of pain, and observations of behaviors that reflect pain (crying, grimacing, and pulling away). It is sometimes possible to apply more than one measurement of the dependent variable with little increase in time, effort, or cost.

Experimenter Expectancies (Rosenthal Effect)

The expectancies of the researcher can bias the data. For example, experimenter expectancy occurs if a researcher expects a particular intervention to relieve pain. The data that he or she collects may be biased to reflect this expectation. If another researcher who does not believe the intervention would be effective had collected the data, results could have been different. The extent to which this effect actually influences studies is not known. Because of their concern about experimenter expectancy, some researchers are not involved in the data collection process. In other studies, data collectors do not know which subjects are assigned to treatment and control groups, which means that they were blinded to group assignment.

External Validity

External validity is concerned with the extent to which study findings can be generalized beyond the sample used in the study (Shadish et al., 2002). With the most serious threat, the findings would be meaningful only for the group studied. To some extent, the significance of the study depends on the number of types of people and situations to which the findings can be applied. Sometimes, the factors influencing external validity are subtle and may not be reported in research reports; however, the researcher must be responsible for these factors. Generalization is usually narrower for a single study than for multiple replications of a study using different samples, perhaps from different populations in different settings. Some of the threats to the ability to generalize the findings (external validity) in terms of study design are described here and summarized in Table 8-1.

Interaction of Selection and Treatment

Seeking subjects who are willing to participate in a study can be difficult, particularly if the study requires extensive amounts of time or some other investment by subjects. If a large number of persons approached to participate in a study decline to participate, the sample actually selected will be limited in ways that might not be evident at first glance. Only the researcher knows the subjects well. Subjects might be volunteers, "do-gooders", or those with nothing better to do. In this case, generalizing the findings to all members of a population, such as all nurses, all hospitalized patients, or all persons experiencing diabetes, is not easy to justify.

The study must be planned to limit the investment demands on subjects and thereby improve participation. For example, the researchers would select instruments that are valid and reliable but have fewer items to decrease subject burden. The researcher must report the number of persons who were approached and refused to participate in the study (refusal rate) so that those who examine the study can judge any threats to external validity. As the percentage of those who decline to participate increases, external design validity decreases. Sufficient data need to be collected on the subjects to allow the researcher to be familiar with the characteristics of subjects and, to the greatest extent possible, the characteristics of those who decline to participate (see Chapter 9).

Interaction of Setting and Treatment

Bias exists in regard to the types of settings and organizations that agree to participate in studies. This bias has been particularly evident in nursing studies. For example, some hospitals welcome nursing studies and encourage employed nurses to conduct studies. Others are resistant to the conduct of nursing research. These two types of hospitals may be different in important ways; thus there might be an interaction of setting and treatment that limits the generalizability of the findings. Researchers must consider this factor when making statements about the population to which their findings can be generalized.

Interaction of History and Treatment

The circumstances occurring when a study is conducted might influence the treatment, which could affect the generalization of the findings. Logically, one can never generalize to the future; however, replicating the study during various time periods strengthens the usefulness of findings over time. In critically appraising studies, you need to consider the effects of nursing practice and societal events that occur during the period of the reported findings.

ELEMENTS OF DESIGNS EXAMINING CAUSALITY

Quasi-experimental and experimental designs are implemented in studies to obtain an accurate representation of cause and effect by the most efficient means. That is, the design should provide the greatest amount of control, with the least error possible. The effects of some extraneous variables are controlled in a study by using specific sampling criteria, a structured independent variable or intervention, and a highly controlled setting. Randomized controlled trials (RCTs) are also designed to examine causality and are considered by some sources to be one of the strongest designs to examine cause and effect (Hoare & Hoe, 2013; Schulz, Altman, & Moher, 2010). RCTs are discussed later in this chapter. The essential elements of research to examine causality are:

- Random assignment of subjects to groups
- Precisely defined independent variable or intervention
- Researcher-controlled manipulation of the intervention
- Researcher control of the experimental situation and setting

- Inclusion of a control or comparison group in the study
- Clearly identified sampling criteria (see Chapter 9)
- Carefully measured dependent or outcome variables (see Chapter 10)

Examining Interventions in Nursing Studies

In studies examining causality, investigators develop an intervention that is expected to result in differences in post-test measures between the treatment and control or comparison groups. An intervention might also be called a treatment or an independent variable in a study. Interventions may be physiological, psychosocial, educational, or a combination of these. The therapeutic nursing intervention implemented in a nursing study needs to be carefully designed, clearly described, and appropriately linked to the outcomes (dependent variables) to be measured in the study. The intervention needs to be provided consistently to all subjects. A published study needs to document intervention fidelity, which includes a detailed description of the essential elements of the intervention and the consistent implementation of the intervention during the study (Morrison et al., 2009; Santacroce, Maccarelli & Grey, 2004). Sometimes, researchers provide a table of the intervention content and/or the protocol used to implement the intervention to each subject consistently. A research report also needs to indicate who implemented the intervention and what training was conducted to ensure consistent intervention implementation. Some studies document the monitoring of intervention fidelity (completeness and consistency of the intervention implementation) during the conduct of the study (Carpenter et al., 2013).

Kim, Chung, Park, and Kang (2012) implemented an aquarobic exercise program to determine its effects on the self-efficacy, pain, body weight, blood lipid levels, and depression of patients with osteoarthritis. These researchers detailed the components of their aquarobic exercise program (intervention) in a table in their published study. Table 8-2 identifies the categories, session composition, physical fitness factors, and exercise content for the exercise program to promote the consistent and complete implementation of the intervention to each of the study subjects. Kim and colleagues (2012, p. 183) indicated that "the aquarobic exercise program consisted of both patient education and aquarobic exercise. A professor of exercise physiology, medical specialist of sports medicine, professor of mental health nursing, professor of adult nursing, professor of senior nursing, and public-health nurse assessed the validity of the aquarobic exercise program." The osteoarthritis patients were educated in the exercise program and led in the exercises by a trained instructor to promote intervention fidelity in this study. The details of the design of this quasi-experimental study are presented in the next section.

Experimental and Control or Comparison Groups

The group of subjects who received the study intervention is referred to as the experimental or treatment group. The group that is not exposed to the intervention is referred to as the control or comparison group. Although control and comparison groups traditionally have received no intervention, adherence to this expectation is not possible in many nursing studies. For example, it would be unethical not to provide preoperative teaching to a patient. Furthermore, in many studies, it is possible that just spending time with a patient or having a patient participate in activities that he or she considers beneficial may in itself cause an effect. Therefore the study often includes a comparison group nursing action.

This nursing action is usually the standard care that the patient would receive if a study were not being conducted. The researcher must describe in detail the standard care that the control or

convenience, in which the subjects are included in the study because they are at the right place at the right time (see Chapter 9). The subjects selected are then randomly assigned to receive the experimental treatment or standard care. The group who receives standard care is usually referred to as a comparison group versus a control group, who would receive no treatment or standard care (Shadish et al., 2002). However, the terms *control group* and *comparison group* are frequently used interchangeably in nursing studies.

In many studies, subjects from the original sample are randomly assigned to the experimental or comparison group, which is an internal design validity strength. Occasionally, comparison and treatment groups may evolve naturally. For example, groups may include subjects who choose a treatment as the experimental group and subjects who choose not to receive a treatment as the comparison group. These groups cannot be considered equivalent, because the subjects who select to be in the comparison group probably differ in important ways from those who select to be in the treatment group. For example, if researchers were implementing an intervention of an exercise program to promote weight loss, the subjects should not be allowed to select whether they are in the experimental group receiving the exercise program or the comparison group not receiving an exercise program. Subjects' self-selecting to be in the experimental or comparison group is a threat to the internal design validity of a study.

Pretest and Post-test Designs with Comparison Group

Quasi-experimental study designs vary widely. The most frequently used design in social science research is the untreated comparison group design, with pretest and post-test (Figure 8-9). With this design, the researcher has a group of subjects who receive the experimental treatment (or intervention) and a comparison group of subjects who receive standard care.

Another commonly used design is the post-test–only design with a comparison group, shown in Figure 8-10. This design is used in situations in which a pretest is not possible. For example, if the

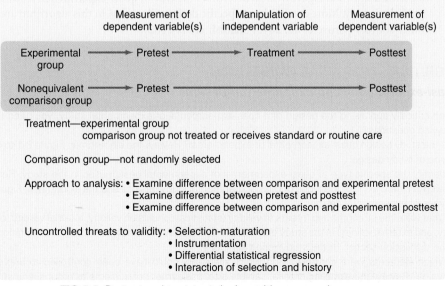

FIG 8-9 Pretest and post-test design with a comparison group.

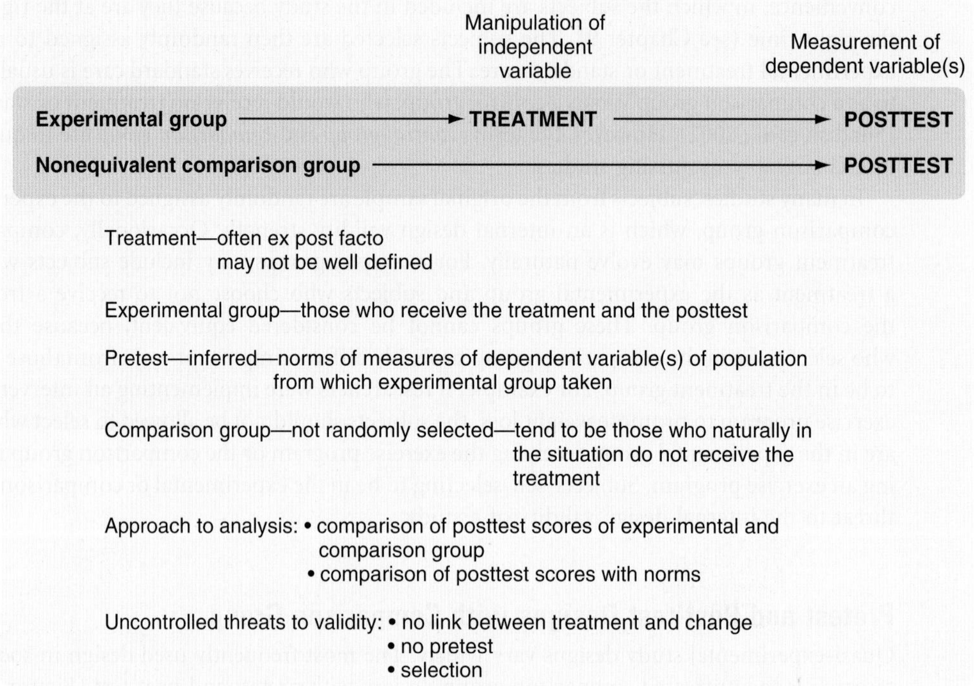

	Manipulation of independent variable	Measurement of dependent variable(s)
Experimental group	→ TREATMENT	→ POSTTEST
Nonequivalent comparison group		→ POSTTEST

Treatment—often ex post facto
    may not be well defined

Experimental group—those who receive the treatment and the posttest

Pretest—inferred—norms of measures of dependent variable(s) of population
    from which experimental group taken

Comparison group—not randomly selected—tend to be those who naturally in
    the situation do not receive the
    treatment

Approach to analysis: • comparison of posttest scores of experimental and
    comparison group
    • comparison of posttest scores with norms

Uncontrolled threats to validity: • no link between treatment and change
    • no pretest
    • selection

FIG 8-10 Post-test–only design with a comparison group.

researcher is examining differences in the amount of pain a subject feels during a painful procedure, and a nursing intervention is used to reduce pain for subjects in the experimental group, it might not be possible (or meaningful) to pretest the amount of pain before the procedure. This design incorporates a number of threats to validity because of the lack of a pretest. You can use the algorithm shown in Figure 8-11 to determine the type of quasi-experimental study design used in a published study. More details about specific designs identified in this algorithm are available from other sources (Grove et al., 2013; Shadish et al., 2002).

? CRITICAL APPRAISAL GUIDELINES

Quasi-experimental and Experimental Designs

When critically appraising the design of a quasi-experimental or experimental study, you need to address the following questions:
1. Is the study design quasi-experimental or experimental? Review the algorithm in Figure 8-1 to determine the type of study design.
2. Identify the specific type of quasi-experimental or experimental design used in the study. Review the algorithm in Figure 8-11 for the types of quasi-experimental study designs and the algorithm in Figure 8-12 for the types of experimental designs.
3. What were the strengths and threats to validity (statistical conclusion validity, internal validity, construct validity, and external validity) in the study (see Table 8-1)? Review the methods section and limitations identified in the discussion section of the study report for ideas.
4. Which elements were controlled and which elements could have been controlled to improve the study design? Review the sampling criteria, sample size, assignment of subjects to groups, and study setting.

5. Was the study intervention described in detail? Was a protocol developed to ensure consistent or reliable implementation of the intervention with each subject throughout the study? Did the study report indicate who implemented the intervention? If more than one person implemented the treatment, how were they trained to ensure consistency in the delivery of the treatment? Was intervention fidelity achieved in the study?
6. Were the study dependent variables measured with reliable and valid measurement methods?

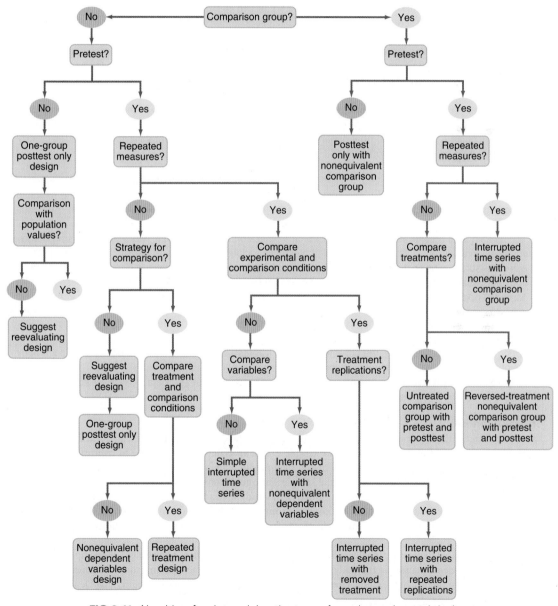

FIG 8-11 Algorithm for determining the type of quasi-experimental design.

⚡ RESEARCH EXAMPLE

Quasi-experimental Pretest–Post-test Design with a Comparison Group

Research Study Excerpt

Kim and associates (2012) conducted a quasi-experimental study to examine the effect of an aquarobic exercise program on the self-efficacy, pain, body weight, blood lipid levels, and depression of patients with osteoarthritis. The intervention for this study was introduced in the previous section, and we encourage you to locate this article on the website for this text and critically appraise the design of this study. The critical appraisal of this study was conducted using the Guidelines for Critically Appraising Quasi-experimental and Experimental Designs. The key elements of the Kim and co-workers' (2012) study design are presented in the following excerpt:

"A nonequivalent control group and a pre- and posttest quasi-experimental design were used. The independent variables were thirty-six 60-minute sessions of an aquarobic exercise program three times a week. The dependent variables were self-efficacy, pain, body weight, blood lipids, and depression level.... The inclusion criteria for this study consisted of the following: (a) women, (b) 60 years and older, (c) osteoarthritis.... The exclusion criteria were the following: (a) previous knee or hip joint replacement surgery, (b) any other surgical procedure of the lower limbs in the previous 6 months, (c) rheumatoid arthritis, (d) mental or physical disorders, and (e) participation in a similar intervention in the past.... A total of 80 patients were initially recruited and randomly assigned to either a control or an experimental group (40 patients in each).... The final number of participants was 35 in the experimental group and 35 in the control group...." (Kim et al., 2012, pp.182-183)

Instruments

"Self-efficacy is the attitude of self-confidence and the competency of oneself to continue the exercise under any situation. A questionnaire consisting of 14 items on a 10-point Likert-type scale that measures self-efficacy for patients with arthritis was previously developed. ... Cronbach's alpha in this study was .90. ... Pain was measured with a VAS [visual analog scale]. ... Body weight was assessed using a body composition analyzer. ... Blood lipids (total cholesterol, triglycerides, and high density lipoproteins [HDLs]) were measured using enzymatic methods... Blood samples were sent for analysis immediately after collection" (Kim et al. 2012, p. 185). Depression was measured with the Zung Depression Scale that consists of 20 items (10 positive and 10 negative) with 4-point Liker-type scale. The Cronbach's alpha found in this study was .75.

Procedure

"Prior to the start of the study, we collected baseline (pretest) data that included...self-efficacy, pain, body weight, blood lipid levels, and levels of depression from the experimental and control groups. The experimental group underwent an aquarobic exercise program for 12 weeks. Post-test data ...were collected following completion of the exercise program." (Kim et al., 2012, p. 185).

Critical Appraisal

Kim and colleagues (2012) clearly identified the quasi-experimental design used in their study, and this design was appropriate to address the study purpose. The sample exclusion criteria were selected to control the effects of extraneous variables, such as joint replacements or rheumatoid arthritis, on the study dependent or outcome variables (internal validity strength). The initial sample was one of convenience (threat to internal and external validity), and the researchers recommended conducting the study with a larger, random sample. The subjects were randomly assigned to the experimental and control groups, with 40 subjects in each group (internal validity strength). The attrition was 12.5% for each group, which is an internal design validity strength for a 12-week study.

The instruments used to measure the dependent variables—self-efficacy, pain, body weight, blood lipid levels, and depression levels—were discussed in the study and were appropriate and reliable, adding to the statistical conclusion and construct design validity of the study. However, the validity of the self-efficacy scale and Zung Depression Scale were not addressed, and more detail might have been provided on the accuracy of the physiological measures of body weight and blood lipid levels.

The aquarobic exercise program was detailed in the published study (see Table 8-2) and was consistently implemented, promoting the fidelity of the intervention and adding to the design statistical conclusion validity and external validity. The setting for the exercises was highly controlled, which also adds to the external validity of the design. The researchers noted that the study participants were recruited from a single public health center, which limits the generalization of the findings. The design of the Kim et al. (2012) study was extremely strong and demonstrated statistical conclusion, and internal, construct, and external validity with few threats to design validity.

Implications for Practice

Kim and associates (2012) found that the experimental group had significant improvement in self-efficacy, pain, body weight, blood lipid levels, and depression levels when compared with the control group. The researchers recommended the use of this intervention in patients with osteoarthritis. The QSEN implications are that this exercise intervention for patients with osteoarthritis is supported by research. Nurses and students are encouraged to provide this type of evidence-based exercise intervention to their patients with osteoarthritis.

EXPERIMENTAL DESIGNS

A variety of experimental designs, some relatively simple and others very complex, have been developed for studies focused on examining causality. In some cases, researchers may combine characteristics of more than one design to meet the needs of their study. Names of designs vary from one text to another. When reading and critically appraising a published study, determine the author's name for the design (some authors do not name the design used) and/or read the description of the design to determine the type of design used in the study. Use the algorithm shown in Figure 8-12 to determine the type of experimental design used in a published study. More details about the specific designs identified in Figure 8-12 are available in other texts (Grove et al., 2013; Shadish et al., 2002).

Classic Experimental Pretest and Post-test Designs with Experimental and Control Groups

A common experimental design used in healthcare studies is the pretest–post-test design with experimental and control groups (Campbell & Stanley, 1963; Shadish et al., 2002). This design is shown in Figure 8-13; it is similar to the quasi-experimental design in Figure 8-9, except that the experimental study is more tightly controlled in the areas of intervention, setting, measurement, and/or extraneous variables, resulting in fewer threats to design validity. The experimental design is stronger if the initial sample is randomly selected; however, most studies in nursing do not include a random sample but do randomly assign subjects to the experimental and control groups. Most studies in nursing use the quasi-experimental design shown in Figure 8-9 because of the inability to control selected extraneous and environmental variables.

Multiple groups (both experimental and control) can be used to great advantage in experimental designs. For example, one control group might receive no treatment, another control group might receive standard care, and another control group might receive a placebo or intervention

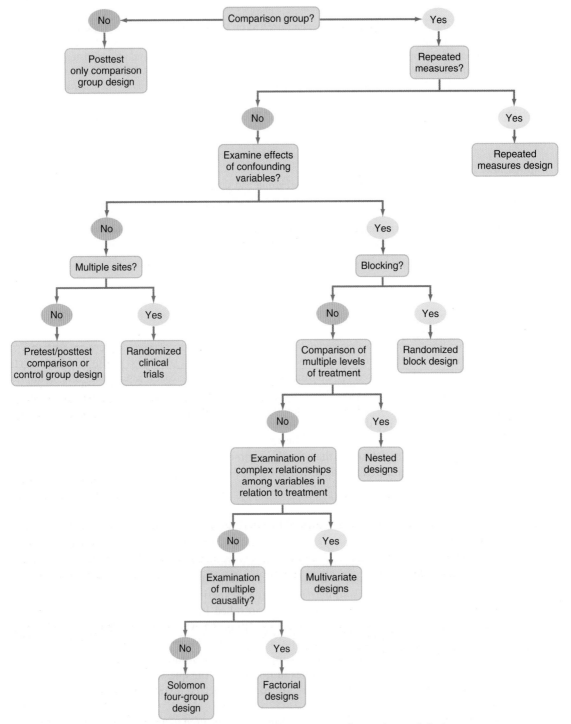

FIG 8-12 Algorithm for determining the type of experimental design.

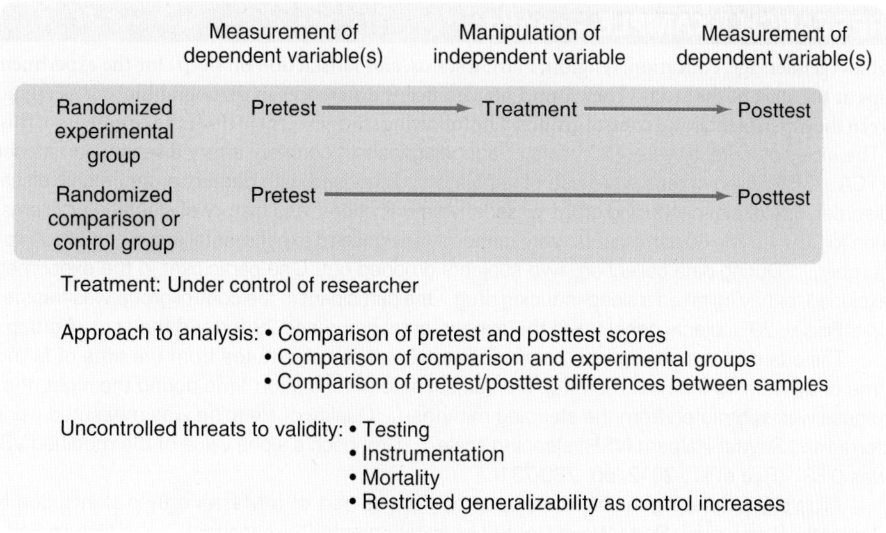

	Measurement of dependent variable(s)	Manipulation of independent variable	Measurement of dependent variable(s)
Randomized experimental group	Pretest ⟶	Treatment ⟶	Posttest
Randomized comparison or control group	Pretest ⟶		Posttest

Treatment: Under control of researcher

Approach to analysis: • Comparison of pretest and posttest scores
• Comparison of comparison and experimental groups
• Comparison of pretest/posttest differences between samples

Uncontrolled threats to validity: • Testing
• Instrumentation
• Mortality
• Restricted generalizability as control increases

FIG 8-13 Pretest–post-test control group design.

with no effect like a sugar pill in a drug study. Each one of multiple experimental groups can receive a variation of the treatment, such as a different frequency, intensity, or duration of nursing care measures. For example, different frequency, intensity, or duration of massage treatments might be implemented in a study to determine their effect(s) on patients' muscle pain. These additions greatly increase the generalizability of study findings when the sample is representative of the target population and the sample size is strong.

Post-test–Only with Control Group Design

The experimental post-test–only control group design is also frequently used in healthcare studies when a pretest is not possible or appropriate. This design is similar to the design in Figure 8-13, with the pretest omitted. The characteristics of the experimental and control groups are usually examined at the start of the study to ensure that the groups are similar. The lack of a pretest does, however, increase the potential for error that might affect the findings. Additional research is recommended before generalization of findings. Ryu, Park, and Park (2012) conducted an experimental study with post-test–only control group design that is presented here as an example.

RESEARCH EXAMPLE

Experimental Post-test–Only Control Group Design

Research Study Excerpt

Ryu and co-workers (2012) conducted an experimental study to examine the effect of sleep-inducing music on sleep in persons who had undergone percutaneous transluminal coronary angiography (PTCA) in the cardiac care unit (CCU). These researchers used a post-test–only control group design in their study because the patients were usually only in the CCU 24 hours or less after their PTCA procedure. Ryu and colleagues collected data on the demographic

Continued

variables (gender, age, education, religion, marital status, and satisfaction on sleep) for the experimental and control groups at the start of the study. They found no significant differences in demographic and sleeping characteristics between the experimental and control groups. The following study excerpt includes key elements of this study's design:

"The inclusion criteria were ≥ 20 years of age, diagnosis of coronary artery disease, admittance to CCU after PTCA.... Exclusion criteria were use of ventilators; diagnosed with dementia, neurologic disease, or sensory disorder; use of sleep-inducing drugs or sedative medications; and history of sleeping problems before admission to CCU.... The 60 participants were randomly assigned to experimental group or control group using a card number.... During data collection, two subjects dropped out. One participant in the experimental group was excluded for having taken a sleep-inducing drug. One participant in the control group was transferred to another unit. Finally, 29 subjects constituted the experimental group and 29 formed the control group....

The quantity of sleeping was counted as total number of minutes from the time of falling asleep to the time of awakening the next morning. If a subject awoke for a short time during the night, the time of wakefulness was subtracted from the sleeping minutes.... Quality of sleeping was measured using the modified Verran and Snyder-Halpern (VSH) sleeping scale.... Cronbach's alpha value of the modified VSH in this study was 0.83" (Ryu et al., 2012, pp. 730-731).

"The sleep-inducing music [developed by Park as part of a Master's thesis] included Nature Sounds (2 minutes 8 seconds), Delta Wave Control Music (5 minutes 21 seconds)... and Nature Sounds (2 minutes 25 seconds). The MP3 music was supplied through earphones to the participants from 10:00-10:53 PM. If a subject fell asleep with the music still in progress, the earphone was not removed intentionally until 5 AM the next morning. Eye bandage CS-204 (CS Berea Korea) was also applied to the participants at 10 PM and was removed at 5 AM.... No music was offered to the control group participants, but ear plugs 370 Bilsom No. 303 were applied from 10 PM-5 AM the next morning. The same eye bandage used in the experimental group was also applied to the control participants." (Ryu et al., 2012, p. 731)

Critical Appraisal

Ryu and colleagues (2012) identified their design as experimental in their study abstract but did not identify the specific type of design as a post-test–only control group design. This design was appropriate for addressing the study purpose and hypotheses. The sample exclusion criteria controlled possible extraneous variables, and the random assignment of subjects to the experiment and control groups increased the internal and external validity of the study design. The subject attrition was very low (one subject per group, for total of 3.3% for the study), and the reasons for their dropping out of the study were documented and seemed usual (internal validity strength).

A trained data collector measured the dependent variable quantity of sleeping in a structured, consistent way. The quality of sleeping variable was measured with a VSH sleeping scale that had established reliability in previous studies and strong reliability in this study, with Cronbach's alpha = 0.83 (83% reliable and 17% error). More detail was needed about the validity of this scale and its ability to measure quality of sleeping. For the most part, quality instruments were used in this study, adding to the statistical conclusion and construct validity of the study.

The experimental group received a structured sleep-inducing music intervention that was delivered consistently using an MP3 player for each subject, which ensured intervention fidelity. Both groups of subjects received the standard care of eye bandages, and the control group was also provided with standard earplugs. The study was in the CCU setting, so the researchers were able to control the environment of the subjects. The intervention fidelity and controlled study setting strengthen the study's external and statistical conclusion validity. The detailed control of the intervention, setting, and data collection process are consistent with implementing an experimental study design. This study's design included several strengths and a few weaknesses, which increased the validity of the findings and their potential usefulness for practice.

Implications for Practice

Ryu and associates (2012) found that the sleep-inducing music intervention significantly improved the quantity and quality of sleeping for the experimental group over that of the control group. The researchers recommended that offering CCU patients sleep-inducing music might be an easy, cost-effective intervention for improving sleep for these patients.

RANDOMIZED CONTROLLED TRIALS

Currently, in medicine and nursing, the randomized controlled trial (RCT) is noted to be the strongest methodology for testing the effectiveness of a treatment because of the elements of the design that limit the potential for bias. Subjects are randomized to the treatment and control groups to reduce selection bias (Carpenter et al., 2013; Hoare & Hoe, 2013; Schulz et al., 2010). In addition, blinding or withholding of study information from data collectors, participants, and their healthcare providers can reduce the potential for bias. RCTs, when appropriately conducted, are considered the gold standard for determining the effectiveness of healthcare interventions. RCTs may be carried out in a single setting or in multiple geographic locations to increase sample size and obtain a more representative sample.

The initial RCTs conducted in medicine demonstrated inconsistencies and biases. Consequently, a panel of experts—clinical trial researchers, medical journal editors, epidemiologists, and methodologists—developed guidelines to assess the quality of RCTs reports. This group initiated the Standardized Reporting of Trials (SORT) statement that was revised and became the CONsolidated Standards for Reporting Trials (CONSORT). This current guideline includes a checklist and flow diagram that might be used to develop, report, and critically appraise published RCTs (CONSORT, 2012). Nurse researchers need to follow the CONSORT 2010 statement recommendations in the conduct of RCTs and in their reporting (Schulz et al., 2010). You might use the flow diagram in Figure 8-14 to critically appraise the RCTs reported in nursing journals. An RCT needs to include the following elements:

1. The study was designed to be a definitive test of the hypothesis that the intervention caused the defined dependent variables or outcomes.
2. The intervention is clearly described and its implementation is consistent to ensure intervention fidelity (CONSORT, 2012; Santacroce et al., 2004; Schulz et al., 2010; Yamada, Stevens, Sidani, Watt-Watson, & De Silva, 2010).
3. The study is conducted in a clinical setting, not in a laboratory.
4. The design meets the criteria of an experimental study (Schulz et al., 2010).
5. Subjects are drawn from a reference population through the use of clearly defined criteria. Baseline states are comparable in all groups included in the study. Selected subjects are then randomly assigned to treatment and comparison groups (see Figure 8-14)—thus, the term *randomized controlled trial* (CONSORT, 2012; Schulz et al., 2010).
6. The study has high internal validity. The design is rigorous and involves a high level of control of potential sources of bias that will rule out possible alternative causes of the effect (Shadish et al., 2002). The design may include blinding to accomplish this purpose. With blinding the patient, those providing care to the patient, and/or the data collectors are unaware of whether the patient is in the experimental group or in the control group.
7. Dependent variables or outcomes are measured consistently with quality measurement methods (Waltz et al., 2010).
8. The intervention is defined in sufficient detail so that clinical application can be achieved (Schulz et al., 2010).
9. The subjects lost to follow-up are identified with their rationale for not continuing the study. The attrition from the experimental and control groups needs to be addressed, as well as the overall sample attrition.
10. The study has received external funding sufficient to allow a rigorous design with a sample size adequate to provide a definitive test of the intervention.

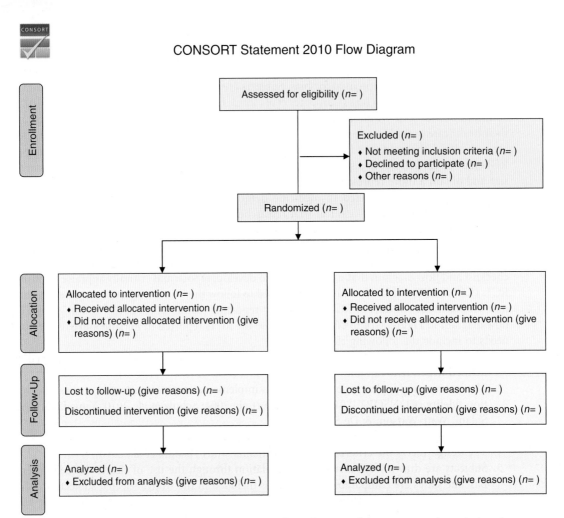

CONSORT Statement 2010 Flow Diagram

FIG 8-14 CONSORT 2010 statement showing a flow diagram of the progress through the phases of a parallel randomized trial of two groups (enrollment, intervention allocation, follow-up, and data analysis). (From CONSORT. [2012]. The CONSORT statement. Retrieved May 6, 2013 from http://www.consort-statement.org/consort-statement; and Schulz, K. F., Altman, D. G., & Moher, D. [2010]. CONSORT 2010 statement: Updated guidelines for reporting parallel group randomized trials. *Annals of Internal Medicine, 152*[11], 726-733.)

RESEARCH EXAMPLE

Randomized Controlled Trial (RCT)

Research Study Excerpt

Jones, Duffy, and Flanagan (2011) conducted a RCT to test the efficacy of a nurse-coached intervention (NCI) on the outcomes of patients undergoing ambulatory arthroscopic surgery. The NCI was developed to improve the postoperative experiences of patients and families following ambulatory surgery. This study was funded by the National Institute of Nursing Research. The following study excerpt identifies the study hypothesis, design, and major findings:

"This study was conducted to test the hypothesis that ambulatory arthroscopic surgery patients who receive a nurse-coached telephone intervention will have significantly less symptom distress and better functional health status than a comparable group who receive usual practice.…

The study sample in this *randomized controlled trial* with repeated measures was 102 participants (52 in the intervention group and 50 in the usual practice group) drawn from a large academic medical center in the Northeast United States. Symptom distress was measured using the Symptom Distress Scale, and functional health was measured using the Medical Outcomes Study 36-Item Short-Form Health Survey General Health Perceptions and Mental Health subscales." (Jones et al., 2011, p. 92)

Critical Appraisal

Jones and co-workers (2011) detailed their study intervention and the steps taken by the researchers to promote fidelity in the implementation of the NCI. The nurses were trained in the delivery of the NCI by the study team using a video. Each nurse coach was provided with a packet of guidelines for management of the participants' symptoms.

"The guidelines addressed common patient problems associated with postoperative recovery after arthroscopy with general anesthesia (e.g., nausea, vomiting, pain, immobility). The guidelines contained five areas to evaluate: (a) assessment (self-report), (b) current management of symptoms, (c) evaluation by the coach of the adequacy of the intervention, (d) additional intervention strategies to address the presenting symptoms, and (e) proposed outcome (self-report)" (Jones et al., 2011, p. 95).

The sample criteria were detailed to identify the target population. Once the patients consented to be in the study, they were randomly assigned to the NCI group or the usual care group using the sealed envelope method (Maxwell & Delaney, 2004). The steps of this study followed the steps outlined in the CONSORT flow diagram in Figure 8-14. However, the sample size and group sizes were small for a RCT, and the study was implemented in only one setting, decreasing the generalizability of the findings.

Implications for Practice

Jones and colleagues (2011) found that the NCI delivered by telephone postoperatively to arthroscopic surgery patients significantly reduced their symptom distress and improved their physical and mental health. The findings for this study were consistent with previous research in this area and have potential use in practice. The NCI was provided in a format that might be implemented in clinical settings. The QSEN implications are that the NCI is an appropriate way for nurses to provide patient-centered care to individuals following arthroscopic surgery to improve their recovery.

INTRODUCTION TO MIXED-METHODS APPROACHES

There is controversy among nurse researchers about the relative validity of various approaches or designs needed to generate knowledge for nursing practice. Designing quantitative experimental studies with rigorous controls may provide strong external validity but sometimes have limited internal validity. Qualitative studies may have strong internal validity but questionable external validity. A single approach to measuring a concept may be inadequate to justify the claim that it is a valid measure of a theoretical concept. Testing a single theory may leave the results open to the challenge of rival hypotheses from other theories (Creswell, 2014).

As research methodologies continue to evolve, mixed-methods approaches offer investigators the ability to use the strengths of qualitative and quantitative research designs. Mixed-methods research is characterized as research that contains elements of both qualitative and quantitative approaches (Creswell, 2014; Grove et al., 2013; Marshall & Rossman, 2011; Morse, 1991; Myers & Haase, 1989).

There has been debate about the philosophical underpinnings of mixed-methods research and which paradigm best fits this method. It is recognized that all researchers bring assumptions to their research, consciously or unconsciously, and investigators decide whether they are going to view their study from a postpositivist (quantitative) or constructivist (qualitative) perspective (Fawcett & Garity, 2009; Munhall, 2012).

Over the last few years, many researchers have departed from the idea that one paradigm or one research strategy is right and have taken the perspective that the search for truth requires the use of all available strategies. To capitalize on the representativeness and generalizability of quantitative research and the in-depth, contextual nature of qualitative research, mixed methods are combined in a single research study (Creswell, 2014). Because phenomena are complex, researchers are more likely to capture the essence of the phenomenon by combining qualitative and quantitative methods.

The idea of using mixed-methods approaches to conduct studies has a long history. More than 50 years ago, quantitative researchers Campbell and Fiske (1959) recommended mixed methods to measure a psychological trait more accurately. This mixed methodology was later expanded into what Denzin (1989) identified as "triangulation." Denzin believed that combining multiple theories, methods, observers, and data sources can assist researchers in overcoming the intrinsic bias that comes from single-theory, single-method, and single-observer studies. Triangulation evolved to include using multiple data collection and analysis methods, multiple data sources, multiple analyses, and multiple theories or perspectives. Today, the studies including both quantitative and qualitative design strategies are identified as mixed-methods designs or approaches (Creswell, 2014). More studies with mixed-methods designs have been appearing in nursing journals. You need to recognize studies with mixed-methods designs and be able to appraise the quantitative and qualitative aspects of these designs critically.

RESEARCH EXAMPLE

Mixed-Methods Approaches

Research Study Excerpt

Piamjariyakul, Smith, Russell, Werkowitch, and Elyachar (2013) conducted a mixed-methods study to examine the feasibility and effects of a telephone coaching program on family caregivers' home management of family members with heart failure (HF). The major elements of this study's design are presented in the following excerpt.

Research Design

"This pilot study employed a mixed methods design. The measures of caregiver burden, confidence, and preparedness were compared pre- and post-intervention. Also overall cost analysis was used to determine the expenses for educational materials and the cost of the nurse's time to administer the coaching program [quantitative quasi-experimental single group pre-test and posttest design]. Focus group and content analysis research methods were used to evaluate the feasibility and helpfulness of the program [exploratory-descriptive qualitative design]. Caregivers in this study were recruited from a group of HF patients receiving care at a large Midwestern University Medical Center who were recently hospitalized due to HF exacerbation [sample of convenience]. . . . All 12 family caregivers completed baseline data, and 10 subjects completed the four-session program. Two caregivers completed only the first weekly session (one was too ill and the other was too busy to continue)." (Piamjariyakul et al., 2013, pp. 33-34)

Caregiver Telephone Heart Failure Home Management Coaching Program [intervention]

"The coaching program for family caregivers was nurse-administered and conducted in four telephone sessions. The content in the program and the need for the four coaching sessions was based on previous study results, the American Heart Association HF national clinical guidelines, and the Heart Failure Society of America (HFSA) information for family and friends.... The content was presented in a detailed table.... For fidelity of the intervention implementation, a 2-hour training session...was provided for the 5 nurse interventionists" (Piamjariyakul et al., 2013, p. 34)

"Coaching program cost data was collected for all costs related to implementation of the program.... All nurse interventionists shared their experiences in a focus group that was held after delivery of the coaching program." (Piamjariyakul et al., 2013, p. 36)

Critical Appraisal

Piamjariyakul and associates (2013) clearly described their study as a mixed-methods design. The major focus of this study was the development and evaluation of the telephone HF home management coaching program intervention that was tested using a quasi-experimental, pretest–post-test, one-group design. This is a weak design that includes no control group for comparison of study outcomes but might be considered acceptable for this pilot study focused on intervention development. The qualitative part of the design included conducting a focus group with the nurses who delivered the coaching intervention and doing content analysis of the focus group transcript. The researchers might have provided more detail on the qualitative part of this design.

The subjects were selected with a sample of convenience, and the sample size was small (12 subjects, with a 15% attrition to a final sample of 10). However, the researchers did indicate that this was a pilot study, and they recommended the coaching program should be further tested with a larger sample. The HF home management coaching program was presented in great detail. The content of the intervention was presented in a table in the research report and was based on previous research and national evidence-based guidelines. The implementation of the intervention with trained nurse interventionists ensured the fidelity of the intervention. The measurement methods (Caregiving Burden Scale, confidence in providing HF care scale, and preparedness scale) were briefly described, but more detail is needed about the scales' reliability and validity.

Implications for Practice

Piamjariyakul and co-workers (2013) found that the caregiver burden scores were significantly reduced by the implementation of the HF home management coaching program, and the confidence and preparedness for HF home management scores improved 3 months after the intervention. The qualitative part of the study described the coaching program as feasible to implement and helpful to the caregivers. This study provided a quality HF home management coaching program intervention, but more research is needed to determine the effectiveness of this intervention for clinical practice (Brown, 2014; Craig & Smyth, 2012).

▌ KEY CONCEPTS

- A research design is a blueprint for conducting a quantitative study that maximizes control over factors that could interfere with the validity of the findings.
- Four common types of quantitative designs are used in nursing—descriptive, correlational, quasi-experimental, and experimental.
- Descriptive and correlational designs are conducted to describe and examine relationships among variables. These types of designs are also called nonexperimental designs.
- Cross-sectional design involves examining a group of subjects simultaneously in various stages of development, levels of educational, severity of illness, or stages of recovery to describe changes in a phenomenon across stages.
- Longitudinal design involves collecting data from the same subjects at different points in time and might also be referred to as repeated measures.

- Correlational designs are of three different types: (1) descriptive correlational, in which the researcher can seek to describe a relationship; (2) predictive correlational, in which the researcher can predict relationships among variables; and (3) the model testing design, in which all the relationships proposed by a theory are tested simultaneously.
- Elements central to the study design include the presence or absence of a treatment, number of groups in the sample, number and timing of measurements to be performed, method of sampling, time frame for data collection, planned comparisons, and control of extraneous variables.
- The concepts important to examining causality include multicausality, probability, bias, control, and manipulation.
- Study validity is a measure of the truth or accuracy of the findings obtained from a study. Four types of validity are covered in this text—statistical conclusion validity, internal validity, construct validity, and external validity.
- The essential elements of experimental research are (1) the random assignment of subjects to groups; (2) the researcher's manipulation of the independent variable; and (3) the researcher's control of the experimental situation and setting, including a control or comparison group.
- Interventions or treatments are implemented in quasi-experimental and experimental studies to determine their effect on selected dependent variables. Interventions may be physiological, psychosocial, education, or a combination of these.
- Critically appraising a design involves examining the study setting, sample, intervention or treatment, measurement of dependent variables, and data collection procedures.
- Randomized controlled trial (RCT) design is noted to be the strongest methodology for testing the effectiveness of an intervention because of the elements of the design that limit the potential for bias.
- As research methodologies continue to evolve in nursing, mixed-methods approaches are being conducted to use the strengths of both qualitative and quantitative research designs.

REFERENCES

Battistelli, A., Portoghese, I., Galletta, M., & Pohl, S. (2013). Beyond the tradition: Test of an integrative conceptual model on nurse turnover. *International Nursing Review, 60*(1), 103–111.

Brown, S. J. (2014). *Evidence-based nursing: The research-practice connection* (3rd ed.). Sudbury, MA: Jones & Bartlett.

Buet, A., Cohen, B., Marine, M., Scully, F., Alper, P., Simpser, E., et al. (2013). Hand hygiene opportunities in pediatric extended care facilities. *Journal of Pediatric Nursing, 28*(1), 72–76.

Burns, K., Murrock, C. J., & Graor, C. H. (2012). Body mass index and injury severity in adolescent males. *Journal of Pediatric Nursing, 27*(5), 508–513.

Campbell, D. T., & Fiske, D. W. (1959). Convergent and discriminate validation by the multitrait-multimethod matrix. *Psychological Bulletin, 56*(2), 81–105.

Campbell, D. T., & Stanley, J. C. (1963). *Experimental and quasi-experimental designs for research*. Chicago: Rand McNally.

Carpenter, J. S., Burns, D. S., Wu, J., Yu, M., Ryker, K., Tallman, E., et al. (2013). Methods: Strategies used and data obtained during treatment fidelity monitoring. *Nursing Research, 62*(1), 59–65.

Cohen, J. (1988). *Statistical power analysis for the behavioral sciences* (2nd ed.). New York: Academic Press.

CONSORT, (2012). The CONSORT statement. Retrieved May 6, 2013 from, http://www.consort-statement.org/consort-statement.

Coyle, M. K. (2012). Depressive symptoms after a myocardial infarction and self-care. *Archives of Psychiatric Nursing, 26*(2), 127–134.

Craig, J., & Smyth, R. (2012). *The evidence-based practice manual for nurses* (3rd ed.). Edinburgh: Churchill Livingstone Elsevier.

Creswell, J. W. (2014). *Research design: Qualitative, quantitative and mixed methods approaches* (4th ed.). Thousand Oaks, CA: Sage.

Denzin, N. K. (1989). *The research act: A theoretical introduction to sociological methods* (3rd ed.). New York: McGraw-Hill.

Fawcett, J., & Garity, J. (2009). *Evaluating research for evidence-based nursing practice.* Philadelphia: F. A. Davis.

Grove, S. K., Burns, N., & Gray, J. R. (2013). *The practice of nursing research: Appraisal, synthesis, and generation of evidence* (7th ed.). St. Louis: Elsevier Saunders.

Hoare, Z., & Hoe, J. (2013). Understanding quantitative research: Part 2. *Nursing Standard, 27*(18), 48–55.

Hoe, J., & Hoare, Z. (2012). Understanding quantitative research: Part 1. *Nursing Standard, 27*(15–17), 52–57.

Jones, D., Duffy, M. E., & Flanagan, J. (2011). Randomized clinical trial testing efficacy of a nurse-coached intervention in arthroscopy patients. *Nursing Research, 60*(2), 92–99.

Kerlinger, F. N., & Lee, H. B. (2000). *Foundations of behavioral research* (4th ed.). Fort Worth, TX: Harcourt College Publishers.

Kim, I., Chung, S., Park, Y., & Kang, H. (2012). The effectiveness of an aquarobic exercise program for patients with osteoarthritis. *Applied Nursing Research, 25*(3), 181–189.

Maloni, J. A., Przeworski, A., & Damato, E. G. (2013). Web recruitment and Internet use and preferences reported by women with postpartum depression after pregnancy complications. *Archives of Psychiatric Nursing, 27*(2), 90–95.

Marshall, C., & Rossman, G. B. (2011). *Designing qualitative research* (5th ed.). Thousand Oaks, CA: Sage.

Maxwell, S. E., & Delaney, H. D. (2004). *Designing experiments and analyzing data: A model comparison perspective* (2nd ed.). Mahway, NJ: Lawrence Erlbaum Associates.

Morrison, D. M., Hoppe, M. J., Gillmore, M. R., Kluver, C., Higa, D., & Wells, E. A. (2009). Replicating an intervention: The tension between fidelity and adaptation. *AIDS Education and Prevention, 21*(2), 128–140.

Morse, J. M. (1991). Approaches to qualitative-quantitative methodological triangulation. *Nursing Research, 40*(1), 120–123.

Munhall, P. L. (2012). *Nursing research: A qualitative perspective* (5th ed.). Sudbury, MA: Jones & Bartlett.

Myers, S. T., & Haase, J. E. (1989). Guidelines for integration of quantitative and qualitative approaches. *Nursing Research, 38*(5), 299–301.

Piamjariyakul, U., Smith, C. E., Russell, C., Werkowitch, M., & Elyachar, A. (2013). The feasibility of a telephone coaching program on heart failure home management for family caregivers. *Heart & Lung, 42*(1), 32–39.

Quality and Safety Education for Nurses (QSEN), (2013). *Pre-licensure knowledge, skills, and attitudes (KSAs).* Retrieved February 11, 2013 from, http://qsen.org/competencies/pre-licensure-ksas/.

Ryu, M., Park, J. S., & Park, H. (2012). Effect of sleep-inducing music on sleep in persons with percutaneous transluminal coronary angiography in the cardiac care unit. *Journal of Clinical Nursing, 21*(5/6), 728–735.

Santacroce, S. J., Maccarelli, L. M., & Grey, M. (2004). Methods: Intervention fidelity. *Nursing Research, 53*(1), 63–66.

Schulz, K. F., Altman, D. G., & Moher, D. (2010). CONSORT 2010 statement: Updated guidelines for reporting parallel group randomized trials. *Annals of Internal Medicine, 152*(11), 726–733.

Shadish, W. R., Cook, T. D., & Campbell, D. T. (2002). *Experimental and quasi-experimental designs for generalized causal inference.* Chicago: Rand McNally.

Sherwood, G., & Barnsteiner, J. (2012). *Quality and safety in nursing: A competency approach to improving outcomes.* Ames, IA: Wiley-Blackwell.

Waltz, C. F., Strickland, O. L., & Lenz, E. R. (2010). *Measurement in nursing and health research* (4th ed.). New York: Springer.

World Health Organization (WHO), (2009). *Guidelines for hand hygiene in health care.* Retrieved May 6, 2013 from, http://whqlibdoc.who.int/publications/2009/9789241597906_eng.pdf.

Yamada, J., Stevens, B., Sidani, S., Watt-Watson, J., & De Silva, N. (2010). Content validity of a process evaluation checklist to measure intervention implementation fidelity of the EPIC Intervention. *Worldviews of Evidence-Based Nursing, 7*(3), 158–164.

CHAPTER

9

Examining Populations and Samples in Research

CHAPTER OVERVIEW

LEARNING OUTCOMES

After completing this chapter, you should be able to:

1. Describe sampling theory, including the concepts of population, target population, sampling criteria, sampling frame, subject or participant, sampling plan, sample, representativeness, sampling error, and systematic bias.
2. Critically appraise the sampling criteria (inclusion and exclusion criteria) in published studies.

3. Identify the specific type of probability and nonprobability sampling methods used in published quantitative, qualitative, and outcomes studies.
4. Describe the elements of power analysis used to determine sample size in selected studies.
5. Critically appraise the sample size of quantitative and qualitative studies.

6. Critically appraise the sampling processes used in quantitative, qualitative, and outcomes studies.

7. Critically appraise the settings used in quantitative, qualitative, and outcomes studies.

KEY TERMS

Acceptance rate, p. 253
Accessible population, p. 250
Cluster sampling, p. 261
Convenience sampling, p. 264
Effect size, p. 267
Elements, p. 250
Exclusion sampling criteria, p. 251
Generalization, p. 250
Heterogeneous, p. 251
Highly controlled setting, p. 278
Homogeneous, p. 251
Inclusion sampling criteria, p. 251
Intraproject sampling, p. 274
Natural (or field) setting, p. 277
Network sampling, p. 271
Nonprobability sampling, p. 263

Partially controlled setting, p. 277
Participants, p. 250
Population, p. 250
Power, p. 266
Power analysis, p. 266
Probability sampling, p. 257
Purposeful or purposive sampling, p. 270
Quota sampling, p. 265
Random sampling, p. 255
Random variation, p. 252
Refusal rate, p. 253
Representativeness, p. 252
Research setting, p. 276
Sample, p. 249
Sample attrition, p. 253
Sample retention, p. 254

Sample size, p. 266
Sampling, p. 249
Sampling frame, p. 255
Sampling method or plan, p. 255
Sampling or eligibility criteria, p. 251
Saturation, p. 274
Simple random sampling, p. 259
Stratified random sampling, p. 260
Subjects, p. 250
Systematic sampling, p. 262
Systematic variation, p. 252
Target population, p. 250
Theoretical sampling, p. 273
Verification, p. 274

Students often enter the field of research with preconceived notions about samples and sampling methods. Many of these notions come from exposure to television advertisements, public opinion polls, and newspaper reports of research findings. A television spokesperson boasts that four of five doctors recommend a particular pain medication, a newscaster announces that John Jones will win the senate election by a margin of 10%, and a newspaper reporter writes that research has shown that aggressive treatment of hypertension to maintain a blood pressure of 120/80 mm Hg or lower significantly reduces the risk for coronary artery disease and stroke.

All these examples include a sampling technique or method. Some of the outcomes from these sampling methods are more valid than others, based on the sampling method used and the sample size achieved. When critically appraising a study, you need to examine the sampling process and determine its quality. The sampling process is usually described in the methods section of a published research report. This chapter was developed to assist you in understanding and critically appraising the sampling processes implemented in quantitative, qualitative, and outcomes studies. Initially, the concepts of sampling theory are introduced, including sampling criteria, sampling frame, and representativeness of a sample. The nonprobability and probability sampling methods and sample sizes for quantitative and qualitative studies are detailed. The chapter concludes with a discussion of the natural, partially controlled, and highly controlled settings used in conducting research.

UNDERSTANDING SAMPLING CONCEPTS

Sampling involves selecting a group of people, events, objects, or other elements with which to conduct a study. A sampling method or plan defines the selection process, and the sample defines the selected group of people (or elements). A sample selected in a study should represent an identified population of people. The population might be all people who have diabetes, all patients who have had abdominal surgery, or all persons who receive care from a registered nurse. In most cases, however, it would be impossible for researchers to study an entire population. Sampling theory was developed to determine the most effective way to acquire a sample that accurately reflects the population under study. Key concepts of sampling theory include populations, target population, sampling or eligibility criteria, accessible population, elements, representativeness, sampling frames, and sampling methods or plans. The following sections describe these concepts and include relevant examples from published studies.

Populations and Elements

The population is a particular group of individuals or elements, such as people with type 2 diabetes, who are the focus of the research. The target population is the entire set of individuals or elements who meet the sampling criteria (defined in the next section), such as female, 18 years of age or older, new diagnosis of type 2 diabetes confirmed by the medical record, and not on insulin. Figure 9-1 demonstrates the link of the population, target population, and accessible population in a study. An accessible population is the portion of the target population to which the researcher has reasonable access. The accessible population might include elements within a country, state, city, hospital, nursing unit, or primary care clinic, such as the individuals with diabetes who were provided care in a primary care clinic in Arlington, Texas. Researchers obtain the sample from the accessible population by using a particular sampling method or plan, such as simple random sampling. The individual units of the population and sample are called elements. An element can be a person, event, object, or any other single unit of study. When elements are persons, they are referred to as participants or subjects (see Figure 9-1). Quantitative and outcomes researchers refer to the people they study as subjects or participants. Qualitative researchers refer to the individuals they study as participants.

Generalization extends the findings from the sample under study to the larger population. In quantitative and outcomes studies, researchers obtain a sample from the accessible population with the goal of generalizing the findings from the sample to the accessible population and then, more abstractly, to the target population (see Figure 9-1). The quality of the study and consistency of the study's findings with the findings from previous research in this area influence the extent of the generalization. If a study is of high quality, with findings consistent with previous research,

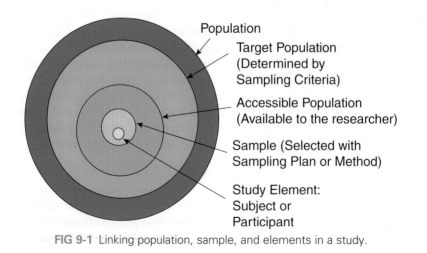

Population

Target Population
(Determined by
Sampling Criteria)

Accessible Population
(Available to the researcher)

Sample (Selected with
Sampling Plan or Method)

Study Element:
Subject or
Participant

FIG 9-1 Linking population, sample, and elements in a study.

then researchers can be more confident in generalizing their findings to the target population. For example, the findings from the study of female patients with a new diagnosis of type 2 diabetes in a primary care clinic in Arlington, Texas, may be generalized to the target population of women with type 2 diabetes managed in primary care clinics. With this information, you can decide whether it is appropriate to use this evidence in caring for the same type of patients in your practice, with the goal of moving toward evidence-based practice (EBP; Brown, 2014; Melnyk & Fineout-Overholt, 2011).

Sampling or Eligibility Criteria

Sampling or eligibility criteria include the list of characteristics essential for eligibility or membership in the target population. For example, researchers may choose to study the effect of pre-operative teaching about early ambulation on the outcome of length of hospital stay for adults having knee joint replacement surgery. In this study, the sampling criteria may include (1) age of at least 18 years of age or older (adults), (2) able to speak and read English, (3) surgical replacement of one knee joint, (4) no history of previous joint replacement surgery, (5) no diagnosis of dementia, and (6) no debilitating chronic muscle diseases. The sample is selected from the accessible population that meets these sampling criteria. Sampling criteria for a study may consist of inclusion or exclusion sampling criteria, or both. Inclusion sampling criteria are the characteristics that the subject or element must possess to be part of the target population. In the example, the inclusion criteria are age 18 years of age or older, able to speak and read English, and surgical replacement of one knee joint. Exclusion sampling criteria are those characteristics that can cause a person or element to be excluded from the target population. For example, any subjects with a history of previous joint replacement surgery, diagnosis of dementia, and diagnosis of a debilitating chronic muscle disease were excluded from the preoperative teaching study. Researchers should state a sample criterion only once and should not include it as both an inclusion and exclusion criterion. Thus, researchers should not have an inclusion criterion of no diagnosis of dementia *and* an exclusion criterion of diagnosis of dementia.

When the quantitative or outcomes study is completed, the findings are often generalized from the sample to the target population that meets the sampling criteria (Fawcett & Garity, 2009). Researchers may narrowly define the sampling criteria to make the sample as homogeneous (or similar) as possible to control for extraneous variables. Conversely, the researcher may broadly define the criteria to ensure that the study sample is heterogeneous, with a broad range of values or scores on the variables being studied. If the sampling criteria are too narrow and restrictive, researchers may have difficulty obtaining an adequately sized sample from the accessible population, which can limit the generalization of findings.

In discussing the generalization of quantitative study findings in a published research report, investigators sometimes attempt to generalize beyond the sampling criteria. Using the example of the early ambulation preoperative teaching study, the sample may need to be limited to subjects who speak and read English because the preoperative teaching is in English and one of the measurement instruments requires that subjects be able to read English. However, the researchers may believe that the findings can be generalized to non–English-speaking persons. When reading studies, you need to consider carefully the implications of using these findings with a non–English-speaking population. Perhaps non–English-speaking persons, because they come from another culture, do not respond to the teaching in the same way as that observed in the study population. When critically appraising a study, examine the sample inclusion and exclusion criteria, and determine whether the generalization of the study findings is appropriate based on the study sampling criteria. (Chapter 11 provides more detail on generalizing findings from studies.)

REPRESENTATIVENESS OF A SAMPLE IN QUANTITATIVE AND OUTCOMES RESEARCH

Representativeness means that the sample, accessible population, and target population are alike in as many ways as possible (see Figure 9-1). In quantitative and outcomes research, you need to evaluate representativeness in terms of the setting, characteristics of the subjects, and distribution of values on variables measured in the study. Persons seeking care in a particular setting may be different from those who seek care for the same problem in other settings or those who choose to use self-care to manage their problems. Studies conducted in private hospitals usually exclude low-income patients. Other settings may exclude older adults or those with less education. People who do not have access to care are usually excluded from studies. Subjects in research centers and the care that they receive are different from patients and the care that they receive in community hospitals, public hospitals, veterans' hospitals, or rural hospitals. People living in rural settings may respond differently to a health situation from those who live in urban settings. Thus the setting identified in published studies does influence the representativeness of the sample. Researchers who gather data from subjects across a variety of settings have a more representative sample of the target population than those limiting the study to a single setting.

A sample must be representative in terms of characteristics such as age, gender, ethnicity, income, and education, which often influence study variables. These are examples of demographic or attribute variables that might be selected by researchers for examination in their study. Researchers analyze data collected on the demographic variables to produce the sample characteristics—characteristics used to provide a picture of the sample. These sample characteristics must be reasonably representative of the characteristics of the population. If the study includes groups, the subjects in the groups must have comparable demographic characteristics (see Chapter 5 for more details on demographic variables and sample characteristics).

Studies that obtain data from large databases have more representative samples. For example, Monroe, Kenaga, Dietrich, Carter, and Cowan (2013) examined the prevalence of employed nurses enrolled in substance use monitoring programs by examining data from the National Council of State Boards of Nursing (NCSBN) 2010 Survey of Regulatory Boards Disciplinary Actions on Nurses. This NCSBN survey included the United States and its territories and found that 17,085 (0.51%) of the employed nurses were enrolled in substance use monitoring programs. This study examined data from multiple sites (United States and its territories) and included a large national population of nurses (all employed nurses), resulting in a representative sample.

Random and Systematic Variation of Subjects' Values

Measurement values also need to be representative. Measurement values in a study often vary randomly among subjects. Random variation is the expected difference in values that occurs when different subjects from the same sample are examined. The difference is random because some values will be higher and others lower than the average (mean) population value. As sample size increases, random variation decreases, improving representativeness.

Systematic variation, or systematic bias—a serious concern in sampling—is a consequence of selecting subjects whose measurement values differ in some specific way from those of the population. This difference usually is expressed as a difference in the average (or mean) values between the sample and population. Because the subjects have something in common, their values tend to be similar to those of others in the sample but different in some way from those of the population as a whole. These values do not vary randomly around the population mean. Most of the variation from the mean is in the same direction; it is systematic. Thus the sample mean may be higher than or lower than the mean of the target population. Increasing the sample size has no effect on systematic variation. For example, if all the subjects in a study examining some type of knowledge level have an intelligence quotient (IQ) above 120, then all their test scores in the study are likely to be higher than those of the population mean, which includes people with a wide variation in IQ scores (but with a mean IQ of 100). The IQs of the subjects will introduce a systematic bias. When systematic bias occurs in quasi-experimental or experimental studies, it can lead the researcher to conclude that the treatment has made a difference, when in actuality the values would have been different, even without the treatment.

Acceptance and Refusal Rates in Studies

The probability of systematic variation increases when the sampling process is not random. Even in a random sample, however, systematic variation can occur when a large number of the potential subjects declines participation. As the number of subjects declining participation increases, the possibility of a systematic bias in the study becomes greater. In published studies, researchers may identify a *refusal rate*, which is the percentage of subjects who declined to participate in the study, and the subjects' reasons for not participating (Grove, Burns, & Gray, 2013). The formula for calculating the refusal rate in a study is as follows:

$$\text{Refusal rate} = (\text{Number refusing participation}$$
$$\div \text{ number meeting sampling criteria approached}) \times 100\%$$

For example, if 80 potential subjects meeting sampling criteria are approached to participate in the hypothetical study about the effects of early ambulation preoperative teaching on length of hospital stay, and 4 patients refuse, then the refusal rate would be:

$$\text{Refusal rate} = (4 \div 80) \times 100\% = 0.5 \times 100\% = 5\%$$

Other studies record an *acceptance rate*, which is the percentage of subjects meeting sampling criteria consenting to participate in a study. However, researchers will report the refusal or acceptance rate, but not both. The formula for calculating the acceptance rate in a study is as follows:

$$\text{Acceptance rate} = (\text{Number accepting participation}$$
$$\div \text{ number meeting sampling criteria approached}) \times 100\%$$

In the hypothetical preoperative teaching study, 4 of 80 potential subjects refused to participate—so $80 - 4 = 76$ accepted. Plugging the following numbers into the stated formula gives:

$$\text{Acceptance rate} = (76 \div 80) \times 100\% = 0.95 \times 100\% = 95\%$$

You can also calculate the acceptance and refusal rates as follows:

$$\text{Acceptance rate} = 100\% - \text{refusal rate}$$

Or:

$$\text{Refusal rate} = 100\% - \text{acceptance rate}$$

In this example, the acceptance rate was $100\% - 5\%$ (refusal rate) $= 95\%$, which is high or strong. In studies with a high acceptance rate or a low refusal rate reported, the chance for systematic variation is less, and the sample is more likely to be representative of the target population. Researchers usually report the refusal rate, and it is best to provide rationales for the individuals refusing to participate.

Sample Attrition and Retention Rates in Studies

Systematic variation also may occur in studies with high sample attrition. *Sample attrition* is the withdrawal or loss of subjects from a study that can be expressed as a number of subjects withdrawing or a percentage. The percentage is the sample attrition rate and it is best if researchers include both the number of subjects withdrawing and the attrition rate. The formula for calculating the sample attrition rate in a study is as follows:

$$\text{Sample attrition rate} = (\text{Number of subjects withdrawing from a study} \div \text{sample size of study}) \times 100\%$$

For example, in the hypothetical study of preoperative teaching, 31 subjects—12 from the treatment group and 19 from the comparison group—withdraw, for various reasons. Loss of 31 subjects means a 41% attrition rate:

$$\text{Sample attrition rate} = (31 \div 76) \times 100\% = 0.418 \times 100\% = 40.8\% = 41\%$$

In this example, the overall sample attrition rate was considerable (41%), and the rates differed for the two groups to which the subjects were assigned. You can also calculate the attrition rates for the groups. If the two groups were equal at the start of the study and each included 38 subjects, then the attrition rate for the treatment group was $(12 \div 38) \times 100\% = 0.316 \times 100\% = 31.6\% = 32\%$. The attrition for the comparison group was $(19 \div 38) \times 100\% = 0.5 \times 100\% = 50\%$. Systematic variation is greatest when a large number of subjects withdraw from the study before data collection is completed or when a large number of subjects withdraw from one group but not the other(s) in the study. In studies involving a treatment, subjects in the comparison group who do not receive the treatment may be more likely to withdraw from the study. However, sometimes the attrition is higher for the treatment group if the intervention is complex and/or time-consuming (Kerlinger & Lee, 2000). In the early ambulation preoperative teaching example, there is a strong potential for systematic variation because the sample attrition rate was large (41%) and the attrition rate in the comparison group (50%) was larger than the attrition rate in the treatment group (32%). The increased potential for systematic variation results in a sample that is less representative of the target population.

The opposite of sample attrition is the **sample retention**, which is the number of subjects who remain in and complete a study. You can calculate the sample retention rate in two ways:

$$\text{Sample retention rate} = (\text{Number of subjects completing the study} \div \text{sample size}) \times 100\%$$

Or:

$$\text{Sample retention rate} = 100\% - \text{sample attrition rate}$$

In the example, early ambulation preoperative teaching study, 45 subjects were retained in the study that had an original sample of 76 subjects:

$$\text{Sample retention rate} = (45 \div 76) \times 100\% = 0.59 \times 100\% = 59.2\% = 59\%$$

Or:

$$\text{Sample retention rate} = 100\% - 41\% = 59\%$$

The higher the retention rate, the more representative the sample is of the target population and the more likely the study results are an accurate reflection of reality. Often, researchers will identify the attrition rate or retention rate, but not both. It is best to provide a rate in addition to the number of subjects withdrawing from a study, as well as the subjects' reasons for withdrawing.

Sampling Frames

From a sampling theory perspective, each person or element in the population should have an opportunity to be selected for the sample. One method of providing this opportunity is referred to as random sampling. For everyone in the accessible population to have an opportunity for selection in the sample, each person in the population must be identified. To accomplish this, the researcher must acquire a list of every member of the population, using the sampling criteria to define eligibility. This list is referred to as the sampling frame. In some studies, the complete sampling frame cannot be identified because it is not possible to list all members of the population. The Health Insurance Portability and Accountability Act (HIPAA) has also increased the difficulty in obtaining a complete sampling frame for many studies because of its requirements to protect individuals' health information (see Chapter 4 for more information on HIPAA). Once a sampling frame is identified, researchers select subjects for their studies using a sampling plan or method.

Sampling Methods or Plans

Sampling methods or plans outline strategies used to obtain samples for studies. Like a design, a sampling plan is not specific to a study. The sampling plan may include probability (random) or nonprobability (nonrandom) sampling methods. Probability sampling methods are designed to

---

? CRITICAL APPRAISAL GUIDELINES

Adequacy of the Sampling Criteria, Acceptance or Refusal Rate, and Sample Attrition or Retention Rate

When critically appraising the samples of quantitative and outcomes studies, address the following questions:
1. Does the researcher define the target and accessible populations for the study?
2. Are the sampling inclusion criteria, sampling exclusion criteria, or both clearly identified and appropriate for the study?
3. Is either the refusal or acceptance rate identified in the study? Are reasons provided for the potential subjects who refused to participate?
4. Is the sample attrition or retention rate addressed in the study? Are reasons provided for those who withdrew from the study?

⚡ RESEARCH EXAMPLE

Sampling Criteria, Acceptance or Refusal Rate, and Sample Attrition or Retention Rate

Research Excerpt

Giakoumidakis and colleagues (2013) conducted a randomized controlled trial (RCT) to investigate the effects of intensive blood glucose control (120 to 150 mg/dL) on cardiac surgery patient outcomes, such as mortality (in-hospital and 30-day postdischarge), length of intensive care unit (ICU) stay, length of postoperative hospital stay, duration of tracheal intubation, presence of severe hypoglycemic events, and incidence of postoperative infections. The sampling criteria, acceptance rate, and sample retention rate from this study are presented here as an example. Giakoumidakis and associates (2013) provided a description of their study sampling criteria and documented the participants enrolled in their study using a flow diagram (see Figure 9-2 of this example). This flow diagram is based on the CONsolidated Standards of Reporting Trials (CONSORT) Statement that is the international standard for reporting the sampling process in RCTs (CONSORT Group, 2010; see Chapter 13 for more information on the CONSORT statement).This study is critically appraised using the questions designated earlier in the Critical Appraisal Guidelines box.

"The study was a randomized quasi-experimental trial. We treated blood glucose levels during the first 24 hours postoperatively [independent variable] in patients of the therapy group and compared them with the control group. The inclusion criteria were: (1) open heart surgery, (2) surgery requiring CPB

Continued

[cardio-pulmonary bypass], (3) patient age ≥ 18 years old, and (4) the patient's informed consent for participation in our study. The exclusion criteria included: (1) renal dysfunction or failure (preoperative creatinine > 1.5 mg/dL), (2) neurological or mental disorder, (3) chronic obstructive pulmonary disease, (4) preoperative use of any type of antibiotics, (5) emergency and urgent surgeries, (6) history of previous cardiac surgery, (7) ICU length of stay < 24 hours, (8) mediastinal re-exploration for bleeding, (9) hemodynamic support with intra-aortic balloon pump (IABP) intraoperatively and/or during the first 24 hours postoperatively, and (10) use of cardioversion for severe ventricular arrhythmias (ventricular tachycardia and/or fibrillation) within the first 24 hours of ICU hospitalization. These criteria were established in an effort to ensure a more homogenous sample for our study....

Over a period of 5 months (from September 2011 to January 2012), 298 patients were admitted to the 8-bed cardiac surgery ICU... and were eligible for enrollment in the study. Two hundred and twelve out of 298 (71.1%) patients met the inclusion criteria and simultaneously did not meet the exclusion criteria and consequently constituted our study sample (see Figure 9-2).

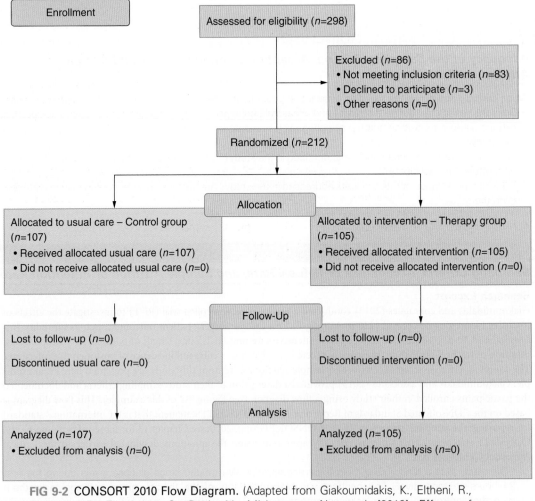

FIG 9-2 CONSORT 2010 Flow Diagram. (Adapted from Giakoumidakis, K., Eltheni, R., Patelarou, E., Theologou, S., Patris, V., Michopanou, N., et al. [2013]. Effects of intensive glycemic control on outcomes of cardiac surgery. *Heart & Lung, 42*[2], p. 148.)

One of the researchers, the same each time, randomly assigned patients, immediately postoperatively, to the (odd numbers into the control group and the evens into the therapy group): (1) control group ($n = 107$) with a targeted blood glucose levels of 161-200 mg/dL, or (2) therapy group ($n = 105$) with blood glucose target of 120-160 mg/dL, or during the first 24 hours postoperatively. (see Figure 9-2)." (Giakoumidakis et al., 2013, p. 147)

Critical Appraisal

Giakoumidakis and co-workers (2013) identified specific inclusion and exclusion sampling criteria to designate the subjects in the target population selectively. As the researchers indicated, the sampling criteria were narrowly defined by the researchers to promote the selection of a homogeneous sample of cardiac surgery patients. These sampling criteria were appropriate for this study to reduce the effects of possible extraneous variables on the implementation of the treatment (blood glucose control) and the measurement of the dependent variables or outcomes (mortality, length of ICU and hospital stays, duration of tracheal intubation, presence of severe hypoglycemic events, and incidence of postoperative infection). The increased controls imposed by the sampling criteria strengthened the likelihood that the study outcomes were caused by the treatment and not by extraneous variables.

These researchers assessed 298 patients for eligibility in the study, but 83 of them did not meet the sampling criteria. Thus 215 patients met the sampling criteria. However, three of these patients declined or refused to participate in the study, resulting in a 1.4% ($3 \div 215 \times 100\% = 0.014 \times 100\% = 1.4\%$) refusal rate. Figure 9-2 indicates that the sample of 212 patients was equally randomized into the control group ($n = 107$) and therapy group ($n = 105$). There was no attrition of subjects from this study, as indicated in Figure 9-2, in which the starting group sizes were the same at the end and all subjects ($N = 212$) were included in the data analyses. This study had very rigorous sampling criteria, low refusal rate of 1.4% (acceptance rate of 98.6%), and 0% attrition rate, which increased the representativeness of the sample of the accessible and target populations. The study would have been strengthened by the researchers including not only the numbers but also the sample refusal rate and the reasons for the three patients refusing to participate in the study.

Implications for Practice

Giakoumidakis and colleagues (2013) found that only the in-hospital mortality rate was significantly affected by the intensive blood glucose control. The postoperative glycemic control did not affect the other patient outcomes that were studied. However, the researchers recognized that the sample size was small for a RCT, which limited the numbers of patients in the control and therapy groups. In addition, the study was conducted using only the patients from one hospital. Therefore the researchers recommended that future studies include larger samples obtained from a variety of hospitals. This initial research indicates that intensive blood glucose control is important to cardiac patients' mortality and might have other beneficial effects on patient outcomes in future research. The Quality and Safety Education for Nurses (QSEN) importance is that these research findings provide knowledge to address patient-centered care and safety competencies to promote quality care to patients and families (QSEN, 2013; Sherwood & Barnsteiner, 2012).

increase representativeness and decrease systematic variation or bias in quantitative and outcomes studies. When critically appraising a study, identify the study sampling plan as probability or non-probability, and determine the specific method or methods used to select the sample. The different types of probability and nonprobability sampling methods are introduced next.

PROBABILITY SAMPLING METHODS

In **probability sampling**, each person or element in a population has an opportunity to be selected for a sample, which is achieved through random sampling. Probability or random sampling methods increase the sample's representativeness of the target population. All the subsets of the population, which may differ from each other but contribute to the parameters (e.g., the means and standard deviations) of the population, have a chance to be represented in the sample. The opportunity for systematic bias is less when subjects are selected randomly, although it is possible for a systematic bias to occur by chance.

Without random sampling strategies, researchers, who have a vested interest in the study, might tend (consciously or unconsciously) to select subjects whose conditions or behaviors are consistent with the study hypotheses. For example, researchers may exclude potential subjects because they are too sick, not sick enough, coping too well, not coping adequately, uncooperative, or noncompliant. By using random sampling, however, researchers leave the selection to chance, thereby increasing the validity of their study findings.

There are four sampling designs that achieve probability sampling included in this text—simple random sampling, stratified random sampling, cluster sampling, and systematic sampling. Table 9-1 identifies the common probability and nonprobability sampling methods used in nursing studies,

TABLE 9-1   PROBABILITY AND NONPROBABILITY SAMPLING METHODS

SAMPLING METHOD	COMMON APPLICATION(S)	REPRESENTATIVENESS
Probability		
Simple random sampling	Quantitative and outcomes research	Strong representativeness of the target population that increases with sample size
Stratified random sampling	Quantitative and outcomes research	Strong representativeness of the target population that increases with control of stratified variable(s)
Cluster sampling	Quantitative and outcomes research	Less representative of the target population than simple random sampling and stratified random sampling
Systematic sampling	Quantitative and outcomes research	Less representative of the target population than simple random sampling and stratified random sampling methods
Nonprobability		
Convenience sampling	Quantitative, qualitative, and outcomes research	Questionable representativeness of the target population that improves with increasing sample size; may be representative of the phenomenon, process, or cultural elements in qualitative research
Quota sampling	Quantitative and outcomes research and, rarely, qualitative research	Use of stratification for selected variables in quantitative research makes the sample more representative than convenience sampling. In qualitative research, stratification might be used to provide greater understanding and increase the representativeness of the phenomenon, processes, or cultural elements.
Purposeful or purposive sampling	Qualitative and sometimes quantitative research	Focus is on insight, description, and understanding of a phenomenon or process with specially selected study participants.
Network or snowball sampling	Qualitative and sometimes quantitative research	Focus is on insight, description, and understanding of a phenomenon or process in a difficult to access population.
Theoretical sampling	Qualitative research	Focus is on developing a theory in a selected area.

their applications, and their representativeness for the study. Probability and nonprobability sampling methods are used in quantitative and outcomes studies, and nonprobability sampling methods are used in qualitative studies (Fawcett & Garity, 2009; Munhall, 2012).

Simple Random Sampling

Simple random sampling is the most basic of the probability sampling plans. It is achieved by randomly selecting elements from the sampling frame. Researchers can accomplish random selection in a variety of ways; it is limited only by the imagination of the researcher. If the sampling frame is small, researchers can write names on slips of paper, place them into a container, mix them well, and then draw them out one at a time until they have reached the desired sample size. The most common method for randomly selecting subjects for a study is use of a computer program. The researcher can enter the sampling frame (list of potential subjects) into a computer, which will then randomly select subjects until the desired sample size is achieved.

Another method for randomly selecting a study sample is use of a table of random numbers. Table 9-2 displays a section from a random numbers table. To use a table of random numbers, the researcher places a pencil or finger on the table with eyes closed. That number is the starting place. Then, by moving the pencil or finger up, down, right, or left, numbers are identified in order until the desired sample size is obtained. For example, you want to select five subjects from a population of 100, and the number 58 is initially selected as a starting point (fourth column from the left, fourth row down), your subject numbers would be 58, 25, 15, 55, and 38. Table 9-2 is useful only when the population number is less than 100. Full tables of random numbers are available from other sources (Grove et al., 2013).

TABLE 9-2   SECTION FROM A RANDOM NUMBERS TABLE

06	84	10	22	56	72	25	70	69	43
07	63	10	34	66	39	54	02	33	85
03	19	63	93	72	52	13	30	44	40
77	32	69	58	25	15	55	38	19	62
20	01	94	54	66	88	43	91	34	28

RESEARCH EXAMPLE

Simple Random Sampling

Research Excerpt

Lee, Faucett, Gillen, Krause, and Landry (2013) conducted a predictive correlational study to determine critical care nurses' perception of the risk of musculoskeletal (MSK) injury. The researchers randomly selected (sampling method) 1000 critical care nurses from the 2005 American Association of Critical Care (AACN) membership list (sampling frame). "A total of 412 nurses returned completed questionnaires (response rate = 41.5%, excluding eight for whom mailing addresses were incorrect). Of these, 47 nurses who did not meet the inclusion criteria were excluded: not currently employed ($n=5$); not employed in a hospital ($n=1$); not employed in critical care ($n=8$); not a staff or charge nurse ($n=28$); or not performing patient-handling tasks ($n=5$). In addition, four nurses employed in a neonatal ICU were excluded because of the different nature of their physical workload. The final sample for data analysis comprised 361 [sample size] critical care nurses." (Lee et al., 2013, p. 38)

Critical Appraisal

Lee and associates (2013) clearly identified that a random sampling method was used to select study participants from a population of critical care nurses. The 41.5% response rate for mailed questionnaires is considered adequate,
Continued

because the response rate to questionnaires averages 25% to 50% (Grove et al., 2013). The 47 nurses who did not meet sample criteria and the four nurses working in a neonatal ICU were excluded, ensuring a more homogeneous sample and decreasing the potential effect of extraneous variables. These sampling activities limit the potential for systematic variation or bias and increase the likelihood that the study sample is representative of the accessible and target populations. The study would have been strengthened if the researchers had indicated how the nurses were randomly selected from the AACN membership list, but this was probably a random selection by a computer.

Implications for Practice

Lee and co-workers (2013, p. 43) identified the following findings from their study: "Improving the physical and psychosocial work environment may make nursing jobs safer, reduce the risk of MSK injury, and improve nurses' perceptions of job safety. Ultimately, these efforts would contribute to enhancing safety in nursing settings and to maintaining a healthy nursing workforce. Future research is needed to determine the role of risk perception in preventing MSK injury." The QSEN importance is that the findings from this study contribute to the safety competencies in which strategies are used to reduce the risk of harm to nurses and others (QSEN, 2013).

Stratified Random Sampling

Stratified random sampling is used in situations in which the researcher knows some of the variables in the population that are critical for achieving representativeness. Variables commonly used for stratification include age, gender, race and ethnicity, socioeconomic status, diagnosis, geographic region, type of institution, type of care, type of registered nurse, nursing area of specialization, and site of care. Stratification ensures that all levels of the identified variables are adequately represented in the sample. With stratification, researchers can use a smaller sample size to achieve the same degree of representativeness relative to the stratified variable than can be derived from using a larger sample acquired through simple random sampling. One disadvantage is that a large population must be available from which to select subjects.

If researchers have used stratification, they must define categories (strata) of the variables selected for stratification in the published report. For example, using race and ethnicity for stratification, the researcher may define four strata—white, non-Hispanic; black; Hispanic; and other. The population may be 60% white, non-Hispanic; 20% black; 15% Hispanic; and 5% other. Researchers may select a random sample for each stratum equivalent to the target population proportions of that stratum. Thus a sample of 100 subjects would need to include approximately 60 white, non-Hispanic; 20 black; 15 Hispanic; and 5 other. Alternatively, equal numbers of subjects may be randomly selected for each stratum. For example, if age is used to stratify a sample of 100 adult subjects, the researcher may obtain 25 subjects 18 to 34 years of age, 25 subjects 35 to 50 years of age, 25 subjects 51 to 66 years of age, and 25 subjects older than 66 years of age.

Stratified Random Sampling

Research Excerpt

Toma, Houck, Wagnild, Messecar, and Jones (2013, p. 16) conducted a predictive correlational study "to identify predictors of physical function in older adults living with fibromyalgia (FM) and to examine the influence of resilience on the relationship between fibromyalgia pain and physical function." This study included a stratified random sample that is described in the following study excerpt:

"An age-stratified random sample [sampling method] of 400 community-dwelling older adults was created from a database of FM patients [population] at a large academic medical center in the Pacific Northwest.

The database included over 5,000 community-dwelling FM patients who had been diagnosed with FM (ICD-9 729.1) in clinical practice or as a participant in FM clinical trials [sampling frame]. Limits were set on the database to extract only those persons 50 years of age and older who had participated in FM studies in the last 2 years [sampling criteria and target population]. An age of 50 years was selected as the lower limit because FM often begins in the third and fourth decade of life and can impact PF [physical function].... Those persons extracted were then placed into an Excel spreadsheet and stratified into five age groups (50-54, 55-59, 60-64, 65-69, 70+ years). Eighty persons were selected randomly from each group and invited to participate in the study." (Toma et al., 2013, p. 17). Of the 400 invited to participate in the study, 224 returned the completed questionnaires, for a response rate of 56%.

Critical Appraisal

Toma and colleagues (2013) clearly identified their population as community-dwelling FM patients and the sampling frame was large, including 5000 FM patients in a national database. The researchers provided a sound rationale for limiting the sample to FM patients 50 years of age and older. Stratification by age groups seemed important in this study to control extraneous variables that could affect physical function. Most of the categories for stratification were equal, with each age group including 5 years, except for the last category. The random selection of 80 FM patients for each of the age groups increased the representativeness of the strata in the sample. In summary, this study included a rigorous stratified random sampling method that resulted in a large sample ($n=224$) of FM patients who were fairly equally distributed among the five age groups. This sampling process increased the representativeness of the sample and decreased the potential for systematic error or bias.

Implications for Practice

Toma and associates (2013) found that resilience was a predictor of physical function in this sample of community-dwelling FM patients. However, they recommended further research to promote understanding of the relationships among resilience, FM impact, and the aging process.

Cluster Sampling

In cluster sampling, a researcher develops a sampling frame that includes a list of all the states, cities, institutions, or organizations with which elements of the identified population can be linked. A randomized sample of these states, cities, institutions, or organizations can then be used in the study. In some cases this randomized selection continues through several stages and is then referred to as multistage sampling. For example, the researcher may first randomly select states and then randomly select cities within the sampled states. Next, the researcher may randomly select hospitals within the randomly selected cities. Within the hospitals, nursing units may be randomly selected. At this level, all the patients on the nursing unit who fit the criteria for the study may be included, or patients can be randomly selected.

Cluster sampling is commonly used in two types of research situations. In the first situation, the researcher considers it necessary to obtain a geographically dispersed sample but recognizes that obtaining a simple random sample will require too much travel time and expense. In the second, the researcher cannot identify the individual elements making up the population and therefore cannot develop a sampling frame. For example, a complete list of all people in the United States who have had open heart surgery does not exist. Nevertheless, it is often possible to obtain lists of institutions or organizations with which the elements of interest are associated—in this example, perhaps large medical centers, university hospitals with cardiac surgery departments, and large cardiac surgery practices—and then randomly select institutions from which the researcher can acquire subjects.

⚡ RESEARCH EXAMPLE

Cluster Sampling

Research Excerpt

Fouladbakhsh and Stommel (2010, p. E8) used multistage cluster sampling in their study of the "complex relationships among gender, physical and psychological symptoms, and use of specific CAM [complementary and alternative medicine] health practices among individuals living in the United States who have been diagnosed with cancer." These researchers described their sampling method in the following excerpt and the particular aspects of the sample have been identified in [brackets].

"The NHIS [National Health Interview Survey] methodology employs a multistage probability cluster sampling design [sampling method] that is representative of the NHIS target universe, defined as 'the civilian noninstitutionalized population' [sampling frame] (Botman, Moore, Moriarty, & Parsons, 2000, p. 14; National Center for Health Statistics). In the first stage, 339 primary sampling units were selected from about 1,900 area sampling units representing counties, groups of adjacent counties, or metropolitan areas covering the 50 states and the District of Columbia [1st stage cluster sampling]. The selection includes all of the most populous primary sampling units in the United States and stratified probability samples (by state, area poverty level, and population size) of the less populous ones. In a second step, primary sampling units were partitioned into substrata (up to 21) based on concentrations of African American and Hispanic populations [2nd stage cluster sampling]. In a third step, clusters of dwelling units form the secondary sampling units selected from each substratum [3rd stage cluster sampling]. Finally, within each secondary sampling unit, all African American and Hispanic households were selected for interviews, whereas other households were sampled at differing rates within the substrata. Therefore, the sampling design of the NHIS includes oversampling of minorities." (Fouladbakhsh & Stommel, 2010, pp. E8-E9)

Critical Appraisal

These researchers detailed their use of multistage cluster sampling and clearly identified the three stages of cluster sampling implemented and the rationale for each stage. The study had a large national sample that seemed representative of all 50 states and the District of Columbia, with an oversampling of minorities to accomplish the purpose of the study. The complex cluster sampling method used in this study provided a representative sample, which decreases the likelihood of sampling error and increases the validity of the study findings.

Implications for Practice

Their findings (Fouladbakhsh and Stommel, 2010, p. E7) indicated that "CAM practice use was more prevalent among female, middle-aged, Caucasian, and well-educated subjects. Pain, depression, and insomnia were strong predictors of practice use, with differences noted by gender and practice type." Nurses need to be aware of the CAM practices of their cancer patients and incorporate this information when managing their care. The QSEN importance is that this research-based knowledge encourages nurses to deliver patient-centered care to patients and families (QSEN, 2013).

Systematic Sampling

Systematic sampling is used when an ordered list of all members of the population is available. The process involves selecting every kth individual on the list, using a starting point selected randomly. If the initial starting point is not random, the sample is a nonprobability or nonrandom sample. To use this design, the researcher must know the number of elements in the population and the size of the sample desired. The population size is divided by the desired sample size, giving k, the size of the gap between elements selected from the list. For example, if the population size is $N = 1200$ and the desired sample size is $n = 100$, then $k = 12$. Thus the researcher would include every 12th person on the list in the sample. You obtain this value by using the following formula:

$$k = \text{Population size} \div \text{by the desired sample size}$$

Example:

$$k = 1200 \text{ subjects in the population} \div 100 \text{ desired sample size} = 12$$

Some argue that this procedure does not actually give each element of a population an opportunity to be included in the sample and does not provide as representative a sample as simple random sampling and stratified random sampling. Systematic sampling provides a random but not equal chance for inclusion of participants in a study (Kerlinger & Lee, 2000).

RESEARCH EXAMPLE

Systematic Sampling

Research Excerpt

De Silva, Hanwella, and de Silva (2012) used systematic sampling in their outcomes study of the direct and indirect costs of care incurred by patients with schizophrenia (population) in a tertiary care psychiatric unit.

"Systematic sampling [sampling method] selected every second patient with an ICD-10 clinical diagnosis of schizophrenia [target population] presenting to the clinic during a two-month period [sampling frame].... Sample consisted of 91 patients [sample size]. Direct cost was defined as cost incurred by the patient (out-of-pocket expenditure) for outpatient care." (De Silva, et al., 2012, p. 14)

Critical Appraisal

De Silva and co-workers (2012) clearly identified that systematic sampling was used in their study. The population and target population were appropriate for this study. Using systematic sampling increased the representativeness of the sample, and the sample size of 91 schizophrenic patients seems adequate for the focus of this study. However, the sampling frame was identified as only the patients presenting over 2 months, and k was small (every second patient) in this study. The researchers might have provided more details on how they implemented the systematic sampling method to ensure that the start of the sampling process was random (Grove et al., 2013).

IMPLICATIONS FOR PRACTICE

De Silva and colleagues (2012, p. 14) concluded that "despite low direct cost of care, indirect cost and cost of informal treatment results in substantial economic impact on patients and their families. It is recommended that economic support should be provided for patients with disabling illnesses such as schizophrenia, especially when patients are unable to engage in full-time employment."

NONPROBABILITY SAMPLING METHODS COMMONLY USED IN QUANTITATIVE RESEARCH

In nonprobability sampling, not every element of a population has an opportunity to be selected for a study sample. Although this approach decreases a sample's representativeness of a target population, it commonly is used in nursing studies because of the limited number of patients available for research. Thus it is important to be able to discriminate among the various nonprobability sampling plans used in nursing research. The five nonprobability sampling plans used most frequently in nursing research are convenience sampling, quota sampling, purposive or purposeful sampling, network sampling, and theoretical sampling. Convenience sampling is frequently used in quantitative, qualitative, and outcomes nursing studies. Quota sampling is occasionally used in quantitative and outcomes studies. Purposive, network, and theoretical sampling are used more frequently in qualitative research and are discussed later in this chapter. Table 9-1 provides a list of the common applications of these sampling methods and the representativeness achieved by them.

Convenience Sampling

Convenience sampling, also called *accidental sampling*, is a weak approach because it provides little opportunity to control for biases; subjects are included in the study merely because they happen to be in the right place at the right time (Grove et al., 2013; Kerlinger & Lee, 2000). A classroom of students, patients who attend a clinic on a specific day, subjects who attend a support group, and patients hospitalized with specific medical diagnoses or nursing problems are examples of convenience samples. The researcher simply enters available subjects into the study until the desired sample size is reached. Multiple biases may exist in the sample, some of which may be subtle and unrecognized. However, serious biases are not always present in convenience samples. According to Kerlinger and Lee (2000), a convenience sample is acceptable when it is used with reasonable knowledge and care in implementing a study.

Convenience samples are inexpensive, accessible, and usually less time-consuming to obtain than other types of samples. This type of sampling provides a means to conduct studies on nursing interventions when researchers cannot use probability sampling methods. Convenience sampling method is commonly used in healthcare studies because most researchers have limited access to patients who meet study sample criteria. Probability or random sampling is not possible when the pool of potential patients is limited. Researchers often think it best to include all patients who meet sample criteria (sample of convenience) to increase the sample size.

For some healthcare studies, the sampling frames for some populations are not available, so researchers often use a sample of convenience. Many researchers are now conducting quasi-experimental studies and clinical trials in medicine and nursing, and these types of studies frequently require the use of the convenience sampling method. As a component of these study designs, subjects usually are randomly assigned to groups. This random assignment to groups, which is not a sampling method but a design strategy, does not alter the risk of biases resulting from convenience sampling but does strengthen the equivalence of the study groups. With these potential biases and the narrowly defined sampling criteria used to select subjects in most clinical trials, representativeness of the sample is a concern. To strengthen the representativeness of a sample, researchers often increase the sample size for clinical trials (Parent & Hanley, 2009). Sample size is discussed later in this chapter.

⚓ RESEARCH EXAMPLE

Convenience Sampling

Research Excerpt

Long and associates (2013, p. 17) conducted a quasi-experimental study to test "the effectiveness of using cell phones with digital pictures to prompt memory and use of mypyramidtracker.gov to estimate self-reported fruit and vegetable intake in 69 college students." The intervention involved study participants taking pictures of what they had eaten to review later when reporting dietary intake on a government website that calculated the nutritional value of the intake. The website during the study was mypyramidtracker.gov and is now https://www.supertracker.usda.gov/default.aspx. The following excerpt describes their sampling process.

"After obtaining approval from the institutional review board, a convenience sample of college-age students [population] was recruited from a local university through campus and class announcements.... A sample of 146 college-age students [sample size] from various majors who were enrolled in coursework in the Department of Exercise and Sports Sciences was obtained [target population]. After study attrition, 69 subjects remained in the study." (Long et al., 2013, p. 20)

Critical Appraisal

Long and co-workers (2013) clearly identified their sampling method and indicated that college students from various majors were included in the sample, which increases the representativeness of the sample of university students. The original sample was strong, with 146 students included in the study, but the attrition was high, with 77 students withdrawing from the study, leaving a sample of 69 (146 − 69 = 77). The researchers needed to provide more details about the students withdrawing from this study. Because this study used a nonprobability sampling method and had a high attrition rate (53%), the sample had decreased representativeness of the target population, which increased the potential for error and decreased the ability to generalize the findings.

Implications for Practice

Long and colleagues (2013, p. 17) found a significant difference between the use of cell phone versus short-term memory in recording diet information. "Cell phone pictures improved memory and accuracy of recall when using an online self-reported interactive diet record and was considered an easy, relevant, and accessible way to record diet." The researchers encouraged nurses to provide nutrition counseling that included technology, such as the use of cell phone to help improve diet management.

Quota Sampling

Quota sampling uses a convenience sampling technique with an added feature—a strategy to ensure the inclusion of subject types likely to be underrepresented in the convenience sample, such as females, minority groups, older adults, and the poor, rich, and undereducated. The goal of quota sampling is to replicate the proportions of subgroups present in the target population. This technique is similar to that used in stratified random sampling. Quota sampling requires that the researcher be able to identify subgroups and their proportions in the target population in order to achieve representativeness for the problem being studied. Quota sampling offers an improvement over convenience sampling and tends to decrease potential biases.

RESEARCH EXAMPLE

Quota Sampling

Research Excerpt

Pieper, Templin, Kirsner, and Birk (2010) used quota sampling to examine the impact of vascular leg disorders, such as chronic venous disorders (CVDs) and peripheral arterial disease (PAD), on the physical activity levels of opioid-addicted adults in a methadone maintenance program. The following excerpt describes their sampling process:

"The sample ($n = 713$) was obtained from September 2005 to December 2007 from 12 methadone treatment clinics [settings] located in a large urban area [convenience sampling]. The sample was stratified on four variables: age (25-39 years, 40-49 years, 50-65 years); gender (male, female); ethnicity (African American, white); and drug use (non-IDU [injection drug use], arm/upper body injection only, or legs ± upper body injection [quota sampling].... The purpose of the stratification was to allow comparisons of type of drug use with minimal confounding by age, gender, or ethnicity. Additional inclusion criteria included presence of both legs, able to walk, and able to speak and understand English. The analyses reported here are on the 569 participants who completed the revised LDUQ [Legs in Daily Use Questionnaire], which were edited after examining the test-retest data from 104 participants, not included in the 569, who were tested first." (Pieper et al., 2010, p. 429)

Critical Appraisal

Pieper and associates (2010) clearly identified that the original sample was one of convenience because it was people attending 12 methadone treatment clinics who were willing to participate in the study. The quota sampling involved

Continued

SAMPLING IN QUALITATIVE RESEARCH

Qualitative research is conducted to gain insights and discover meaning about a particular phenomenon, situation, cultural element, or historical event (Fawcett & Garity, 2009; Munhall, 2012). The intent of qualitative research is an in-depth understanding of a phenomenon or topic in a specially selected sample, not on the generalization of findings from a randomly selected sample to a target population, as in quantitative research. The sampling in qualitative research focuses more on experiences, events, incidents, and settings than on people (Sandelowski, 1995). In ethnography studies, qualitative researchers often select the setting and site and then the population and phenomenon of interest (Marshall & Rossman, 2011). In other types of qualitative research, researchers often select the phenomenon or population of interest and then identify potential participants for their studies. Qualitative researchers attempt to select participants who have experience or are knowledgeable in the area of study and are willing to share rich, in-depth information about the phenomenon, situation, culture, or event being studied. For example, if the goal of the study is to describe the phenomenon of living with chronic pain, the researcher will select individuals who are articulate and reflective, have a history of chronic pain, and are willing to share their chronic pain experience (Coyne, 1997; Munhall, 2012).

Common sampling methods used in qualitative nursing research are purposive or purposeful sampling, network or snowball sampling, theoretical sampling, and convenience sampling (described earlier). These sampling methods are summarized in Table 9-1. These sampling methods enable researchers to select information-rich cases or participants who they believe will provide them the best data for their studies. The sample selection process can have a profound effect on the quality of the study; researchers need to describe this in enough depth to promote interpretation of the findings and replication of the study.

Purposeful or Purposive Sampling

With **purposeful or purposive sampling**, sometimes referred to as "judgmental" or "selective" sampling, the researcher consciously selects certain participants, elements, events, or incidents to include in the study. Researchers may try to include typical or atypical participants or similar or varied situations. Qualitative researchers may select participants who are of various age categories, those who have different diagnoses or illness severity, or those who received an ineffective rather than an effective treatment for their illness. For example, researchers describing grief following the loss of a child might include parents who lost a child in the previous 6, 12, and 24 months, and the children who were lost might be varying ages (<5 years old, 5 to 10 years old, and >10 years old). The ultimate goal of purposeful sampling is selecting information-rich cases from which researchers can obtain in-depth information needed for their studies.

Some have criticized the purposeful sampling method because it is difficult to evaluate the accuracy or relevance of the researcher's judgment. Therefore researchers must indicate the characteristics that they desired in study participants and provide a rationale for selecting these types of individuals to obtain essential data for their study. In qualitative studies, purposive sampling seems the best way to gain insights into a new area of study, discover new meaning, or obtain in-depth understanding of a complex experience, situation, or event (Fawcett & Garity, 2009; Marshall & Rossman, 2011; Munhall, 2012).

RESEARCH EXAMPLE

Purposeful or Purposive Sampling

Research Excerpt

Lapidus-Graham (2012) conducted a phenomenological study to describe the lived experience of participation in student nursing associations (SNAs) by students in New York. This researcher used purposive sampling to select her study participants.

> "The purposive sample consisted of 15 nursing graduates from five Long Island nursing programs who were members of a SNA within the past five years.... Former nursing students were chosen from the downstate Long Island area via contact with faculty SNA advisors and through input from nursing department chairs. It was determined from the sample that only one of the five schools required mandatory membership in the SNA. The participants ranged in age from approximately 21 to 50 years and included two male and 13 female students." (Lapidus-Graham, 2012, p. 7)

Critical Appraisal

Lapidus-Graham (2012) clearly identified the use of a purposive sampling method to select the 15 participants for her study. Using purposive sampling, she was able to obtain participants from five different settings. The students were a broad age range and included males and females, which increased the richness of the data collected. During data analysis, the final themes were determined only after 12 or more of the participants had described an experience related to a specific concept or idea. The purposive sampling method using SNA advisors and nursing department chairs seemed to identify participants who were rich with information about SNA. In addition, the sample size seemed adequate to provide rich, quality data for this study.

Implications for Practice

Lapidus-Graham (2012) identified the themes generated by the study, implications for practice, and recommendations for further research in the following study excerpt.

> "Six themes of the lived experiences of the participants in SNA emerged: (1) leadership: communication, collaboration, and resolving conflict; (2) mentoring and mutual support; (3) empowerment and ability to change practice; (4) professionalism; (5) sense of teamwork; and (6) accountability and responsibility. Recommendations from the study included an orientation and mentoring of new students to the SNA by senior students and faculty. Additionally nursing faculty could integrate SNA activities within the classroom and clinical settings to increase the awareness of the benefits of participation in a student nursing organization. Recommendations for future research include a different sample and use of different research designs" (Lapidus-Graham, 2012, p. 4).

The QSEN (2013) implications from this study are that participation in SNAs provides experiences in teamwork, collaboration, and leadership, which are important competencies for delivering quality, safe, patient-centered care in nursing.

Network Sampling

Network sampling, sometimes referred to as "snowball," "chain," or "nominated" sampling holds promise for locating participants who would be difficult or impossible to obtain in other ways or who have not been previously identified for study (Marshall & Rossman, 2011; Munhall, 2012). Network sampling takes advantage of social networks and the fact that friends tend to have characteristics in common. This strategy is also particularly useful for finding subjects in socially devalued populations, such as persons who are dependent on alcohol, abuse children, commit sexual offenses, are addicted to drugs, or commit criminal acts. These persons seldom are willing to make themselves known. Other groups, such as widows, grieving siblings, or persons successful at lifestyle changes, also may be located using network sampling. They are typically outside the existing healthcare system and are difficult to find. When researchers have found a few participants who meet the sampling criteria, they ask for their assistance in finding others with similar characteristics.

Researchers often obtain the first few study participants through a purposeful sampling method and expand the sample size using network sampling. This sampling method is used in quantitative studies but is more common in qualitative studies. In qualitative research, network sampling is an effective strategy for identifying subjects who can provide the greatest insight and essential information about an experience or event that is being studied. For example, if a study were being conducted to describe the lives of adolescents who are abusing substances, network sampling would enable researchers to find participants who have a prolonged history of substance abuse and who could provide rich information about their lives in an interview (Fawcett & Garity, 2009).

RESEARCH EXAMPLE
Network Sampling

Research Excerpt

Milroy, Wyrick, Bibeau, Strack, and Davis (2012) conducted an exploratory-descriptive qualitative study to investigate student physical activity promotion on college campuses. The study included 14 of 15 (93%) universities recruited, and 22 employees from these universities participated in the study interviews. Milroy and colleagues (2012) implemented purposive and snowball (network) sampling to recruit individuals into their study and described their sampling process in the following excerpt:

"Participants were recruited from a southeastern state university system [study settings].... Initially, non-probabilistic purposive sampling [sampling method] was used to identify one potential participant from each university. Individuals selected for recruitment were identified to be most likely responsible for student physical activity promotion [study participants].... Snowball sampling [sampling method] followed the non-probabilistic purposive sampling to identify additional individuals on each campus who were engaged in promoting physical activity to students. Guidelines of snowball sampling prescribe that each interview participant be asked to identify any other individuals on their campus who are also responsible for promoting physical activity to students. Using snowball sampling helps to reduce the likelihood of omitting key participants. This technique was initiated during each interview until all those responsible for student physical activity promotion on each campus were identified and interviewed." (Milroy et al., 2012, p. 306)

Critical Appraisal

Milroy and associates (2012) clearly identified that the focus of their purposive sample was to obtain study participants who had extensive experience with and knowledge of the study topic. The rationale for using snowball sampling was described, and the process for implementing it was detailed. The study was conducted in multiple settings with knowledgeable participants who provided in-depth information about the health promotion physical activities on university campuses. The researchers indicated that they continued snowball sampling until all those responsible for student physical activity promotion on the different campuses were identified and interviewed. This study demonstrates a quality sampling process for addressing the study purpose.

Implications for Practice

Milroy and co-workers (2012) concluded that great efforts were put forth to encourage students to attend fitness classes or join incentive programs, but the students' involvement in physical activities was limited. Thus new methods are needed to promote physical activity on college campuses, and the administration is important in creating a culture that supports and values physical activity. Milroy and colleagues (2012, p. 305) recommended that "replication of this study is needed to compare these findings with other types of universities, and to investigate the relationship between promotion of activities (type and exposure) and physical activity behaviors of college students."

Theoretical Sampling

Theoretical sampling is used in qualitative research to develop a selected theory through the research process (Munhall, 2012). This type of sampling strategy is used most frequently with grounded theory research, because the focus of this type of research is theory development. The researcher gathers data from any person or group who is able to provide relevant, varied, and rich information for theory generation. The data are considered relevant and rich if they include information that generates, delimits, and saturates the theoretical codes in the study needed for theory generation (Huberman & Miles, 2002). A code is saturated if it is complete and the researcher can see how it fits in the theory. The researcher continues to seek sources and gather data until the codes are saturated, and the theory evolves from the codes and data. Diversity in the sample is encouraged so that the theory developed covers a wide range of behaviors in varied situations and settings (Munhall, 2012; Strauss & Corbin, 1998).

RESEARCH EXAMPLE

Theoretical Sampling

Research Excerpt

Beaulieu, Kools, Kennedy, and Humphreys (2011, p. 41) conducted a qualitative study using grounded theory methods to "explore and better understand the reasons for the apparent underuse of emergency contraceptive pills (ECPs) in young people in coupled relationships." These researchers applied three sampling methods: (1) convenience sampling, (2) snowball sampling, and (3) theoretical sampling. They described their sampling methods in the following study excerpt:

"A convenience sample was recruited via public notices and snowball sampling [sampling methods]. Inclusion criteria were women 18 to 25 years of age, English speaking, with basic knowledge of ECPs, and currently involved in a sexual relationship with a partner who was also willing to participate in the study... . Analysis began simultaneously with data collection as dictated by the tenets of grounded theory. The initial analysis of interviews and filed notes consisted of strategies of open coding and memoing (Glaser & Strauss, 1967). . . . As new categories emerged, the original interview guide was revised and additional couples were recruited to allow for theoretical sampling [sampling method]—that is, sampling specifically to fill in theoretical gaps, strengthen categories and their relationships, and verify or challenge emerging conceptualizations (Strauss & Corbin, 1998) and forced coding." (Beaulieu et al., 2011, p. 43)

Critical Appraisal

Beaulieu and associates (2011) clearly identified their sampling methods that were appropriate for a qualitative study conducted with grounded theory methodology. Both convenience and snowball sampling methods were applied since the researchers wanted an adequate number of couples to participate in their study and discuss the decision making regarding ECPs. Beaulieu and co-workers (2011) also provided detailed rationale for their use of theoretical sampling to develop a theory about young couples' decision making related to ECPs. The sampling methods provided a quality sample of 22 couples, who provided the essential information for grounded theory development. The number of participants allowed a broader view of the use of ECP, a complex and sensitive topic. More details on this study are presented later in this chapter in the discussion of sample size in qualitative studies.

Implications for Practice

Beaulieu and colleagues (2011) discussed the following implications for practice based on their study findings:

"Nurses whose practice includes young people, especially young women, need to be aware of possible couple dynamics when discussing contraception. Clinicians should first assess the characteristics of the relationship before trying to involve the partner. Those young women who exhibit a capacity for intimacy and are supportive relationships should be encouraged to engage in open communications with their partners about their contraception needs, including possible ECP use." (Beaulieu et al., 2011, p. 47)

They also recommended that further research should include more diverse groups, as well as couples who were in agreement regarding the use of ECP.

SAMPLE SIZE IN QUALITATIVE STUDIES

In quantitative research, the sample size must be large enough to identify relationships among variables or determine differences between groups. The larger the sample size and effect size, the greater the power to detect relationships and differences in quantitative and outcomes studies. However, qualitative research focuses on the quality of information obtained from the person, situation, or event sampled, rather than on the size of the sample (Creswell, 2014; Huberman & Miles, 2002; Munhall, 2012; Sandelowski, 1995).

The purpose of the study determines the sampling plan and initial sample size. The depth of information that is obtained and needed to gain insight into a phenomenon, describe a cultural element, develop a theory, describe an important healthcare concept or issue, or understand a historical event determines the final number of people, sites, artifacts, or documents sampled. Morse (2000) refers to this as intraproject sampling, or the additional sampling that is done during data collection and analysis to promote the development of quality study findings. The sample size can be too small when the data collected lack adequate depth or richness, and an inadequate sample size can reduce the quality and credibility of the research findings.

The number of participants in a qualitative study is adequate when saturation and verification of information are achieved in the study area. Saturation of study data occurs when additional sampling provides no new information, only redundancy of previous collected data. Verification of study data occurs when researchers are able to confirm hunches, relationships, or theoretical models further. With grounded theory research, "sampling for verification occurs when linkages are made between categories and/or concepts in the developing analysis. In other words, as theory emerges, data collection continues" (Morse, 2007, p. 537). The theory linkages developed need to be based on data, regardless of how abstract they are. Important factors that need to be considered in determining sample size are (1) scope of the study, (2) nature of the topic, (3) quality of the data, and (4) design of the study (Morse, 2000, 2007; Munhall, 2012).

Scope of the Study

If the scope of the study is broad, researchers will need extensive data to address the study purpose, and it will take longer to reach saturation. Therefore a study with a broad scope requires more sampling of participants, events, or documents than what is needed for a study with a narrow scope (Morse, 2000). For example, a qualitative study of the experience of living with chronic illness in older adulthood would require a large sample because of the broad scope of the problem. A study that has a clear purpose and provides focused data collection usually has richer, more credible findings. In contrast to the study of chronic illness experiences of older adults, researchers exploring the lived experience of adults older than 70 years who have rheumatoid arthritis could obtain credible findings with a smaller sample. When critically appraising a qualitative study, determine whether the sample size was adequate for the identified scope of the study.

Nature of the Topic

If the topic of study is clear and easily discussed by the subjects, then fewer subjects are needed to [collect] the essential data. If the topic is difficult to define and awkward for people to discuss, then [more par]ticipants are often needed to achieve data saturation (Morse, 2000; Munhall, 2012). For [a] phenomenological study of the experience of an adult living with a history of child sexual abuse is a very sensitive, complex topic to investigate. This type of topic probably will require increased participants and interview time to collect essential data. When critically appraising published studies, be sure to consider whether the sample size was adequate based on the complexity and sensitivity of the topic studied.

✗ Quality of the Information

The quality of information obtained from an interview, observation, or document review influences the sample size. When the quality of the data is high, with a rich content, few participants are needed to achieve saturation of data in the area of study. Quality data are best obtained from articulate, well-informed, and communicative participants (Munhall, 2012; Sandelowski, 1995). Such participants are able to share richer data in a clear and concise manner. In addition, participants who have more time to be interviewed usually provide data with greater depth and breadth. The researchers will continue sampling until saturation and verification of data are achieved to produce the best study results. Remember to consider these factors in your critical appraisal of a qualitative study:

- The quality of the information available from the participants, events, or documents
- The richness of the data collected
- The adequacy of the sample based on the findings obtained

Study Design

Some studies are designed to increase the number of interviews with each participant. When researchers conduct multiple interviews with a person, they probably will collect higher quality, richer data. For example, with a study design that includes an interview before and after an event, more data are produced than with a single-interview design. Designs that involve interviewing families usually produce more data than designs with single-participant interviews (Munhall, 2012).

🔘 CRITICAL APPRAISAL GUIDELINES

Adequacy of the Sampling Processes in Qualitative Studies

When critically appraising the sampling processes in qualitative studies, you need to address the following questions:

1. Is the sampling plan adequate to address the purpose of the study? If purposive sampling is used, does the researcher provide a rationale for the sample selection process? If network or snowball sampling is used, does the researcher identify the networks used to obtain the sample and provide a rationale for their selection? If theoretical sampling is used, does the researcher indicate how participants are selected to promote the generation of a theory?
2. Are the sampling criteria identified?
3. Does the researcher identify the study setting and discuss the entry into the setting?
4. Does the researcher discuss the quality of the data provided by the study participants? Were the participants articulate, well informed, and willing to share information relevant to the study topic?
5. Did the sampling process produce saturation and verification of data in the area of the study?
6. Is the sample size adequate based on the scope of the study, nature of the topic, quality of the data, and study design?

RESEARCH EXAMPLE

Qualitative Study Sample

Research Excerpt

Beaulieu and associates (2011) conducted a grounded theory study that was introduced earlier in the discussion of theoretical sampling. This study focused on developing a theory about young adult couples' decision making regarding their use of emergency contraceptive pills (ECPs). The sample was obtained with convenience, snowball, and theoretical sampling and resulted in a sample size of 22 couples. The following study excerpt provides the researchers' rationale for the final sample size of their study:

"A convenience sample was recruited via public notices and snowball sampling.... All interested young women initiated the first contact with the researcher by e-mail or telephone.... At the first meeting, which also included partners, study procedures were reviewed with participants, after which written consent and demographic information were obtained....

Analysis began simultaneously with data collection as dictated by the tenets of grounded theory.... As these processes progressed, axial coding was performed to identify core categories and their relationships. As new categories emerged, the original interview guide was revised and additional couples were recruited to allow for theoretical sampling—that is, sampling specifically to fill in theoretical gaps, strengthen categories and their relationships, and verify or challenge emerging conceptualizations (Strauss & Corbin, 1998) and focused coding.... Member checking occurred throughout the analysis by sharing the preliminary findings with subsequent couples to meet the requirements of confirmability of developing conceptualizations.... Saturation—when no new categories emerge (Strauss & Corbin, 1998)—was reached after interviewing 18 couples, but five more couples were included to ensure comprehensive analysis as well as theoretical verification. As the analysis continued through the processes of grounded theorizing, salient categories consistent with contemporary grounded theory principles were constructed to characterize the experience of young couples regarding ECPs." (Beaulieu et al., 2011, p. 43)

Critical Appraisal

Beaulieu and co-workers' (2011) study has many strengths in the area of sampling, including quality sampling methods (convenience, snowball, and theoretical), conscientious, information-rich participants, and robust sample size ($N = 22$ couples), which allowed for multiple perspectives on ECP use. The researchers provided extensive details of the theoretical sampling conducted to ensure saturation was achieved, with no new categories emerging. The saturation occurred after 18 couples but the researchers interviewed five more couples to ensure depth and breadth in the data for theoretical verification. They described how they were able to successfully develop a theoretical model of young couples' experiences regarding ECPs. The study would have been strengthened by knowing how many study participants were obtained by each of the sampling methods (convenience, snowball, and theoretical). Also, the researchers mentioned that saturation was obtained with 18 couples but five more couples were included, or $N = 23$, but the sample size identified was $N = 22$. A rationale is needed for the attrition of one of the couples from the study.

Implications for Practice

The implications for practice for the Beaulieu and colleagues' (2011) study were presented earlier in this chapter in the section on theoretical sampling.

RESEARCH SETTINGS

The research setting is the site or location used to conduct a study. Three common settings for conducting nursing studies are natural, partially controlled, and highly controlled (Grove et al., 2013). Chapter 2 initially introduced the types of settings for quantitative research. Some studies are strengthened by having more than one setting, making the sample more representative of the target population. The selection of a setting in quantitative and qualitative research is based on the purpose of the study, accessibility of the setting(s) or site(s), and number and type of participants or subjects available in the settings. The setting needs to be clearly described in the research report, with a rationale for selecting it. If the setting is partially or highly controlled, researchers should include a discussion of how they manipulated the setting. The following sections describe the three types of research settings, with examples provided from some of the studies discussed earlier.

Natural Setting

A natural or field setting is an uncontrolled, real-life situation or environment. Conducting a study in a natural setting means that the researcher does not manipulate or change the environment for the study. Descriptive and correlational quantitative studies and qualitative studies are often conducted in natural settings.

🔊 RESEARCH EXAMPLE

Natural Setting

Research Excerpt

Beaulieu and associates (2011) conducted a grounded theory study to describe young adult couples' decision making regarding the use of ECPs (see earlier). The researchers conducted their study in natural settings that were convenient for the study participants. "The study design included three semistructured interviews conducted with each couple-dyad; individual interviews were scheduled consecutively, lasting 30 to 45 minutes, and a 45- to 60-minute couple interview was scheduled approximately 1 week later. The interviews took place in various public settings or the couples' homes" (Beaulieu et al., 2011, p. 43).

Critical Appraisal

Beaulieu and co-workers (2011) clearly described their natural study settings, which were selected for the convenience of the study participants. These settings were natural, with no attempts by the researchers to manipulate the settings. The three interviews (for each study participant and as a couple) were scheduled at a time and place that facilitated the involvement of the participants in the study. Because of the sensitive nature of the topic, it was important to make the participants as comfortable as possible.

Partially Controlled Setting

A partially controlled setting is an environment that is manipulated or modified in some way by the researcher. An increasing number of nursing studies, usually correlational, quasi-experimental, and experimental studies, are being conducted in partially controlled settings. Manipulation of a study environment is very uncommon in qualitative research; however, qualitative researchers might manipulate a setting to promote the most effective environment to obtain the information that they need.

🔊 RESEARCH EXAMPLE

Partially Controlled Setting

Research Excerpt

Giakoumidakis and colleagues (2013) used a partially controlled setting to conduct their randomized quasi-experimental trial of the effects of intensive glycemic control on the outcomes of cardiac surgery patients. The study was conducted over 5 months, from September 2011 to January 2012, in an eight-bed cardiac surgery ICU in a general hospital. The structure of the ICU environment enabled the researchers to implement the treatment of an insulin infusion protocol to tightly control the experimental subjects' blood glucose level (120 to 160 mg/dL).

Critical Appraisal

This partially controlled environment made it possible to collect data consistently and accurately on the outcome variables of mortality, length of ICU stay, length of postoperative hospital stay, duration of tracheal intubation, presence of severe hypoglycemia events, and incidence of postoperative infections.

Highly Controlled Setting

A highly controlled setting is an artificially constructed environment developed for the sole purpose of conducting research. Laboratories, research or experimental centers, and test units in hospitals or other healthcare agencies are highly controlled settings in which experimental studies often are conducted. This type of setting reduces the influence of extraneous variables, which enables researchers to examine the effects of independent variables on dependent variables accurately.

RESEARCH EXAMPLE

Highly Controlled Setting

Research Excerpt

Sharma, Ryals, Gajewski, and Wright (2010) conducted an experimental study of the effects of aerobic exercise on analgesia and neurotrophin-3 (NT-3) synthesis in an animal model of chronic widespread pain. The aim of this study was to gain a cellular understanding of the impact of aerobic exercise on chronic pain to increase the understanding of the impact of exercise on the chronic pain of fibromyalgia (FM) patients. This study was conducted in a laboratory setting; the setting is briefly described in the following excerpt:

"All experiments were approved by the Institutional Animal Care and Use Committee of the University of Kansas Medical Center and adhered to the university's animal care guidelines. Forty CF-1 female mice (weight = 25 g) were used to examine the effects of moderately intense exercise on primary (muscular) and secondary (cutaneous) hyperalgesia and NT-3 synthesis. Because women develop widespread pain syndromes at a greater rate than age-matched men, hyperalgesia was induced in female mice. The mice were exposed to 12-hour light/dark cycle and had access to food and water *ad libitum*. The mice received two 20-µl injections of either acidic saline... or normal saline... 2 days apart into the right gastrocnemius muscle to induce chronic widespread hyperalgesia or pain-like behavior." (Sharma et al., 2010, p. 715)

Critical Appraisal

Sharma and associates (2010) used a highly controlled laboratory setting in their study in terms of the housing of the mice, light and temperature of the environment, implementation of the treatments, and measurements of the dependent variables. This type of setting control can only be achieved with animals, and the researchers documented that the animals were treated humanely, according to national guidelines. This type of highly controlled setting removes the impact of numerous extraneous variables, so that the researchers can clearly determine the effects of the independent variables on the dependent variables.

Implications for Practice

This experimental study provides basic knowledge about the biological processes of mice exposed to chronic pain and provides a basis for applied human research to examine the effects of aerobic exercise on chronic widespread pain, such as the pain experienced by FM patients. Because this study was conducted on animals, the findings cannot be generalized to humans, and additional research is needed to determine the effects of the independent variables on the dependent variables in clinical settings.

KEY CONCEPTS

- Sampling involves selecting a group of people, events, behaviors, or other elements to study.
- Sampling theory was developed to determine the most effective way of acquiring a sample that accurately reflects the population under study.
- Important sampling theory concepts include population, sampling criteria, target population, accessible population, study elements, representativeness, randomization, sampling frame, and sampling method or plan.

- In quantitative research, a sampling plan is developed to increase representativeness of the target population and decrease systematic bias and sampling error.
- In qualitative research, a sampling plan is developed to increase representativeness of the findings related to the phenomenon, processes, or cultural elements being studied.
- The two main types of sampling plans are probability and nonprobability.
- The common probability sampling methods used in nursing research include simple random sampling, stratified random sampling, cluster sampling, and systematic sampling.
- The five nonprobability sampling methods discussed in this chapter are convenience sampling, quota sampling, purposeful or purposive sampling, network sampling, and theoretical sampling.
- Convenience sampling is used frequently in quantitative, qualitative, and outcomes studies.
- Quota sampling is used more commonly in quantitative and outcomes research and rarely in qualitative research.
- Purposive, network, and theoretical sampling are used more often in qualitative research.
- Factors to consider in making decisions about sample size in quantitative studies include the type of study, number of variables, sensitivity of measurement methods, data analysis techniques, and expected effect size.
- Power analysis is an effective way to determine an adequate sample size for quantitative and outcomes studies. In power analysis, effect size, level of significance (alpha $= 0.05$), and standard power (0.8, or 80%) are used to determine sample size for a prospective study and evaluate the sample size of a completed study.
- The number of participants in a qualitative study is adequate when saturation and verification of data are achieved in the study area.
- Important factors to consider in determining sample size for qualitative studies include (1) scope of the study, (2) nature of the topic, (3) quality of the data collected, and (4) design of the study.
- Three common settings for conducting nursing research are natural, partially controlled, and highly controlled.

REFERENCES

Aberson, C. L. (2010). *Applied power analysis for the behavioral sciences.* New York: Routledge Taylor & Francis Group.

Beaulieu, R., Kools, S. M., Kennedy, H. P., & Humphreys, J. (2011). Young adult couples' decision making regarding emergency contraceptive pills. *Journal of Nursing Scholarship, 43*(1), 41–48.

Botman, S. L., Moore, T. F., Moriarty, C. L., & Parsons, V. L. (2000). Design and estimation for the National Health Interview Survey, 1995-2004. *National Center for Health Statistics, Vital Health Statistics, Series 2, No. 130,* 1–32.

Brown, S. J. (2014). *Evidence-based nursing: The research-practice connection* (3rd ed.). Sudbury, MA: Jones & Bartlett.

Cohen, J. (1988). *Statistical power analysis for the behavioral sciences* (2nd ed.). New York: Academic Press.

CONSORT Group. (2010). *CONSORT statement.* Retrieved March 29, 2013 from, http://www.consort-statement.org/consort-statement.

Coyne, I. T. (1997). Sampling in qualitative research. Purposeful and theoretical sampling: Merging or clear boundaries. *Journal of Advanced Nursing, 26*(3), 623–630.

Creswell, J. W. (2014). *Research design: Qualitative, quantitative, and mixed methods approaches* (3rd ed.). Thousand Oaks, CA: Sage.

De Silva, J., Hanwella, R., & de Silva, V. A. (2012). Direct and indirect cost of schizophrenia in outpatients treated in a tertiary care psychiatry unit. *Ceylon Medical Journal, 57*(1), 14–18.

Fawcett, J., & Garity, J. (2009). *Evaluating research for evidence-based nursing practice.* Philadelphia: F. A. Davis.

Fouladbakhsh, J. M., & Stommel, M. (2010). Gender, symptom experience, and use of complementary and alternative medicine practices among cancer survivors in the U.S. cancer population. *Oncology Nursing Forum, 37*(1), E7–E15. http://dx.doi.org/10.1188/10.ONR.E7-E15.

Giakoumidakis, K., Eltheni, R., Patelarou, E., Theologou, S., Patris, V., Michopanou, N., et al. (2013). Effects of intensive glycemic control on outcomes of cardiac surgery. *Heart & Lung, 42*(2), 146–151.

Glaser, B. G., & Strauss, A. L. (1967). *The discovery of grounded theory: Strategies for qualitative research.* Chicago: Aldine.

Grove, S. K., Burns, N., & Gray, J. R. (2013). *The practice of nursing research: Appraisal, synthesis, and generation of evidence* (7th ed.). St. Louis: Elsevier Saunders.

Hodgins, M. J., Ouellet, L. L., Pond, S., Knorr, S., & Geldart, G. (2008). Effect of telephone follow-up on surgical orthopedic recovery. *Applied Nursing Research, 21*(4), 218–226.

Huberman, A. M., & Miles, M. B. (2002). *The qualitative researcher's companion.* Thousand Oaks, CA: Sage.

Kerlinger, F. N., & Lee, H. B. (2000). *Foundations of behavioral research.* New York: Harcourt Brace.

Kraemer, H. C., & Theimann, S. (1987). *How many subjects? Statistical power analysis in research.* Newbury Park, CA: Sage.

Lapidus-Graham, J. (2012). The lived experience of participation in student nursing associations and leadership behaviors: A phenomenological study. *Journal of the New York State Nurses Association, 43*(1), 4–12.

Lee, S., Faucett, J., Gillen, M., Krause, N., & Landry, L. (2013). Risk perception of musculoskeletal injury among critical care nurses. *Nursing Research, 62*(1), 36–44.

Long, J. D., Boswell, C., Rogers, T. J., Littlefield, L. A., Estep, G., Shriver, B. J., et al. (2013). Effectiveness of cell phones and mypyramidtracker.gov to estimate fruit and vegetable intake. *Applied Nursing Research, 26*(1), 17–23.

Marshall, C., & Rossman, G. B. (2011). *Designing qualitative research* (5th ed.). Los Angeles: Sage.

Melnyk, B. M., & Fineout-Overholt, E. (2011). *Evidence-based practice in nursing & healthcare: A guide to best practice* (2nd ed.). Philadelphia: Lippincott, Williams, & Wilkins.

Milroy, J. H., Wyrick, D. L., Bibeau, D. L., Strack, R. W., & Davis, P. G. (2012). A university system-wide qualitative investigation into student physical activity promotion conducted on college campuses. *American Journal of Health Promotion, 26*(5), 305–312.

Monroe, T. B., Kenaga, H., Dietrich, M. S., Carter, M. A., & Cowan, R. L. (2013). The prevalence of employed nurses identified or enrolled in substance use monitoring programs. *Nursing Research, 62*(1), 10–15.

Morse, J. M. (2000). Determining sample size. *Qualitative Health Research, 10*(1), 3–5.

Morse, J. M. (2007). Strategies of intraproject sampling. In P. L. Munhall (Ed.), *Nursing research: A qualitative perspective* (pp. 529–539) (4th ed.). Sudbury, MA: Jones & Bartlett.

Munhall, P. L. (2012). *Nursing research: A qualitative perspective* (5th ed.). Sudbury, MA: Jones & Bartlett Learning.

Parent, N., & Hanley, J. A. (2009). Assessing quality of reports on randomized clinical trials in nursing journals. *Canadian Journal of Cardiovascular Nursing, 19*(2), 25–31.

Pieper, B., Templin, T. N., Kirsner, R. S., & Birk, T. J. (2010). The impact of vascular leg disorders on physical activity in methadone-maintained adults. *Research in Nursing & Health, 33*(5), 426–440.

Quality and Safety Education for Nurses (QSEN), (2013). *Pre-licensure knowledge, skills, and attitudes (KSAs).* Retrieved February 11, 2013 from, http://qsen.org/competencies/pre-licensure-ksas.

Sandelowski, M. (1995). Focus on qualitative methods: Sample size in qualitative research. *Research in Nursing & Health, 18*(2), 179–183.

Sharma, N. K., Ryals, J. M., Gajewski, B. J., & Wright, D. E. (2010). Aerobic exercise alters analgesia and neurotrophin-3 synthesis in an animal model of chronic widespread pain. *Physical Therapy, 90*(5), 714–725.

Sherwood, G., & Barnsteiner, J. (2012). *Quality and safety in nursing: A competency approach to improving outcomes.* Ames, IA: Wiley-Blackwell.

Strauss, A., & Corbin, J. (1998). *Basics of qualitative research, techniques, and procedures for developing grounded theory* (2nd ed.). Thousand Oaks, CA: Sage.

Toma, L. M., Houck, G. M., Wagnild, G. M., Messecar, D., & Jones, K. D. (2013). Growing old with fibromyalgia. *Nursing Research, 62*(1), 16–24.

Clarifying Measurement and Data Collection in Quantitative Research

CHAPTER OVERVIEW

LEARNING OUTCOMES

After completing this chapter, you should be able to:

1. Describe measurement theory and its relevant concepts of directness of measurement, levels of measurement, measurement error, reliability, and validity.
2. Determine the levels of measurement—nominal, ordinal, interval, and ratio—achieved by measurement methods in published studies.
3. Identify possible sources of measurement error in published studies.
4. Critically appraise the reliability and validity of measurement methods in published studies.

5. Critically appraise the accuracy, precision, and error of physiological measures used in studies.
6. Critically appraise the sensitivity, specificity, and likelihood ratios of diagnostic tests.
7. Critically appraise the measurement approaches—physiological measures, observations, interviews, questionnaires, and scales—used in published studies.
8. Critically appraise the use of existing databases in studies.
9. Critically appraise the data collection section in published studies.

KEY TERMS

Measurement is a very important part of the quantitative research process. When quality measurement methods are used in a study, it improves the accuracy or validity of study outcomes or findings. Measurement is the process of assigning numbers or values to individuals' health status, objects, events, or situations using a set of rules (Kaplan, 1963). For example, we measure a patient's blood pressure (BP) using a measurement method such as a stethoscope, cuff, and sphygmomanometer. Then a number or value is assigned to that patient's BP, such as 120/80 mm Hg. In research, variables are measured with the best possible measurement method available to produce trustworthy data that can be used in statistical analyses. Trustworthy data are essential if a study is to produce useful findings to guide nursing practice (Brown, 2014; Fawcett & Garity, 2009).

In critically appraising studies, you need to judge the trustworthiness of the measurement methods used. To produce trustworthy measurements, rules have been established to ensure that numbers, values, or categories will be assigned consistently from one subject (or event) to another and, eventually, if the measurement method or strategy is found to be meaningful, from one study to another. The rules of measurement established for research are similar to those used in nursing practice. For example, measuring a BP requires that the patient be allowed to rest for 5 minutes and then should be sitting, legs uncrossed, arm relaxed on a table at heart level, cuff of accurate size placed correctly on the upper arm that is free of restrictive clothing, and stethoscope correctly placed over the brachial artery at the elbow. Following these rules ensures that the patient's BP is accurately and precisely measured and that any change in the BP reading can be attributed to a change in BP, rather than to an inadvertent error in the measurement technique.

Understanding the logic of measurement is important for critically appraising the adequacy of measurement methods in nursing studies. This chapter includes a discussion of the key concepts of measurement theory—directness of measurement, levels of measurement, measurement error, reliability, and validity. The accuracy and precision of physiological measures and sensitivity and specificity of diagnostic and screening tests are also addressed. Some of the most common measurement methods or strategies used in nursing research are briefly described. The chapter concludes with guidelines for critically appraising the data collection processes used in studies.

CONCEPTS OF MEASUREMENT THEORY

Measurement theory guides the development and use of measurement methods or tools in research. Measurement theory was developed many years ago by mathematicians, statisticians, and other scholars and includes rules that guide how things are measured (Kaplan, 1963). These rules allow individuals to be consistent in how they perform measurements; thus a measurement method used by one person will consistently produce similar results when used by another person. This section discusses some of the basic concepts and rules of measurement theory, including directness of measurement, levels of measurement, measurement error, reliability, and validity.

Directness of Measurement

To measure, the researcher must first identify the object, characteristic, element, event, or situation to be measured. In some cases, identifying the object to measure and determining how to measure it are quite simple, such as when the researcher measures a person's weight and height. These are referred to as direct measures. Direct measures involve determining the value of concrete factors such as weight, waist circumference, temperature, heart rate, BP, and respiration. Technology is available to measure many bodily functions, biological indicators, and chemical characteristics. The focus of measurement in these instances is on the accuracy and precision of the measurement method and process. If a patient's BP is to be accurate, it must be measured with a quality stethoscope and sphygmomanometer and must be precisely or consistently measured, as discussed earlier in the introduction. In research, three BP measurements are usually taken and averaged to determine the most accurate and precise BP reading. Nurse researchers are also experienced in gathering direct measures of demographic variables such as age, gender, ethnic origin, and diagnosis.

However, in many cases in nursing, the thing to be measured is not a concrete object but an abstract idea, characteristic, or concept such as pain, stress, caring, coping, depression, anxiety, and adherence. Researchers cannot directly measure an abstract idea, but they can capture some of its elements in their measurements, which are referred to as indirect measures or indicators of the concepts. Rarely, if ever, can a single measurement strategy measure all aspects of an abstract concept. Therefore multiple measurement methods or indicators are needed, and even then they cannot be expected to measure all elements of an abstract concept. For example, multiple measurement methods might be used to describe pain in a study, which decreases the measurement error and increases the understanding of pain. The measurement methods of pain might include the FACES Pain Scale, observation (rubbing and/or guarding the area that hurts, facial grimacing, and crying), and physiological measures, such as pulse and blood pressure. Figure 10-1

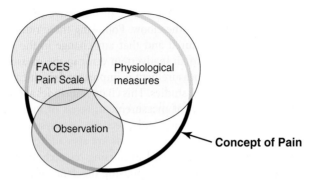

FIG 10-1 Multiple measures of the concept of pain.

demonstrates multiple measures of the concept of pain and demonstrates how having more measurement methods increases the understanding of the concept. The bold, black-rimmed largest circle represents the concept of pain and the pale-colored smaller circles represent the measurement methods. A larger circle is represented by physiological measures indicating these measures (pulse, blood pressure, and respirations) add more to the objective measurement of pain. Even with three different types of measurement methods being used, the entire concept of pain is not completely measured, as indicated by the white areas within the black-rimmed large circle.

Levels of Measurement

Various measurement methods produce data that are at different levels of measurement. The traditional levels of measurement were developed by Stevens (1946), who organized the rules for assigning numbers to objects so that a hierarchy in measurement was established. The levels of measurement, from low to high, are nominal, ordinal, interval, and ratio.

Nominal-Level Measurement

Nominal-level measurement is the lowest of the four measurement categories. It is used when data can be organized into categories of a defined property but the categories cannot be rank-ordered. For example, you may decide to categorize potential study subjects by diagnosis. However, the category "kidney stone," for example, cannot be rated higher than the category "gastric ulcer"; similarly, across categories, "ovarian cyst" is no closer to "kidney stone" than to "gastric ulcer." The categories differ in quality but not quantity. Therefore, it is not possible to say that subject A possesses more of the property being categorized than subject B. (RULE: The categories must not be orderable.) Categories must be established in such a way that each datum will fit into only one of the categories. (RULE: The categories must be exclusive.) All the data must fit into the established categories. (RULE: The categories must be exhaustive.) Data such as gender, race and ethnicity, marital status, and diagnoses are examples of nominal data. The rules for the four levels of measurement are summarized in Figure 10-2.

Ordinal-Level Measurement

With ordinal-level measurement, data are assigned to categories that can be ranked. (RULE: The categories can be ranked [see Figure 10-2].) To rank data, one category is judged to be (or is ranked) higher or lower, or better or worse, than another category. Rules govern how the data

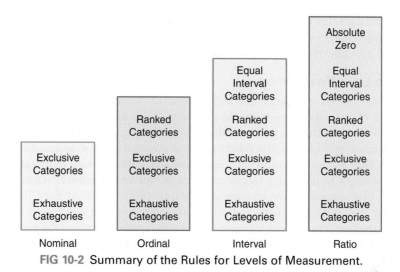

FIG 10-2 Summary of the Rules for Levels of Measurement.

are ranked. As with nominal data, the categories must be exclusive (each datum fits into only one category) and exhaustive (all data fit into at least one category). With ordinal data, the quantity also can be identified (Stevens, 1946). For example, if you are measuring intensity of pain, you may identify different levels of pain. You probably will develop categories that rank these different levels of pain, such as excruciating, severe, moderate, mild, and no pain. However, in using categories of ordinal measurement, you cannot know with certainty that the intervals between the ranked categories are equal. A greater difference may exist between mild and moderate pain, for example, than between excruciating and severe pain. Therefore ordinal data are considered to have unequal intervals.

Many scales used in nursing research are ordinal levels of measurement. For example, it is possible to rank degrees of coping, levels of mobility, ability to provide self-care, or levels of dyspnea on an ordinal scale. For dyspnea with activities of daily living (ADLs), the scale could be:

0 = no shortness of breath with ADLs
1 = minimal shortness of breaths with ADLs
2 = moderate shortness of breath with ADLs
3 = extreme shortness of breath with ADLs
4 = shortness of breath so severe the person is unable to perform ADLs without assistance

The measurement is ordinal because it is not possible to claim that equal distances exist between the rankings. A greater difference may exist between the ranks of 1 and 2 than between the ranks of 2 and 3.

Interval-Level Measurement

Interval-level measurement uses interval scales, which have equal numerical distances between intervals. These scales follow the rules of mutually exclusive, exhaustive, and ranked categories and are assumed to represent a continuum of values. (RULE: The categories must have equal intervals between them [see Figure 10-2].) Therefore the magnitude of the attribute can be more precisely defined. However, it is not possible to provide the absolute amount of the attribute, because the interval scale lacks a zero point. Temperature is the most commonly used example of an interval scale. The difference between the temperatures of 70° F and 80° F is 10° F and is the same as the difference between the temperatures of 30° F and 40° F. Changes in temperature can be measured precisely. However, a temperature of 0° F does not indicate the absence of temperature.

Ratio-Level Measurement

Ratio-level measurement is the highest form of measurement and meets all the rules of other forms of measurement—mutually exclusive categories, exhaustive categories, ordered ranks, equally spaced intervals, and a continuum of values. Interval- and ratio-level data can be added, subtracted, multiplied, and divided because of the equal intervals and continuum of values of these data. Thus interval and ratio data can be analyzed with statistical techniques of greater precision and strength to determine significant relationships and differences (Grove, 2007). In addition, ratio-level measures have absolute zero points. (RULE: The data must have absolute zero [see Figure 10-2].) Weight, length, and volume are commonly used as examples of ratio scales. All three have absolute zeros, at which a value of zero indicates the absence of the property being measured; zero weight means the absence of weight. Because of the absolute zero point, such statements as "Subject A weighs 25 more pounds than subject B" or "Medication container A holds two times as much as container B" can be justified (Stevens, 1946).

In critically appraising a study, you need to determine the level of measurement achieved for each measurement method. Researchers try to achieve the highest level of measurement possible for a variable because more rigorous statistical analyses can be conducted on interval- and ratio-level data to describe variables, determine relationships among variables, and examine differences among groups.

Measurement Error

The ideal perfect measure is referred to as the true measure or score. However, some error is always present in any measurement strategy. Measurement error is the difference between the true measure and what is actually measured (Grove, Burns, & Gray, 2013). The amount of error in a measure varies from considerable error in one measurement to very little in another. Measurement error exists with direct and indirect measures. With direct measures, both the object and measurement method are visible. Direct measures, which generally are expected to be highly accurate, are subject to error. For example, a weight scale may be inaccurate for 0.5 pound, precisely calibrated BP equipment might decrease in precision with use, or a tape measure may not be held at exactly the same tension in measuring the waist of each patient. A subject in a study may be 65 years old but may write illegibly on the demographic form. As a result, the age may be entered inaccurately into the study database.

With indirect measures, the element being measured cannot be seen directly. For example, you cannot see pain. You may observe behaviors or hear words that you think represent pain, but pain is a sensation that is not always clearly recognized or expressed by the person experiencing it. The measurement of pain is usually conducted with a scale but can also include observation and physiological measures as shown in Figure 10-1. Efforts to measure concepts such as pain usually result in measuring only part of the concept. Sometimes measures may identify some aspects of the concept but may include other elements that are not part of the concept. In Figure 10-1, the measurement methods of scale, observation, and physiological measures include factors other than pain, as indicated by the parts of the circles that are outside the black-rimmed circle of the concept pain. For example, measurement methods for pain might be measuring aspects of anxiety and fear in addition to pain. However, using multiple methods to measure a concept or variable usually decreases the measurement error and increases the understanding of the concept being measured.

Two types of error ar~
ference between random ~
ment error, the difference
direction (random). In one
value, whereas in the next
true value. A number of chan
that can result in random error
the measurements may not use t
pencil scale may accidentally mar
puter may punch the wrong key. Th
combining a number of values and c
closer estimate of the true measureme
of the estimate decreases.

Measurement error that is not randoi
ment error, the variation in measureme.
same direction. For example, most of the
was calculated. Systematic error occurs beca
concept. For example, a paper and pencil rat
be measuring perceived support. When meas
that are 2 pounds over the true weights will giv
weights will be high, and as a result the mean w
used. Some systematic error occurs in almost any
of error in a study, researchers spend considerable
minimize systematic measurement error (Waltz et

CHAPTER 10   Clarifying Measurement and

Center for Epidemiologi

These questions are about how
As I read this way in the l
behaved this way: (Interviewer
this way:

288

~uts
~ measured
~ weight scale were
~.ie importance of this type
~ort refining their instruments to
~10).

In critically appraising a published study, you will not be able to judge the extent of measurement error directly. However, you may find clues about the amount of measurement error in the published report. For example, if the researchers have described the method of measurement in great detail and provided evidence of accuracy and precision of the measurement, then the probability of error typically is reduced. The measurement errors for BP readings can be minimized by checking the BP cuff and sphygmomanometer for accuracy and recalibrating them periodically during data collection, obtaining three BP readings and averaging them to determine one BP reading for each subject, and having a trained nurse using a protocol to take the BP readings. If a checklist of pain behaviors is developed for observation, less error occurs than if the observations for pain are unstructured. Measurement will also be more precise if researchers use a well-developed, reliable, and valid scale, such as the FACES Pain Scale, instead of developing a new pain scale for their study. In published studies, look for the steps that researchers have taken to decrease measurement error and increase the quality of their study findings.

Reliability

Reliability is concerned with the consistency of a measurement method. For example, if you are using a paper and pencil scale to measure depression, it should indicate similar depression scores each time a subject completes it within a short period of time. A scale that does not produce similar scores for a subject with repeat testing is considered unreliable and results in increased measurement error (Kerlinger & Lee, 2000; Waltz et al., 2010). For example, the Center for Epidemiologic Studies Depression Scale (CES-D) was developed to diagnose depression in mental health patients (Radloff, 1977). The CES-D has proven to be a quality measure of depression in research over the last 40 years. Figure 10-3 illustrates this 20-item Likert scale. If the items on this scale consistently

Studies Depression Scale

DEPA

you have been feeling lately.
ents, please tell me how often you felt or
st week. (Hand card). **For each statement, did you feel**
You may help respondent focus on the whichever "style" answer is easier)

0 = Rarely or none of the time (or less than 1 day)?
1 = Some or a little of the time (or 1–2 days)?
2 = Occasionally or a moderate amount of time (or 3–4 days)?
3 = Most or all of the time (or 5–7 days)?

		R	S	O	M	NR
1.	I was bothered by things that usually don't bother me.	0	1	2	3	--
2.	I did not feel like eating; my appetite was poor.	0	1	2	3	--
3.	I felt that I could not shake off the blues even with help from my family and friends.	0	1	2	3	--
4.	I felt that I was just as good as other people.	0	1	2	3	--
5.	I had trouble keeping my mind on what I was doing.	0	1	2	3	--
6.	I felt depressed.	0	1	2	3	--
7.	I felt that everything I did was an effort.	0	1	2	3	--
8.	I felt hopeful about the future.	0	1	2	3	--
9.	I thought my life had been a failure.	0	1	2	3	--
10.	I felt fearful.	0	1	2	3	--
11.	My sleep was restless.	0	1	2	3	--
12.	I was happy.	0	1	2	3	--
13.	I talked less than usual.	0	1	2	3	--
14.	I felt lonely.	0	1	2	3	--
15.	People were unfriendly.	0	1	2	3	--
16.	I enjoyed life.	0	1	2	3	--
17.	I had crying spells.	0	1	2	3	--
18.	I felt sad.	0	1	2	3	--
19.	I felt people disliked me.	0	1	2	3	--
20.	I could not get going.	0	1	2	3	--

FIG 10-3 Center of Epidemiologic Studies Depression Scale (CES-D). (Radloff, L. S. [1977]. The CES-D scale: A self report depression scale for research in the general population. *Applied Psychological Measures, 1,* 385-394.)

measure what it was developed to measure, depression, then this scale is considered to be both reliable and valid. The different types of reliability and validity testing are discussed in the next sections (outlined in Table 10-1).

Reliability Testing

Reliability testing is a measure of the amount of random error in the measurement technique. It takes into account such characteristics as dependability, precision, stability, consistency, and reproducibility (Grove et al., 2013; Waltz et al., 2010). Because all measurement techniques contain some random error, reliability exists in degrees and usually is expressed as a correlation coefficient (*r*).

TABLE 10-1	DETERMINING THE QUALITY OF MEASUREMENT METHODS
QUALITY INDICATOR	**DESCRIPTION**
Reliability	**Test-retest reliability:** Repeated measures with a scale or instrument to determine the consistency or *stability* of the instrument in measuring a concept
	Alternate forms reliability: Comparison of two paper and pencil instruments to determine their *equivalence* in measuring a concept
	Interrater reliability: Comparison of two observers or judges in a study to determine their *equivalence* in making observations or judging events
	Homogeneity or internal consistency reliability: Reliability testing used primarily with multi-item scales in which each item on the scale is correlated with all other items to determine the consistency of the scale in measuring a concept
Validity	**Content validity:** Examines the extent to which a measurement method includes all the major elements relevant to the concept being measured.
	Evidence of validity from contrasting groups: Instrument or scale given to two groups expected to have opposite or contrasting scores; one group scores high on the scale and the other scores low.
	Evidence of validity from convergence: Two scales measuring the same concept are administered to a group at the same time, and the subjects' scores on the scales should be positively correlated. For example, subjects completing two scales to measure depression should have positively correlated scores.
	Evidence of validity from divergence: Two scales that measure opposite concepts, such as hope and hopelessness, are administered to subjects at the same time and should result in negatively correlated scores on the scales.
Readability	**Readability level:** Conducted to determine the participants' ability to read and comprehend the items on an instrument. Researchers need to report the level of education that subjects need to read the instrument. Readability must be appropriate to promote reliability and validity of an instrument.
Precision	**Precision of physiological measure:** Degree of consistency or reproducibility of the measurements made with physiological instruments or equipment; comparable to reliability for paper and pencil scales.
Accuracy	**Accuracy of physiological measure:** Addresses the extent to which the physiological instrument or equipment measures what it is supposed to measure in a study; comparable to validity for paper and pencil scales.

Cronbach's alpha coefficient is the most commonly used measure of reliability for scales with multiple items (see the following discussion of homogeneity for more details). *Estimates of reliability are specific to the sample being tested.* Thus high reliability values reported for an established instrument do not guarantee that reliability will be satisfactory in another sample or with a different population. Researchers need to perform reliability testing on each instrument used in a study to ensure that it is reliable for that study (Bialocerkowski, Klupp, & Bragge, 2010; DeVon et al., 2007).

Reliability testing focuses on the following three aspects of reliability—stability, equivalence, and homogeneity (see Table 10-1). Stability is concerned with the consistency of repeated measures of the same attribute with the use of the same scale or instrument. It is usually referred to as test-retest reliability. This measure of reliability is generally used with physical measures, technological measures, and paper and pencil scales. Use of the technique requires an assumption that the factor to be measured remains the same at the two testing times and that any change in the value or score is a consequence of random error. For example, physiological measures such as BP equipment can be tested and then immediately retested, or the equipment can be used for a time and then retested to determine the necessary frequency of recalibration. Researchers need to include test-retest reliability results in their published studies to document the reliability of their measurement methods. For example, the CES-D (see Figure 10-3) has been used frequently in nursing studies over the years and has demonstrated test-retest reliability ranging from $r=0.51$ to 0.67 in 2- to 8-week intervals. This is very solid test-retest reliability for this scale, indicating that it is consistently measuring depression with repeat testing and recognizing that subjects' levels of depression vary somewhat over time (Locke & Putnam, 2002; Sharp & Lipsky, 2002).

Reliability testing can also include equivalence, which involves the comparison of two versions of the same paper and pencil instrument or of two observers measuring the same event. Comparison of two observers or two judges in a study is referred to as interrater reliability. Studies that include collecting observational data or the making of judgments by two or more data gatherers require the reporting of interrater reliability. There is no absolute value below which interrater reliability is unacceptable. However, any value below 0.80 should generate serious concern about the reliability of the data, data gatherer, or both. The interrater reliability value is best to be 0.90 or 90%, which means 90% reliability and 10% random error, or higher.

Comparison of two paper and pencil instruments is referred to as alternate forms reliability, or parallel forms reliability. Alternative forms of instruments are of more concern in the development of normative knowledge testing such as the Scholastic Aptitude Test (SAT), which is used as a college entrance requirement. The SAT has been used for decades, and there are many forms of this test, with a variety of items included on each. These alternate forms of the SAT were developed to measure students' knowledge consistently and protect the integrity of the test.

Homogeneity is a type of reliability testing used primarily with paper and pencil instruments or scales to address the correlation of each question to the other questions within the scale. Questions on a scale are also called items. The principle is that each item should be consistently measuring a concept such as depression and so should be highly correlated with the other items. Homogeneity testing examines the extent to which all the items in the instrument consistently measure the construct and is a test of internal consistency. The statistical procedure used for this process is Cronbach's alpha coefficient for interval- and ratio-level data. On some scales, the person responding selects between two options, such as yes and no. The resulting data are dichotomous, and the Kuder-Richardson formula (K-R 20) is used to estimate internal consistency. A Cronbach alpha coefficient of 1.00 indicates perfect reliability, and a coefficient of 0.00 indicates no reliability (Waltz et al., 2010). A reliability of 0.80 is usually considered a strong coefficient for a scale that has documented reliability and has been used in several studies, such as the CES-D (Grove et al., 2013; Radloff, 1977). The CES-D has strong internal consistency reliability, with Cronbach's alphas ranging from 0.84 to 0.90 in field studies (Locke & Putnam, 2002; Sharp & Lipsky, 2002). For relatively new scales, a reliability of 0.70 is considered acceptable because the scale is being refined and used with a variety of samples. The stronger correlation coefficients, which are closer to 1.0, indicate less random error and a more reliable scale. A research report needs to include the results from stability, equivalence, and/or homogeneity reliability testing done on a measurement method from previous research and in the present study (Grove et al., 2013). A measurement method must be reliable if it is to be considered a valid measure for a study concept.

Validity

The validity of an instrument is a determination of how well the instrument reflects the abstract concept being examined. Validity, like reliability, is not an all or nothing phenomenon; it is measured on a continuum. No instrument is completely valid, so researchers determine the degree of validity of an instrument rather than whether validity exists (DeVon et al., 2007; Waltz et al., 2010). Validity will vary from one sample to another and one situation to another; therefore validity testing evaluates the use of an instrument for a specific group or purpose, rather than the instrument itself. An instrument may be valid in one situation but not another. For example, the CES-D was developed to measure the depression of patients in mental health settings. Will the same scale be valid as a measure of the depression of cancer patients? Researchers determine this by pilot-testing the scale to examine the validity of the instrument in a new population. In addition, the original CES-D (see Figure 10-3) was developed for adults, but the scale has been refined and tested with young children (4 to 6 years of age), school-age children, adolescents, and older adults. Thus different versions of this scale can be used with those of all ages, ranging from 4 years old to geriatric age (Sharp & Lipsky, 2002).

In this text, validity is considered a single broad method of measurement evaluation, referred to as **construct validity**, and includes content and predictive validity (Rew, Stuppy, & Becker, 1988). **Content validity** examines the extent to which the measurement method or scale includes all the major elements or items relevant to the construct being measured. The evidence for content validity of a scale includes the following: (1) how well the items of the scale reflect the description of the concept in the literature; (2) the content experts' evaluation of the relevance of items on the scale that might be reported as an index (Grove et al., 2013); and (3) the potential subjects' responses to the scale items.

Paper and pencil and electronic instruments or scales must be at a level that potential study subjects can read and understand. **Readability level** focuses on the study participants' ability to read and comprehend the content of an instrument or scale. Readability is essential if an instrument is to be considered valid and reliable for a sample (see Table 10-1). Assessing the level of readability of an instrument is relatively simple and takes about 10 to 15 minutes. More than 30 readability formulas are available. These formulas use counts of language elements to provide an index of the probable degree of difficulty of comprehending the scale (Grove et al., 2013). Readability formulas are now a standard part of word-processing software.

Three common types of validity presented in published studies include evidence of validity from (1) contrasting groups, (2) convergence, and (3) divergence. An instrument's **evidence of validity from contrasting groups** can be tested by identifying groups that are expected (or known) to have contrasting scores on an instrument. For example, researchers select samples from a group of individuals with a diagnosis of depression and a group that does not have this diagnosis. You would expect these two groups of individuals to have contrasting scores on the CES-D. The group with the diagnosis of depression would be expected to have higher scores than those without the depression diagnosis, which would add to the construct validity of this scale.

Evidence of validity from convergence is determined when a relatively new instrument is compared with an existing instrument(s) that measures the same construct. The instruments, the new and existing ones, are administered to a sample at the same time, and the results are evaluated with correlational analyses. If the measures are strongly positively correlated, the validity of each instrument is strengthened. For example, the CES-D has shown positive correlations ranging from 0.40 to 0.80 with the Hamilton Rating Scale for Depression, which supports the convergent validity of both scales (Locke & Putnam, 2002; Sharp & Lipsky, 2002).

Sometimes instruments can be located that measure a concept opposite to the concept measured by the newly developed instrument. For example, if the newly developed instrument is a measure of hope, you could make a search for an instrument that measures hopelessness or despair. Having study participants complete both these scales is a way to examine **evidence of validity from** divergence. Correlational procedures are performed with the measures of the two concepts. If the divergent measure (hopelessness scale) is negatively correlated (such as −0.4 to −0.8) with the other instrument (hope scale), validity for each of the instruments is strengthened (Waltz et al., 2010).

The evidence of an instrument's validity from previous research and the current study needs to be included in the published report. In critically appraising a study, you need to judge the validity of the measurement methods that were used. However, you cannot consider validity apart from reliability (see Table 10-1). If a measurement method does not have acceptable reliability or is not consistently measuring a concept, then it is not valid.

ACCURACY, PRECISION, AND ERROR OF PHYSIOLOGICAL MEASURES

Physiological measures are measurement methods used to quantify the level of functioning of living beings (Ryan-Wenger, 2010). The precision, accuracy, and error of physiological and biochemical measures tend not to be reported or are minimally covered in published studies. These routine physiological measures are assumed to be accurate and precise, an assumption that is not always correct. Some of the most common physiological measures used in nursing studies include BP, heart rate, weight, body mass index, and laboratory values. Sometimes researchers obtain these measures from the patient's record, with no consideration given to their accuracy. For example, how many times have you heard a nurse ask a patient his or her height or weight, rather than measuring or weighing the patient? Thus researchers using physiological measures need to provide evidence of the measures' accuracy, precision, and potential for error (see Table 10-1; Gift & Soeken, 1988; Ryan-Wenger, 2010).

Accuracy

Accuracy is comparable to validity in that it addresses the extent to which the instrument measures what it is supposed to measure in a study (Ryan-Wenger, 2010). For example, oxygen saturation measurements with pulse oximetry are considered comparable with measures of oxygen saturation with arterial blood gases. Because pulse oximetry is an accurate measure of oxygen saturation, it has been used in studies because it is easier, less expensive, less painful, and less invasive for research participants. Researchers need to document that previous research has been conducted to determine the accuracy of pulse oximetry for the measurement of individuals' oxygen saturation levels in their study.

Precision

Precision is the degree of consistency or reproducibility of measurements made with physiological instruments. Precision is comparable to reliability. The precision of most physiological equipment depends on following the manufacturer's instructions for care and routine testing of the equipment. Test-retest reliability is appropriate for physiological variables that have minimal fluctuations, such as cholesterol (lipid) levels, bone mineral density, or weight of adults (Ryan-Wenger, 2010). Test-retest reliability can be inappropriate if the variables' values frequently fluctuate with various activities, such as with pulse, respirations, and BP. However, test-retest is a good measure of precision if the measurements are taken in rapid succession. For example, the national BP guidelines encourage taking three BP readings 1 to 2 minutes apart and then averaging them to obtain the most precise and accurate measure of BP (http://www.nhlbi.nih.gov/guidelines/hypertension).

Error

Sources of error in physiological measures can be grouped into the following five categories: environment, user, subject, equipment, and interpretation. The environment affects the equipment and subject. Environmental factors might include temperature, barometric pressure, and static electricity. User errors are caused by the person using the equipment and may be associated with variations by the same user, different users, or changes in supplies or procedures used to operate the equipment. Subject errors occur when the subject alters the equipment or the equipment alters the subject. In some cases, the equipment may not be used to its full capacity. Equipment error may be related to calibration or the stability of the equipment. Signals transmitted from the equipment are also a source of error and can result in misinterpretation (Gift & Soeken, 1988). Researchers need to report the protocols followed or steps taken to prevent errors in their physiological and biochemical measures in their published studies (Ryan-Wenger, 2010; Stone & Frazier, 2010).

? CRITICAL APPRAISAL GUIDELINES

Directness, Level of Measurement, Reliability, and Validity of Scales, Accuracy, Precision, and Error of Physiological Measures

In critically appraising a published study, you need to determine the directness and level of measurement, reliability and validity of scales, accuracy and precision of physiological measures, and potential measurement error for the different measurement methods used in a study. In most studies, the methods section includes a discussion of measurement methods, and you can use the following questions to evaluate them:

1. What measurement method(s) were used to measure each study variable?
2. Was the type of measurement direct or indirect?
3. What level of measurement was achieved for each of the study variables?
4. Was reliability information provided from previous studies and for this study?
5. Was the validity of each measurement method adequately described? In some studies, researchers simply state that the measurement method has acceptable validity based on previous research. This statement provides insufficient information for you to judge the validity of an instrument.
6. Did the researchers address the accuracy, precision, and potential for errors with the physiological measures?
7. Was the process for obtaining, scoring, and/or recording data described?
8. Did the researchers provide adequate description of the measurement methods to judge the extent of measurement error?

✦ RESEARCH EXAMPLE

Directness, Level of Measurement, Reliability, and Validity of Scales, Accuracy, Precision, and Error of Physiological Measures

Research Excerpt

Whittenmore, Melkus, Wagner, Dziura, Northrup, and Grey (2009) studied the effects of a lifestyle change program on the outcomes for patients with type 2 diabetes. The lifestyle program was delivered by nurse practitioners (NPs) in primary care settings. The following excerpt describes some of the measurement methods used in this study.

Outcome Measures

"Data were collected at the individual (participant) and organizational (NP and site) levels at scheduled time points throughout the study. … All data were collected by trained research assistants blinded to group assignment, with the exception of … lipids, which were collected by experienced laboratory personnel at each site and sent to one laboratory for analysis." (Whittenmore et al., 2009, p. 5)

Continued

RESEARCH EXAMPLE—cont'd

"Efficacy data were collected on clinical outcomes on (weight loss, waist circumference, and lipid profiles); behavioral outcomes (nutrition and exercise); and psychological outcomes (depressive symptoms). . . . All data were collected at baseline, 3 months, and 6 months, with the exception of the laboratory data, which were collected at baseline and 6 months. . . . Efficacy data collection measures and times were based on the DPP [diabetes prevention program] study and modified for the short duration of this pilot study.

Weight loss was the primary outcome and was calculated as a percentage of weight loss from baseline to 6 months. . . . Waist circumference and lipid profiles were secondary clinical outcomes. Waist circumference was measured by positioning a tape measure snugly midway between the upper hip bone and the uppermost border of the iliac crest. In very overweight participants, the tape was placed at the level of the umbilicus (Klein et al., 2007). Lipid profiles (LDL [low-density lipoproteins], HDL [high-density lipoproteins], total cholesterol, and total triglycerides) were determined using fasting venous blood.

Diet and exercise health-promoting behaviors were measured with the exercise and nutrition subscales of the Health-Promoting Lifestyle Profile II (eight and nine items, respectively), which has items constructed on a 4-point Likert scale and measures patterns of diet and exercise behavior (Walker, Sechrist, & Pender, 1987). This instrument has been used in diverse samples, and demonstrates adequate internal consistency ($r = .70$ to .90 for subscales; Jefferson, Melkus, & Spollett, 2000). The alpha coefficients for the exercise and nutrition subscales in this study were .86 and .76, respectively. . . .

Psychosocial data were collected on depressive symptoms, as measured by the Center for Epidemiologic Studies Depression Scale (CES-D), a widely used scale (Radloff, 1977). The CES-D consists of 20 items that address depressed mood, guilt or worthlessness, helplessness or hopelessness, psychomotor retardation, loss of appetite, and sleep disturbance [see Figure 10-3]. Each item is rated on a scale of 0 to 3 in terms of frequency during the past week. The total score may range from 0 to 60, with a score of 16 or more indicating impairment. High internal consistency, acceptable test-retest reliability, and good construct validity have been demonstrated (Posner et al., 2001). The alpha coefficient was .93 for the CES-D in this sample." (Whittenmore et al., 2009, p. 6)

Critical Appraisal

Whittenmore and colleagues (2009) detailed their measurement methods and data collection process in their research report. The outcomes of weight loss, waist circumference, and lipid profiles were measured directly with physiological measures that provided ratio-level data. Weight loss was calculated as a percentage, but the researchers did not describe the precision and accuracy of the weight scales used to determine the patients' weights. Waist circumference was measured with a tape measure according to national guidelines and included a plan for measuring very overweight individuals. Following a national measurement protocol increased the precision and accuracy of the waist measurements and decreased the potential for error. The subjects' blood samples were collected by experienced laboratory personnel at each site and sent to one laboratory for analysis, which increases the precision and accuracy of the lipid values.

Diet and exercise health-promoting behaviors were measured with the subscales from an established, quality Likert scale, Health-Promoting Lifestyle Profile II. The subscales had strong reliability ($r = 0.70$ to 0.90) when used in previous research and the reliability for the subscales in this study were strong (0.86 for diet and 0.76 for exercise). The Health-Promoting Lifestyle Profile II has been used to collect data from diverse samples, which adds to the scale validity. However, the discussion of this measurement method would have been strengthened by expanding on the scale's validity testing from previous studies.

The CES-D is an indirect measure of depression producing interval-level data. This scale has been widely used in research, which adds to its construct validity. The researchers also identified the focus of the 20 items of the scale, which addresses the scale's content validity. The scale was reported to have good construct validity but no further specific information was provided to support this statement. The CES-D has a history of acceptable test-retest reliability and high internal consistency. In addition, the Cronbach alpha coefficient for this sample was very strong, at $r = 0.93$.

The research assistants were trained and blinded to group assignment, decreasing the potential for error and bias during data collection. However, the study would have been strengthened by including the interrater reliability percentage achieved during the training of the data collectors. In summary, Whittenmore and associates (2009) selected quality measurement methods that were consistently implemented. However, expanding the validity discussions of the scales used would have strengthened the study.

Implications for Practice

Whittenmore and co-workers (2009) stated that

"the results of this study support the feasibility of implementing a DPP by NPs in a primary care setting to adults at risk of T2D [type 2 diabetes]. . . . Preliminary efficacy results of the lifestyle program indicate modest improvements with respect to clinical and behavioral outcomes. Twenty-five percent of the lifestyle participants achieved a 5% weight loss goal compared with 11% of participants in standard care." (Whittenmore et al., 2009, pp. 8-9)

The study results indicated that the lifestyle program was effective for the target population of adults at risk for T2D. Further research is needed, however, to determine the long-term effects of such a program. These study findings provide knowledge to help you achieve the Quality and Safety Education for Nurses (QSEN, 2013; Sherwood & Barnsteiner, 2012) competencies for evidence-based practice (EBP) for prelicensure nursing students. Research indicates that this patient-centered lifestyle program has the potential to improve the outcomes of patients with T2D.

USE OF SENSITIVITY, SPECIFICITY, AND LIKELIHOOD RATIOS TO DETERMINE THE QUALITY OF DIAGNOSTIC AND SCREENING TESTS

Sensitivity and Specificity

An important part of evidence-based practice (EBP) is the use of quality diagnostic and screening tests to determine the presence or absence of disease (Sackett, Straus, Richardson, Rosenberg, & Haynes, 2000). Clinicians want to know which laboratory or imaging study to order to help screen for or diagnose a disease. When the test is ordered, are the results valid or accurate? The accuracy of a screening test or a test used to confirm a diagnosis is evaluated in terms of its ability to assess the presence or absence of a disease or condition correctly as compared with a gold standard. The gold standard is the most accurate means of currently diagnosing a particular disease and serves as a basis for comparison with newly developed diagnostic or screening tests. If the test is positive, what is the probability that the disease is present? If the test is negative, what is the probability that the disease is not present? When nurses, nurse practitioners, and physicians talk to their patients about the results of their tests, how sure are they that the patient does or does not have the disease? Sensitivity and specificity are the terms used to describe the accuracy of a screening or diagnostic test. You will see these terms used in studies and other healthcare literature, and we want you to be aware of their definitions and usefulness for practice and research.

There are four possible outcomes of a screening test for a disease: (1) true positive, which is an accurate identification of the presence of a disease; (2) false positive, which indicates that a disease is present when it is not; (3) true negative, which indicates accurately that a disease is not present; or (4) false negative, which indicates that a disease is not present when it is. Table 10-2 is commonly used to visualize sensitivity, specificity, and these four outcomes (Grove, 2007; Melnyk & Fineout-Overholt, 2011; Sackett et al., 2000).

You can calculate sensitivity and specificity based on research findings and clinical practice outcomes to determine the most accurate diagnostic or screening tool to use when identifying the presence or absence of a disease for a population of patients. The calculations for sensitivity and specificity are provided as follows:

TABLE 10-2   RESULTS OF SENSITIVITY AND SPECIFICITY OF SCREENING TESTS

DIAGNOSTIC TEST RESULT	DISEASE PRESENT	DISEASE NOT PRESENT OR ABSENT	TOTAL
Positive test	*a* (true positive)	*b* (false positive)	*a* + *b*
Negative test	*c* (false negative)	*d* (true negative)	*c* + *d*
Total	*a* + *c*	*b* + *d*	*a* + *b* + *c* + *d*

a, Number of people who have the disease and the test is positive (true positive); *b*, number of people who do not have the disease and the test is positive (false positive); *c*, number of people who have the disease and the test is negative (false negative); *d*, number of people who do not have the disease and the test is negative (true negative).
From Grove, S. K. (2007). *Statistics for health care research: A practical workbook* (p. 335). Philadelphia: Saunders.

$$Sensitivity\ calculation = probability\ of\ disease = a/(a+c) = true\ positive\ rate$$
$$Specificity\ calculation = probability\ of\ no\ disease = d/(b+d) = true\ negative\ rate$$

Sensitivity is the proportion of patients with the disease who have a positive test result, or true positive. The CES-D (see Figure 10-3) with a score of 15 or higher has 89% sensitivity for diagnosing depression in adults and 92% sensitivity in older adults. The researcher or clinician might refer to the test sensitivity in the following ways:

- A highly sensitive test is very good at identifying the disease in a patient.
- If a test is highly sensitive, it has a low percentage of false negatives.

Specificity is the proportion of patients without the disease who have a negative test result, or true negative. The CES-D with a score of 15 or higher has 70% specificity for diagnosing depression in adults and 87% specificity in older adults. The researcher or clinician might refer to the test specificity in the following ways:

- A highly specific test is very good at identifying the patients without a disease.
- If a test is very specific, it has a low percentage of false positives.

? CRITICAL APPRAISAL GUIDELINES

Sensitivity and Specificity of Diagnostic and Screening Tests

When critically appraising a study, you need to judge the sensitivity and specificity of the diagnostic and screening tests used in the study.
1. Was a diagnostic or screening test used in a study?
2. Are the sensitivity and specificity values provided for the diagnostic or screening test from previous studies and for this study's population?

RESEARCH EXAMPLE

Sensitivity and Specificity

Research Excerpt
Sarikaya, Aktas, Ay, Cetin, and Celikmen (2010) conducted a study to determine the sensitivity and specificity of the rapid antigen detection testing for diagnosing pharyngitis in emergency department (ED) patients. Acute pharyngitis is primarily a viral infection, but in 10% of cases it is caused by bacteria. Most of the bacterial pharyngitis cases are caused by group A beta-hemolytic streptococci (GABHS). One laboratory method for diagnosing GABHS is

rapid antigen diagnostic testing (RADT), which has become more popular than a throat culture because it can be processed rapidly during an ED and primary care visit. The following study excerpt describes the quality of the RADT in this sample:

"We conducted a study to define the sensitivity and specificity of RADT, using throat culture results as the gold standard, in 100 emergency department patients who presented with symptoms consistent with streptococcal pharyngitis. We found that RADT had a sensitivity of 68.2% (15 of 22), a specificity of 89.7% (70 of 78), a positive predictive value of 65.2% (15 of 23), and a negative predictive value of 90.9% (70 of 77)." (Sarikaya, et al., p. 180)

The results of Sarikaya and colleagues' (2010) study are shown in Table 10-3, so you can see how the sensitivity and specificity were calculated.

TABLE 10-3	RESULTS OF SENSITIVITY AND SPECIFICITY OF RAPID ANTIGEN DIAGNOSTIC TESTING (RADT)		
RADT DIAGNOSTIC TEST RESULT	GABHS PHARYNGITIS PRESENT	GABHS PHARYNGITIS ABSENT	TOTAL
Positive	a (true positive) = 15	b (false positive) = 8	a+b=15+8=23
Negative	c (false negative) = 7	d (true negative) = 70	c+d=7+70=77
Total	a+c=15+7=22	b+d=8+70=78	a+b+c+d=100

a, Number of people who have group A beta-hemolytic streptococci (GABHS) pharyngitis and the test is positive (true positive); b, number of people who do not have GABHS pharyngitis and the test is positive (false positive); c, number of people who have GABHS pharyngitis and the test is negative (false negative); d, number of people who do not have GABHS pharyngitis and the test is negative (true negative).

Sensitivity calculation = probability of disease = a/(a + c) = true-positive rate
Sensitivity = probability of GABHS pharyngitis = $15/(15 + 7) = 15/22 = 68.18\% = 68.2\%$
Specificity calculation = probability of no disease = d/(b + d) = true negative rate
Specificity = probability of no GABHS pharyngitis = $70/(8 + 70) = 70/78 = 89.74\% = 89.7\%$

The sensitivity of 68.2% indicates the percentage of patients with a positive RADT who had GABHS pharyngitis (true positive rate). The specificity of 89.7% indicates the percentage of the patients with a negative RADT who did not have GABHS pharyngitis (true negative rate).

Critical Appraisal

Sarikaya and associates (2010) provided a quality discussion about sensitivity and specificity of RADT in identifying GABHS pharyngitis in ED patients. They detailed sensitivity and specificity information in their narrative and in a table.

Implications for Practice

Sarikaya and co-workers (2010, p. 180) concluded that "RADT is useful in the ED when the clinical suspicion is GABHS pharyngitis, but results should be confirmed with a throat culture in patients whose RADT results are negative." In developing a diagnostic or screening test, researchers need to achieve the highest sensitivity and specificity possible. In selecting screening tests to diagnose illnesses, clinicians need to determine the most sensitive and specific screening test but also need to examine cost and ease of access to these tests when making their final decision for practice (Craig & Smyth, 2012).

Likelihood Ratios

Likelihood ratios (LRs) are additional calculations that can help researchers determine the accuracy of diagnostic or screening tests, which are based on the sensitivity and specificity results. The LRs are calculated to determine the likelihood that a positive test result is a true positive and that a negative test result is a true negative. The ratio of the true-positive results to false-positive results is known as the positive likelihood ratio (Campo, Shiyko, & Lichtman, 2010; Craig & Smyth, 2012). The positive LR is calculated as follows, using the data from the Sarikaya et al. (2010) study:

$$\textbf{Positive LR} = \textbf{sensitivity} \div (\textbf{100\%} - \textbf{specificity})$$

Positive LR for GABHS pharyngitis $= 68.2\% \div (100\% - 89.7\%) = 68.2\% \div 10.3\% = 6.62$

The negative likelihood ratio is the ratio of true-negative results to false-negative results and is calculated as follows:

$$\textbf{Negative LR} = (\textbf{100\%} - \textbf{sensitivity}) \div \textbf{specificity}$$

Negative LR for GABHS pharyngitis $= (100\% - 68.2\%) \div 89.7\% = 31.8\% \div 89.7\% = 0.35$

The very high LRs (or those that are >10) rule in the disease or indicate that the patient has the disease. The very low LRs (or those that are <0.1) almost rule out the chance that the patient has the disease (Campo et al., 2010; Melnyk & Fineout-Overholt, 2011). Understanding sensitivity, specificity, and LR increases your ability to read clinical studies and determine the most accurate diagnostic test to use in clinical practice.

MEASUREMENT STRATEGIES IN NURSING

Nursing studies examine a wide variety of phenomena and thus require an extensive array of measurement methods. Some nursing phenomena have not been examined because no one has thought of a way to measure them, which has implications for clinical practice and research. This section describes some of the most common measurement methods used in nursing research, including physiological measures, observational measurement, interviews, questionnaires, and scales.

Physiological Measures

Some of the first physiological nursing studies examined basic care activities, such as mouth care, pressure ulcer care, and infection control related to urinary bladder catheterization, intravenous therapy, and tracheotomy care. Even at this fairly basic level, developing valid methods to measure the variables of interest was difficult and required considerable time and expense. Creativity and attention to detail are also important for the development of physiological measures currently used in research and practice (Ryan-Wenger, 2010).

An increased need for ways to measure the outcomes of nursing care has generated more nursing studies that include physiological measures. The outcome of interest may be the outcome of all nursing care received for a particular care episode or the outcome of a particular nursing intervention. An important focus of physiological measurement is finding a means to quantify changes, directly or indirectly, that occur in physiological variables as a result of nursing care. This upsurge of interest in outcome measures has broadened the base of physiological research beyond nurse physiologists to include nurse clinicians (Brown, 2014; Doran, 2011).

A variety of approaches for obtaining physiological measures are possible. Some measurements are relatively easy to obtain and are an extension of the measurement methods used in nursing practice, such as those used to obtain weight and BP. Other measurements are not difficult to obtain, but the methods sometimes require an imaginative approach. For example, some physiological measures are obtained by using self-report with diaries, scales, or observation checklists, and other physiological measures are obtained using laboratory tests and electronic monitoring.

The availability of electronic monitoring equipment has greatly increased the possibilities of physiological measurement in nursing studies, particularly in critical care environments. Electronic monitoring requires placing sensors on or within the subject, such as electrocardiogram leads and arterial lines. The sensors measure changes in bodily functions, such as electrical energy. Some electronic equipment provides simultaneous recording of multiple physiological measures that are displayed on a monitor, such as equipment that records BP, pulse, heart rhythm, and arterial pressure. The equipment is often linked to a computer, which allows review and analysis of the complex data (Pugh & DeKeyser, 1995; Stone & Frazier, 2010).

RESEARCH EXAMPLE

Physiological Measures

Research Excerpt

Lu, Lin, Chen, Tsang, and Su (2013) conducted a quasi-experimental study to determine the effect of acupressure on the sleep quality of psychogeriatric inpatients. Acupressure was performed for each study participant in the psychiatric hospital's examination room. Sleep quality was measured indirectly or subjectively by the patients' self-report of their sleep and directly or objectively using actigraphy, a method that uses an electronic device to detect and record movement. The following study excerpt describes these two types of physiological measures:

"Sleep quality was assessed subjectively and objectively. Subjective data were measured by the PSQI [Pittsburg Sleep Quality Index] developed by Buysse, Reynolds, Monk, Berman, and Kupfer (1989). The PSQI is a 19-item questionnaire used to measure sleep quality and disturbances for the previous 4 weeks leading up to administration. Seven component scores (sleep latency, sleep duration, habitual sleep efficiency, sleep disturbances, the use of sleeping medications, daytime dysfunction, and perceived sleep quality) are generated and are summed to yield one global score. The higher the score is, the worse the sleep quality. The sensitivity and specificity of a global score over 5 (*poor sleeper*) is 90% and 87%, respectively (Buysse et al., 1989)." (Lu et al., 2013, p. 132)

The PSQI has documented reliability and validity from previous studies and the internal consistency for this sample was Cronbach's $\alpha = 0.87$.

"Objective data were measured using actigraphy (Lenience No.: 019678), a standardized, noninvasive, ambulatory device equipped with a sensor (piezoelectric accelerometer) that is worn by participants to monitor and record gross motor activities continuously over an extended period of time. Actigraphy is useful to assess sleep-wake cycles and circadian rhythms and offers reliable results with an average accuracy over 90%, which approximates that of the polysomnography... Participants wore the device all day, every day for 4 weeks, except when showering. The participant elected to wear the device on either the nondominant wrist or ankle. To enhance the data accuracy and prevent the device from being incidentally dislodged, an external wrapper was used during the wearing. Data were read, transferred, stored, and analyzed using Acti-Web software.... [T]he actigraphical data were translated into meaningful information used to assess the participants' sleep latency, total sleep time, sleep efficiency, number of sleep interruptions (wake episodes), and minutes of wake time after the onset of sleep." (Lu et al., 2013, pp. 132-133)

Continued

Critical Appraisal

Lu and colleagues (2013) used two strong physiological measures of self-report (PSQI) and electronic monitoring (actigraphy) to measure their dependent variable of sleep quality. The PSQI has strong sensitivity (90%) and specificity (87%) in determining sleep problems and was reliable in this sample (Cronbach's $\alpha = 0.87$). The discussion of this scale would have been strengthened by providing reliability and validity information from previous studies (Waltz et al., 2010). The actigraphy used to electronically monitor sleep activities was described in detail. The researchers compared this device to the polysomnography and indicated that it was 90% as accurate. When wearing the device, the participants took actions to promote the accuracy and precision of the data. The processes for transferring and analyzing the data were also detailed, indicating that the results were strong in describing sleep quality, with limited potential for measurement error.

Implications for Practice

Lu and associates (2013) found that sleep quality was significantly improved after acupressure, as measured by PSQI and actigraphy. Because acupressure is noninvasive, low-risk, and low cost, the researchers recommended that it might be an effective intervention to treat insomnia. QSEN implications indicate that acupressure might be a safer, evidence-based intervention to use to promote sleep than hypnotic agents for the psychogeriatic inpatient. This type of research-based knowledge is essential for the delivery of EBP (QSEN, 2013; Sherwood & Barnsteiner, 2012).

Observational Measurement

Observational measurement involves an interaction between the study participants and observer(s), in which the observer has the opportunity to watch the participant perform in a specific setting (Waltz et al., 2010). Observation is often used to collect data in qualitative studies, and it is usually unstructured (see Chapter 3). Unstructured observations involve spontaneously observing and recording what is seen in words. The analysis of these data may lead to a more structured observation and an observational checklist (Creswell, 2014; Marshall & Rossman, 2011; Munhall, 2012).

In structured observational measurement, the researcher carefully defines what he or she will observe and how the observations are to be made, recorded, and coded as numbers (Waltz et al., 2010). For observations to be structured, researchers will develop a category system for organizing and sorting the behaviors or events being observed. Checklists are often used to indicate whether a behavior occurred. Rating scales allow the observer to rate the behavior or event. This provides more information for analysis than dichotomous data, which indicate only whether or not the behavior occurred. Because observation tends to be more subjective than other types of measurement, it is often considered less credible. In many cases, observation may be the only approach for obtaining important data for nursing's body of knowledge. As with any means of measurement, consistency is very important. As a result, reporting interrater reliability of those doing the observations is essential.

CRITICAL APPRAISAL GUIDELINES

Observational Measurement

When critically appraising observational measures, consider the following questions:
1. Is the object of observation clearly identified and defined?
2. Are the techniques for recording observations described?
3. Is interrater reliability for the observers described?

RESEARCH EXAMPLE

Observational Measurement

Research Excerpt

Liaw, Yang, Chang, Chou, and Chao (2009) conducted a study to determine the effects of an educational program for nurses in a neonatal unit on how to provide developmental supportive care (DSC) to preterm infants during bathing. They provided an extensive description of their use of observational measurement to identify infant and nurse behaviors during the bathing process. The following excerpt includes part of their description of their observational measurement methods:

"Nurse caregiving and infant behaviors were measured from the time that a nurse put her hands through an isolette porthole to the stage when she completed the bath and removed her hands from an incubator and left. Researchers developed two coding schemes: one was the preterm infant behavioral coding scheme for assessing preterm infant behavior responses during bath, and the other one was the nursing behavioral coding scheme for assessing nurse caregiving behavior during bath. The behaviors included in this coding scheme were only those that could be reliably recorded and observed from videotapes and with which another expert (Dr. Evelyn Thoman) agreed as being behaviors and states that could be consistently observed on video recordings [see Table 10-4]. Time-triggered coding was used to measure all behaviors and states. There were four observers watching the videotapes. Two were responsible for recording infant behavior, and the other two observed nurse behavior. All behavior data were coded at 10-second intervals on a continuous basis with an electronic auditory device, and codes were typed in a Microsoft Word file. "(Liaw et al., 2009, pp. 87-88)

TABLE 10-4   DEFINITIONS OF INFANT BEHAVIORS AND CODES FOR SCORING VIDEOTAPES

BEHAVIOR	CODE	DEFINITION
Startle	J	Sudden movement in which the arms extend quickly outward and then return toward midline: leg may flex or extend
Jerk	J	Sudden movement of at least a whole limb, one arm, or one leg
Tremor	J	Fine rhythmic movement of the extremities
Extension	S	Stiff extensor positioning of extremities—salute, airplane, sitting on air, leg bracing, or other hypertonic behaviors
Arching	S	Movement of all limbs and trunk showing labored stretching and struggling
Squirming	S	Truncal extension into an arch or head extension in prone, supine, or upright position
Finger splay	H	Sudden stiff extension of fingers and hand
Grasping	H	Grasping movement, with hands directed at baby's own face or baby's own body, at midair, or a caregiver's hands, finger, or body, tubing, or bedding
Fisting	H	Strong hand holding by flexing the baby's fingers and forming a fist
Grimace	G	Cry face or frown
Sucking	K	Infant sucks on one's own hands, fingers, swabs, or pacifier (although coders cannot see the baby's face, it is assumed that the baby is sucking)
Unknown	D	It is not known whether the eyes are open or closed because the coder cannot see the baby's eyes for the whole epoch.
Eyes closed	C	Eyes are closed during all 10 seconds or at any time during the epoch that the baby's eyes can be seen.
Eyes open	O	Eyes are open at any time during the 10 seconds.
Fussing or crying	F	Intermittent fussy or sustained vocal sound of distress

From Liaw, J., Yang, L., Chang, L., Chou, H., & Chao, S. (2009). Improving neonatal caregiving through a developmentally supportive care training program. *Applied Nursing Research, 22*(2), 88.   *Continued*

RESEARCH EXAMPLE—cont'd

"Validity and Reliability

The preterm infant behaviors included in this study have been studied in other reports (Becker et al., 1999; Peters, 1998). Researchers have reported that stress behaviors, such as finger splay, leg extension, and grimace, are significantly related to ongoing caregiving procedures (Peters, 1998). . . . These studies are cited as evidence to support validity of the behaviors included in this study. . . . Selected nurse caregiving behaviors are based on the concepts and principles of DSC from the literature (Als, 1999; Als et al., 2003; Becker et al., 1999). Moreover, these behaviors have also been tested in other studies and could refer to behaviors that have been found to be key components of DSC. Some negative nursing behaviors, such as inappropriate position and exposure to light, which often occurred during real bathing procedures, were also included.

Interrater reliability was examined by two observers through video observations and coding. Thirty tapes were randomly selected and scored. Pearson correlation coefficients were used to calculate interrater reliability between the observers' scores. Correlation coefficients of the infant behavioral coding scheme between two observers ranged from 0.82 to 0.99, and correlation coefficients of the nursing behavior coding scheme between the other two scorers were from 0.91 to 0.98." (Liaw et al., 2009, pp. 88-89)

Critical Appraisal

Liaw and co-workers (2009) provided an excellent description of the observations to be recorded and the process for recoding them by the observers. The coding and recoding processes were very structured to improve the validity and reliability of the observations made in the study. They provided two tables that documented the behaviors observed and the codes used when reviewing the videotapes of the infants and nurses (see Table 10-4 for the infant behaviors and codes). The behaviors selected for coding were based on previous research, which strengthens the validity of the observation measures for infant and nurse. The study included two observers coding the preterm infant behaviors from a video, and they had very strong interrater reliability (0.82 to 0.99). The interrater reliability for the two observers for the nurse behaviors was also very strong, with coefficients ranging from 0.91 to 0.98. In summary, Liaw and colleagues (2009) provided a quality description of the highly valid and reliable observation methods used in their study.

Implications for Practice

Liaw and associates (2009) found that the infants were less stressed and the nurses were more supportive following their DSC training. The researchers identified the following implications for practice:

"Preterm infants need gentle and sensitive care to support the healthy development of their body systems, especially the brain. To significantly improve nurses' caregiving skills, they need to initially receive DSC training and to repeat the training at regular intervals—about twice a year." (Liaw et al., 2009, p. 91)

The researchers also recommended that additional studies be conducted to extend the DSC- type training to other nursing caregiving activities for neonates. QSEN (2013) implications are that critically appraising studies promotes EBP and the delivery of safe, patient-centered care to neonates.

Interviews

An interview involves verbal communication between the researcher and subject, during which information is provided to the researcher. Although this data collection strategy is most commonly used in qualitative and descriptive studies, it also can be used in other types of quantitative studies. You can use a variety of approaches to conduct an interview, ranging from a totally unstructured interview (see Chapter 3), in which the content is controlled by the study participant, to a structured interview, in which the content is similar to that of a questionnaire, with the possible responses to questions carefully designed by the researcher (Creswell, 2014; Waltz et al., 2010). During structured interviews, researchers use strategies to control the content of the interview. Usually, researchers ask specific questions and enter the participant's responses onto a rating scale or paper and pencil instrument during the interview. For example, researchers could use an in-person or telephone interview to obtain responses to an instrument. Researchers might also enter responses into an electronic database.

Because nurses frequently use interviewing techniques in nursing assessment, the dynamics of interviewing are familiar. However, using the technique for measurement in research requires greater sophistication and needs to be discussed in the study's methods section. The response rate for interviews is higher than for questionnaires, which usually allows a more representative sample to be obtained. Interviewing also allows collection of data from participants who are unable or unlikely to complete questionnaires, such as those who are very ill or may have limited ability to read, write, and express themselves. Interviews are a form of self-report, and it must be assumed that the information provided is accurate. Because of time and cost, sample size is usually limited. Participant bias is always a threat to the validity of the findings, as is inconsistency in data collection from one subject to another (Waltz et al., 2010).

CRITICAL APPRAISAL GUIDELINES
Structured Interviews

When critically appraising interviews conducted in studies, you need to consider the following questions:
1. For structured interviews, what guided the interview process?
2. Are the interview questions relevant for the research purpose?
3. Does the design indicate the process for conducting the interviews?
4. If multiple interviewers are used to gather data, how were these individuals trained, and what consistency was achieved for the interview process?
5. Do the questions tend to bias subjects' responses?

RESEARCH EXAMPLE
Structured Interview

Research Excerpt

Dickson, Buck, and Riegel (2013) used a structured interview format to determine the comorbid conditions of a sample of patients with heart failure (HF). The focus of the study was to examine how multiple comorbid conditions challenge HF patients' self-care. The following excerpt describes the structured interview process used in this study.

"The interview format of the Charlson Comorbidity Index (CCI) was used to gather data about comorbid conditions (Charlson, Pompei, Ales, & MacKenzie, 1987). Participants were asked about preexisting diseases (e.g., diabetes), most of which are scored with 1 point, although some (e.g., cirrhosis) are assigned >1 point. Scores on the CCI can range from 0 to 34, with each study participant having a score ≥ 1 because of the HF. Responses were summed, weighted, and indexed into one of three categories: 0-1 = *low*, 2-3 = *moderate*, and ≥ 4 = *high*, according to the published methods....The ability of the CCI to predict mortality, complications, acute care resource use, length of hospital stay, discharge disposition, and cost (Charlson et al., 1987) provide evidence for the criterion-related validity." (Dickson et al., 2013, p. 4)

Critical Appraisal

Dickson and co-workers (2013) clearly identified the CCI as the structure for their interviews with HF patients. The interview process seemed to be consistently implemented and produced a score for each HF patient, who was then assigned to a low, moderate, or high category for comorbid conditions. The CCI had criterion-related validity and

Continued

included nonbiased questions. In summary, Dickson and colleagues (2013) implemented a reliable structured interview using the CCI, a valid and unbiased index, to address the purpose of their study.

Implications for Practice

Dickson et al. (2013) found that multiple comorbid conditions decreased HF patients' self-efficacy, which reduced the patients' ability to provide self-care. The researchers stressed the importance of delivering self-care education that integrated the patients' comorbid conditions. In addition, studies are needed to develop and test interventions that foster self-efficacy and focus on self-care for patients across multiple chronic conditions. QSEN implications are that these evidence-based findings have the potential to improve the care and outcomes for patients with HF (QSEN, 2013).

Questionnaires

A questionnaire is a self-report form designed to elicit information through written, verbal, or electronic responses of the subject. Questionnaires may be printed and distributed in person or mailed, available on a computer, or accessed online. Questionnaires are sometimes referred to as surveys, and a study using a questionnaire may be referred to as survey research. The information obtained from questionnaires is similar to that obtained by an interview, but the questions tend to have less depth. The subject is not permitted to elaborate on responses or ask for clarification of questions, and the data collector cannot use probing strategies. However, questions are presented in a consistent manner to each subject, and opportunity for bias is less than in an interview.

Questionnaires often are used in descriptive studies to gather a broad spectrum of information from subjects, such as facts about the subject or facts about persons, events, or situations known by the subject. It is also used to gather information about beliefs, attitudes, opinions, knowledge, or intentions of the subjects. Questionnaires are often developed for a particular study to enable researchers to gather data from a selected population in a new area of study. Like interviews, questionnaires can have various structures. Some questionnaires have open-ended questions, which require written responses (qualitative data) from the subject. Other questionnaires have closed-ended questions, which have limited options from which participants can select their answers.

Although you can distribute questionnaires to very large samples face to face, through the mail, or via the Internet, the response rate for questionnaires generally is lower than that for other forms of self-report, particularly if the questionnaires are mailed. If the response rate is lower than 50%, the representativeness of the sample is seriously in question. The response rate for mailed questionnaires is usually small (25% to 40%), so researchers frequently are unable to obtain a representative sample, even with random sampling methods. Questionnaires distributed via the Internet are more convenient for subjects, which may result in a higher response rate than questionnaires that are mailed. Many researchers are choosing the Internet format if they have access to the potential subjects' e-mail addresses (Grove et al., 2013; Waltz et al., 2010).

Respondents commonly fail to mark responses to all the questions, especially on long questionnaires. The incomplete nature of the data can threaten the validity of the instrument. Thus it is important for researchers to describe how missing data were managed in their study report. With most questionnaires, researchers analyze data at the level of individual items, rather than adding the items together and analyzing the total scores. Responses to items are usually measured at the nominal or ordinal level.

CRITICAL APPRAISAL GUIDELINES

Questionnaires

When critically appraising a questionnaire in a published study, consider the following questions:

1. Does the questionnaire address the focus of the study outlined in the study purpose and/or objective, questions, or hypotheses? Examine the description of the contents of the questionnaire in the measurement section of the study.
2. Does the study provide information on content-related validity for the questionnaire?
3. Was the questionnaire implemented consistently from one subject to another?

RESEARCH EXAMPLE

Questionnaires

Research Excerpt

Lucas, Anderson, and Hill (2012) conducted a study to determine the knowledge of elementary school teachers concerning the care of children with asthma. They developed a questionnaire to gather their study data, described in the following excerpt:

"After reviewing numerous existing instruments measuring asthma knowledge, the first author determined that there was not a single tool that adequately assessed each aspect of asthma. Therefore, a two-part questionnaire was developed for this study by the first author. Part 1 of the Basic Facts About Asthma Questionnaire (Box 10-1) was developed to assess the teacher's knowledge of asthma.... The content for the questionnaire was based on the literature. This tool is a self-administered questionnaire consisting of 25 questions, 14 true-false questions, and 11 multiple-choice questions. The questionnaire comprised 7 questions that focused on signs and symptoms, 6 questions that focused on general asthma knowledge, 5 items that focused on treatment management, 32 questions that focused on asthma triggers, and 4 questions regarding knowledge of medication administration. Each question was allowed one point for each correct answer....The higher the total score, the greater the knowledge level of the participant.

BOX 10-1 BASIC FACTS ABOUT ASTHMA QUESTIONNAIRE (EXAMPLE)

Part 1

Directions: This survey is a combination of true-false and multiple-choice questions. Please circle the best answer for each question.

1. Asthma is a disease characterized by:
   a. Inflamed airways
   b. Chronic airway obstruction
   c. Increased mucus production within the airways
   d. Hyperresponsive or sensitive airways
   e. All of the above
   f. None of the above
2. Which symptom(s) are indicative of a child experiencing a severe asthma attack?
   a. Inability to talk in sentences or walk
   b. Excessively rapid and shallow breathing
   c. Restlessness
   d. Preoccupation with breathing
   e. All of the above
   f. a, b, and d

Continued

RESEARCH EXAMPLE—cont'd

3. Which of the following is most likely to cause an asthma attack in a child with asthma?
   a. Too much medication that morning
   b. Not getting enough sleep the night before
   c. Extreme changes in humidity or temperature
   d. Too much caffeine or sugar in their diet
   e. All of the above
   f. None of the above
4. What are the most common symptoms associated with asthma?
   a. Coughing
   b. Wheezing
   c. Ear aches
   d. Shortness of breath
   e. All of the above
   f. a, b, and d

From Lucas, T., Anderson, M. A., & Hill, P. D. (2012). What level of knowledge do elementary school teachers possess concerning the care of children with asthma? A pilot study. *Journal of Pediatric Nursing, 27*(5), 524.

Part 2 of the questionnaire consisted of eight multiple-choice questions that queried the teachers regarding years of experience, level of education, teaching specialty, and prior training on chronic illness.... Content validity of the evidence-based questionnaire was accomplished by an expert in the field, namely a pediatric pulmonologist, who reviewed the questionnaire assessing for adequate coverage of content focusing on general asthma knowledge. Test-retest reliability was accomplished by administering the questionnaire to a group of elementary teachers, not involved in this project, on two separate occasions and comparing the results. The percentage of agreement for 25-item test and three elementary teachers was 90.7%." (Lucas et al., 2012, p. 524)

Critical Appraisal

Lucas and associates (2012) documented the need to develop a questionnaire to gather their study data. The items of the Basic Facts About Asthma Questionnaire were based on current literature, with examples of these items provided in the research report (see Box 10-1). The questionnaire items focused on determining elementary school teachers' knowledge about the care of children with asthma, which addressed the purpose of the study. The researchers documented the content validity of the questionnaire that was achieved by an expert review and evidence obtained from the literature review. The test-retest reliability of the questionnaire was also strong (90.7%), supporting this questionnaire as a reliable and valid measurement method for this study.

Implications for Practice

Lucas and co-workers (2012) found that the elementary school teachers had a knowledge deficit regarding the care of children with asthma. Teachers with exposure and/or experience with asthma scored significantly higher than those with limited exposure. The QSEN implications are that these research findings support the need for additional education of teachers and school personnel to assist them in providing safe, evidence-based care to children with asthma in the classroom (QSEN, 2013).

Scales

The scale, a form of self-report, is a more precise means of measuring phenomena than a questionnaire. Most scales are developed to measure psychosocial variables, but researchers also use scaling techniques to obtain self-reports on physiological variables such as pain, nausea, or functional capacity. The various items on most scales are summed to obtain a single score. These are termed *summated scales*. Fewer random and systematic errors occur when the total score of a scale is used (Nunnally & Bernstein, 1994). The various items in a scale increase the dimensions of the concept that are measured by the instrument. The three types of scales described in this section that are commonly used in nursing research are rating scales, Likert scales, and visual analog scales.

Rating Scales

Rating scales are the crudest form of measurement involving scaling techniques. A rating scale lists an ordered series of categories of a variable that are assumed to be based on an underlying continuum. A numerical value is assigned to each category, and the fineness of the distinctions between categories varies with the scale. Rating scales are commonly used by the general public. In conversations, one can hear statements such as "On a scale of 1 to 10, I would rank that. . . ." Rating scales are fairly easy to develop, but researchers need to be careful to avoid end statements that are so extreme that no subject will select them. You can use a rating scale to rate the degree of cooperativeness of the patient or the value placed by the subject on nurse-patient interactions. Rating scales are also used in observational measurement to guide data collection.

Some rating scales are more valid than others because they were constructed in a structured way and used in a variety of studies with different populations. For example, the FACES Pain Scale is a commonly used rating scale to assess the pain of children in clinical practice and has proven to be valid and reliable over the years (Figure 10-4). Nurses often assess pain in adults with a numeric rating scale (NRS) similar to the one in Figure 10-5. Using the NRS is more valid and reliable than asking a patient to rate her or his pain on a scale from 1 to 10.

Likert Scale

The Likert scale is designed to determine the opinions or attitudes of study subjects. This scale contains a number of declarative statements, with a scale after each statement. The Likert scale is the most commonly used of the scaling techniques. The original version of the scale included five response

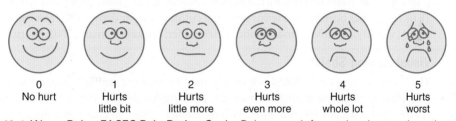

0	1	2	3	4	5
No hurt	Hurts little bit	Hurts little more	Hurts even more	Hurts whole lot	Hurts worst

FIG 10-4 Wong-Baker FACES Pain Rating Scale. Point to each face using the words to describe the pain intensity. Ask the child to choose the face that best describes the child's own pain and record the appropriate number. *(From Hockenberry, M.J., & Wilson, D. [2013]. Wong's essentials of pediatric nursing [9th ed., p. 148]. St. Louis, MO: Mosby.)*

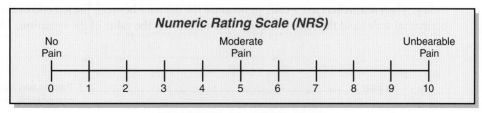

FIG 10-5 Numeric Rating Scale.

categories. Each response category was assigned a value, with a value of 0 or 1 given to the most negative response and a value of 4 or 5 given to the most positive response (Kerlinger & Lee, 2000; Nunnally & Bernstein, 1994). Response choices in a Likert scale usually address agreement, evaluation, or frequency. Agreement options may include statements such as *strongly disagree, disagree, uncertain, agree, and strongly agree.* Evaluation responses ask the respondent for an evaluative rating along a bad-good dimension, such as negative to positive or terrible to excellent. Frequency responses may include statements such as *never, rarely, sometimes, frequently,* and *all the time.* The terms used are versatile and are selected based on the content of the questions or items in the scale. For example, an item such as "Describe the nursing care you received during your hospitalization" could have a response scale of *unsatisfactory, below average, average, above average,* and *excellent.*

Sometimes seven options are given on a response scale, sometimes only four. When the response scale has an odd number of options, the middle option is usually an uncertain or neutral category. Using a response scale with an odd number of options is controversial because it allows the subject to avoid making a clear choice of positive or negative statements. To avoid this, researchers may choose to provide only four or six options, with no middle point or uncertain category. This type of scale is referred to as a *forced choice version* (Nunnally & Bernstein, 1994).

A Likert scale usually consists of 10 to 20 items, each addressing an element of the concept being measured. Usually, the values obtained from each item in the instrument are summed to obtain a single score for each subject. Although the values of each item are technically ordinal-level data, the summed score is often analyzed as interval-level data. The CES-D is a Likert scale used to assess the level of depression in patients in clinical practice and research (see Figure 10-3). Whittenmore and colleagues (2009) used the CES-D in their study (see earlier). This scale has four response options—*Rarely or none of the time (less than 1 day)* = 0, *Some or a little of the time (1 to 2 days)* = 1, *Occasionally or a moderate amount of time (3 to 4 days)* = 2, and *Most or all of the time (5 to 7 days)* = 3. Subjects are instructed on the scale: "Below is a list of the ways you might have felt or behaved. Please tell me how often you have felt this way during the past week" (see Figure 10-3; Radloff, 1977). The scores on the scale can range from 0 to 60, with the higher scores indicating more depressive symptoms. A score of 16 or higher has been used extensively as the cutoff point for depression. The scale has strong reliability, validity, sensitivity, and specificity (see earlier; Locke & Putnam, 2002; Sharp & Lipsky, 2002).

Visual Analog Scales

The visual analog scale (VAS) is typically used to measure strength, magnitude, or intensity of individuals' subjective feelings, sensations, or attitudes about symptoms or situations. The VAS is a line that is usually 100 mm long, with right angle "stops" at either end. Researchers can present the line horizontally or vertically, with bipolar anchors or descriptors beyond either end of the line (Waltz et al., 2010). These end anchors must include the entire range of sensations possible for the phenomenon being measured (e.g., all and none, best and worst, no pain, and most severe pain possible). An example of a VAS for measuring pain is presented in Figure 10-6.

Subjects are asked to place a mark through the line to indicate the intensity of the sensation or feeling. Then researchers use a ruler to measure the distance between the left end of the line (on a horizontal scale) and the subject's mark. This measure is the value of the sensation. The VAS has

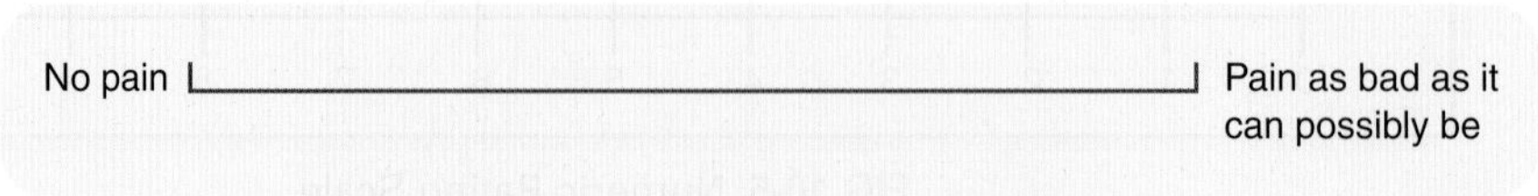

No pain |_____| Pain as bad as it can possibly be

FIG 10-6 Example of a visual analog scale.

been used to measure pain, mood, anxiety, alertness, craving for cigarettes, quality of sleep, attitudes toward environmental conditions, functional abilities, and severity of clinical symptoms.

The reliability of the VAS is usually determined by the test-retest method. The correlations between the two administrations of the scale need to be moderate or strong to support the reliability of the scale (Wewers & Lowe, 1990). Because these scales are used to measure phenomena that are dynamic or erratic over time, test-retest reliability is sometimes not appropriate, and the low correlation is then caused by the change in sensation versus a problem with the scale. Because the VAS contains a single item, other methods of determining reliability such as homogeneity cannot be used. The validity of the VAS is usually determined by correlating the VAS scores with other measures, such as rating or Likert scales, that measure the same phenomenon, such as pain (Waltz et al., 2010).

CRITICAL APPRAISAL GUIDELINES

Scales

When critically appraising a rating scale, Likert scale, or VAS in a study, ask the following questions:
1. Is the rating scale, Likert scale, or VAS clearly described in the research report?
2. Are the techniques used to administer and score the scale provided?
3. Is information about validity and reliability of the scale described from previous studies and for this study?

RESEARCH EXAMPLE

Scales

Research Excerpt

Brenner and associates (2013) conducted a randomized controlled trial (RCT) to determine the effectiveness of a topical anesthetic applied 15 minutes before venipuncture on children's perception of pain and anxiety. The study included 120 children ages 5 to 18 years who were randomly assigned to the liposomal 4% lidocaine or placebo cream groups. The scales included in this study were critically appraised using the questions in the critical appraisal guidelines (see earlier).

"Participant anxiety was measured by the study participant and the objective observer before (anticipatory), during (venipuncture), and after (recovery) venipuncture using a validated visual analog (VAS) with a range of 0 to 100, with the higher scores indicating higher anxiety levels.... The VAS is usually a 100-mm-long scale that measures the extremes of a patient experience or subjective phenomena. Research has shown that lines shorter than 100 mm tend to produce greater error variance. When the VAS is used appropriately, it is a valid, reliable, and sensitive tool for studying subjective phenomena..... Pain was measured immediately after the venipuncture by the study participant using the 6-point validated FACES pain scale, which has been validated in patients aged 5 to 18 years, with the higher scores indicating higher pain levels. For analysis, we used a mean FACES score." (Brenner et al., 2013, p. 22)

Critical Appraisal

Brenner and co-workers (2013) clearly identified that they used a six-point FACES scale, as shown in Figure 10-4, to measure pain and a VAS, similar to Figure 10-5, to measure anxiety. The researchers stressed the importance of the VAS being 100 mm long to decrease the potential for error. They also indicated that the VAS was a valid, reliable, and sensitive tool for measuring anxiety in this study. However, the discussion of these scales would have been stronger if specific reliability and validity information about the VAS and FACES scales had been provided from previous research. In addition, the researchers did not conduct interrater reliability testing between raters in this study to ensure that the VAS was consistently used in measuring the children's anxiety.

Continued

> **⬧ RESEARCH EXAMPLE—cont'd**
>
> **Implications for Practice**
> Brenner and colleagues (2013) found no significant differences between the experimental group receiving liposomal 4% lidocaine and the group receiving the placebo cream for pain or anxiety during venipuncture. The researchers thought that the varying ages of the children and their previous experiences with venipuncture might have affected the study outcomes. They did confirm that anxiety negatively affected the children's perception of pain and requires additional research to manage both these perceptions.

DATA COLLECTION PROCESS

Data collection is the process of acquiring subjects and collecting the data for a study. The actual steps of collecting the data are specific to each study and depend on the research design and measurement techniques. During the data collection process, researchers initially train the data collectors, recruit study participants, implement the study intervention (if applicable), collect data in a consistent way, and protect the integrity (or validity) of the study.

Researchers need to describe their data collection process clearly in their research report. Often, the data collection process is addressed in the methods section of the report in a subsection entitled "Procedure." The strategies used to approach potential subjects who meet the sampling criteria need to be described (see Chapter 9). Researchers should also specify the number and characteristics of subjects who decline to participate in the study. If the study includes an intervention, the details about the intervention and how it was implemented should be described (see Chapter 8). The approaches used to perform measurements and the time and setting for the measurements are also described. The desired result is a step by step description of exactly how, where, and in what sequence the researchers collected the study data. The following sections discuss some of the common data collections tasks described in research reports, such as recruitment of study participants, consistency of data collection, and control in implementing the study design. Nurse researchers are also conducting studies using data from existing databases, and it is important to critically appraise data obtained from these databases.

Recruitment of Study Participants

The research report needs to describe the study participant recruitment process. Study participants or subjects may be recruited only at the initiation of data collection or throughout the data collection period. The design of the study determines the method of selecting the participants. Recruiting the number of subjects originally planned is critical because data analysis and interpretation of findings depend on having an adequate sample size.

Consistency in Data Collection

The key to accurate data collection in any study is consistency. Consistency involves maintaining the data collection pattern for each collection event as it was developed in the research plan. A good plan will facilitate consistency and maintain the validity of the study. Researchers should note deviations, even if they are minor, and report their impact on the interpretation of the findings in their final study report. If a study uses data collectors, researchers need to report the training process and the interrater reliability achieved during training and data collection.

Control in the Study Design

Researchers build controls into their study plan to minimize the influence of intervening forces on the findings. Control is very important in quasi-experimental and experimental studies to ensure that the intervention is consistently implemented (Shadish, Cook, & Campbell, 2002). The research report needs to reflect the controls implemented in a study and any problems that needed to be managed during the study. In addition to maintaining the controls identified in the plan, researchers continually look for previously unidentified, extraneous variables that might have an impact on the data being collected. An extraneous variable often is specific to a study and tends to become apparent during the data collection period and needs to be discussed in the research report. For example, Lu and associates (2013) examined the effects of acupressure on sleep quality and controlled the environment in which the intervention was implemented to decrease the effects of any extraneous variables, such as noise, temperature, or lighting that might influence the study findings. The subjects did not receive sleeping medications during this study to prevent the influence of this extraneous variable. Researchers need to consider the extraneous variables identified during data collection, data analysis, and interpretation. They should also note these variables in the research report so that future researchers can be aware of and attempt to control them.

Studies Obtaining Data from Existing Databases

Nurse researchers are increasing their use of existing databases to address the research problems they have identified as being essential for generating evidence for practice. The reasons for using these databases in studies are varied. With the computerization of healthcare information, more databases have been developed internationally, nationally, regionally, at the state level, and within clinical agencies. These databases include large amounts of information that have relevance in developing research evidence needed for practice (Brown, 2014; Melnyk & Fineout-Overholt, 2011). The costs and technology for storage of data have improved over the last 10 years, making these databases more reliable and accessible. Using existing databases makes it possible to conduct complex analyses to expand our understanding of healthcare outcomes (Doran, 2011). Another reason is that the primary collection of data in a study is limited by the availability of research participants and expense of the data collection process. By using existing databases, researchers are able to have larger samples, conduct more longitudinal studies, have lower costs during the data collection process, and limit the burdens placed on the study participants (Johantgen, 2010).

The existing healthcare data consist of two types, secondary and administrative. Data collected for a particular study are considered primary data. Data collected from previous research and stored in a database are considered secondary data when used by other researchers to address their study purposes. Because these data were collected as part of research, details can be obtained about the data collection and storage processes. In the methodology section of their research report, researchers usually clearly indicate when secondary data analyses were conducted as part of their study (Johantgen, 2010).

Data collected for reasons other than research are considered administrative data. Administrative data are collected within clinical agencies, obtained by national, state, and local professional organizations, and collected by federal, state, and local agencies. The processes for collection and storage of administrative data are more complex and often more unclear than the data collection process for research (Johantgen, 2010). The data in administrative databases are collected by different people in different sites using different methods. However, the data elements collected for most administrative databases include demographics, organizational characteristics, clinical diagnosis and treatment, and geographic information. These database elements were standardized by the Health Insurance Portability and Accountability Act (HIPAA) of 1996, which improved the quality of the databases (see Chapter 4).

When secondary data and administrative data from existing databases are used in a study, they need to be critically appraised to determine the quality of the study findings. The type of database used in a study needs to be clearly described. The data in the database needs to address the researchers' study purpose and their objectives, questions, or hypotheses. The validity and reliability of the data in the existing database need to be described in the research report.

CRITICAL APPRAISAL GUIDELINES

Data Collection

When critically appraising the data collection process, consider the following questions:
1. Were the recruitment and selection of study participants or subjects clearly described and appropriate?
2. Were the data collected in a consistent way?
3. Were the study controls maintained as indicated by the design? Did the design include an intervention that was consistently implemented?
4. Was the integrity of the study protected, and how were any problems resolved?
5. Did the researchers obtain data from an existing database? If so, did the data obtained address the study problem and objectives, questions, or hypotheses? Were the reliability and validity of the database addressed in the research report?

RESEARCH EXAMPLE

Data Collection

Research Excerpt

Whittenmore and associates (2009) developed a study to determine the effectiveness of a Diabetes Prevention Program (DPP) delivered by NPs in primary care settings to adults who were at risk for type 2 diabetes (T2D). This study was discussed earlier, and the measurement methods were described. The data collection process for this study is presented in the following excerpt.

"Procedure

The NPs recruited a convenience sample of 58 adults at risk of T2D from their practices (31 treatment and 27 control group participants). The sample size for this pilot study was determined by a power analysis, recruiting 20% of what would be necessary for a clinical trial testing the intervention.

Intervention
Enhanced Standard Care

After informed consent was obtained and baseline data were collected, all participants (regardless of group assignment) received culturally relevant written information about diabetes prevention, a 20- to 30-minute individual session with their NP on the importance of a healthy lifestyle for the prevention of T2D, and a 45-minute individual session with a nutritionist hired for the study.

Lifestyle Change Program

The lifestyle change program for this pilot study was based on the protocol for the DPP (Diabetes Prevention Research Group, 1999). The goals for this program were identical to enhanced standard care, yet the approach was more intensive and based on behavioral science evidence which recognizes the difficulty inherent in diet and exercise lifestyle change.

Outcome Measures

Data were collected at the individual (participant) and organization (NP and site) levels at scheduled time points throughout the study to evaluate the reach, implementation, and preliminary efficacy of the lifestyle program. All data were collected by trained research assistants blinded to group assignment, with exception of the GTT [glucose tolerance test]. . . . and lipids, which were collected by experienced laboratory personnel at each site and sent to one laboratory for analysis.

Reach

Recruitment rates were documented for each NP practice. Demographic and clinical data (e.g., age, gender, socioeconomic status, ethnicity, and health history) were collected using a standard form.

Implementation

Participant measures of implementation consisted of attendance, attrition, and a satisfaction survey. The satisfaction survey was a 7-item summated scale modified from the Diabetes Treatment Satisfaction Survey to evaluate a DPP.... Adequate internal consistency has been reported with the original scale ($\alpha = .82$) and was demonstrated with the modified scale in this study ($\alpha = .86$).

Organizational measures of implementation consisted of NP and nutrition session documentation forms, which were created with components of each session itemized. The percentage of protocol implementation was calculated by dividing the number of protocol items by the number of items completed per session. The NPs were also interviewed at 3 and 6 months to address issues of implementation.

Data Analysis

Data were entered into databases (Microsoft Access or Excel) via an automated Teleform (Cardiff, Vista, CA) system. Mean substitution was employed for missing data of individual items on instruments (up to 15%). If more than 15% of the items were missing (rare), the subscale or scale was coded as missing data." (Whittenmore et al., 2009, p. 4-6)

Critical Appraisal

As can be seen in this study excerpt, Whittenmore and co-workers (2009) took careful steps to maintain the rigor and control of their data collection by implementing a detailed plan. The recruit process, recruitment rates, selection of study participants, and informed consent process were described and appropriate. The sample size was adequate for a pilot study based on a power analysis. The researchers clearly described their implementation of the lifestyle change program intervention to the experimental group and of standard care to both groups. The design included scheduled pretests and post-tests, and the outcome measures were collected by trained research assistants using a structured protocol. The percentage of protocol implemented was also calculated, ensuring the quality of the data collection process. The reliability values of the scales used were strong but the researchers might have expanded on the description of the scales' validity. The physiological measures were precise and accurate. The researchers indicated how the data were entered into the computer to promote accuracy and the actions that were taken for consistent management of missing data. In summary, Whittenmore and colleagues (2009) provided a detailed description of their data collection process that was extremely strong. Their highly structured data collection plan and process of implementation decreased the potential for error and increased the likelihood that the study findings were an accurate reflection of reality.

Implications for Practice

The implications of this study's findings for practice were discussed earlier in this chapter.

KEY CONCEPTS

- The purpose of measurement is to produce trustworthy data or evidence that can be used in examining the outcomes of research.
- The rules of measurement ensure that the assignment of values or categories is performed consistently from one subject (or event) to another and, eventually, if the measurement strategy is found to be meaningful, from one study to another.
- The levels of measurement from low to high are nominal, ordinal, interval, and ratio.

- Reliability in measurement is concerned with the consistency of the measurement technique; reliability testing focuses on equivalence, stability, and homogeneity.
- The validity of an instrument is a determination of the extent to which the instrument reflects the abstract concept being examined. Construct validity includes content-related validity and evidence of validity from examining contrasting groups, convergence, and divergence.
- Readability level focuses on the study participants' ability to read and comprehend the content of an instrument, which adds to the reliability and validity of the instrument.
- Physiological measures are examined for precision, accuracy, and error in research reports.
- Diagnostic and screening tests are examined for sensitivity, specificity, and likelihood ratios.
- Common measurement approaches used in nursing research include physiological measures, observation, interviews, questionnaires, and scales.
- The scales discussed in this chapter include rating scales, Likert scales, and visual analog scales.
- Researchers are using existing databases when conducting their studies, and the quality of these databases need to be addressed in the research report.
- The data collection tasks that need to be critically appraised in a study include (1) recruit of study participants, (2) consistent collection of data, and (3) maintenance of controls in the study design.
- It is important to critically appraise the measurement methods and data collection process of a published study for threats to validity.

REFERENCES

Als, H. (1999). Reading the premature infant. In E. Goldson (Ed.), *Nurturing the premature infant: Developmental interventions in neonatal intensive care nursery* (pp. 18–85). New York: Oxford University Press.

Als, H., Gilkerson, L., Duffy, F. H., McAnulty, G. B., Buehler, D. M., Vandenberg, K., et al. (2003). A three-center, randomized, controlled trial of individualized developmental care for very low birth weight preterm infants: Medical neurodevelopmental, parenting and caregiving effects. *Journal of Developmental and Behavioral Pediatrics, 24*(6), 399–408.

Becker, P. T., Grunwald, P. C., & Brazy, J. E. (1999). Motor organization in very low birth weight infants during caregiving: Effects of a developmental intervention. *Journal of Developmental and Behavioral Pediatrics, 20* (5), 344–354.

Bialocerkowski, A., Klupp, N., & Bragge, P. (2010). Research methodology series: How to read and critically appraise a reliability article. *International Journal of Therapy and Rehabilitation, 17* (3), 114–120.

Brenner, S. M., Rupp, V., Boucher, J., Weaver, K., Dusza, S. W., & Bokovoy, J. (2013). A randomized, controlled trial to evaluate topical anesthetic for 15 minutes before venipuncture in pediatrics. *American Journal of Emergency Medicine, 31*(1), 20–25.

Brown, S. J. (2014). *Evidence-based nursing: The research-practice connection* (3rd ed.). Sudbury, MA: Jones & Bartlett.

Buysse, D. L., Reynolds, C. F., 3rd., Monk, T. H., Berman, S. R., & Kupfer, D. J. (1989). The Pittsburgh Sleep Quality Index: A new instrument for psychiatric practice and research. *Psychiatry Research, 28*(2), 193–213.

Campo, M., Shiyko, M. P., & Lichtman, S. W. (2010). Sensitivity and specificity: A review of related statistics and controversies in the context of physical therapist education. *Journal of Physical Therapy Education, 24*(3), 69–78.

Charlson, M. E., Pompei, P., Ales, K. L., & MacKenzie, C. R. (1987). A new method of classifying prognostic comorbidity in longitudinal studies: Development and validation. *Journal of Chronic Diseases, 40*(5), 373–383.

Craig, J., & Smyth, R. (2012). *The evidence-based practice manual for nurses* (3rd ed.). Edinburgh: Churchill Livingstone Elsevier.

Creswell, J. W. (2014). *Research design: Qualitative, quantitative and mixed methods approaches* (4th ed.). Thousand Oaks, CA: Sage.

DeVon, H. A., Block, M. E., Moyle-Wright, P., Ernst, D. M., Hayden, S. J., Lazzara, D. J., et al. (2007). A psychometric toolbox for testing validity and reliability. *Journal of Nursing Scholarship, 39*(2), 155–164.

Diabetes Prevention Research Group. (1999). Design and methods for a clinical trial in the prevention of type 2 diabetes. *Diabetes Care, 22*(4), 623–634.

Dickson, V. V., Buck, H., & Riegel, B. (2013). Multiple comorbid conditions challenge heart failure self-care by decreasing self-efficacy. *Nursing Research, 62*(1), 2–9.

Doran, D. M. (2011). *Nursing outcomes: The state of the science* (2nd ed.). Sudbury, MA: Jones & Bartlett.

Fawcett, J., & Garity, J. (2009). *Evaluating research for evidence-based nursing practice.* Philadelphia: F. A. Davis.

Gift, A. G., & Soeken, K. L. (1988). Assessment of physiologic instruments. *Heart & Lung, 17*(2), 128–133.

Grove, S. K. (2007). *Statistics for health care research: A practical workbook.* Philadelphia: Elsevier Saunders.

Grove, S. K., Burns, N., & Gray, J. R. (2013). *The practice of nursing research: Appraisal, synthesis, and generation of evidence* (7th ed.). St. Louis: Elsevier Saunders.

Jefferson, V. W., Melkus, G. D., & Spollett, G. R. (2000). Health promotion practices of young black women at risk for diabetes. *Diabetes Educator, 26*(2), 295–302.

Johantgen, M. (2010). Using existing administrative and national databases. In C. F. Waltz, O. L. Strickland, & E. R. Lenz (Eds.), *Measurement in nursing and health research* (pp. 241–250) (4th ed.). New York: Springer.

Kaplan, A. (1963). *The conduct of inquiry: Methodology for behavioral science.* New York: Harper & Row.

Kerlinger, F. N., & Lee, H. B. (2000). *Foundations of behavioral research* (4th ed.). Fort Worth, TX: Harcourt.

Klein, S., Allison, D. B., Heymsfield, S. B., Kelley, D. E., Leibel, R. L., Nonas, C., et al. (2007). Waist circumference and cardiometabolic risk: A consensus statement from Shaping America's Health: Association for Weight Management and Obesity Prevention; NAASO, The Obesity Society; the American Society for Nutrition and the American Diabetes Association. *Obesity, 15*(5), 1061–1067.

Liaw, J., Yang, L., Chang, L., Chou, H., & Chao, S. (2009). Improving neonatal caregiving through a developmentally supportive care training program. *Applied Nursing Research, 22*(2), 86–93.

Locke, B. Z., & Putnam, P. (2002). *Center for Epidemiologic Studies Depression Scale (CES-D Scale).* Bethesda, MD: National Institute of Mental Health.

Lu, M., Lin, S., Chen, K., Tsang, H., & Su, S. (2013). Acupressure improves sleep quality of psychogeriatric inpatients. *Nursing Research, 62*(2), 130–137.

Lucas, T., Anderson, M. A., & Hill, P. D. (2012). What level of knowledge do elementary school teachers possess concerning the care of children with asthma? A pilot study. *Journal of Pediatric Nursing, 27*(5), 523–527.

Marshall, C., & Rossman, G. B. (2011). *Designing qualitative research* (5th ed.). Thousand Oaks, CA: Sage.

Melnyk, B. M., & Fineout-Overholt, E. (2011). *Evidence-based practice in nursing & healthcare: A guide to best practice* (2nd ed.). Philadelphia: Lippincott, Williams, & Wilkins.

Munhall, P. L. (2012). *Nursing research: A qualitative perspective* (5th ed.). Sudbury, MA: Jones & Bartlett.

Nunnally, J. C., & Bernstein, I. H. (1994). *Psychometric theory* (3rd ed.). New York: McGraw-Hill.

Peters, K. (1998). Bathing premature infants: Physiological and behavioral consequences. *American Journal of Critical Care, 7*(2), 90–100.

Posner, S. F., Stewart, A. L., Marin, G., & Perez-Stable, E. J. (2001). Factor variability of the Center for Epidemiological Studies Depression Scale (CES-D) among urban Latinos. *Ethnicity & Health, 6*(2), 137–144.

Pugh, L. C., & DeKeyser, F. G. (1995). Use of physiologic variables in nursing research. *Image—Journal of Nursing Scholarship, 27*(4), 273–276.

Quality and Safety Education for Nurses (QSEN). (2013). *Pre-licensure knowledge, skills, and attitudes (KSAs).* Retrieved July 5, 2013 from http://qsen.org/competencies/pre-licensure-ksas.

Radloff, L. S. (1977). The CES-D scale: A self report depression scale for research in the general population. *Applied Psychological Measurement, 1*, 385–394.

Rew, L., Stuppy, D., & Becker, H. (1988). Construct validity in instrument development: A vital link between nursing practice, research, and theory. *Advances in Nursing Science, 10*(4), 10–22.

Ryan-Wenger, N. A. (2010). Evaluation of measurement precision, accuracy, and error in biophysical data for clinical research and practice. In C. F. Waltz, O. L. Strickland, & E. R. Lenz (Eds.), *Measurement in nursing and health research* (pp. 371–383) (4th ed.). New York: Springer.

Sackett, D. L., Straus, S. E., Richardson, W. S., Rosenberg, W., & Haynes, R. B. (2000). *Evidence-based medicine: How to practice and teach EBM* (2nd ed.). London: Churchill Livingstone.

Sarikaya, S., Aktas, C., Ay, D., Cetin, A., & Celikmen, F. (2010). Sensitivity and specificity of rapid antigen detection testing for diagnosing pharyngitis in emergency department. *Ear, Nose, & Throat Journal, 89* (4), 180–182.

Shadish, W. R., Cook, T. D., & Campbell, D. T. (2002). *Experimental and quasi-experimental designs for generalized causal inference.* Chicago: Rand McNally.

Sharp, L. K., & Lipsky, M. S. (2002). Screening for depression across the lifespan: A review of measures for use in primacy care settings. *American Family Physician, 66*(6), 1001–1008.

Sherwood, G., & Barnsteiner, J. (2012). *Quality and safety in nursing: A competency approach to improving outcomes.* Ames, IA: Wiley-Blackwell.

Stevens, S. S. (1946). On the theory of scales of measurement. *Science, 103*(2684), 677–680.

Stone, K. S., & Frazier, S. K. (2010). Measurement of physiological variables using biomedical instrumentation. In C. F. Waltz, O. L. Strickland, & E. R. Lenz (Eds.), *Measurement in nursing and health research* (pp. 335–370) (4th ed.). New York: Springer.

Walker, S. N., Sechrist, K. R., & Pender, N. J. (1987). The Health-Promoting Lifestyle Profile: Development and psychometric characteristics. *Nursing Research, 36*(2), 76–81.

Waltz, C. F., Strickland, O. L., & Lenz, E. R. (2010). *Measurement in nursing and health research* (4th ed.). New York: Springer Publishing Company.

Wewers, M. E., & Lowe, N. K. (1990). A critical review of visual analogue scales in the measurement of clinical phenomena. *Research in Nursing & Health, 13*(4), 227–236.

Whittenmore, R., Melkus, G., Wagner, J., Dziura, J., Northrup, V., & Grey, M. (2009). Translating the diabetes prevention program to primary care: A pilot study. *Nursing Research, 58*(1), 2–12.

chapter 11

Understanding Statistics in Research

CHAPTER OVERVIEW

LEARNING OUTCOMES

After completing this chapter, you should be able to:

1. Identify the purposes of statistical analyses.
2. Describe the process of data analysis: (a) management of missing data; (b) description of the sample; (c) reliability of the measurement methods; (d) exploratory analysis of the data; and (e) use of inferential statistical analyses

guided by study objectives, questions, or hypotheses.

3. Describe probability theory and decision theory that guide statistical data analysis.

4. Describe the process of inferring from a sample to a population.

5. Discuss the distribution of the normal curve.

6. Compare and contrast type I and type II errors.

7. Identify descriptive analyses, such as frequency distributions, percentages, measures of central tendency, and measures of dispersion, conducted to describe the samples and study variables in research.

8. Describe the results obtained from the inferential statistical analyses conducted to examine relationships (Pearson product-moment correlation and factor analysis) and make predictions (linear and multiple regression analysis).

9. Describe the results obtained from inferential statistical analyses conducted to examine differences, such as chi-square analysis, *t*-test, analysis of variance, and analysis of covariance.

10. Describe the five types of results obtained from quasi-experimental and experimental studies that are interpreted within a decision theory framework: (a) significant and predicted results; (b) nonsignificant results; (c) significant and unpredicted results; (d) mixed results; and (e) unexpected results.

11. Compare and contrast statistical significance and clinical importance of results.

12. Critically appraise statistical results, findings, limitations, conclusions, generalization of findings, nursing implications, and suggestions for further research in a study.

KEY TERMS

Analysis of covariance, p. 353

Analysis of variance, p. 351

Between-group variance, p. 351

Bimodal distribution, p. 333

Bivariate correlation, p. 340

Causality, p. 347

Chi-square test of independence, p. 347

Clinical importance, p. 355

Coefficient of multiple determination, p. 345

Conclusions, p. 355

Confidence interval, p. 334

Decision theory, p. 325

Degrees of freedom, p. 329

Descriptive statistics, p. 319

Effect size, p. 329

Explained variance, p. 341

Exploratory analysis, p. 323

Factor, p. 343

Factor analysis, p. 343

Findings, p. 354

Frequency distribution, p. 330

Generalization, p. 326

Grouped frequency distributions, p. 330

Implications for nursing, p. 356

Independent groups, p. 338

Inference, p. 326

Inferential statistics, p. 319

Level of statistical significance, p. 325

Limitations, p. 355

Line of best fit, p. 344

Mean, p. 333

Measures of central tendency, p. 331

Measures of dispersion, p. 333

Median, p. 333

Mixed results, p. 354

Mode, p. 331

Multiple regression, p. 344

Negative relationship, p. 341

Nonparametric analyses, p. 338

Nonsignificant results, p. 353

Normal curve, p. 326

One-tailed test of significance, p. 327

Outliers, p. 323

Paired groups or dependent groups, p. 338

Parametric analyses, p. 338

Pearson product-moment correlation, p. 340

Percentage distribution, p. 331

Positive relationship, p. 341

Posthoc analyses, p. 347

Power, p. 329

Power analysis, p. 329

Probability theory, p. 324

Range, p. 333

Recommendations for further study, p. 356

Regression analysis, p. 344

Scatterplot, p. 335

Significant and unpredicted results, p. 354

Significant results, p. 353

Simple linear regression, p. 344

Standard deviation, p. 334

Standardized scores, p. 335

Statistical techniques, p. 319

Symmetrical, p. 341

Total variance, p. 351

The expectation that nursing practice be based on research evidence has made it important for students and clinical nurses to acquire skills in reading and evaluating the results from statistical analyses (Brown, 2014; Craig & Smyth, 2012). Nurses probably have more anxiety about data analysis and statistical results than they do about any other aspect of the research process. We hope that this chapter will dispel some of that anxiety and facilitate your critical appraisal of research reports. The statistical information in this chapter is provided from the perspective of reading, understanding, and critically appraising the results sections in quantitative studies rather than on selecting statistical procedures for data analysis or performing statistical analyses.

To appraise the results from quantitative or outcomes studies critically, you need to be able to (1) identify the statistical procedures used, (2) judge whether these procedures were appropriate for the purpose and the hypotheses, questions, or objectives of the study and level of measurement of the variables, (3) determine whether the researchers' interpretations of the results are appropriate, and (4) evaluate the clinical importance of the study's findings. This chapter was developed to provide you with a background for critically appraising the results and discussion sections of quantitative studies.

The elements of the statistical analysis process are discussed at the beginning of this chapter. Relevant theories and concepts of statistical analyses are described to provide a background for understanding the results included in research reports. Some of the common statistical procedures used to describe variables, examine relationships among variables, predict outcomes, and test causal hypotheses are introduced. Strategies are identified for determining the appropriateness of the statistical analysis techniques included in the results sections of published studies. Guidelines are provided for critically appraising the statistical results of studies. The chapter concludes with guidelines for critically appraising the following study outcomes—findings, limitations, conclusions, generalizations, implications for nursing practice, and suggestions for further study. Examples from current studies are provided throughout this chapter to promote your understanding of the content.

UNDERSTANDING THE ELEMENTS OF THE STATISTICAL ANALYSIS PROCESS

Statistical techniques are analysis procedures used to examine, reduce, and give meaning to the numerical data gathered in a study. In this textbook, statistics are divided into two major categories, descriptive and inferential. Descriptive statistics are summary statistics that allow the researcher to organize data in ways that give meaning and facilitate insight. Descriptive statistics are calculated to describe the sample and key study variables. Inferential statistics are designed to address objectives, questions, and hypotheses in studies to allow inference from the study sample to the target population. Inferential analyses are conducted to identify relationships, examine predictions, and determine group differences in studies.

In critically appraising a study, it may be helpful to understand the process that researchers use to perform data analyses. The statistical analysis process consists of several stages: (1) management of missing data; (2) description of the sample; (3) examination of the reliability of measurement methods; (4) conduct of exploratory analyses of study data; and (5) conduct of inferential analyses guided by the study hypotheses, questions, or objectives. Although not all of these stages are equally reflected in the final published report of the study, they all contribute to the insights that can be gained from analysis of the study data.

Management of Missing Data

Except in very small studies, researchers almost always use computers for data analyses. The first step of the process is entering the data into the computer using a systematic plan designed to reduce errors. Missing data points are identified during data entry. If enough data are missing for certain variables, researchers may have to determine whether the data are sufficient to perform analyses using those variables. In some cases, subjects must be excluded from an analysis because data considered essential to that analysis are missing. In examining the results of a published study, you might note that the number of subjects included in the final analyses is less than the original sample; this could be a result of attrition and/or subjects with missing data being excluded from the analyses. It is important for researchers to discuss missing data and its management in the study.

Description of the Sample

Researchers obtain as complete a picture of the sample as possible for their research report. Variables relevant to the sample are called demographic variables and might include age, gender, ethnicity, educational level, and number of chronic illnesses (see Chapter 5). Demographic variables measured at the nominal and ordinal levels, such as gender, ethnicity, and educational level, are analyzed with frequencies and percentages. Estimates of central tendency (e.g., the mean) and dispersion (e.g., the standard deviation) are calculated for variables such as age and number of chronic illnesses that are measured at the ratio level. Analysis of these demographic variables produces the sample characteristics for the study participants or subjects. When a study includes more than one group (e.g., treatment group and control or comparison group), researchers often compare the groups in relation to the demographic variables. For example, it might be important to know whether the groups' distributions of age and chronic illnesses were similar. When demographic variables are similar for the treatment (intervention) and comparison groups, the study is stronger because the outcomes are more likely to be caused by the intervention rather than by group differences at the start of the study.

? CRITICAL APPRAISAL GUIDELINES

Description of the Sample

When critically appraising a study, you need to examine the sample characteristics and judge the representativeness of the sample using the following questions.
1. What variables were used to describe the sample?
2. What statistical techniques were used to descriptively analyze the demographic variables, and were these techniques appropriate based on the level of measurement of these variables? Figure 10-2 covers the rules for the nominal, ordinal, interval, and ratio levels of measurement.
3. Was the sample representative of the study target population? For example, was this study's sample similar to the samples of other studies in this area that were cited in the literature review or the discussion section of the study?
4. If the sample is divided into groups for data analyses, was the similarity or homogeneity of the groups discussed? (See Chapter 9.)

RESEARCH EXAMPLE

Description of the Sample

Research Study

Kim, Chung, Park, and Kang (2012) conducted a quasi-experimental study to examine the effectiveness of an aquarobic exercise program on the self-efficacy, pain, body weight, blood lipid levels, and depression of patients with osteoarthritis. The study included 70 subjects, with 35 patients randomly assigned to the experimental group and 35 to the control group. We recommend that you obtain this article, and review this study. The results from this study are presented as examples several times in this chapter to facilitate your understanding of statistical techniques.

The demographic variables used to describe the sample in the Kim and colleagues' (2012) study included age, educational level, marital status, religion, occupation, income, and health status. Descriptive statistics of frequency and percentage (%) were used to analyze the demographic data, and the experimental and control groups were compared for similarities. The results from these analyses are presented in Table 11-1

TABLE 11-1   Homogeneity Test of General Characteristics Between Experimental and Control Groups

Characteristics	Experimental Group $n=35$ $n(\%)$	Control Group $n=35$ $n(\%)$	p
Age (yr)			
55-59	0 (0.0)	2 (5.7)	0.545*
60-64	11 (31.4)	9 (25.7)	
65-69	15 (42.9)	17 (48.6)	
≥ 70	9 (25.7)	7 (20.0)	
Educational Level			
None	4 (11.4)	1 (2.9)	0.373*
Elementary	5 (14.3)	11 (31.4)	
Middle school	15 (42.9)	14 (40.0)	
High school	5 (14.3)	5 (14.3)	
College or more	6 (17.1)	4 (11.4)	
Marital Status			
Married	22 (62.9)	22 (62.9)	1.000*
Bereavement	11 (31.4)	12 (34.3)	
Other	2 (5.7)	1 (2.9)	
Religion			
Christian	8 (22.9)	7 (20.0)	0.907*
Catholic	12 (34.3)	15 (42.9)	
Buddhist	9 (25.7)	9 (25.7)	
None	5 (14.3)	4 (11.4)	
Occupation			
Yes	4 (11.4)	3 (8.6)	1.000*
None	31 (88.6)	32 (91.4)	

Continued

RESEARCH EXAMPLE—cont'd

TABLE 11-1   **Homogeneity Test of General Characteristics Between Experimental and Control Groups—cont'd**

Characteristics	Experimental Group $n=35$ n(%)	Control Group $n=35$ n(%)	p
Income (per/mo)			
<100	18 (51.4)	18 (51.4)	0.496*
100-200	5 (14.3)	9 (25.7)	
201-300	7 (20.0)	6 (17.1)	
>300	5 (14.3)	2 (5.7)	
Health Status			
Good	5 (14.7)	5 (14.3)	0.649
Fair	16 (47.1)	16 (45.7)	
Bad	13 (38.2)	14 (40.0)	

*Fisher's exact test.
From Kim, I., Chung, S., Park, Y., & Kang, H. (2012). The effectiveness of an aquarobic exercise program for patients with osteoarthritis. *Applied Nursing Research, 25*(3), p. 186 (Table 2 from the article).

Critical Appraisal

Kim and associates (2012) developed a table that clearly presented the results of their analysis of demographic variables, and they discussed this table in the results section of their research report. The demographic variables of age, educational level, marital status, occupation, and income are commonly used in many studies to describe the samples. The descriptive analysis techniques of frequency and percentage were appropriate for the demographic variables measured at the nominal or ordinal level. Age, educational level, income, and health status were measured at the ordinal level, and marital status, religion, and occupation were measured at the nominal level.

The study included two groups (experimental and control), and differences between these two groups were examined for each of the demographic variables using the chi-square or Fisher's exact tests. These analytical procedures are appropriate for examining group differences for nominal-level variables and are discussed in more depth later in this chapter. The *p* values (probabilities in this study) were all greater than 0.05, indicating no significant differences between the experimental and control groups for the demographic variables. Therefore the groups could be considered demographically similar in this study, so any significant differences noted are more likely to be caused by the study intervention than by differences in the groups at the start of the study.

Implications for Practice

Kim and co-workers (2012) implemented a structured aquarobic exercise program that included two educational sessions, followed by selected aerobic exercises. The aquarobic exercises are detailed in a table in the article and involved an instructor leading the patients with osteoarthritis through various aerobic exercises in the water for 1 hour, three times a week, for a total of 36 sessions over 12 weeks. The researchers found that the "Aquarobic Exercise Program was effective in enhancing self-efficacy, decreasing pain, and improving depression levels, body weight, and blood lipid levels in patients with osteoarthritis" (Kim et al., 2012, p. 181). They recommended the use of this program in managing patients with osteoarthritis but also recognized the need for additional research to determine the long-term benefits of this program for these patients. The Quality and Safety Education for Nursing Institute (QSEN, 2013) provides competencies for prelicensure nurses. The QSEN implication of this research report is the evidence-based intervention of an aquarobic exercise program, which improved the health outcomes for these patients with osteoarthritis. Nurses and students are encouraged to use research findings in promoting an evidence-based practice (EBP) for nursing.

Reliability of Measurement Methods

Researchers need to report the reliability of the measurement methods used in their study. The reliability of observational or physiological measures is usually determined during the data collection phase and needs to be noted in the research report. If a scale was used to collect data, the Cronbach alpha procedure needs to be applied to the scale items to determine the reliability of the scale for this study (Waltz, Strickland, & Lenz, 2010). If the Cronbach alpha coefficient is unacceptably low (<0.70), the researcher must decide whether to analyze the data collected with the instrument. A value of 0.70 is considered acceptable, especially for newly developed scales. A Cronbach alpha coefficient value of 0.80 to 0.89 from previous research indicates that a scale is sufficiently reliable to use in a study (see Chapter 10). The t-test or Pearson's correlation statistics may be used to determine test-retest reliability (Grove, Burns, & Gray, 2013). In critically appraising a study, you need to examine the reliability of the measurement methods and the statistical procedures used to determine these values. Sometimes researchers examine the validity of the measurement methods used in their studies, and this content also needs to be included in the research report (see Chapter 10).

An example is presented from the Kim and colleagues' (2012) study (see earlier). They measured self-efficacy with a 14-item Likert-type scale that had been previously developed for patients with arthritis. The higher scores indicated greater levels of self-efficacy. The calculated Cronbach alpha for this scale in this study was 0.90, indicating 90% reliability or consistency in the measurement of self-efficacy and 10% error. Kim and associates (2012) measured depression with the Zung Self-Rating Depression Scale, which "consisted of 20 items (10 positive and 10 negative) on a 4-point Likert-type scale. Negative responses were converted into scores, and higher scores indicated greater levels of depression. Cronbach's alpha in this study was 0.75" (75% reliability and 25% error; Kim et al., 2012, p. 185). This study included a concise description of the scales used to collect psychosocial data and documented the scales' reliability using Cronbach alpha values. The reliability of the self-efficacy scale was strong at 0.90, but the Zung Self-Rating Depression Scale reliability (0.75) was a little low for an established scale.

Exploratory Analyses

The next step, exploratory analysis, is used to examine all the data descriptively. This step is discussed in more detail later (see later, "Using Statistics to Describe"). Data on each study variable are examined using measures of central tendency and dispersion to determine the nature of variation in the data and identify outliers. Outliers are subjects or data points with extreme values (values that lie far from other plotted points on a graph) that seem unlike the rest of the sample. Researchers usually indicate whether outliers are identified during data analysis and how these were managed. In critically appraising a study's results, note any discussion of outliers and determine how they were managed and might have affected the study results.

Inferential Statistical Analyses

The final phase of data analysis involves conducting inferential statistical analyses for the purpose of generalizing findings from the study sample to appropriate accessible and target populations. To justify generalization of the results from inferential statistical analyses, a rigorous research methodology is needed, including a strong research design (Shadish, Cook, Campbell, 2002), reliable and valid measurement methods (Waltz et al., 2010), and a large sample size (Cohen, 1988).

Most researchers include a section in their research report that identifies the statistical analysis techniques conducted on the study data and the program used to calculate them. This discussion includes the inferential analysis techniques (e.g., those focused on relationships, prediction, and differences) and sometimes the descriptive analysis techniques (e.g., frequencies, percentages, and measures of central tendency and dispersion) conducted in the study. The identification of data analysis techniques conducted in a study are usually presented just prior to the study's results section. Kim and co-workers (2012) had a strong pretest and post-test quasi-experimental design with experimental and control groups (see Chapter 8). The study variables were measured with fairly reliable scales and accurate and precise physiological instruments. The inferential statistical analyses conducted were clearly identified and focused on addressing the study purpose. This study excerpt identifies the analysis techniques:

"Data Analysis

Data analysis was performed using SPSS [Statistical Package for the Social Sciences] version 12.0. Homogeneity of the two groups was assessed using Fisher's exact test, the chi-square test, and independent t-tests [discussed later in this chapter]. Comparisons of posttest values for the experimental and control groups were then made using independent t-tests." (Kim et al., 2012, p. 185)

UNDERSTANDING THEORIES AND CONCEPTS OF THE STATISTICAL ANALYSIS PROCESS

One reason that nurses tend to avoid statistics is that many were taught only the mathematical procedures of calculating statistical equations, with little or no explanation of the logic behind those procedures or the meaning of the results. Computation is a mechanical process usually performed by a computer, and information about the calculation procedure is not necessary to begin understanding statistical results. Here we present an approach to data analysis that will enhance your understanding of the statistical analysis process. You can then use this understanding to appraise data analysis techniques critically in the results section of research reports.

This section presents a brief explanation of some of the theories and concepts important in understanding the statistical analysis process. Probability theory and decision theory are discussed, and the concepts of hypothesis testing, level of significance, inference, generalization, the normal curve, tailedness, type I and type II errors, power, and degrees of freedom are described. More extensive discussion of these topics can be found in other sources, and we recommend our own textbooks (Grove, 2007; Grove et al., 2013) and a quality statistical text by Plichta and Kelvin (2013).

Probability Theory

Probability theory is used to explain the extent of a relationship, the probability that an event will occur in a given situation, or the probability that an event can be accurately predicted. The researcher might want to know the probability that a particular outcome will result from a nursing intervention. For example, the researcher may want to know how likely it is that urinary catheterization during hospitalization will lead to a urinary tract infection (UTI) after discharge from the hospital. The researcher also may want to know the probability that subjects in the experimental group are members of the same larger population from which the comparison or control group subjects were taken. Probability is expressed as a lower case letter p, with values expressed as percentages or as a decimal value, ranging from 0 to 1. For example, if the probability is 0.23, then it is expressed as $p = 0.23$. This means that there is a 23% probability that a particular outcome (e.g., a UTI) will occur. Probability values also can be stated as less than a specific value, such as 0.05, expressed as $p < 0.05$. (The symbol $<$ means less than.) A study may indicate the probability that the experimental group subjects were members of the same larger population as the comparison group subjects was less than or equal to 5% ($p \leq 0.05$). In other words, it is not very likely that the comparison group and the experimental group are from the same population. Put another way, you might say that there is a 5% chance that the two groups are from the same population, and a 95% chance that they are not from the same population. The inference is that the experimental group is different from the comparison group because of the effect of the intervention in the study. Probability values often are stated with the results of inferential statistical analyses. In critically appraising studies, it is useful to recognize these symbols and understand what they mean.

Decision Theory, Hypothesis Testing, and Level of Significance

Decision theory assumes that all of the groups in a study (e.g., experimental and comparison groups) used to test a particular hypothesis are components of the same population relative to the variables under study. This expectation (or assumption) traditionally is expressed as a null hypothesis, which states that there is no difference between (or among) the groups in a study, in terms of the variables included in the hypothesis (see Chapter 5 for more details of types of hypotheses). It is up to the researcher to provide evidence for a genuine difference between the groups. For example, the researcher may hypothesize that the frequency of UTIs that occurred after discharge from the hospital in patients who were catheterized during hospitalization is no different from the frequency of such infections in those who were not catheterized. To test the assumption of no difference, a cutoff point is selected before data collection. The cutoff point, referred to as alpha (α), or the level of statistical significance, is the probability level at which the results of statistical analysis are judged to indicate a statistically significant difference between the groups. The level of significance selected for most nursing studies is 0.05. If the p value found in the statistical analysis is less than or equal to 0.05, the experimental and comparison groups are considered to be significantly different (members of different populations).

Decision theory requires that the cutoff point selected for a study be absolute. Absolute means that even if the value obtained is only a fraction above the cutoff point, the samples are considered to be from the same population, and no meaning can be attributed to the differences. It is inappropriate when using decision theory to state that the findings approached significance at $p = 0.051$ if the alpha level was set at 0.05. Using decision theory rules, this finding indicates that the groups tested are not significantly different, and the null hypothesis is accepted. On the other hand, once the level of significance has been set at 0.05 by the researcher, if the analysis reveals a significant difference of 0.001, this result is not considered more significant than the 0.05 originally proposed (Slakter, Wu, & Suzaki-Slakter, 1991). The level of significance is dichotomous, which means that the difference is significant or not significant; there are no "degrees" of significance. However, some people, not realizing that their reasoning has shifted from decision theory to probability theory, indicate in their research report that the 0.001 result makes the findings more significant than if they had obtained only a 0.05 level of significance.

From the perspective of probability theory, there is considerable difference in the risk of occurrence of a type I error (saying something is significant when it is not) when the probability is between 0.05 and 0.001. If $p = 0.001$, the probability that the two groups are components of the same population is 1 in 1000; if $p = 0.05$, the probability that the groups belong to the same population is 5 in 100. In other words, if $p = 0.05$, then in 5 times out of 100, groups with statistical values such as those found in these statistical analyses actually are members of the same population, and the conclusion that the groups are different is erroneous.

In computer analysis, the probability value obtained from each data analysis (e.g., $p = 0.03$ or $p = 0.07$) frequently is provided on the printout and is often reported by the researcher in the published study, along with the level of significance set before data analysis was conducted. In summary, the probability (p) value reveals the risk of a type I error in a particular study. The alpha (α) value, set prior to the study, usually at $\alpha = 0.05$, reveals whether the probability value for a particular analysis in a study met the cutoff point for a significant difference between groups or a significant relationship between variables.

Inference and Generalization

An inference is a conclusion or judgment based on evidence. Statistical inferences are made cautiously and with great care. The decision theory rules used to interpret the results of statistical procedures increase the probability that inferences are accurate. A generalization is the application of information that has been acquired from a specific instance to a general situation. Generalizing requires making an inference; both require the use of inductive reasoning. An inference is made from a specific case and extended to a general truth, from a part to the whole, from the concrete to the abstract, and from the known to the unknown. In research, an inference is made from the study findings obtained from a specific sample and applied to a more general target population, using the results from statistical analyses. For example, a researcher may conclude in a research report that a significant difference was found in the number of UTIs between two samples, one in which the subjects had been catheterized during hospitalization and another in which the subjects had not. The researcher also may conclude that this difference can be expected in all patients who have received care in hospitals. The findings are generalized from the sample in the study to all previously hospitalized patients. Statisticians and researchers can never prove something using inference; they can never be certain that their inferences and generalizations are correct. The researcher's generalization of the incidence of UTIs may not have been carefully thought out—the findings may have been generalized to a population that was overly broad. It is possible that in the more general population, there is no difference in the incidence of UTIs based on whether the patient was catheterized or not. Generalizing study findings are part of the discussion section of a research report (see later).

Normal Curve

A normal curve is a theoretical frequency distribution of all possible values in a population; however, no real distribution exactly fits the normal curve (Figure 11-1). The idea of the normal curve was developed by an 18-year-old mathematician, Johann Gauss, in 1795. He found that data from variables (e.g., the mean of each sample) measured repeatedly in many samples from the same population can be combined into one large sample. From this large sample, a more accurate representation can be developed of the pattern of the curve in that population than is possible with only one sample. Surprisingly, in most cases, the curve is similar, regardless of the specific variables examined or the population studied.

Levels of significance and probability are based on the logic of the normal curve. The normal curve presented in Figure 11-1 shows the distribution of values for a single population. Note that 95.5% of the values are within 2 standard deviations (SDs) of the mean, ranging from −2 to +2 SDs. (Standard deviation is described later in this chapter; see "Using Statistics to Describe.") Thus there is approximately a 95% probability that a given measured value (e.g., the mean of a group) would fall within approximately 2 SDs of the mean of the population, and there is a 5% probability that the value would fall in the tails of the normal curve (the extreme ends of the normal curve, below −2 (−1.96 exactly) SDs [2.5%] or above +2 (+1.96 exactly) SDs [2.5%]). If the groups being

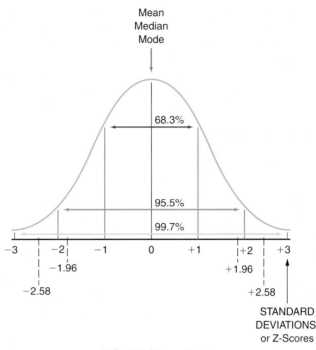

FIG 11-1 Normal curve.

compared are from the same population (not significantly different), you would expect the values (e.g., the means) of each group to fall within the 95% range of values on the normal curve. If the groups are from (significantly) different populations, you would expect one of the group values to be outside the 95% range of values. An inferential statistical analysis performed to determine differences between groups, using a level of significance (α) set at 0.05, would test that expectation. If the statistical test demonstrates a significant difference (the value of one group does not fall within the 95% range of values), the groups are considered to belong to different populations. However, in 5% of statistical tests, the value of one of the groups can be expected to fall outside the 95% range of values but still belong to the same population (a type I error).

Tailedness

Nondirectional hypotheses usually assume that an extreme score (obtained because the group with the extreme score did not belong to the same population) can occur in either tail of the normal curve (Figure 11-2). The analysis of a nondirectional hypothesis is called a two-tailed test of significance. In a one-tailed test of significance, the hypothesis is directional, and extreme statistical values that occur in a single tail of the curve are of interest (see Chapter 5 for a discussion of directional and nondirectional hypotheses). The hypothesis states that the extreme score is higher or lower than that for 95% of the population, indicating that the sample with the extreme score is not a member of the same population. In this case, 5% of statistical values that are considered significant will be in one tail, rather than two. Extreme statistical values occurring in the other tail of the curve are not considered significantly different. In Figure 11-3, which shows a one-tailed figure, the portion of the curve in which statistical values will be considered significant is the right tail. Developing a one-tailed hypothesis requires that the researcher have sufficient knowledge

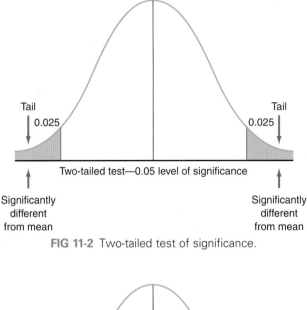

Tail
0.025

Tail
0.025

Two-tailed test—0.05 level of significance

Significantly
different
from mean

Significantly
different
from mean

FIG 11-2 Two-tailed test of significance.

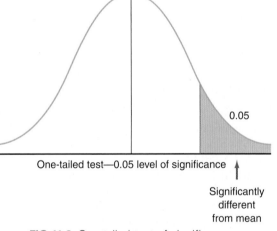

0.05

One-tailed test—0.05 level of significance

Significantly
different
from mean

FIG 11-3 One-tailed test of significance.

of the variables to predict whether the difference will be in the tail above the mean or in the tail below the mean. One-tailed statistical tests are uniformly more powerful than two-tailed tests, decreasing the possibility of a type II error (saying something is not significant when it is).

Type I and Type II Errors

According to decision theory, two types of error can occur when a researcher is deciding what the result of a statistical test means, type I and type II (Table 11-2). A **type I error** occurs when the null hypothesis is rejected when it is true (e.g., when the results indicate that there is a significant difference, when in reality there is not). The risk of a type I error is indicated by the level of significance. There is a greater risk of a type I error with a 0.05 level of significance (5 chances for error in 100) than with a 0.01 level of significance (1 chance for error in 100).

TABLE 11-2 **TYPE I AND TYPE II ERRORS**		
	IN REALITY, THE NULL HYPOTHESIS* IS:	
DATA ANALYSIS INDICATES	**TRUE**	**FALSE**
Results significant, null hypothesis rejected	Type I error (α)	Correct decision (power)
Results not significant, null hypothesis not rejected	Correct decision	Type II error (β)

*The null hypothesis is stating that no difference or relationship exists.

A type II error occurs when the null hypothesis is regarded as true but is in fact false. For example, statistical analyses may indicate no significant differences between groups, but in reality the groups are different (see Table 11-2). There is a greater risk of a type II error when the level of significance is 0.01 than when it is 0.05. However, type II errors are often caused by flaws in the research methods. In nursing research, many studies are conducted with small samples and with instruments that do not accurately and precisely measure the variables under study (Grove et al., 2013; Waltz et al., 2010). In many nursing situations, multiple variables interact to cause differences within populations. When only a few of the interacting variables are examined, small differences between groups may be overlooked. This leads to nonsignificant study results, which can cause researchers to conclude falsely that there are no differences between the samples when there actually are. Thus the risk of a type II error is often high in nursing studies.

Power: Controlling the Risk of a Type II Error

Power is the probability that a statistical test will detect a significant difference that exists (see Table 11-2). The risk of a type II error can be determined using power analysis. Cohen (1988) has identified four parameters of a power analysis: (1) the level of significance; (2) sample size; (3) power; and (4) effect size. If three of the four are known, the fourth can be calculated using power analysis formulas. The minimum acceptable power level is 0.80 (80%). The researcher determines the sample size and the level of significance (usually set at $\alpha = 0.05$). (Chapter 9 provides a detailed discussion of power analysis.) Effect size is "the degree to which the phenomenon is present in the population, or the degree to which the null hypothesis is false" (Cohen, 1988, pp. 9-10). For example, if changes in anxiety level are measured in a group of patients before surgery, with the first measurement taken when the patients are still at home, and the second taken just before surgery, the effect size will be large if a great change in anxiety occurs in the group between the two points in time. If the effect of a preoperative teaching program on the level of anxiety is measured, the effect size will be the difference in the post-test level of anxiety in the experimental group compared with that in the comparison group. If only a small change in the level of anxiety is expected, the effect size will be small. In many nursing studies, only small effect sizes can be expected. In such a study, a sample of 200 or more is often needed to detect a significant difference (Cohen, 1988). Small effect sizes occur in nursing studies with small samples, weak study designs, and measurement methods that measure only large changes. The power level should be discussed in studies that fail to reject the null hypothesis (or have nonsignificant findings). If the power level is below 0.80, you need to question the validity of the nonsignificant findings.

Degrees of Freedom

The concept of degrees of freedom (*df*) is important for calculating statistical procedures and interpreting the results using statistical tables. Degrees of freedom involve the freedom of a score value to vary given the other existing scores' values and the established sum of these scores (Grove et al., 2013). Degrees of freedom are often reported with statistical results.

USING STATISTICS TO DESCRIBE

Descriptive statistics, introduced earlier, allow researchers to organize numerical data in ways that give meaning and facilitate insight. In any study in which the data are numerical, data analysis begins with descriptive statistics. For some descriptive studies, researchers limit data analyses to descriptive statistics. For other studies, researchers use descriptive statistics primarily to describe the characteristics of the sample and describe values obtained from the measurement of dependent or research variables. Descriptive statistics presented in this book include frequency distributions, percentages, measures of central tendency, measures of dispersion, and standardized scores.

Frequency Distributions

Frequency distribution describes the occurrence of scores or categories in a study. For example, the frequency distribution for gender in a study might be 42 males and 58 females. A frequency distribution usually is the first method used to organize the data for examination. There are two types of frequency distributions, ungrouped and grouped.

Ungrouped Frequency Distributions

Most studies have some categorical data that are presented in the form of an ungrouped frequency distribution, in which a table is developed to display all numerical values obtained for a particular variable. This approach is generally used on discrete rather than continuous data. Examples of data commonly organized in this manner are gender, ethnicity, marital status, diagnoses of study subjects, and values obtained from the measurement of selected research and dependent variables. Table 11-3 is an example table developed for this text; it includes nine different scores obtained by 50 subjects. This is an example of ungrouped frequencies because each score is represented in the table with the number of subjects receiving this score.

Grouped Frequency Distributions

Grouped frequency distributions are used when continuous variables are being examined. Many measures taken during data collection, including body temperature, vital lung capacity, weight, age, scale scores, and time, are measured using a continuous scale. Any method of grouping results in loss of information. For example, if age is grouped, a breakdown into two groups, younger than 65 years and older than 65 years, provides less information about the data than groupings of

TABLE 11-3   EXAMPLE OF AN UNGROUPED FREQUENCY TABLE

SCORE	FREQUENCY	PERCENTAGE	CUMULATIVE FREQUENCY (f)	CUMULATIVE PERCENTAGE
1	4	8	4	8
3	6	12	10	20
4	8	16	18	36
5	14	28	32	64
7	8	16	40	80
8	6	12	46	92
9	4	8	$N = 50$	100

10-year age spans. As with levels of measurement, rules have been established to guide classification systems. There should be at least five but not more than 20 groups. The classes established must be exhaustive; each datum must fit into one of the identified classes. The classes must be exclusive; each datum must fit into only one (Grove et al., 2013). A common mistake occurs when the ranges contain overlaps that would allow a datum to fit into more than one class. For example, a researcher may classify age ranges as 20 to 30, 30 to 40, 40 to 50, and so on. By this definition, subjects aged 30, 40, and so on can be classified into more than one category. The range of each category must be equivalent. For example, if 10 years is the age range, each age category must include 10 years of ages. This rule is violated in some cases to allow the first and last categories to be open-ended and worded to include all scores above or below a specified point. Table 11-4 is an example of a grouped frequency distribution for income for registered nurses (RNs), in which the categories are exhaustive and mutually exclusive.

Percentage Distributions

A percentage distribution indicates the percentage of subjects in a sample whose scores fall into a specific group and the number of scores in that group. Percentage distributions are particularly useful for comparing the present data with findings from other studies that have different sample sizes. A cumulative distribution is a type of percentage distribution in which the percentages and frequencies of scores are summed as one moves from the top of the table to the bottom. Consequently, the bottom category would have a cumulative frequency equivalent to the sample size and a cumulative percentage of 100 (see Table 11-3). Frequency distributions are also displayed using tables or graphs (e.g., pie chart, bar chart, line graph). Graphic displays of the frequency distribution of data from Table 11-3 are presented in Figure 11-4. You might note in the bar and line graphs that the data distribution forms a normal curve.

Measures of Central Tendency

Measures of central tendency frequently are referred to as the midpoint in the data or as an average of the data. The measures of central tendency are the most concise statement of the nature of the data in a study. The three measures of central tendency that are commonly used in statistical analyses are the mode, median, and mean. For a data set that has a normal distribution, these values are equal (see Figure 11-1); however, they usually are different for data obtained from real samples.

Mode

The mode is the numerical value or score that occurs with greatest frequency; it does not necessarily indicate the center of the data set. The mode can be determined by examination of an

TABLE 11-4 INCOME OF FULL-TIME REGISTERED NURSES ($n=100$)	
INCOME	FREQUENCY (%)
Below $60,000	5 (5%)
$60,000-69,999	20 (20%)
$70,000-79,999	35 (35%)
$80,000-90,000	25 (25%)
Above $90,000	15 (15%)

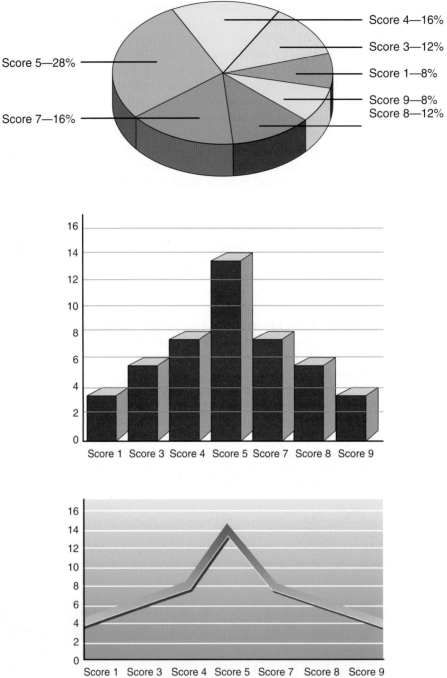

FIG 11-4 Commonly used graphic displays of frequency distribution.

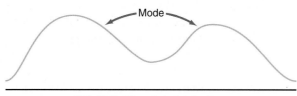

FIG 11-5 Bimodal distribution.

ungrouped frequency distribution of the data. In Table 11-3, the mode is the score of 5, which occurred 14 times in the data set. The mode can be used to describe the typical subject or identify the most frequently occurring value on a scale item. The mode is the appropriate measure of central tendency for nominal data. A data set can have more than one mode. If two modes exist, the data set is referred to as bimodal distribution (Figure 11-5). A data set with more than two modes is said to be multimodal.

Median

The median is the midpoint or the score at the exact center of the ungrouped frequency distribution—the 50th percentile. The median is obtained by rank-ordering the scores. If the number of scores is uneven, exactly 50% of the scores are above the median, and 50% are below it. If the number of scores is even, the median is the average of the two middle scores; thus the median may not be one of the scores in the data set. Unlike the mean, the median is not affected by extreme scores in the data (outliers). The median is the most appropriate measure of central tendency for ordinal data. The median for the data in Table 11-3 is 5.

Mean

The most commonly used measure of central tendency is the mean. The mean is the sum of the scores divided by the number of scores being summed. Like the median, the mean may not be a member of the data set. The mean is the appropriate measure of central tendency for interval- and ratio-level data. However, if the study has outliers, the mean is most affected by these, and the median might be the measure of central tendency included in the research report. The mean for the data in Table 11-3 is 5.28.

Measures of Dispersion

Measures of dispersion, or variability, are measures of individual differences of the members of the sample. They give some indication of how scores in a sample are dispersed or spread around the mean. These measures provide information about the data that is not available from measures of central tendency. The measures of dispersion indicate how different the scores are or the extent to which individual scores deviate from one another. If the individual scores are similar, measures of variability are small, and the sample is relatively homogeneous, or similar, in terms of those scores. A heterogeneous sample has a wide variation in scores. The measures of dispersion generally used are range, variance, and standard deviation. Standardized scores may be used to express measures of dispersion. Scatterplots frequently are used to illustrate the dispersion in the data (discussed later).

Range

The simplest measure of dispersion is the range, which is obtained by subtracting the lowest score from the highest score. The range for the scores in Table 11-3 is calculated as $9 - 1 = 8$. The range is a difference score, which uses only the two extreme scores for the comparison. It is a very crude measure of dispersion but is sensitive to outliers. The range might also be expressed as the lowest to the highest scores. For the data in Table 11-3, the range might also be expressed as the scores from 1 to 9.

Variance

The variance for scores in a study is calculated with a mathematical equation and indicates the spread or dispersion of the scores (see Grove et al., 2013, for the equation). The variance can only be calculated on data at the interval or ratio level of measurement. The numerical value obtained from the calculation depends on the measurement scale used, such as the laboratory measurement of fasting blood glucose values or the scale measurement of weights. The calculated variance value has no absolute value and can be compared only with data obtained using similar measures. Generally, however, the larger the variance value, the greater the dispersion of scores. The variance for the data in Table 11-3 is 4.94.

Standard Deviation

The standard deviation (*SD*) is the square root of the variance. Just as the mean is the average value, the *SD* is the average difference (deviation) value. The *SD* provides a measure of the average deviation of a value from the mean in that particular sample. It indicates the degree of error that would result if the mean alone were used to interpret the data. In the normal curve, 68% of the values will be within 1 *SD* above or below the mean, 95% will be within 1.96 *SDs* above or below the mean, and 99% will be within 2.58 *SDs* above or below the mean (see Figure 11-1; Grove, 2007).

The *SD* for the example data presented in Table 11-3 of Kim and colleagues' (2012) study is 2.22. The mean is 5.28, so the value of a subject 1 *SD* below the mean would be $5.28 - 2.22$, or 3.06. The value of a subject 1 *SD* above the mean would be $5.28 + 2.22$, or 7.50. Therefore approximately 68% of the sample (and perhaps the population from which it was derived) can be expected to have values in the range of 3.06 to 7.50, which is expressed as (3.06, 7.50). Extending this calculation further, the value of a subject 2 *SDs* below the mean would be $5.28 - 2.22 - 2.22 = 0.84$ and the value of a subject 2 *SDs* above the mean would be $5.28 + 2.22 + 2.22 = 9.72$. The values for 2 *SDs* below and above the mean would be expressed as (0.84, 9.72). Using this strategy, the entire distribution of values can be estimated (Grove, 2007). The value of a single individual can be compared with the value calculated for the total sample (e.g., mean, median, or mode). Standard deviation is an important measure, both for understanding dispersion within a distribution and interpreting the relationship of a particular value to the distribution.

Confidence Interval

When the probability of including the value of the population within an interval estimate is known, it is referred to as a confidence interval (CI). Calculating a CI involves the use of two formulas to identify the upper and lower ends of the interval (see Grove et al., 2013, for the formulas). For example, the CI for a study might include a lower value of 15.34 and an upper value of 20.56 and would be expressed as "(15.34, 20.56)." CIs are usually calculated for 95% and 99% intervals. The 95% CI indicates that 95% of the time, the population mean would fall within this interval. Theoretically, we can produce a confidence interval for any population value or parameter of a distribution. It is a generic statistical procedure. For example, confidence intervals can also be developed around correlation coefficients and *t*-test values. Estimation can be used for a single population or for multiple populations. You will see the use of CIs when reading the results section of studies.

Standardized Scores

Because of differences in the characteristics of various distributions, comparing a value in one distribution with a value in another is difficult. For example, perhaps you want to compare test scores from two classroom examinations. The highest possible score in one test is 100 and in the other it is 70; the scores will be difficult to compare. To facilitate this comparison, a mechanism was developed to transform raw scores into standardized scores. Numbers that make sense only within the framework of measurements used within a specific study are transformed into numbers (standardized scores) that have a more general meaning. Transformation into standardized scores allows an easy conceptual grasp of the meaning of the score. A common standardized score is called a Z-score. It expresses deviations from the mean (difference scores) in terms of SD units (see Figure 11-1). A score that falls above the mean will have a positive Z-score, whereas a score that falls below the mean will have a negative Z-score. The mean expressed as a Z-score is zero. The SD is equal to the Z-score. Thus a Z-score of 2 indicates that the score from which it was obtained is 2 SDs above the mean. A Z-score of −0.5 indicates that the score is 0.5 SD below the mean.

Scatterplots

A scatterplot has two scales, horizontal and vertical. Each scale is referred to as an axis. The vertical scale is called the y-axis; the horizontal scale is the x-axis. A scatterplot can be used to illustrate the dispersion of values on a variable. In this case, the x-axis represents the possible values of the variable. The y-axis represents the number of times each value of the variable occurred in the sample. Scatterplots also can be used to illustrate the relationship between values on one variable and values on another. Then each axis will represent one variable. For example, if a graph is developed to illustrate the relationship between subjects' anxiety and depression scores measured with Likert scales, the horizontal axis could represent anxiety and the vertical axis could represent depression. For each unit or subject, there is a value for x and a value for y. The point at which the values of x and y for a single subject intersect is plotted on the graph (Figure 11-6). When the values for each

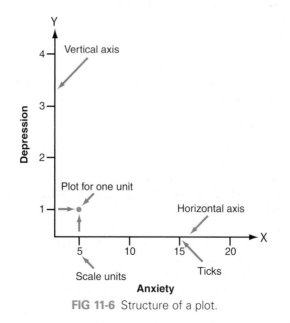

FIG 11-6 Structure of a plot.

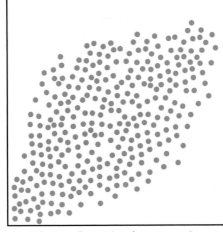

FIG 11-7 Example of a scatterplot.

subject in the sample have been plotted, the degree of relationship between the variables is revealed (Figure 11-7). If the scatterplot in Figure 11-7 was an example of the relationship between anxiety and depression, the plot is positive and indicates that as anxiety increases so does depression in the study subjects.

Understanding Descriptive Statistical Results

In published studies, investigators report descriptive statistics in tables and in the narrative of the results section. Descriptive statistics are used to describe the sample (see earlier) and study variables. Measures of central tendency (mode, median, and mean) and measures of dispersion (range and *SD*) are usually calculated to describe study variables. Also, descriptive and inferential statistics might be presented together to describe differences or similarities between groups at the start of the study. Inferential statistical procedures often used for this purpose include the chi-square test for nominal-level data and the *t*-test for interval- and ratio-level data. From a perspective of descriptive analyses, the purpose is not to test for causality, but rather to describe the differences or similarities between the groups in a study.

RESEARCH EXAMPLE
Description of Study Variables

Research Study

Kim and colleagues' (2012) study, presented as an example earlier in this chapter, focused on determining the effectiveness of an aquarobic exercise program (independent variable) for patients with osteoarthritis. The dependent or outcome variables in this study were self-efficacy, pain, body weight, blood lipids, and depression. These variables were described at the start of the study using means and *SD*s, and these variables were examined for differences between the experimental and control groups using the *t*-test. Table 11-5 presents the results from these analyses, which indicate that none of the *t*-tests were significant (p values all > 0.05).

TABLE 11-5 Homogeneity Test of Dependent Variables Between Experimental and Control Groups

Variable	Experimental Group (n = 35) M ± SD	Control Group (n = 35) M ± SD	t	p
Self-efficacy	1,124.87 ± 206.75	1,166.00 ± 152.31	−0.95	0.345
Pain	6.83 ± 1.92	7.03 ± 1.99	−0.43	0.670
Body weight	60.86 ± 9.48	59.19 ± 5.87	0.86	0.392
Blood lipid levels				
Total cholesterol (mg)	212.94 ± 43.47	218.20 ± 39.51	−0.53	0.598
Triglycerides (mg/dL)	157.34 ± 121.25	123.34 ± 60.21	1.49	0.142
HDL cholesterol (mg/dL)	57.06 ± 25.09	64.03 ± 27.47	−1.11	0.272
Depression	32.66 ± 6.78	32.26 ± 7.81	0.22	0.827

HDL, High-density-lipoprotein.
From Kim, I., Chung, S., Park, Y., & Kang, H. (2012). The effectiveness of an aquarobic exercise program for patients with osteoarthritis. *Applied Nursing Research, 25*(3), 186.

Critical Appraisal

The descriptive analysis techniques (mean [*M*] and *SD*) were appropriate for the level of measurement of the variables, which were interval or ratio. Self-efficacy and depression were measured with Likert scales, and the totals of these scales are often considered interval-level data (Grove et al., 2013; Waltz et al., 2010). Pain was measured with a visual analog scale that produces at least interval-level data (see Chapter 10); the physiological variables of body weight and lipids are ratio-level data. These descriptive results were clearly presented in a table and discussed in the narrative of the results section. However, it would have been helpful to include the range for these variables to examine for outliers.

The study included two groups (experimental and control), and differences between these two groups were examined for each of the dependent variables. Differences between the groups were appropriately analyzed with *t*-tests. The experimental and control groups were found to have no significant differences in the dependent variables at the start of the study (*p* values > 0.05). Thus these groups are considered homogeneous or similar for these variables. These results strengthen the study because the groups need to be as similar as possible for the dependent variables at the start of the study. Thus any significant differences noted at the end of the study are more likely to be a result of the study intervention than of error.

Implications for Practice

The implications of the study findings for practice were discussed earlier in this chapter.

DETERMINING THE APPROPRIATENESS OF INFERENTIAL STATISTICS IN STUDIES

Multiple factors are involved in determining the appropriateness or suitability of inferential statistical procedures conducted in a study. Inferential statistics are conducted to examine relationships, make predictions, and determine causality or differences in studies. The inferential statistics used in a study are determined by the study's (1) purpose, (2) hypotheses, questions, or objectives, (3) design, and (4) level of measurement of the variables. Determining the suitability of various inferential statistical procedures for a particular study is not straightforward. Regrettably, there is not usually one "right" statistical procedure for a study.

Evaluating statistical procedures requires that you make a number of judgments about the nature of the data and what the researcher wanted to know. You need to determine (1) whether the data for analysis were treated as nominal, ordinal, or interval or ratio (see Figure 10-2 in Chapter 10), (2) how many groups were in the study, and (3) whether the groups were paired (dependent) or independent. You might see statistical techniques identified as parametric or non-parametric, based on the level of measurement of the study variables. If the variables are measured at the nominal and ordinal levels, nonparametric analyses are conducted. If variables are at the interval or ratio level of measurement, and the values of the subjects for the variable are normally distributed, parametric analyses are conducted (Grove, 2007). Researchers run a computer program to determine if the data for variables are normally distributed. Interval and ratio levels of data are often included together because the analysis techniques are the same whether the data are at the interval or ratio level of measurement.

In independent groups, the selection of one subject is unrelated to the selection of other subjects. For example, if subjects are randomly assigned to treatment and control groups, the groups are independent. In paired groups (also called dependent groups), subjects or observations selected for data collection are related in some way to the selection of other subjects or observations. For example, if subjects serve as their own control by using the pretest as a control group, the observations (and therefore the groups) are paired. Also, if matched pairs of subjects are used for the comparison and treatment groups, the observations are paired or dependent (see Chapter 8). Researchers sometimes match groups on age and level of illness to control the effect of these demographic variables in a study. In a study of twins, one twin may be placed in the control group and the other in the experimental or treatment group. Because they are twins, they are matched on several variables.

One approach for judging the appropriateness of an analysis technique in a study is to use a decision tree or algorithm. The algorithm directs you by gradually narrowing the number of appropriate statistical procedures as you make judgments about the nature of the study and the data. An algorithm for judging the appropriateness of statistical procedures is presented in Figure 11-8. This algorithm identifies four factors related to the appropriateness of a statistical procedure—nature of the research question, level of measurement of the dependent and research variables, number of groups, and research design. To use the decision tree or algorithm in Figure 11-8, you would (1) determine whether the research question focuses on differences or associations (relationships), (2) determine the level of measurement (nominal, ordinal, or interval/ratio) of the study variables, (3) select the number of groups that are included in the study, and (4) determine the design, with independent or paired (dependent) samples, that most closely fits the study you are critically appraising. The lines on the algorithm are followed through each selection to identify the appropriate statistical procedure listed at the far right in the figure.

Critical Appraisal Guidelines for Inferential Statistical Analyses

When critically appraising the appropriateness of inferential statistical procedures used in published studies, you must not only be familiar with the statistical procedure used in the study, but you also must be able to compare that procedure with others that could have been used, perhaps to greater advantage. Figure 11-8 can be used to determine the appropriateness of the inferential statistical procedures included in a study. The following critical appraisal guidelines will assist you in assessing the quality of the results presented in published studies.

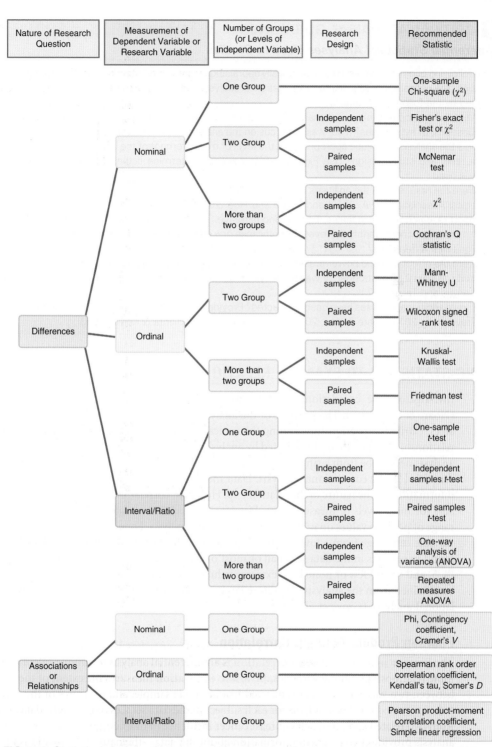

FIG 11-8 Statistical decision tree or algorithm for identifying an appropriate analysis technique. (Modified from Grove, S. K., Burns, N., & Gray, J. R. [2013]. *The practice of nursing research: Appraisal, synthesis, and generation of evidence* [7th ed.]. St. Louis: Elsevier Saunders, p. 547.)

Inferential Statistical Analyses Used in Studies

The following questions will assist you in critically appraising the inferential statistical analyses and their results in studies. The critical appraisals of inferential statistical analysis techniques provided in the rest of this chapter are guided by the following questions:

1. Were the appropriate inferential analysis techniques performed to address the study purpose or objectives, questions, or hypotheses? If so, was the focus on the analyses' relationships, prediction, and/or differences?
2. Was the analysis technique appropriate for the level of measurement of the data (nominal, ordinal, or interval or ratio) and study design? Use Figure 11-8 to help you determine if the appropriate analysis technique was used.
3. Were the results from the analyses clearly presented and appropriately interpreted? The American Psychological Association (APA, 2010) and Hoare and Hoe (2013) have provided detailed discussions on how to report research results in tables, figures, and narrative.
4. Did the researchers identify the level of significance or α used in the study? Did the findings show statistically significant differences?
5. Were the effect size and power presented for each nonsignificant finding? Was the power adequate for the study, at least 0.80 or stronger, or was there a potential for a type II error? (See earlier discussion of types I and II errors and Table 11-2.)
6. Should additional analyses have been conducted? Provide a rationale for your answer (Fawcett & Garity, 2009; Grove et al., 2013; Hoare & Hoe, 2013; Hoe & Hoare, 2012; Plichta & Kelvin, 2013).

USING STATISTICS TO EXAMINE RELATIONSHIPS

Investigators use correlational analyses to identify relationships between or among variables (Hoare & Hoe, 2013). The purpose of the analysis may be to describe relationships between variables, clarify the relationships among theoretical concepts, or assist in identifying possible causal relationships, which then can be tested by analyses examining group differences. All the data for the analysis need to be from a single population from which values were available on all variables to be examined in the correlational analysis. Data measured at interval or ratio levels provide the best information on the nature of the relationship. However, correlational analysis procedures are available for most levels of measurement. Data for a correlational analysis also need to span the full range of possible values on each variable used in the analysis. For example, if values for a particular variable can range from a low of 1 to a high of 9, each of the values from 1 to 9 will probably be found in subjects in the data set. If all or most of the values are in the middle of that scoring range (4, 5, and 6) and few or none have extreme values, a full understanding of the relationship cannot be obtained from the analysis. Therefore large samples with diverse scores are desirable for correlational analyses (Grove et al., 2013).

Pearson Product-Moment Correlation

The Pearson product-moment correlation is an inferential analysis technique calculated to determine relationships among variables. Bivariate correlation measures the extent of the relationship between two variables. Data are collected from a single sample, and measures of the two variables to be examined must be available for each subject in the data set. Less commonly, data are obtained from two related subjects, such as breast cancer incidence in mothers and daughters. Correlational analysis provides two pieces of information about the data—the nature of a relationship (positive or negative) between the two variables and the magnitude (or strength) of the relationship.

Scatterplots sometimes are presented to illustrate the relationship graphically (see Figure 11-7). The outcomes of correlational analyses are symmetrical, rather than asymmetrical. Symmetrical means that the analysis gives no indication of the direction of the relationship. It is not possible to establish from correlational analysis whether variable A leads to or causes variable B, or that B causes A. Thus the focus of correlational analysis techniques is examining relationships, not determining cause and effect.

Interpreting Pearson Correlation Analysis Results

The outcome of the Pearson product-moment correlation analysis is a correlation coefficient (r) with a value between -1 and $+1$. This r value indicates the degree of relationship between the two variables. A value of 0 indicates no relationship. A value of $r = -1$ indicates a perfect negative (inverse) correlation. In a negative relationship, a high score on one variable is correlated with a low score on the other variable. A value of $r = +1$ indicates a perfect positive relationship. In a positive relationship, a high score on one variable is correlated with a high score on the other variable. A positive correlation also exists when a low score on one variable is correlated with a low score on the other variable. The variables vary or change in the same direction, either increasing or decreasing together. As the negative or positive values of r approach 0, the strength of the relationship decreases (Grove, 2007).

Traditionally, an r value of less than 0.3 or -0.3 is considered to indicate a weak relationship and a value between 0.3 and 0.5 or -0.3 and -0.5 indicates a moderate relationship; if the r value is above 0.5 or -0.5, it is considered a strong relationship (Grove et al., 2013). However, this interpretation of the r value depends to a great extent on the variables being examined and the situation in which they were measured. Therefore interpretation requires some judgment on the part of the researcher.

When Pearson's correlation coefficient is squared (r^2), the resulting number is the percentage of variance explained by the relationship. Even when two variables are related, values of the two variables will not be a perfect match. For example, if two variables show a strong positive relationship, a high score on one variable can be expected to be associated with a high score on the other variable. However, a subject who has the highest score on one value will not necessarily have the highest score on the other variable. Thus r^2 indicates the variance that is known by correlating two variables (Grove, 2007).

There will be some variation in the relationship between values for the two variables for individual subjects. Some of the variation in values is explained by the relationship between the two variables and is called explained variance, which is indicated by r^2 and is expressed as a percentage. For example, researchers may state that the relationship of the two variables anxiety and depression in their study is $r = 0.6$, and $r^2 = 0.36 \times 100\% = 36\%$. Thus the explained variance is 36% for the variables anxiety and depression, which means that patients' anxiety scores can explain 36% of the variance in their depression scores. However, part of the variation is the result of factors other than the relationship and is called unexplained variance. In the example provided, $100\% - 36\%$ (explained variance) $= 64\%$ (unexplained variance). Therefore 64% of the variation in scores is a result of something other than the relationship studied, perhaps variables not examined in the study. A strong correlation has less unexplained variance than a weak correlation.

There has been a tendency to disregard weak correlations in nursing research. This approach can result in overlooking a relationship that may actually have some meaning within nursing knowledge if the relationship is examined in the context of other variables. Three common reasons for this situation, which is similar to that of a type II error, have been recognized. First, many nursing measurements are not powerful enough to detect fine discriminations. Some instruments may not detect extreme scores, and a relationship may be stronger than that indicated by the crude measures available. Second, correlational studies must have a wide range of scores for relationships to be detected. If the study scores are homogeneous or the sample is small, relationships that exist in the population may not show up as clearly in the sample. Third, in many cases, bivariate analysis does not provide a clear picture of the dynamics in the situation. A number of variables can be linked through weak correlations, but together they provide increased insight into situations of interest. Statistical procedures (e.g., regression analysis [see later]) are available for examining the relationships among multiple variables simultaneously (Plichta & Kelvin, 2013).

Testing the Significance of a Correlation Coefficient

Before inferring that the sample correlation coefficient applies to the population from which the sample was taken, statistical analysis must be performed to determine whether the coefficient is significantly different from zero (no correlation). With a small sample, a very high correlation coefficient can be nonsignificant. With a very large sample, the correlation coefficient can be statistically significant when the degree of association is too small to be clinically important. Therefore in judging the significance of the coefficient, both the size of the coefficient and its statistical significance need to be considered.

RESEARCH EXAMPLE

Correlation Results

Research Study

Bingham and colleagues (2009) conducted a descriptive correlational study examining the relationships of obesity and cholesterol in a sample of 4013 fourth-grade children in three different countries. The purpose of this study was to describe, correlate, and compare "two risk factors for future CVD [cardiovascular disease] in United States (U.S.), French, and Japanese children. Total serum cholesterol and two measures of overweight, including BMI [body mass index] and body fat percentage, were examined in children 9 to 10 years of age from Japan, France, and the U.S. (Whites and Blacks)" (Bingham et al., 2009, p. 316). The researchers correlated BMI with total cholesterol for males and females in the three countries and presented their results in a table (Table 11-6).

TABLE 11-6　Correlation of Body Mass Index with Total Cholesterol

	France (N=570)	Japan (N=1865)	U.S. White (N=1226)	U.S. Black (N=324)
Males				
Pearson r	0.02	0.17	0.24	0.29
p Value	0.6960	0.0001	0.0001	0.0002
Females				
Pearson r	0.12	0.12	0.22	-0.14
p Value	0.0494	0.0004	0.0001	0.0822

NOTE: The number of subjects varies slightly for each variable because of some missing data.
From Bingham, M. O., Harrell, J. S., Takada, H., Washino, K., Bradley, C., Berry, D., et al. (2009). Obesity and cholesterol in Japanese, French, and U.S. children. *Journal of Pediatric Nursing, 24*(4), 318.

Critical Appraisal

Bingham and associates (2009) conducted a Pearson product-moment correlation analysis to determine the relationships between BMI and total cholesterol for males and females from three different countries. This analytical technique was used to address the study purpose of determining the relationship between the BMI and total cholesterol. Because BMI and total cholesterol are both measured at the ratio level, Pearson's correlational analysis is the appropriate technique for examining relationships between these two variables. The researchers clearly presented the results of the correlation of BMI with total cholesterol in a table format (APA, 2010). The table includes the group size *(n)* for each country and the *p* value for each correlation value *(r)*. If the *p* values are less than or equal to $\alpha = 0.05$, then the correlations are significant. Table 11-6 includes six significant correlations and two nonsignificant correlations. The researchers noted that the numbers of subjects varied for each variable because of missing data. They might have expanded on the reasons for the missing data in the narrative of the article.

As part of the critical appraisal, you are also encouraged to interpret the results from this table. Six of the correlations or *r* values are significant, with $\alpha = 0.05$ indicating that there is a statistically significant relationship between BMI and total cholesterol for the three countries. The strongest relationship was for U.S. Black males ($r = 0.29$) and the weakest relationship was for French males ($r = 0.02$; Bingham et al., 2009). However, all the correlation values are small or less than 0.30 (Grove, 2007). Even the largest correlation at $r = 0.29$ only explains 8.4% of the variance between BMI and total cholesterol. This is calculated by $r^2 \times 100\% = 0.29^2 \times 100\% = 0.084 \times 100\% = 8.4\%$. The unexplained variance in this relationship is $100\% - 8.4\% = 91.6\%$. Thus most of the correlational results in Table 11-6 are statistically significant but the clinical importance is still in question. Clinical importance is discussed in greater detail later in this chapter.

Implications for Practice

Bingham and co-workers (2009) reached the following conclusion:

"It appears that the relationship between obesity [BMI] and total cholesterol may vary by culture or ethnicity and by gender, indicating the need for more culture- and gender-specific studies in children to evaluate the relative importance of these common risk factors for developing CVD. A better understanding of the impact of culture and gender on obesity and cholesterol levels in children will help nurse clinicians as they assess children for risk factors for CVD and will provide information that may be used to develop culturally specific interventions to reduce these risk factors. It is important to monitor BMI and cholesterol in children 9-10 years old; however, additional research is needed to determine the impact of these two variables on the future development of CVD." (Bingham et al., 2009, p. 320)

Factor Analysis

Factor analysis examines interrelationships among large numbers of variables and disentangles those relationships to identify clusters of variables that are most closely linked. Intellectually, you might do this by identifying categories and sorting the variables according to your judgment of the most appropriate category. Factor analysis sorts the variables into categories according to how closely related they are to the other variables. Closely related variables are grouped together into a factor. Several factors may be identified within a data set. Once the factors have been identified mathematically, the researcher must interpret the results by explaining why the analysis grouped the variables in a specific way. Statistical results will indicate the amount of variance in the data set that can be explained by a particular factor and the amount of variance in the factor that can be explained by a particular variable.

Factor analysis aids in the identification of theoretical constructs; it is also used to confirm the accuracy of a theoretically developed construct. For example, a theorist may state that the concept (or construct) of "hope" consists of the following elements: (1) anticipation of the future; (2) belief that things will work out for the best; and (3) optimism. Ways to measure these three elements can be developed. The measurement instrument operationalizes the theoretical construct, such as hope. A factor analysis can be conducted on the data to determine whether subject responses clustered into these three groupings identified for the concept hope.

Factor analysis is frequently used in the process of developing measurement instruments, particularly those related to psychological variables, such as attitudes, beliefs, values, and opinions (Grove et al., 2013). Factor analysis is used to examine the construct validity of a scale for the population studied. For example, factor analysis might be used to examine the construct validity of a multi-item Likert scale to measure hope in a group of older adults. We want to provide you with some idea of the meaning of factor analysis when you see it in research reports.

USING STATISTICS TO PREDICT OUTCOMES

The ability to predict future events is becoming increasingly more important worldwide. People are interested in predicting who will win the football game, what the weather will be like next week, or which stocks are likely to increase in value in the near future. In nursing practice, as in the rest of society, the ability to predict is crucial. For example, nurse researchers would like to be able to predict the length of a hospital stay for patients with illnesses of different severity, as well as the responses of patients with a variety of characteristics (e.g., age, gender, level of education) to nursing interventions. Nurses need to know which variables play an important role in predicting health outcomes in patients and families (Doran, 2011). For example, variables of BMI, blood lipid levels, and smoking pack-years (number of years smoking times the number of packs smoked per day) have been used to predict the outcome of the incidence of myocardial infarction (MI). Predictive analyses are based on probability theory, not on decision theory. Prediction is one approach for examining causal relationships between or among variables.

Regression Analysis

Regression analysis is used to predict the value of one variable when the value of one or more other variables is known. The variable to be predicted in a regression analysis is referred to as the dependent or outcome variable. The dependent variable is usually measured at the interval or ratio level. The goal of the analysis is to explain as much of the variance in the dependent variable as possible. In regression analysis, variables used to predict values of the dependent variable are referred to as independent variables. When one independent variable is used to predict a dependent variable, the analytical procedure used is simple linear regression. Multiple regression is used to analyze study data that include two or more independent variables. In regression analysis, the symbol for the dependent variable is Y, and the symbol for the independent variable(s) is X. Scatterplots and a bivariate correlation matrix are often developed before regression analysis is performed to examine the relationships that exist among the variables. The purpose of the regression analysis is to develop a line of best fit that will best reflect the values on the scatterplot. The line of best fit is often illustrated as an overlay on the scatterplot (Figure 11-9). Many regression analysis techniques have been developed to analyze various types of data. One type, logistic regression, was developed to predict values of a dependent variable measured at the nominal level. Logistic regression is being used with increasing frequency in nursing studies. This type of regression can test whether a patient responds or did not respond to the intervention (Grove et al. 2013; Hoare & Hoe, 2013; Plichta & Kelvin, 2013).

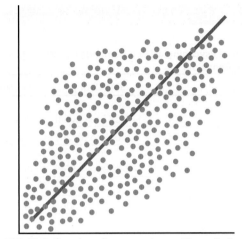

FIG 11-9 Overlay of scatterplot and best-fit line.

Interpreting Results

The outcome of a regression analysis is the regression coefficient, R. When R is squared (R^2), it indicates the amount of variance in the data that is explained by the equation (Grove, 2007). When more than one independent variable is being used to predict values of the dependent variable, R^2 is sometimes referred to as the coefficient of multiple determination. The test statistic used to determine the significance of a regression coefficient may be t (from t-test) or F (from the analysis of variance [ANOVA]). Small sample sizes decrease the possibility of obtaining statistical significance. Values for R^2 and t or F are reported with the results of a regression analysis. The calculated coefficient values may also be expressed as an equation. Many studies using regression analysis are complex, including multiple independent variables and involving more than one regression procedure. Understanding the discussion of complex results requires reading each sentence carefully for comprehension, looking up unfamiliar terms, and determining the statistical significance of the results.

⚡ RESEARCH EXAMPLE

Regression Analysis

Research Study Excerpt

Dickson, Howe, Deal, and McCarthy (2012) conducted a descriptive, predictive correlational study to determine how predictive job characteristics (job demands, job control, workplace support) were of self-care adherence behaviors (adherence to medication, diet, exercise, and symptom monitoring) in older workers with CVD. The steps of this study are presented in Chapter 2, and Figure 2-2 illustrates a copy of the study framework model that was tested using regression analysis. Dickson and colleagues (2012) presented their multiple regression analysis results, as shown in Table 11-7.

Continued

RESEARCH EXAMPLE—cont'd

TABLE 11-7   **Regression of Psychological Job Demands and Workplace Support on Self-Care Adherence Behaviors**

	β	95% CI of β	p Value	Total R^2	Cohen's f^2
Model Controls					
Depression	−.870	(−1.687 to −.054)	0.111	.119	.136*
Physical functioning	.219	(.011 to .447)	0.040		
+ Job Characteristics					
Psychological job demands	−.525	(−1.049 to −.002)	0.049	.214	.272[†]
Job control	.046	(−.321 to .412)	0.803		
Workplace support	1.350	(−.095 to 2.605)	0.035		

CI, confidence interval.
*Considered a medium effect size.
[†]Medium to large effect size.
From Dickson, V. V., Howe, A., Deal, J., & McCarthy, M. M. (2012). The relationship of work, self-care, and quality of life in a sample of older working adults with cardiovascular disease. *Heart & Lung, 41*(1), 10 (Table 2 in the article).

They provided the following discussion of those results:

"Regression analysis was used to assess the relationship among job characteristics (psychological job demands, job control, and workplace support by supervisors) and self-care adherence behaviors, controlling for depression and physical functioning (see Table 11-7). Depression and physical functioning were entered at step 1 [and] explained 11.9% [$R^2 = .119$; see Table 11-7] of the variance in adherence to treatment recommendations. After entry of the job characteristic variables of psychological job demands, job control, and workplace support by supervisors at step 2, the total variance explained was 21.4% ($p < .0001$) [$R^2 = .214$]." (Dickson et al., 2012, pp 9-10)

Critical Appraisal

Dickson and associates (2012) clearly stated their study purpose and objectives that supported the use of regression analysis to examine their use of job characteristics to predict the outcome of self-care adherence behaviors in these older working adults. Regression analysis is appropriate to predict a dependent variable (self-care adherence behaviors) using independent variables (psychological job demands, job control, workplace support, depression, and physical functioning). The results of the multiple regression analysis were clearly presented in Table 11-7 and discussed in the article narrative. The study identified three independent variables, physical functioning ($p = 0.04$), psychological job demands ($p = 0.049$), and workplace supervisor support ($p = 0.035$; see the p value column in Table 11-7) to be significant predictors of the dependent variable of self-care adherence behaviors. The results of the study explained 21.4% ($R^2 \times 100\%$) of the variance in self-care adherence behaviors in older workers with CVD.

Implications for Practice

Dickson and co-workers (2012) identified the following recommendations for further research and implications for practice:

"Research to develop and test interventions to foster worksite programs that facilitate self-care behaviors among older workers with CVD is needed. Research efforts should include the objective measurement of adherence and self-care.... Programs that target general self-care such as diet and exercise...are indicated to address the needs across the working population. Nurses with expertise in occupational health are well suited to champion these efforts. In addition, because job characteristics may interfere with self-care... nurses should assess job demands and include stress reduction as part of patient counseling for workers with CVD during routine office visits." (Dickson et al., 2012, p. 12)

USING STATISTICS TO EXAMINE DIFFERENCES

Inferential statistics are used to examine differences between or among groups, such as examining difference between experimental and control groups on selected demographic variables (see Table 11-1 in this chapter's first research example). Differences are also examined among other types of groups, such as examining differences of blood lipid values between males and females or differences in fasting blood sugar (FBS) and hemoglobin A1c (HgbA1c) levels among Caucasian, African American, American Indian, and Hispanic racial and ethnic groups. Statistical procedures used to examine differences are also conducted to examine causality of the independent variable on the dependent variable. Causality is a way of knowing that one event causes another. Because they can be used to understand the effects of interventions, statistical procedures that examine causality are critical to the development of nursing science. These statistics examine causality by testing for significant differences between or among groups, such as the differences between the experimental and control groups. The statistical procedures used to examine differences included in this text are the chi-square test of independence, *t*-test, ANOVA, and analysis of covariance (ANCOVA). The *t*-test is used to examine differences between two groups and the chi-square test, ANOVA, and ANCOVA can be used to examine differences among three or more groups. The chi-square test is used to analyze nominal or ordinal levels of data, and ANOVA and ANCOVA are conducted to analyze interval and ratio levels of data (Grove et al., 2013; Hoare & Hoe, 2013).

When differences are examined among three groups, posthoc analyses are conducted to determine which of the groups are significantly different. The chi-square test and ANOVA indicate significant differences among the groups but do not specify which groups are different. For example, a study may examine four occupational groups of workers who are smokers to determine differences in smoking behaviors among the groups. Chi-square analysis or ANOVA may show significant differences among the groups, but posthoc analyses are needed to identify which of the four groups are significantly different. If a study has three or more groups being compared for differences, researchers usually identify the type of posthoc analysis conducted and discuss the results.

Chi-Square Test of Independence

The chi-square test of independence determines whether two variables are independent or related; the test can be used with nominal or ordinal data. The procedure examines the frequencies of observed values and compares them with the frequencies that would be expected if the data categories were independent of each other. The procedure is not very powerful; thus, the risk of a type II error is high (outcome of the study is nonsignificant when significant differences actually exist). Large sample sizes are needed to decrease the risk of a type II error. Most studies using this procedure place little importance on results in which no differences are found. Researchers frequently perform multiple chi-square tests in a sample. However, results generally are presented only when a chi-square analysis shows a significant difference.

Interpreting Results

Often, the first reaction to a sentence about "significant differences" by those unfamiliar with reading statistical results is panic. However, a sentence that looks dense with statistics provides a great deal of information in a small amount of space. For example, in the component "(χ^2 [1] = 18.10, $p = 0.001$)," the author is using chi-square (χ^2) analysis to compare two groups on a selected variable, such as the presence or absence of chronic illness. The author provides the degrees of freedom ($df = [1]$), so that the reader can validate the accuracy of the results using a statistical chi-square table (see the text by Grove et al., 2013, p. 683, for a χ^2 statistical table). The numerical value after the first equal sign, 18.10, is the chi-square (χ^2) value obtained from calculating the chi-square equation (probably using a computer). This value has no inherent meaning other than to determine significance on a statistical table. As noted earlier, the symbol p is the abbreviation for probability. The groups were significantly different because $p = 0.001$, which is below the level of significance set at $\alpha = 0.05$. The phrase also indicates that the probability is 1 in 1000 that these groups come from the same population. Therefore the two groups are significantly different because there is only 1 chance in 1000 that the study results are in error.

If a study variable has only two categories, such as the presence or absence of chronic illness, the researchers know the location of the significant difference. However, the exact location of specific differences among more than two categories of variables cannot be determined from chi-square analysis alone. Chi-square analysis identifies whether there is a significant difference, and posthoc analyses can be used to identify the categories in which the significant differences occur.

RESEARCH EXAMPLE

Chi-Square Results

Research Study

Lavoie-Tremblay and colleagues (2008) examined the influence of psychosocial work environment variables on the psychological health of recently educated nurses. The psychosocial work environment variables included effort-reward imbalance, lack of social support from colleagues and superiors, high psychological demand, low decision latitude, and elevated job strain. The nurse participants were divided into two dichotomous groups, those with high psychological distress and those with low psychological distress. The researchers conducted chi-square analysis to determine differences between the two groups of nurses for the psychosocial work environment variables and presented their findings in Table 11-8. Lavoie-Tremblay and associates (2008) noted that the two psychological distress risk groups were significantly different on three psychosocial work environment variables: (1) effort-reward balance ($\chi^2 [1] = 30.471$, $p = 0.000$); (2) high psychological demand ($\chi^2 [1] = 17.625$, $p = 0.000$); and (3) elevated job strain ($\chi^2 [1] = 8.96$, $p = 0.003$).

TABLE 11-8   Chi-Square Analysis of Psychosocial Work Environment Dimensions and Psychological Distress

Psychological Distress and Psychosocial Work Environment Variables	High n	Low n	χ^2	df	p Value
Effort-reward imbalance	101	79	30.471[†]	1	0.000
Lack of social support from colleagues and superiors	84	93	2.443	1	0.118
High psychological demand	87	71	17.625[†]	1	0.000
Low decision latitude	83	96	1.317	1	0.251
Elevated job strain	51	39	8.960[*]	1	0.003

[*]$p = 0.05$
[†]$p = 0.01$
From Lavoie-Tremblay, M., Wright, D., Desforges, N., Gelinas, C., & Marchionni, C., Drevniok, U. (2008). Creating a healthy workplace for new-generation nurses. *Journal of Nursing Scholarship, 40*(3), 294.

Critical Appraisal

Chi-square analysis is appropriate to examine differences between the two groups of nurses that were dichotomized into those with high and low psychological distress. The chi-square results were clearly presented in Table 11-8 and discussed in the text of the article. The chi-square results included the χ^2 values, the df ($df = 1$ for the two groups), and the p values (probability of obtaining each chi-square value). The * or † indicated the level of significance of the chi-square value. Three of the psychosocial work environment variables were significantly linked to psychological distress. Because only two levels or groups of psychological distress risk (high and low) were examined, no posthoc analyses were required.

Implications for Practice

Lavoie-Tremblay and associates (2008) identified the following implications for practice and suggestions for further research:

"As the current worldwide nursing labor shortage is expected to grow worse, retention strategies are needed that will be focused on the psychological health of new generation nurses by targeting the psychosocial work environment. Nursing managers need to revise or develop retention and workplace health-promotion strategies, tailored specifically to next generations, to temper the effect of the nursing shortage. Research is needed on the meaning of reward at work for nurses from Generation Y. How is the effort/reward imbalance perceived? Can the way care is organized be changed to increase perceived rewards in the context of a shortage of healthcare providers and limited financial resources?... Nurse managers play a critical role in continuing to strive towards improving work environments so that new nurses do not forget the heart and soul of nursing and do remain committed to the ideals of caring that led them to the profession in the first place." (Lavoie-Tremblay et al., 2008, p. 296)

t-Test

One of the most common analyses used to test for significant differences between two samples is the *t*-test. The *t*-test is used to examine group differences when the variables are measured at the interval or ratio level of measurement. A variety of *t*-tests have been developed for various types of samples. For example, when independent groups are being compared, the *t*-test for independent samples is used. For paired or dependent groups, the *t*-test for paired samples is used (see Figure 11-8).

Sometimes researchers misuse the *t*-test by conducting multiple *t*-tests to examine differences in various aspects of data collected in a study. This misapplication will result in an escalation of significance that increases the risk of a type I error (saying that something is significant when it is not). The Bonferroni procedure, which controls for the escalation of significance, may be used when multiple *t*-tests must be performed on different aspects of the same data.

Interpreting Results

The result of the mathematical calculation is a *t* statistic. This statistic is compared with the *t* values in a statistical table (see Grove et al., 2013, pp. 677-678). The table is used to identify the critical value of *t*. If the computed statistic is greater than or equal to the critical value, the groups are significantly different.

🔎 RESEARCH EXAMPLE

t-Test

Research Study

Kim and co-workers (2012) conducted *t*-tests for independent samples to determine differences between the experimental and control groups in their study. This study was introduced earlier in this chapter and focused on determining the effects of the independent variable of an aquarobic exercise program on the dependent variables of self-efficacy, pain, body weight, blood lipids, and depression of patients with osteoarthritis. This study was conducted using a quasi-experimental pretest–post-test design with a nonequivalent control group (see Chapter 8 for a model of this design). Study participants were randomly assigned to the experimental or control group, resulting in independent groups. The two groups were not significantly different on the pretest, indicating that the groups were similar for the dependent variables at the start of the study (see Table 11-5 of Kim and associates' study). The experimental group received the exercise program for 12 weeks and then the post-tests were conducted. The results of the *t*-tests are presented in Table 11-9. The experimental and control groups were significantly different on the post-tests for all dependent variables because the *p* values were less than $\alpha = 0.05$.

Continued

RESEARCH EXAMPLE—cont'd

TABLE 11-9   Changes in Dependent Variables between Experimental and Control Groups

Variables	Pretest $M \pm SD$	Post-Test $M \pm SD$	Difference $M \pm SD$	t	p
Self-efficacy					
Experimental (n=35)	1124.87±206.75	1251.46±219.40	126.59±22.77	4.79	0.001
Control (n=35)	1166.00±152.31	1018.65±224.08	−147.35±61.31		
Pain					
Experimental (n=35)	6.83±1.92	6.14±1.80	−0.69±1.7	−2.37	0.021
Control (n=35)	7.03±1.99	7.26±1.92	0.23±1.5		
Body weight					
Experimental (n=35)	60.86±9.48	60.10±8.91	−0.76±1.19	−2.59	0.012
Control (n=35)	59.19±5.87	59.15±5.86	−0.04±1.04		
Blood lipids					
Total cholesterol (mg)					
Experimental (n=35)	212.95±43.47	195.00±33.04	−17.94±5.9	−2.10	0.040
Control (n=35)	218.20±39.51	219.46±40.20	1.26±7.0		
Triglycerides (mg)					
Experimental (n=35)	157.34±121.25	135.94±80.97	−21.40±9.6	−2.26	0.027
Control (n=35)	123.34±60.21	128.51±55.83	5.17±6.8		
HDL Cholesterol (mg)					
Experimental (n=35)	57.06±25.09	58.92±26.01	1.86±1.2	2.54	0.014
Control (n=35)	64.03±27.47	60.60±26.04	−3.43±1.7		
Depression					
Experimental (n=35)	32.66±8.05	29.94±7.25	−2.72±1.5	−3.20	.002
Control (n=35)	32.26±4.93	37.53±9.67	5.27±1.9		

From Kim, I., Chung, S., Park, Y., & Kang, H. (2012). The effectiveness of an aquarobic exercise program for patients with osteoarthritis. *Applied Nursing Research, 25*(3), p. 187 (Table 5 from the article).

Critical Appraisal

Kim and co-workers (2012) clearly presented the results of their *t*-tests for independent samples in tables for the pretests (see Table 11-5) and post-tests (see Table 11-9). The *t*-test analysis technique was appropriate because the focus of the study was to determine differences between the experimental and control groups for selected dependent variables measured at the interval or ratio level (Grove et al., 2013; Plichta & Kelvin, 2013). There were significant differences between the two groups for all dependent variables (self-efficacy, pain, body weight, blood lipids, and depression). The lack of nonsignificant findings indicated adequate power to detect group differences—no type II errors. The significant findings support the effectiveness of the aquarobic exercise program in improving outcomes for patients with osteoarthritis. However, conducting multiple *t*-tests without the Bonferroni procedure raises a concern about an increased risk for a type I error. The study results would have been strengthened by including the Bonferroni correction for multiple *t*-tests.

Implications for Practice

The implications of the study findings for practice were discussed earlier in this chapter.

Analysis of Variance (ANOVA)

Analysis of variance (ANOVA) is a parametric statistical technique used to examine differences among three or more groups. Because this is a parametric analysis, the variables must be measured at the interval or ratio level. There are many types of ANOVA; some are developed for analysis of data from complex experimental designs (Grove et al., 2013; Plichta & Kelvin, 2013). Rather than focusing just on differences between means, ANOVA tests for differences in variance. One source of variance is the variance within each group, because individual scores in the group will vary from the group mean. This variance is referred to as the within-group variance. Another source of variance is the variation of the group means around the grand mean, referred to as the between-group variance. The assumption is that if all the samples are taken from the same population, these two sources of variance will exhibit little difference. When these two types of variance are combined, they are referred to as the total variance.

Interpreting Results

The results of an ANOVA are reported as an F statistic. The F distribution table is used to determine the level of significance of the F statistic. (F statistical tables are provided in the text by Grove et al., 2013, pp. 680-682.) If the F statistic is equal to or greater than the appropriate table value, there is a statistically significant difference between the groups. If only two groups are being examined, the location of a significant difference is clear. However, if more than two groups are under study, it is not possible to determine from the ANOVA where the significant differences occur. Therefore posthoc analyses are conducted to determine the location of the differences among groups. The frequently used posthoc tests are the Bonferroni procedure and the Newman-Keuls', Tukey's honestly significantly difference (HSD), Scheffé's, and Dunnett's tests (Grove et al., 2013).

RESEARCH EXAMPLE

ANOVA

Research Study

In a study introduced earlier in this chapter by Bingham and colleagues (2009), the researchers examined the relationship of obesity and cholesterol in French, Japanese, and U.S. children (see Table 11-6). They also examined differences among their four study groups (French, Japanese, and U.S. White and Black children) for the variables of height, weight, BMI, body fat percentage, and cholesterol using an ANOVA. The researchers reported their findings in Table 11-10, which included the mean and SD for each variable for each of the four groups, along with the ANOVA results. The ANOVA results included an F value and a p value that indicated the significance of the results. For example, for the variable of height, $F = 23.3$ and $p = 0.0001$; this is a statistically significant result because p is less than $\alpha = 0.05$. The ANOVA results demonstrate significant differences among the four groups for all variables (height, weight, BMI, body fat percentage, and cholesterol).

Continued

RESEARCH EXAMPLE—cont'd

TABLE 11-10   BMI, Body Fat, and Cholesterol by Group

Variables	France (n=570)	Japan (n=1865)	U.S. Whites (n=1226)	U.S. Blacks (n=324)	f	p
Height (cm)	137.5±6.6	136.4±6.4	137.3±6.5	139.6±7.4	23.3	0.0001
Weight (kg)	32.3±6.3	32.5±6.6	35.3±9.1	37.9±10.3	71.8	0.0001
BMI (kg/m²)	17.0±2.4	17.3±2.6	18.6±3.6	19.2±3.9	78.6	0.0001
Body fat (%)	17.7±6.8	18.8±5.9	23.1±10.3	22.1±11.4	84.6	0.0001
Cholesterol (mmol/L)	4.73±0.89	4.38±0.66	4.25±0.75	4.47±0.82	54.7	0.001
Cholesterol conversion (mg/dL)	183.0±34.6	169.4±25.5	164.3±29.1	172.7±31.9		

NOTE: Number of subjects varies slightly for each variable because of some missing data.
From Bingham, M. O., Harrell, J. S., Takada, H., Washino, K., Bradley, C., Berry, D., et al. (2009). Obesity and cholesterol in Japanese, French, and U.S. children. *Journal of Pediatric Nursing, 24*(4), 317.

Critical Appraisal

Bingham and associates (2009) conducted their study for the purpose of determining differences among four groups of children (French, Japanese, U.S. Black, and U.S. White) on the variables of height, weight, BMI, body fat percentage, and total cholesterol. These study variables were measured at the ratio level of measurement. ANOVA is the appropriate analysis technique to use with two or more study groups and for variables measured at least at the interval level of measurement. They clearly presented their ANOVA results in table format and discussed these results in the results section of their article.

"The U.S. Black children were the tallest, followed by French, U.S. White, and Japanese participants, with minimal differences in height between the French and U.S. White children. Weight was highest in the U.S. Black children and lowest in French children. BMI was highest in U.S. Black children, followed by U.S. White, Japanese, and French children. Body fat percentage was highest in U.S. White children and lowest in French children. Findings were quite different for total cholesterol, which was highest in French children and lowest in U.S. White children." (Bingham et al., 2009, p. 317)

The researchers did not discuss conducting a posthoc analysis to determine where the significant differences were among the four groups (French, Japanese, and U.S. Black and White children) for the study variables. This study would have been strengthened by a discussion of posthoc analysis to determine where the significant differences occurred among the four groups.

Implications for Practice

Bingham and co-workers (2009) noted the following findings from their study:

"Japanese and French children were significantly leaner than U.S. children (Black and White), with U.S. Black children having the highest BMI (19.2) and U.S. White children the highest body fat percentage (23.1%).... The noted increase in childhood obesity in the United States has been described as resulting from a combination of factors including biological, social, and environmental that may vary and interact differently by country, culture, and race/ethnicity.... The results of our comparison reinforce the need for standards to assess obesity using the same methods of measurement. This uniformity would enable researchers and clinicians to better document and understand differences between countries or ethnic groups and provide more consistency to assess change over time." (Bingham et al., 2009, pp. 318-319)

These researchers recommended using the BMI as the best measure of overweight children, but acknowledged that the cutoff point for risk of or actual clinical complications is still unclear. They recommended additional studies of children in the United States and other countries to determine the link of obesity and total cholesterol with CVD. The QSEN (2013) implication is that the BMI is the best evidence-based measure to identify overweight children and should be monitored by nurses and other healthcare providers.

Analysis of Covariance (ANCOVA)

Analysis of covariance (ANCOVA) allows the researcher to examine the effect of a treatment apart from the effect of one or more potentially confounding variables (see Chapter 5 for a discussion of confounding variables). Potentially confounding variables that are generally of concern include pretest scores, age, education, social class, and anxiety level. These variables would be confounding if they were not measured and if their effects on study variables were not statistically removed by performing regression analysis before performing ANOVA. This strategy removes the effect of differences among groups that is caused by a confounding variable. Once this effect is removed, the effect of the treatment can be examined more precisely. This technique sometimes is used as a method of statistical control when it is not possible to design the study so that potentially confounding variables are controlled. However, control through careful planning of the design is more effective than statistical control.

ANCOVA may be used in pretest–post-test designs in which differences occur in groups on the pretest. For example, people who achieve low scores on a pretest tend to have lower scores on the post-test than those whose pretest scores were higher, even if the treatment had a significant effect on post-test scores. Conversely, if a person achieves a high pretest score, it is doubtful that the post-test will indicate a strong change as a result of the treatment. ANCOVA maximizes the capability to detect differences in such cases. This information was provided so that you might understand why ANCOVA is conducted and are able to identify the confounding variables in a study that you are critically appraising.

INTERPRETING RESEARCH OUTCOMES

To be useful, the evidence from data analysis must be carefully examined, organized, and given meaning. Evaluating the entire research process, organizing the meaning of the results, and forecasting the usefulness of the findings are all part of interpreting research outcomes. Within the process of interpretation of research outcomes are several intellectual activities that can be isolated and explored, including examining findings, exploring the significance of the findings, identifying limitations, forming conclusions, generalizing the findings, considering implications for nursing, and suggesting further studies. This information usually is included in the final section of published studies, which often is entitled "Discussion."

Types of Results

Interpretation of results from quasi-experimental and experimental studies is traditionally based on decision theory, with five possible results: (1) significant results that agree with those predicted by the researcher; (2) nonsignificant results; (3) significant results that are opposite from those predicted by the researcher; (4) mixed results; and (5) unexpected results (Grove et al., 2013; Shadish et al., 2002). In critically appraising a study, you need to identify which types of results are presented in the study.

Significant and Predicted Results

Significant results agree with those predicted by the researcher and support the logical links developed by the researcher among the framework, study questions, hypotheses, variables, and measurement tools. In examining the results, however, you must consider the possibility of alternative explanations for the positive findings. What other elements could possibly have led to the significant results?

Nonsignificant Results

Nonsignificant (or inconclusive) results, often referred to as "negative" results, may be a true reflection of reality. In that case, the reasoning of the researcher or the theory used by the researcher to develop the hypothesis is in error. If it is, the negative findings are an important addition to the body of knowledge. However, the results also may stem from a type II error resulting from inappropriate methodology, a biased or small sample, threats to the design validity (see Chapter 8), inadequate measurement methods, weak statistical measures, or faulty analysis. In such instances, the reported results could introduce faulty information into the body of knowledge (Angell, 1989). Negative results do not mean that no relationships exist among the variables. Negative results indicate only that the study failed to find any. Nonsignificant results provide no evidence of the truth or falsity of the hypothesis.

Significant and Unpredicted Results

Significant and unpredicted results are the opposite of those predicted by the researcher and indicate that flaws are present in the logic of the researcher and theory being tested. If the results are valid, however, they constitute an important addition to the body of knowledge. For example, a researcher may propose that social support and ego strength are positively correlated. If the relevant study shows instead that high social support is correlated with low ego strength, the result is the opposite of that predicted.

Mixed Results

Mixed results probably are the most common outcomes of studies. In this case, one variable may uphold predicted characteristics, whereas another does not, or two dependent measures of the same variable may show opposite results. These differences may be caused by methodology problems, such as differing reliability or sensitivity of two methods of measuring variables. The mixed results may also indicate that existing theory should be modified.

Unexpected Results

Unexpected results usually are relationships found between variables that were not hypothesized and not predicted from the framework being used. Most researchers examine as many elements of data as possible in addition to those directed by the questions. These findings can be useful in the modification of existing theory and development of new theories and later studies. In addition, unexpected or serendipitous results are important evidence for developing the implications of the study. However, serendipitous results must be interpreted carefully, because the study was not designed to examine these results.

Findings

Results in a study are translated and interpreted to become study findings. Although much of the process of developing findings from results occurs in the mind of the researcher, evidence of these thought processes can be found in published research reports.

Exploring the Significance of Findings

The significance of a study is associated with its importance in contributing to nursing's body of knowledge. The significance of study findings is not a dichotomous characteristic (significant or nonsignificant) because studies contribute in varying degrees to the body of knowledge. Significance of study findings may be associated with the amount of variance explained, degree of control in the study design to eliminate unexplained variance, or ability to detect statistically significant differences or relationships. To the extent possible at the time the study is reported, researchers are expected to clarify the significance of the study findings.

The true importance of a particular study may not become apparent for years after publication. Certain characteristics, however, are associated with the significance of studies—significant studies make an important difference in people's lives; it is possible to generalize the findings far beyond the study sample so that the findings have the potential of affecting large numbers of people. The implications of significant studies go beyond concrete facts to abstractions and lead to the generation of theory or revisions of existing theory (Fawcett & Garity, 2009; Hoare & Hoe, 2013; Hoe & Hoare, 2012). A very significant study has implications for one or more disciplines in addition to nursing. The study is accepted by others in the discipline and frequently is referenced in the literature. Over time, the significance of a study is measured by the number of other studies that it generates.

Clinical Importance of Findings

The strongest findings of a study are those that have both statistical significance and clinical importance. **Clinical importance** is related to the practical relevance of the findings. There is no common agreement in nursing about how to evaluate the clinical importance of a finding. The effect size, however, can be used to determine clinical importance. For example, one group of patients may have a body temperature 0.1° F higher than that of another group. Data analysis may indicate that the two groups are statistically significantly different, but the findings have no clinical importance. The difference is not sufficiently important to warrant changing patient care. In many studies, however, it is difficult to judge how much change would constitute clinical importance. In studies testing the effectiveness of a treatment, clinical importance may be demonstrated by the proportion of subjects who showed improvement or the extent to which subjects returned to normal functioning, but how much improvement must subjects demonstrate for the findings to be considered clinically important? Questions also arise regarding who should judge clinical importance—patients and their families, clinicians, researchers, or society at large. At this point in the development of nursing knowledge, clinical importance or relevance is ultimately a value judgment (Fawcett & Garity, 2009; Hoare & Hoe, 2013; LeFort, 1993).

Limitations

Limitations are restrictions or problems in a study that may decrease the generalizability of the findings. Study limitations often include a combination of theoretical and methodological weaknesses. Theoretical weaknesses in a study might include a poorly developed or linked study framework and unclear conceptual definitions of variables. The limited conceptual definitions of the variables might decrease the operationalization or measurement of the study variables. Methodological limitations result from factors such as nonrepresentative samples, weak designs, single setting, limited control over treatment (intervention) implementation, instruments with limited reliability and validity, limited control over data collection, and improper use of statistical analyses. These study limitations can limit the credibility of the findings and conclusions and restrict the population to which the findings can be generalized. Most researchers identify the limitations of their study in the discussion section of the research report and indicate how these limitations might have affected the study findings and conclusions. Identifying study limitations is positive but if these limitations are severe and multiple, the credibility of the findings need to be questioned.

Conclusions

Conclusions are a synthesis of the findings. In forming conclusions, the researcher uses logical reasoning, creates a meaningful whole from pieces of information obtained through data analysis and findings from previous studies, and considers alternative explanations of the data. One of the risks in developing conclusions is going beyond the study results or forming conclusions that are not warranted by the findings.

Generalizing the Findings

Generalization extends the implications of the findings from the sample studied to a larger population (see earlier, "Inference and Generalization"). For example, if the study was conducted on patients with osteoarthritis, it may be possible to generalize the findings from the sample to the larger target population of patients with osteoarthritis or to those with other types of arthritis. Kim and colleagues (2012) were very cautious in making generalizations related to their study findings about the effectiveness of the aquarobic exercise program. They indicated that their study participants were recruited from only one public health center and were most likely not representative of all patients with osteoarthritis. They recommended conducting studies with larger random samples from different settings before generalizing the study findings.

Implications for Nursing

Implications for nursing are the meanings of conclusions from scientific research for the body of nursing knowledge, theory, and practice (Chinn & Kramer, 2011). Implications are based on but are more specific than conclusions; they provide specific suggestions for implementing the findings in nursing. For example, a researcher may suggest how nursing practice should be modified. If a study indicates that a specific solution is effective in decreasing pressure ulcers in hospitalized older patients, the implications will state how the care of older patients needs to be modified to prevent pressure ulcers. Interventions with extensive research support provide the basis for developing EBP guidelines and ensuring quality, safe nursing practice (see Chapter 13).

Recommendations for Further Studies

In every study, the researcher gains knowledge and experience that can be used to design a better study next time. Therefore the researcher often will make suggestions for future studies that emerge logically from the present study. Recommendations for further study may include replications or repeating the design with a different or larger sample, using different measurement methods, or testing a new intervention. Recommendations may also include the formation of hypotheses to further test the framework in use. This section provides other researchers with ideas for future studies needed to develop the knowledge needed for EBP (Brown, 2014; Melnyk & Fineout-Overholt, 2011).

⁇ CRITICAL APPRAISAL GUIDELINES
Research Outcomes

When critically appraising the research outcomes of a study, you need to examine the discussion section of the research report and address the following questions:

1. What are the study findings, and were they appropriate considering the statistical results?
2. Were the study findings linked to previous research findings?
3. Were the findings clinically important?
4. What were the study limitations and how might they have affected the study conclusions?
5. Were the conclusions appropriate based on the study results, findings, and limitations?
6. To what population(s) did the researchers generalize the study findings? Were the generalizations appropriate?
7. What implications for nursing knowledge, theory, and practice were identified?
8. Were the implications for nursing practice appropriate based on the study findings and conclusions?
9. Did the researchers make recommendations for further studies? Were these recommendations based on the study results, findings, limitations, and conclusions?

RESEARCH EXAMPLE

Research Outcomes

Research Study Excerpt

The research outcomes from the discussion section of the study by Lee, Faucett, Gillen, Krause, and Landry (2013) is presented as an example and critically appraised. The purpose of this study was to investigate how "critical care nurses perceived the risk of musculoskeletal [MSK] injury from work and to identify factors associated with their risk perception" (Lee et al., 2013, p. 36). The study sample included 1000 critical care nurses who were randomly selected from the 2005 membership list of the American Association of Critical Care Nurses (AACN). This was a significant study, because nursing is an occupation with a high risk of MSK injury, and how nurses' perceive their risks for injury may be important in preventing work-related injuries. The following study excerpt includes information from the discussion section of this study; the key elements of this section are identified in brackets.

"Critical care nurses, overall, were concerned about ergonomic risks in their work environment. Eighty-three percent of study participants reported that they were more likely than not to experience an MSK injury within 1 year—a relatively short time frame. Particularly, critical care nurses were well aware of risks from manual patient handling, and they felt safer when performing tasks using a lifting device. However, more than half of the participants did not have lifting devices on their units.... Similar findings were shown in a survey by American Nurses Association." [findings compared to previous research].... (Lee et al., 2013, p. 40)

This study identified five significant predictors of risk perception for MSK injury among critical care nurses. Higher overall risk perceptions were associated significantly with greater job strain, higher physical workload index, more frequent patient handling, lack of availability of lift devices or lift teams, and higher MSK symptom index. Of these five variables, job strain and availability of lift devices or lift teams were significant for both risk perception to self and risk perception to others [statistically significant findings]....

Availability of lift devices or lift teams was associated also with all three risk perception measures. Risk perception of MSK injury was lower among nurses who had a lift device or a lift team than those who had neither [clinical importance of findings]. Indeed, actual reduction of risk of MSK injury by the use of lift devices or lift teams has been shown in many studies [findings linked to previous research]....The finding of a significant association between symptom experience and risk perception is meaningful because the ultimate goal of the study is to prevent MSK injury. Determining how risk perception influences injury prevention should be of interest to occupational health researchers, and further research is needed [recommendations for further research]....In addition to the limitations noted above, the representativeness of the sample across critical care nurses may have been limited by the response rates [limitation]. Furthermore, findings about critical care nurses may not generalize to nurses in different clinical settings [generalization of findings]. Also, the use of a single sample survey method may introduce bias related to social desirability or negative affectivity [limitation]."

Conclusions

"In conclusion, critical care nurses' perceptions about risk from their work environment were elucidated and their greater perception of risk for MSK injury was found to be associated with greater job strain, greater physical workload, more frequent patient-handling tasks, the lack of lifting devices or a lifting team, and experience of more severe MSK symptoms [conclusions]. This study provides a framework to assist occupational health professionals and nurse managers to better understand nurses' perceptions about their personal risks.... Occupational health professionals, nurse managers, and nursing organizations should make concerted efforts to ensure the safety of nurses by providing effective preventive measures. Improving the physical and psychosocial work environment may make nursing jobs safer, reduce the risk of MSK injury, and improve nurses' perceptions of job safety. Ultimately, these efforts would contribute to enhancing safety in nursing settings and to maintaining a healthy nursing workforce [implications for nursing]. Future research is needed to determine the role of risk perception in preventing a MSK injury." (Lee et al., 2013, pp. 42-43)

Continued

RESEARCH EXAMPLE—cont'd

Critical Appraisal

Lee and associates (2013) discussed their significant and nonsignificant findings, which were consistent with their study results. The findings were also compared with the findings of previous studies, and possible reasons were provided for nonsignificant findings. However, the researchers did not determine the power achieved with the non-significant results. The findings are clinically important because of the increased understanding provided regarding nurses' perceptions of their risk for MSK injuries.

Lee and co-workers (2013) clearly identified their study limitations, which limited the generalization of the find-ings. The findings were generalized to the accessible population of critical care nurses sampled but were limited by the response rate to the survey from being generalized to the target population of all critical care nurses in the AACN. In addition, the researchers indicated the findings could not be generalized to nurses in other clinical settings.

Lee and colleagues (2013) provided specific conclusions for their study at the end of their research report and clearly labeled the section "Conclusions." The conclusions were consistent with their study results and findings. The researchers' conclusions provided a basis for the implications for nursing practice and recommendations for further research. The implications for practice were clearly expressed and involved enhancing the safety of nurs-ing settings to maintain a healthy nursing workforce. The researchers made recommendations for areas of further research but they might have provided more specific ideas for future studies.

In summary, Lee and associates (2013) provided a comprehensive discussion section that addressed the essential findings, limitations, conclusions, generalizations, implications for nursing, and recommendations for further research. The QSEN (2013) implications are that nurses need a safe work environment to minimize their risk of MSK injury.

KEY CONCEPTS

- In critically appraising a quantitative study, you need to (1) identify the statistical procedures used, (2) judge whether these statistical procedures were appropriate for the hypotheses, ques-tions, or objectives of the study and the data available for analysis, (3) judge whether the authors' interpretation of the results is appropriate, and (4) evaluate the clinical importance of the findings.
- Quantitative data analysis has several stages: (1) management of missing data; (2) description of the study sample; (3) reliability of measurement methods; (4) conduct of exploratory analysis of the data; and (5) conduct of inferential analyses guided by the hypotheses, questions, or objectives.
- Understanding the statistical theories and relevant concepts will assist you in appraising quan-titative studies.
- Probability theory is used to explain a relationship, the probability of an event occurring in a given situation, or the probability of accurately predicting an event.
- Decision theory assumes that all the groups in a study used to test a particular hypothesis are components of the same population in relation to the study variables.
- A type I error occurs when the null hypothesis is rejected when it is true. The researchers con-clude that significant results exist in a study, when in reality they do not. The risk of a type I error is indicated by the level of significance (α).
- A type II error occurs when the null hypothesis is accepted when it is false. The researchers con-clude that the study results are nonsignificant when the results are significant. Type II errors often occur because of flaws in the research methods, and their risk can be examined using power analysis.

- Descriptive or summary statistics covered in this text include frequency distributions, percentages, measures of central tendency, measures of dispersion, and scatterplot.
- Statistical analyses conducted to examine relationships that are covered in this text include Pearson product-moment correlation and factor analysis.
- Regression analysis is conducted to predict the value of one dependent variable using one or more independent variables.
- Statistical analyses conducted to examine group differences and determine causality included in this text are the chi-square test, *t*-test, analysis of variance (ANOVA), and analysis of covariance (ANCOVA).
- Interpretation of results from quasi-experimental and experimental studies is traditionally based on decision theory, with five possible results: (1) significant results predicted by the researcher; (2) nonsignificant results; (3) significant results that are opposite from those predicted by the researcher; (4) mixed results; and (5) unexpected results.
- Research outcomes usually include findings, limitations, conclusions, generalization of findings, implications for nursing, and recommendations for further studies.
- In critically appraising a study, you will need to evaluate the appropriateness and completeness of the researchers' results and discussion sections.

REFERENCES

American Psychological Association (APA). (2010). *Publication manual of the American Psychological Association* (6th ed.). Washington, DC: Author.

Angell, M. (1989). Negative studies. *New England Journal of Medicine, 321*(7), 464–466.

Bingham, M. O., Harrell, J. S., Takada, H., Washino, K., Bradley, C., Berry, D., et al. (2009). Obesity and cholesterol in Japanese, French, and U.S. children. *Journal of Pediatric Nursing, 24*(4), 314–322.

Brown, S. J. (2014). *Evidence-based nursing: The research-practice connection* (3rd ed.). Sudbury, MA: Jones & Bartlett.

Chinn, P. L., & Kramer, M. K. (2011). *Integrated theory and knowledge development in nursing* (8th ed.). St. Louis: Elsevier Mosby.

Cohen, J. (1988). *Statistical power analysis for the behavioral sciences* (2nd ed.). New York: Academic Press.

Craig, J., & Smyth, R. (2012). *The evidence-based practice manual for nurses* (3rd ed.). Edinburgh: Churchill Livingstone Elsevier.

Dickson, V. V., Howe, A., Deal, J., & McCarthy, M. M. (2012). The relationship of work, self-care, and quality of life in a sample of older working adults with cardiovascular disease. *Heart & Lung, 41*(1), 5–14.

Doran, D. M. (2011). *Nursing outcomes: The state of the science* (2nd ed.). Burlington, MA: Jones & Bartlett Learning.

Fawcett, J., & Garity, J. (2009). *Evaluating research for evidence-based nursing practice*. Philadelphia: F. A. Davis.

Grove, S. K. (2007). *Statistics for health care research: A practical workbook*. St. Louis: Elsevier Saunders.

Grove, S. K., Burns, N., & Gray, J. R. (2013). *The practice of nursing research: Appraisal, synthesis, and generation of evidence* (7th ed.). St. Louis: Elsevier Saunders.

Hoare, Z., & Hoe, J. (2013). Understanding quantitative research: Part 2. *Nursing Standard (Royal College of Nursing [Great Britain]), 27*(18), 48–55.

Hoe, J., & Hoare, Z. (2012). Understanding quantitative research: Part 1. *Nursing Standard (Royal College of Nursing [Great Britain]), 27*(15–17), 52–57.

Kim, I., Chung, S., Park, Y., & Kang, H. (2012). The effectiveness of an aquarobic exercise program for patients with osteoarthritis. *Applied Nursing Research, 25*(3), 181–189.

Lavoie-Tremblay, M., Wright, D., Desforges, N., Gelinas, C., Marchionni, C., & Drevniok, U. (2008). Creating a healthy workplace for new-generation nurses. *Journal of Nursing Scholarship, 40*(3), 290–297.

Lee, S., Faucett, J., Gillen, M., Krause, N., & Landry, L. (2013). Risk of perception of musculoskeletal injury among critical care nurses. *Nursing Research, 62*(1), 36–44.

LeFort, S. M. (1993). The statistical versus clinical significance debate. *Image—The Journal of Nursing Scholarship, 25*(1), 57–62.

Melnyk, B. M., & Fineout-Overholt, E. (2011). *Evidence-based practice in nursing & healthcare: A guide to best practice* (2nd ed.). Philadelphia: Lippincott, Williams, & Wilkins.

Plichta, S. B., & Kelvin, E. (2013). *Munro's statistical methods for health care research* (6th ed.). Philadelphia: Lippincott Williams & Wilkins.

Quality and Safety Education for Nurses (QSEN), (2013). *Pre-licensure knowledge, skills, and attitudes (KSAs).* Retrieved February 11, 2013 from, http://qsen.org/ competencies/pre-licensure-ksas.

Shadish, W. R., Cook, T. D., & Campbell, D. T. (2002). *Experimental and quasi-experimental designs for generalized causal inference.* Chicago: Rand McNally.

Slakter, M. H., Wu, Y. B., & Suzaki-Slakter, N. S. (1991). *, **, and ***: Statistical nonsense at the .00000 level. *Nursing Research, 40*(4), 248–249.

Waltz, C. F., Strickland, O. L., & Lenz, E. R. (2010). *Measurement in nursing and health research* (4th ed.). New York: Springer.

CHAPTER 12

Critical Appraisal of Quantitative and Qualitative Research for Nursing Practice

CHAPTER OVERVIEW

LEARNING OUTCOMES

After completing this chapter, you should be able to:

1. Describe when intellectual critical appraisals of studies are conducted in nursing.
2. Implement key principles in critically appraising quantitative and qualitative studies.
3. Describe the three steps for critically appraising a study: (1) identifying the steps of the research process in the study; (2) determining study

strengths and weaknesses; and (3) evaluating the credibility and meaning of the study findings.
4. Conduct a critical appraisal of a quantitative research report.
5. Conduct a critical appraisal of a qualitative research report.

KEY TERMS

Confirmability, p. 392
Credibility, p. 392
Critical appraisal, p. 362
Critical appraisal of qualitative
    studies, p. 389
Critical appraisal of
    quantitative studies, p. 362
Dependability, p. 392

Determining strengths and
    weaknesses in the studies,
    p. 370
Evaluating the credibility and
    meaning of study findings,
    p. 374
Identifying the steps of the
    research process in studies,
    p. 366

Intellectual critical appraisal of
    a study, p. 365
Qualitative research critical
    appraisal process, p. 389
Quantitative research critical
    appraisal process, p. 366
Referred journals, p. 364
Transferable, p. 392
Trustworthiness, p. 392

The nursing profession continually strives for evidence-based practice (EBP), which includes critically appraising studies, synthesizing the findings, applying the scientific evidence in practice, and determining the practice outcomes (Brown, 2014; Doran, 2011; Melnyk & Fineout-Overholt, 2011). Critically appraising studies is an essential step toward basing your practice on current research findings. The term *critical appraisal* or critique is an examination of the quality of a study to determine the credibility and meaning of the findings for nursing. Critique is often associated with criticize, a word that is frequently viewed as negative. In the arts and sciences, however, critique is associated with critical thinking and evaluation—tasks requiring carefully developed intellectual skills. This type of critique is referred to as an intellectual critical appraisal. An intellectual critical appraisal is directed at the element that is created, such as a study, rather than at the creator, and involves the evaluation of the quality of that element. For example, it is possible to conduct an intellectual critical appraisal of a work of art, an essay, and a study.

The idea of the intellectual critical appraisal of research was introduced earlier in this text and has been woven throughout the chapters. As each step of the research process was introduced, guidelines were provided to direct the critical appraisal of that aspect of a research report. This chapter summarizes and builds on previous critical appraisal content and provides direction for conducting critical appraisals of quantitative and qualitative studies. The background provided by this chapter serves as a foundation for the critical appraisal of research syntheses (systematic reviews, meta-analyses, meta-syntheses, and mixed-methods systematic reviews) presented in Chapter 13.

This chapter discusses the implementation of critical appraisals in nursing by students, practicing nurses, nurse educators, and researchers. The key principles for implementing intellectual critical appraisals of quantitative and qualitative studies are described to provide an overview of the critical appraisal process. The steps for critical appraisal of quantitative studies, focused on rigor, design validity, quality, and meaning of findings, are detailed, and an example of a critical appraisal of a published quantitative study is provided. The chapter concludes with the critical appraisal process for qualitative studies and an example of a critical appraisal of a qualitative study.

WHEN ARE CRITICAL APPRAISALS OF STUDIES IMPLEMENTED IN NURSING?

In general, studies are critically appraised to broaden understanding, summarize knowledge for practice, and provide a knowledge base for future research. Studies are critically appraised for class projects and to determine the research evidence ready for use in practice. In addition, critical appraisals are often conducted after verbal presentations of studies, after a published research report, for selection of abstracts when studies are presented at conferences, for article selection for publication, and for evaluation of research proposals for implementation or funding. Therefore nursing students, practicing nurses, nurse educators, and nurse researchers are all involved in the critical appraisal of studies.

Students' Critical Appraisal of Studies

One aspect of learning the research process is being able to read and comprehend published research reports. However, conducting a critical appraisal of a study is not a basic skill, and the content presented in previous chapters is essential for implementing this process. Students usually acquire basic knowledge of the research process and critical appraisal process in their baccalaureate program. More advanced analysis skills are often taught at the master's and doctoral levels. Performing a critical appraisal of a study involves the following three steps, which are detailed in this chapter: (1) identifying the steps or elements of the study; (2) determining the study strengths and limitations; and (3) evaluating the credibility and meaning of the study findings. By critically appraising studies, you will expand your analysis skills, strengthen your knowledge base, and increase your use of research evidence in practice. Striving for EBP is one of the competencies identified for associate degree and baccalaureate degree (prelicensure) students by the Quality and Safety Education for Nurses (QSEN, 2013) project, and EBP requires critical appraisal and synthesis of study findings for practice (Sherwood & Barnsteiner, 2012). Therefore critical appraisal of studies is an important part of your education and your practice as a nurse.

Critical Appraisal of Studies by Practicing Nurses, Nurse Educators, and Researchers

Practicing nurses need to appraise studies critically so that their practice is based on current research evidence and not on tradition or trial and error (Brown, 2014; Craig & Smyth, 2012). Nursing actions need to be updated in response to current evidence that is generated through research and theory development. It is important for practicing nurses to design methods for remaining current in their practice areas. Reading research journals and posting or e-mailing current studies at work can increase nurses' awareness of study findings but are not sufficient for critical appraisal to occur. Nurses need to question the quality of the studies, credibility of the findings, and meaning of the findings for practice. For example, nurses might form a research journal club in which studies are presented and critically appraised by members of the group (Gloeckner & Robinson, 2010).

Skills in critical appraisal of research enable practicing nurses to synthesize the most credible, significant, and appropriate evidence for use in their practice. EBP is essential in agencies that are seeking or maintaining Magnet status. The Magnet Recognition Program was developed by the American Nurses Credentialing Center (ANCC, 2013) to "recognize healthcare organizations for quality patient care, nursing excellence, and innovations in professional nursing," which requires implementing the most current research evidence in practice (see http://www.nursecredentialing.org/Magnet/ProgramOverview.aspx).

Your faculty members critically appraise research to expand their clinical knowledge base and to develop and refine the nursing educational process. The careful analysis of current nursing studies provides a basis for updating curriculum content for use in clinical and classroom settings. Faculty serve as role models for their students by examining new studies, evaluating the information obtained from research, and indicating which research evidence to use in practice. For example, nursing instructors might critically appraise and present the most current evidence about caring for people with hypertension in class and role-model the management of patients with hypertension in practice.

Nurse researchers critically appraise previous research to plan and implement their next study. Many researchers have a program of research in a selected area, and they update their knowledge base by critically appraising new studies in this area. For example, selected nurse researchers have a

Guidelines for Identifying the Components of a Qualitative Study

1. Introduction
    a. Describe the qualifications of the authors to conduct the study. Did the authors acknowledge any potential bias or personal connection related to the study topic and steps taken to reduce bias?
    b. Discuss the clarity of the article title. Is the title clearly focused and does it include the focus and population of the study? Does the title indicate the type of study conducted—phenomenology, grounded theory, ethnography, exploratory-descriptive qualitative, or historical research (Creswell, 2013, 2014; Fawcett & Garity, 2009; Hoe & Hoare, 2012)?
    c. Discuss the quality of the abstract (includes purpose, qualitative approach, sample, and key results; APA, 2010).
2. State the problem.
    a. Significance of the problem
    b. Background of the problem
    c. Problem statement
3. State the purpose.
4. Examine the literature review.
    a. Is the literature review identified as such? In some research articles, the literature review will be identified clearly as a review of the literature; some authors may incorporate the review into the background and significance.
    b. Did the author cite quantitative and qualitative studies relevant to the focus of the study? What other types of literature did the author include?
    c. Identify the disciplines of the authors of studies cited in this paper and the journals in which they published their studies. Does it appear that the author searched databases outside of the *Cumulative Index to Nursing and Allied Health Literature* (CINAHL) for relevant studies?
    d. Are the references current? Are classic or groundbreaking studies included, which may be older?
    e. Did the author evaluate or indicate the weaknesses of the available studies (Grove et al., 2013; Hart, 2009)?
5. Identify the study framework or philosophical orientation of the study.
    a. Did the authors cite primary sources to support the framework or philosophical orientation of the study?
    b. If the study was a grounded theory study, did the researcher develop a theoretical description or diagram as part of the study findings (Creswell, 2013)?
6. List the research objectives (aims) or questions, if identified.
7. Identify the qualitative approach used to answer the research questions (phenomenology, grounded theory, ethnography, exploratory-descriptive, historical, or other approach). If the specific qualitative approach was not identified, what aspects of the method, such as natural settings or coding, indicate that a qualitative approach was used (Creswell, 2013; Munhall, 2012)?
8. Describe the sample and setting.
    a. Identify inclusion and exclusion criteria.
    b. What methods did the researchers use to recruit participants?
    c. Identify the sample size.
    d. Identify the characteristics of the sample.

    e. Discuss the IRB approval. Describe the informed consent process used in the study.
    f. Did the researcher identify that participants might become upset during the collection of data? If so, what measures were in place to address the safety and emotional needs of the participants (Maxwell, 2013)?
    g. Did any potential subjects refuse to participate? Did any of the participants start but not finish the study?
    h. Identify the study setting and indicate whether it is appropriate for the study purpose.
 9. Describe the procedures for data collection.
    a. What methods were used—interviews, focus groups, observation, or other?
    b. Were multiple interviews with the same person conducted or were data collected one time from each participant?
    c. How were data recorded during data collection?
    d. Did the researcher make field notes or journal entries (Creswell, 2014; Miles, Huberman, & Saldana, 2014)?
10. Describe the data analysis processes.
    a. How were the data prepared for analysis?
    b. How were the data analyzed? Did the researcher cite a specific method of analysis and provide a primary source?
    c. Was computer-assisted qualitative data management software used during the analysis?
    d. Which methods were used to increase the trustworthiness of the findings (e.g., verification of the accuracy of transcripts, immersion in the data, documentation of an audit trail, also known as the record of decisions that were made during data collection and analysis, member checking, independent analysis of a portion of the data by another researcher (Cohen & Crabtree, 2008; Miles et al., 2014; Murphy & Yielder, 2010)?
11. Describe the researcher's interpretation of findings.
    a. Are the findings related back to the study framework (if applicable)?
    b. Which findings were not expected?
    c. Are the findings consistent with previous research findings (Fawcett & Garity, 2009)?
12. What study limitations did the researcher identify?
13. What conclusions did the researchers identify based on their interpretation of the study findings?
14. Did the researcher indicate other groups to which these findings might be transferable or applied?
15. What were the implications of the findings for nursing practice?
16. What suggestions were identified for further study?

Step 2: Determining the Strengths and Weaknesses in Studies

At this step, the differences in the critical appraisal processes of quantitative and qualitative studies become more obvious. However, the goal of the critical appraisal remains the same—determining the strengths and weaknesses of the study. Knowledge of the different qualitative approaches and data collection processes is needed to answer the questions during this step. You may want to refer to Chapter 3 and supplement your knowledge with other sources, such as other texts, reference books, and articles (Brown, 2014; Creswell, 2013, 2014; Fawcett & Garity, 2009; Grove et al., 2013; Miles et al., 2014; Munhall, 2012; Petty, Thomson, & Stew, 2012; Sandelowski & Barroso, 2007). The actual methods of the study being appraised are compared to the expectations of qualitative experts, including the original proponents of different qualitative approaches. Because different qualitative experts agree less on the "rules" for implementing qualitative studies, using the guidelines recommended by a specific expert in the method used by the researchers in the study is important. The areas of consistency are strengths of the study, whereas areas of inconsistency may indicate weaknesses of the study. The standards used for appraising the strength of qualitative studies are not quantitative (i.e., reliability of a scale ≥ 0.8); the person conducting the critical appraisal evaluates all aspects of a qualitative study and makes a judgment about its trustworthiness. Trustworthiness is a determination that a qualitative study is rigorous and of high quality. Trustworthiness is the extent to which a qualitative study is dependable, confirmable, credible, and transferable.

A thorough report of a qualitative study should include adequate information so that the reader can assess the report dependability and confirmability of the study (Murphy & Yielder, 2010). Dependability and confirmability are similar to reliability of quantitative studies. Dependability is documentation of steps taken and decisions made during analysis. Remember from Chapter 3 that the researchers' record of the analysis process is called an audit trail. Confirmability is the extent to which other researchers can review the audit trail and agree that the authors' conclusions are logical (Murphy & Yielder, 2010). When a study's findings are appraised to be confirmable and dependable, they have more credibility. Credibility is the confidence of the reader about the extent to which the researchers have produced results that reflect the views of the participants; this is similar to validity in the critical appraisal of quantitative studies (Murphy & Yielder, 2010). Petty and co-workers (2012) have explained that qualitative findings are not generalizable, but are transferable or applicable in other settings with similar participants.

You need to appraise the rigor of the study methods by looking for information about the carefulness of data collection and thoroughness of the data analysis. The questions asked about each component of the study will focus your attention on the rigor of the methods and the logical links among the study elements. Logical links among the study elements are critical to the credibility of the study (Cohen & Crabtree, 2008; Maxwell, 2013). For example, is the purpose of the study consistent with the research questions? Are the purpose and research questions appropriate to address the research problem? Is the selected qualitative approach the best way to answer the research questions? Similar to quantitative research, logical inconsistencies and improperly applied methods are common weaknesses of qualitative studies. Because qualitative research has fewer rules, critically appraising qualitative studies can seem daunting. The following questions provide a structure for you to examine each aspect of the qualitative research process. Remember to consult other references, as needed, to answer each question.

Guidelines for Determining the Strengths and Weaknesses in Studies

1. Research problem and purpose
   a. Is the problem significant to nursing and clinical practice (Cohen & Crabtree, 2008)?
   b. Does the purpose address the focus of the study?
2. Review of literature
   a. Did the researchers provide a broad organized review of the literature that included disciplines other than nursing?
   b. Did the literature review include adequate information to build a logical argument? Did the author provide enough evidence to support the verdict that the study was needed?
   c. Does the literature review summary identify what is known and not known about the research problem and provide direction for the formation of the research purpose?

nursing students, practicing nurses, nurse educators, and nurse researchers are all involved in the critical appraisal of studies.

Students' Critical Appraisal of Studies

One aspect of learning the research process is being able to read and comprehend published research reports. However, conducting a critical appraisal of a study is not a basic skill, and the content presented in previous chapters is essential for implementing this process. Students usually acquire basic knowledge of the research process and critical appraisal process in their baccalaureate program. More advanced analysis skills are often taught at the master's and doctoral levels. Performing a critical appraisal of a study involves the following three steps, which are detailed in this chapter: (1) identifying the steps or elements of the study; (2) determining the study strengths and limitations; and (3) evaluating the credibility and meaning of the study findings. By critically appraising studies, you will expand your analysis skills, strengthen your knowledge base, and increase your use of research evidence in practice. Striving for EBP is one of the competencies identified for associate degree and baccalaureate degree (prelicensure) students by the Quality and Safety Education for Nurses (QSEN, 2013) project, and EBP requires critical appraisal and synthesis of study findings for practice (Sherwood & Barnsteiner, 2012). Therefore critical appraisal of studies is an important part of your education and your practice as a nurse.

Critical Appraisal of Studies by Practicing Nurses, Nurse Educators, and Researchers

Practicing nurses need to appraise studies critically so that their practice is based on current research evidence and not on tradition or trial and error (Brown, 2014; Craig & Smyth, 2012). Nursing actions need to be updated in response to current evidence that is generated through research and theory development. It is important for practicing nurses to design methods for remaining current in their practice areas. Reading research journals and posting or e-mailing current studies at work can increase nurses' awareness of study findings but are not sufficient for critical appraisal to occur. Nurses need to question the quality of the studies, credibility of the findings, and meaning of the findings for practice. For example, nurses might form a research journal club in which studies are presented and critically appraised by members of the group (Gloeckner & Robinson, 2010).

Skills in critical appraisal of research enable practicing nurses to synthesize the most credible, significant, and appropriate evidence for use in their practice. EBP is essential in agencies that are seeking or maintaining Magnet status. The Magnet Recognition Program was developed by the American Nurses Credentialing Center (ANCC, 2013) to "recognize healthcare organizations for quality patient care, nursing excellence, and innovations in professional nursing," which requires implementing the most current research evidence in practice (see http://www.nursecredentialing.org/Magnet/ProgramOverview.aspx).

Your faculty members critically appraise research to expand their clinical knowledge base and to develop and refine the nursing educational process. The careful analysis of current nursing studies provides a basis for updating curriculum content for use in clinical and classroom settings. Faculty serve as role models for their students by examining new studies, evaluating the information obtained from research, and indicating which research evidence to use in practice. For example, nursing instructors might critically appraise and present the most current evidence about caring for people with hypertension in class and role-model the management of patients with hypertension in practice.

Nurse researchers critically appraise previous research to plan and implement their next study. Many researchers have a program of research in a selected area, and they update their knowledge base by critically appraising new studies in this area. For example, selected nurse researchers have a program of research to identify effective interventions for assisting patients in managing their hypertension and reducing their cardiovascular risk factors.

Critical Appraisal of Research Following Presentation and Publication

When nurses attend research conferences, they note that critical appraisals and questions often follow presentations of studies. These critical appraisals assist researchers in identifying the strengths and weaknesses of their studies and generating ideas for further research. Participants listening to study critiques might gain insight into the conduct of research. In addition, experiencing the critical appraisal process can increase the conference participants' ability to evaluate studies and judge the usefulness of the research evidence for practice.

Critical appraisals have been published following some studies in research journals. For example, the research journals *Scholarly Inquiry for Nursing Practice: An International Journal* and *Western Journal of Nursing Research* include commentaries after the research articles. In these commentaries, other researchers critically appraise the authors' studies, and the authors have a chance to respond to these comments. Published research critical appraisals often increase the reader's understanding of the study and the quality of the study findings (American Psychological Association [APA], 2010). A more informal critical appraisal of a published study might appear in a letter to the editor. Readers have the opportunity to comment on the strengths and weaknesses of published studies by writing to the journal editor.

Critical Appraisal of Research for Presentation and Publication

Planners of professional conferences often invite researchers to submit an abstract of a study they are conducting or have completed for potential presentation at the conference. The amount of information available is usually limited, because many abstracts are restricted to 100 to 250 words. Nevertheless, reviewers must select the best-designed studies with the most significant outcomes for presentation at nursing conferences. This process requires an experienced researcher who needs few cues to determine the quality of a study. Critical appraisal of an abstract usually addresses the following criteria: (1) appropriateness of the study for the conference program; (2) completeness of the research project; (3) overall quality of the study problem, purpose, methodology, and results; (4) contribution of the study to nursing's knowledge base; (5) contribution of the study to nursing theory; (6) originality of the work (not previously published); (7) implication of the study findings for practice; and (8) clarity, conciseness, and completeness of the abstract (APA, 2010; Grove, Burns, & Gray, 2013).

Some nurse researchers serve as peer reviewers for professional journals to evaluate the quality of research papers submitted for publication. The role of these scientists is to ensure that the studies accepted for publication are well designed and contribute to the body of knowledge. Journals that have their articles critically appraised by expert peer reviews are called peer-reviewed journals or **referred journals** (Pyrczak, 2008). The reviewers' comments or summaries of their comments are sent to the researchers to direct their revision of the manuscripts for publication. Referred journals usually have studies and articles of higher quality and provide excellent studies for your review for practice.

Critical Appraisal of Research Proposals

Critical appraisals of research proposals are conducted to approve student research projects, permit data collection in an institution, and select the best studies for funding by local, state, national, and international organizations and agencies. You might be involved in a proposal review if you are participating in collecting data as part of a class project or studies done in your clinical agency. More details on proposal development and approval can be found in Grove et al. (2013, Chapter 28).

Research proposals are reviewed for funding from selected government agencies and corporations. Private corporations develop their own format for reviewing and funding research projects

(Grove et al., 2013). The peer review process in federal funding agencies involves an extremely complex critical appraisal. Nurses are involved in this level of research review through national funding agencies, such as the National Institute of Nursing Research (NINR, 2013) and the Agency for Healthcare Research and Quality (AHRQ, 2013).

WHAT ARE THE KEY PRINCIPLES FOR CONDUCTING INTELLECTUAL CRITICAL APPRAISALS OF QUANTITATIVE AND QUALITATIVE STUDIES?

An intellectual critical appraisal of a study involves a careful and complete examination of a study to judge its strengths, weaknesses, credibility, meaning, and significance for practice. A high-quality study focuses on a significant problem, demonstrates sound methodology, produces credible findings, indicates implications for practice, and provides a basis for additional studies (Grove et al., 2013; Hoare & Hoe, 2013; Hoe & Hoare, 2012). Ultimately, the findings from several quality studies can be synthesized to provide empirical evidence for use in practice (O'Mathuna, Fineout-Overholt, & Johnston, 2011).

The major focus of this chapter is conducting critical appraisals of quantitative and qualitative studies. These critical appraisals involve implementing some key principles or guidelines, outlined in Box 12-1. These guidelines stress the importance of examining the expertise of the authors, reviewing the entire study, addressing the study's strengths and weaknesses, and evaluating the credibility of the study findings (Fawcett & Garity, 2009; Hoare & Hoe, 2013; Hoe & Hoare, 2012;

BOX 12-1 KEY PRINCIPLES FOR CRITICALLY APPRAISING QUANTITATIVE AND QUALITATIVE STUDIES

1. *Read and critically appraise the entire study.* A research critical appraisal involves examining the quality of all aspects of the research report.
2. *Examine the organization and presentation of the research report.* A well-prepared report is complete, concise, clearly presented, and logically organized. It does not include excessive jargon that is difficult for you to read. The references need to be current, complete, and presented in a consistent format.
3. *Examine the significance of the problem studied for nursing practice.* The focus of nursing studies needs to be on significant practice problems if a sound knowledge base is to be developed for evidence-based nursing practice.
4. *Indicate the type of study conducted and identify the steps or elements of the study.* This might be done as an initial critical appraisal of a study; it indicates your knowledge of the different types of quantitative and qualitative studies and the steps or elements included in these studies.
5. *Identify the strengths and weaknesses of a study.* All studies have strengths and weaknesses, so attention must be given to all aspects of the study.
6. *Be objective and realistic in identifying the study's strengths and weaknesses.* Be balanced in your critical appraisal of a study. Try not to be overly critical in identifying a study's weaknesses or overly flattering in identifying the strengths.
7. *Provide specific examples of the strengths and weaknesses of a study.* Examples provide evidence for your critical appraisal of the strengths and weaknesses of a study.
8. *Provide a rationale for your critical appraisal comments.* Include justifications for your critical appraisal, and document your ideas with sources from the current literature. This strengthens the quality of your critical appraisal and documents the use of critical thinking skills.
9. *Evaluate the quality of the study.* Describe the credibility of the findings, consistency of the findings with those from other studies, and quality of the study conclusions.
10. *Discuss the usefulness of the findings for practice.* The findings from the study need to be linked to the findings of previous studies and examined for use in clinical practice.

Munhall, 2012). All studies have weaknesses or flaws; if every flawed study were discarded, no scientific evidence would be available for use in practice. In fact, science itself is flawed. Science does not completely or perfectly describe, explain, predict, or control reality. However, improved understanding and increased ability to predict and control phenomena depend on recognizing the flaws in studies and science. Additional studies can then be planned to minimize the weaknesses of earlier studies. You also need to recognize a study's strengths to determine the quality of a study and credibility of its findings. When identifying a study's strengths and weaknesses, you need to provide examples and rationale for your judgments that are documented with current literature.

Critical appraisal of quantitative and qualitative studies involves a final evaluation to determine the credibility of the study findings and any implications for practice and further research (see Box 12-1). Adding together the strong points from multiple studies slowly builds a solid base of evidence for practice. These guidelines provide a basis for the critical appraisal process for quantitative research discussed in the next section and the critical appraisal process for qualitative research (see later).

UNDERSTANDING THE QUANTITATIVE RESEARCH CRITICAL APPRAISAL PROCESS

The quantitative research critical appraisal process includes three steps: (1) identifying the steps of the research process in studies; (2) determining study strengths and weaknesses; and (3) evaluating the credibility and meaning of study findings. These steps occur in sequence, vary in depth, and presume accomplishment of the preceding steps. However, an individual with critical appraisal experience frequently performs two or three steps of this process simultaneously.

This section includes the three steps of the quantitative research critical appraisal process and provides relevant questions for each step. These questions have been selected as a means for stimulating the logical reasoning and analysis necessary for conducting a critical appraisal of a study. Those experienced in the critical appraisal process often formulate additional questions as part of their reasoning processes. We will identify the steps of the research process separately because those new to critical appraisal start with this step. The questions for determining the study strengths and weaknesses are covered together because this process occurs simultaneously in the mind of the person conducting the critical appraisal. Evaluation is covered separately because of the increased expertise needed to perform this step.

Step 1: Identifying the Steps of the Research Process in Studies

Initial attempts to comprehend research articles are often frustrating because the terminology and stylized manner of the report are unfamiliar. Identifying the steps of the research process in a quantitative study is the first step in critical appraisal. It involves understanding the terms and concepts in the report, as well as identifying study elements and grasping the nature, significance, and meaning of these elements. The following guidelines will direct you in identifying a study's elements or steps.

Guidelines for Identifying the Steps of the Research Process in Studies

The first step involves reviewing the abstract and reading the study from beginning to end. As you read, think about the following questions regarding the presentation of the study:

- Was the study title clear?
- Was the abstract clearly presented?
- Was the writing style of the report clear and concise?
- Were relevant terms defined? You might underline the terms you do not understand and determine their meaning from the glossary at the end of this text.

- Were the following parts of the research report plainly identified (APA, 2010)?
  - Introduction section, with the problem, purpose, literature review, framework, study variables, and objectives, questions, or hypotheses
  - Methods section, with the design, sample, intervention (if applicable), measurement methods, and data collection or procedures
  - Results section, with the specific results presented in tables, figures, and narrative
  - Discussion section, with the findings, conclusions, limitations, generalizations, implications for practice, and suggestions for future research (Fawcett & Garity, 2009; Grove et al., 2013)

We recommend reading the research article a second time and highlighting or underlining the steps of the quantitative research process that were identified previously. An overview of these steps is presented in Chapter 2. After reading and comprehending the content of the study, you are ready to write your initial critical appraisal of the study. To write a critical appraisal identifying the study steps, you need to identify each step of the research process concisely and respond briefly to the following guidelines and questions.

1. Introduction
   a. Describe the qualifications of the authors to conduct the study (e.g., research expertise conducting previous studies, clinical experience indicated by job, national certification, and years in practice, and educational preparation that includes conducting research [PhD]).
   b. Discuss the clarity of the article title. Is the title clearly focused and does it include key study variables and population? Does the title indicate the type of study conducted—descriptive, correlational, quasi-experimental, or experimental—and the variables (Fawcett & Garity, 2009; Hoe & Hoare, 2012; Shadish, Cook, & Campbell, 2002)?
   c. Discuss the quality of the abstract (includes purpose, highlights design, sample, and intervention [if applicable], and presents key results; APA, 2010).
2. State the problem.
   a. Significance of the problem
   b. Background of the problem
   c. Problem statement
3. State the purpose.
4. Examine the literature review.
   a. Are relevant previous studies and theories described?
   b. Are the references current (number and percentage of sources in the last 5 and 10 years)?
   c. Are the studies described, critically appraised, and synthesized (Brown, 2014; Fawcett & Garity, 2009)? Are the studies from referred journals?
   d. Is a summary provided of the current knowledge (what is known and not known) about the research problem?
5. Examine the study framework or theoretical perspective.
   a. Is the framework explicitly expressed, or must you extract the framework from statements in the introduction or literature review of the study?
   b. Is the framework based on tentative, substantive, or scientific theory? Provide a rationale for your answer.
   c. Does the framework identify, define, and describe the relationships among the concepts of interest? Provide examples of this.
   d. Is a map of the framework provided for clarity? If a map is not presented, develop a map that represents the study's framework and describe the map.
   e. Link the study variables to the relevant concepts in the map.
   f. How is the framework related to nursing's body of knowledge (Alligood, 2010; Fawcett & Garity, 2009; Smith & Liehr, 2008)?

6. List any research objectives, questions, or hypotheses.
7. Identify and define (conceptually and operationally) the study variables or concepts that were identified in the objectives, questions, or hypotheses. If objectives, questions, or hypotheses are not stated, identify and define the variables in the study purpose and results section of the study. If conceptual definitions are not found, identify possible definitions for each major study variable. Indicate which of the following types of variables were included in the study. A study usually includes independent and dependent variables or research variables, but not all three types of variables.
   a. Independent variables: Identify and define conceptually and operationally.
   b. Dependent variables: Identify and define conceptually and operationally.
   c. Research variables or concepts: Identify and define conceptually and operationally.
8. Identify attribute or demographic variables and other relevant terms.
9. Identify the research design.
   a. Identify the specific design of the study (see Chapter 8).
   b. Does the study include a treatment or intervention? If so, is the treatment clearly described with a protocol and consistently implemented?
   c. If the study has more than one group, how were subjects assigned to groups?
   d. Are extraneous variables identified and controlled? Extraneous variables are usually discussed as a part of quasi-experimental and experimental studies.
   e. Were pilot study findings used to design this study? If yes, briefly discuss the pilot and the changes made in this study based on the pilot (Grove et al., 2013; Shadish et al., 2002).
10. Describe the sample and setting.
    a. Identify inclusion and exclusion sample or eligibility criteria.
    b. Identify the specific type of probability or nonprobability sampling method that was used to obtain the sample. Did the researchers identify the sampling frame for the study?
    c. Identify the sample size. Discuss the refusal number and percentage, and include the rationale for refusal if presented in the article. Discuss the power analysis if this process was used to determine sample size (Aberson, 2010).
    d. Identify the sample attrition (number and percentage) for the study.
    e. Identify the characteristics of the sample.
    f. Discuss the institutional review board (IRB) approval. Describe the informed consent process used in the study.
    g. Identify the study setting and indicate whether it is appropriate for the study purpose.
11. Identify and describe each measurement strategy used in the study. The following table includes the critical information about two measurement methods, the Beck Likert scale and a physiological instrument to measure blood pressure. Completing this table will allow you to cover essential measurement content for a study (Waltz, Strickland, & Lenz, 2010).
    a. Identify each study variable that was measured.
    b. Identify the name and author of each measurement strategy.
    c. Identify the type of each measurement strategy (e.g., Likert scale, visual analog scale, physiological measure, or existing database).
    d. Identify the level of measurement (nominal, ordinal, interval, or ratio) achieved by each measurement method used in the study (Grove, 2007).
    e. Describe the reliability of each scale for previous studies and this study. Identify the precision of each physiological measure (Bialocerkowski, Klupp, & Bragge, 2010; DeVon et al., 2007).
    f. Identify the validity of each scale and the accuracy of physiological measures (DeVon et al., 2007; Ryan-Wenger, 2010).

Variable Measured	Name of Measurement Method (Author)	Type of Measurement Method	Level of Measurement	Reliability or Precision	Validity or Accuracy
Depression	Beck Depression Inventory (Beck)	Likert scale	Interval	Cronbach alphas of 0.82-0.84 for this study; reading level at 6th grade.	Construct validity—content validity from concept analysis, literature review, and reviews of experts; convergent validity of 0.04 with Zung Depression Scale; predictive validity of patients' future depression episodes; successive use validity with the conduct of previous studies and this study.
Blood pressure	Omron blood pressure (BP) equipment (equipment manufacturer)	Physiological measurement method	Ratio	Test-retest values of BPs in previous studies; BP equipment new and recalibrated every 50 BP readings in this study; average three BP readings to determine BP.	Documented accuracy of systolic and diastolic BPs to 1 mm Hg by company developing Omron BP cuff; designated protocol for taking BP average three BP readings to determine BP.

12. Describe the procedures for data collection.
13. Describe the statistical analyses used.
    a. List the statistical procedures used to describe the sample (Grove, 2007).
    b. Was the level of significance or alpha identified? If so, indicate what it was (0.05, 0.01, or 0.001).
    c. Complete the following table with the analysis techniques conducted in the study: (1) identify the focus (description, relationships, or differences) for each analysis technique; (2) list the statistical analysis technique performed; (3) list the statistic; (4) provide the specific results; and (5) identify the probability (p) of the statistical significance achieved by the result (Grove, 2007; Grove et al., 2013; Hoare & Hoe, 2013; Plichta & Kelvin, 2013).

Purpose of Analysis	Analysis Technique	Statistic	Results	Probability (p)
Description of subjects' pulse rate	Mean	M	71.52	
	Standard deviation	SD	5.62	
	Range	range	58-97	
Difference between adult males and females on blood pressure	t-Test	t	3.75	p=0.001
Differences of diet group, exercise group, and comparison group for pounds lost in adolescents	Analysis of variance	F	4.27	p=0.04
Relationship of depression and anxiety in older adults	Pearson correlation	r	0.46	p=0.03

14. Describe the researcher's interpretation of findings.
    a. Are the findings related back to the study framework? If so, do the findings support the study framework?
    b. Which findings are consistent with those expected?
    c. Which findings were not expected?
    d. Are the findings consistent with previous research findings? (Fawcett & Garity, 2009; Grove et al., 2013; Hoare & Hoe, 2013)
15. What study limitations did the researcher identify?
16. What conclusions did the researchers identify based on their interpretation of the study findings?
17. How did the researcher generalize the findings?
18. What were the implications of the findings for nursing practice?
19. What suggestions for further study were identified?
20. Is the description of the study sufficiently clear for replication?

Step 2: Determining the Strengths and Weaknesses in Studies

The second step in critically appraising studies requires determining strengths and weaknesses in the studies. To do this, you must have knowledge of what each step of the research process should be like from expert sources such as this text and other research sources

(Aberson, 2010; Bialocerkowski et al., 2010; Brown, 2014; Creswell, 2014; DeVon et al., 2007; Doran, 2011; Fawcett & Garity, 2009; Grove, 2007; Grove et al., 2013; Hoare & Hoe, 2013; Hoe & Hoare, 2012; Morrison, Hoppe, Gillmore, Kluver, Higa, & Wells, 2009; O'Mathuna et al., 2011; Ryan-Wenger, 2010; Santacroce, Maccarelli, & Grey, 2004; Shadish et al., 2002; Waltz et al., 2010). The ideal ways to conduct the steps of the research process are then compared with the actual study steps. During this comparison, you examine the extent to which the researcher followed the rules for an ideal study, and the study elements are examined for strengths and weaknesses.

You also need to examine the logical links or flow of the steps in the study being appraised. For example, the problem needs to provide background and direction for the statement of the purpose. The variables identified in the study purpose need to be consistent with the variables identified in the research objectives, questions, or hypotheses. The variables identified in the research objectives, questions, or hypotheses need to be conceptually defined in light of the study framework. The conceptual definitions should provide the basis for the development of operational definitions. The study design and analyses need to be appropriate for the investigation of the study purpose, as well as for the specific objectives, questions, or hypotheses. Examining the quality and logical links among the study steps will enable you to determine which steps are strengths and which steps are weaknesses.

Guidelines for Determining the Strengths and Weaknesses in Studies

The following questions were developed to help you examine the different steps of a study and determine its strengths and weaknesses. The intent is not for you to answer each of these questions but to read the questions and then make judgments about the steps in the study. You need to provide a rationale for your decisions and document from relevant research sources, such as those listed previously in this section and in the references at the end of this chapter. For example, you might decide that the study purpose is a strength because it addresses the study problem, clarifies the focus of the study, and is feasible to investigate (Brown, 2014; Fawcett & Garity, 2009; Hoe & Hoare, 2012).

1. Research problem and purpose
   a. Is the problem significant to nursing and clinical practice (Brown, 2014)?
   b. Does the purpose narrow and clarify the focus of the study (Creswell, 2014; Fawcett & Garity, 2009)?
   c. Was this study feasible to conduct in terms of money commitment, the researchers' expertise; availability of subjects, facilities, and equipment; and ethical considerations?
2. Review of literature
   a. Is the literature review organized to demonstrate the progressive development of evidence from previous research (Brown, 2014; Creswell, 2014; Hoe & Hoare, 2012)?
   b. Is a clear and concise summary presented of the current empirical and theoretical knowledge in the area of the study (O'Mathuna et al., 2011)?
   c. Does the literature review summary identify what is known and not known about the research problem and provide direction for the formation of the research purpose?
3. Study framework
   a. Is the framework presented with clarity? If a model or conceptual map of the framework is present, is it adequate to explain the phenomenon of concern (Grove et al., 2013)?
   b. Is the framework related to the body of knowledge in nursing and clinical practice?

   c. If a proposition from a theory is to be tested, is the proposition clearly identified and linked to the study hypotheses (Alligood, 2010; Fawcett & Garity, 2009; Smith & Liehr, 2008)?

4. Research objectives, questions, or hypotheses
   a. Are the objectives, questions, or hypotheses expressed clearly?
   b. Are the objectives, questions, or hypotheses logically linked to the research purpose?
   c. Are hypotheses stated to direct the conduct of quasi-experimental and experimental research (Creswell, 2014; Shadish et al., 2002)?
   d. Are the objectives, questions, or hypotheses logically linked to the concepts and relationships (propositions) in the framework (Chinn & Kramer, 2011; Fawcett & Garity, 2009; Smith & Liehr, 2008)?

5. Variables
   a. Are the variables reflective of the concepts identified in the framework?
   b. Are the variables clearly defined (conceptually and operationally) and based on previous research or theories (Chinn & Kramer, 2011; Grove et al., 2013; Smith & Liehr, 2008)?
   c. Is the conceptual definition of a variable consistent with the operational definition?

6. Design
   a. Is the design used in the study the most appropriate design to obtain the needed data (Creswell, 2014; Grove et al., 2013; Hoe & Hoare, 2012)?
   b. Does the design provide a means to examine all the objectives, questions, or hypotheses?
   c. Is the treatment clearly described (Brown, 2002)? Is the treatment appropriate for examining the study purpose and hypotheses? Does the study framework explain the links between the treatment (independent variable) and the proposed outcomes (dependent variables)? Was a protocol developed to promote consistent implementation of the treatment to ensure intervention fidelity (Morrison et al., 2009)? Did the researcher monitor implementation of the treatment to ensure consistency (Santacroce et al., 2004)? If the treatment was not consistently implemented, what might be the impact on the findings?
   d. Did the researcher identify the threats to design validity (statistical conclusion validity, internal validity, construct validity, and external validity [see Chapter 8]) and minimize them as much as possible (Grove et al., 2013; Shadish et al., 2002)?
   e. If more than one group was used, did the groups appear equivalent?
   f. If a treatment was implemented, were the subjects randomly assigned to the treatment group or were the treatment and comparison groups matched? Were the treatment and comparison group assignments appropriate for the purpose of the study?

7. Sample, population, and setting
   a. Is the sampling method adequate to produce a representative sample? Are any subjects excluded from the study because of age, socioeconomic status, or ethnicity, without a sound rationale?
   b. Did the sample include an understudied population, such as young people, older adults, or minority group?
   c. Were the sampling criteria (inclusion and exclusion) appropriate for the type of study conducted (O'Mathuna et al., 2011)?
   d. Was a power analysis conducted to determine sample size? If a power analysis was conducted, were the results of the analysis clearly described and used to determine the final

sample size? Was the attrition rate projected in determining the final sample size (Aberson, 2010)?

e. Are the rights of human subjects protected (Creswell, 2014; Grove et al., 2013)?

f. Is the setting used in the study typical of clinical settings?

g. Was the rate of potential subjects' refusal to participate in the study a problem? If so, how might this weakness influence the findings?

h. Was sample attrition a problem? If so, how might this weakness influence the final sample and the study results and findings (Aberson, 2010; Fawcett & Garity, 2009; Hoe & Hoare, 2012)?

8. Measurements

a. Do the measurement methods selected for the study adequately measure the study variables? Should additional measurement methods have been used to improve the quality of the study outcomes (Waltz et al., 2010)?

b. Do the measurement methods used in the study have adequate validity and reliability? What additional reliability or validity testing is needed to improve the quality of the measurement methods (Bialocerkowski et al., 2010; DeVon et al., 2007; Roberts & Stone, 2003)?

c. Respond to the following questions, which are relevant to the measurement approaches used in the study:

1) Scales and questionnaires
   (a) Are the instruments clearly described?
   (b) Are techniques to complete and score the instruments provided?
   (c) Are the validity and reliability of the instruments described (DeVon et al., 2007)?
   (d) Did the researcher reexamine the validity and reliability of the instruments for the present sample?
   (e) If the instrument was developed for the study, is the instrument development process described (Grove et al., 2013; Waltz et al., 2010)?

2) Observation
   (a) Is what is to be observed clearly identified and defined?
   (b) Is interrater reliability described?
   (c) Are the techniques for recording observations described (Waltz et al., 2010)?

3) Interviews
   (a) Do the interview questions address concerns expressed in the research problem?
   (b) Are the interview questions relevant for the research purpose and objectives, questions, or hypotheses (Grove et al., 2013; Waltz et al., 2010)?

4) Physiological measures
   (a) Are the physiological measures or instruments clearly described (Ryan-Wenger, 2010)? If appropriate, are the brand names of the instruments identified, such as Space Labs or Hewlett-Packard?
   (b) Are the accuracy, precision, and error of the physiological instruments discussed (Ryan-Wenger, 2010)?
   (c) Are the physiological measures appropriate for the research purpose and objectives, questions, or hypotheses?
   (d) Are the methods for recording data from the physiological measures clearly described? Is the recording of data consistent?

9. Data collection
   a. Is the data collection process clearly described (Fawcett & Garity, 2009; Grove et al., 2013)?
   b. Are the forms used to collect data organized to facilitate computerizing the data?
   c. Is the training of data collectors clearly described and adequate?
   d. Is the data collection process conducted in a consistent manner?
   e. Are the data collection methods ethical?
   f. Do the data collected address the research objectives, questions, or hypotheses?
   g. Did any adverse events occur during data collection, and were these appropriately managed?
10. Data analysis
   a. Are data analysis procedures appropriate for the type of data collected (Grove, 2007; Hoare & Hoe, 2013; Plichta & Kelvin, 2013)?
   b. Are data analysis procedures clearly described? Did the researcher address any problem with missing data, and explain how this problem was managed?
   c. Do the data analysis techniques address the study purpose and the research objectives, questions, or hypotheses (Fawcett & Garity, 2009; Grove et al., 2013; Hoare & Hoe, 2013)?
   d. Are the results presented in an understandable way by narrative, tables, or figures or a combination of methods (APA, 2010)?
   e. Is the sample size sufficient to detect significant differences, if they are present?
   f. Was a power analysis conducted for nonsignificant results (Aberson, 2010)?
   g. Are the results interpreted appropriately?
11. Interpretation of findings
   a. Are findings discussed in relation to each objective, question, or hypothesis?
   b. Are various explanations for significant and nonsignificant findings examined?
   c. Are the findings clinically important (O'Mathuna et al., 2011)?
   d. Are the findings linked to the study framework (Smith & Liehr, 2008)?
   e. Are the findings consistent with the findings of previous studies in this area?
   f. Do the conclusions fit the findings from this study and previous studies?
   g. Does the study have limitations not identified by the researcher?
   h. Did the researcher generalize the findings appropriately?
   i. Were the identified implications for practice appropriate based on the study findings and on the findings from previous research (Brown, 2014; Fawcett & Garity, 2009; Hoe & Hoare, 2012)?
   j. Were quality suggestions made for future research (O'Mathuna et al., 2011)?

Step 3: Evaluating the Credibility and Meaning of Study Findings

Evaluating the credibility and meaning of study findings involves determining the validity, significance, and meaning of the study by examining the relationships among the steps of the study, study findings, and previous studies. The steps of the study are evaluated in light of previous studies, such as an evaluation of present hypotheses based on previous hypotheses, present design based on previous designs, and present methods of measuring variables based on previous methods of measurement. The findings of the present study are also examined in light of the findings of previous studies. Evaluation builds on conclusions reached during the first two stages of the critical appraisal so the credibility, validity, and meaning of the study findings can be determined.

Guidelines for Evaluating the Credibility and Meaning of Study Findings

You need to reexamine the findings, conclusions, and implications sections of the study and the researchers' suggestions for further study. Using the following questions as a guide, summarize your evaluation of the study and document your responses.

1. What rival hypotheses can be suggested for the findings?
2. Do the findings from this study build on the findings of previous studies? You need to read some of the other relevant studies cited by the researchers to address this question.
3. When the findings are examined in light of previous studies, what is now known and not known about the phenomenon under study?
4. Do you believe the study findings are valid? How much confidence can be placed in the study findings (Fawcett & Garity, 2009)?
5. Could the limitations of the study have been corrected?
6. To what populations can the findings be generalized?
7. What questions emerge from the findings, and does the researcher identify them?
8. What implications do the findings have for nursing practice? (Brown, 2014; Craig & Smyth, 2012; Hoe & Hoare, 2012; O'Mathuna et al., 2011)?

The evaluation of a research report should also include a final discussion of the quality of the report. This discussion should include an expert opinion of the study's quality and contribution to nursing knowledge and practice (Brown, 2014; Hoare & Hoe, 2013; O'Mathuna et al., 2011).

EXAMPLE OF A CRITICAL APPRAISAL OF A QUANTITATIVE STUDY

A critical appraisal was conducted of the quasi-experimental study by Shipowick, Moore, Corbett, & Bindler (2009) and is presented as an example in this chapter. The research report, "Vitamin D and Depressive Symptoms in Women During the Winter: A Pilot Study," is included in this section. This study examined the effects of a vitamin D_3 supplement on depressive symptoms in women with low vitamin D levels. This study is followed by the three steps for critically appraising a quantitative study:

- Step 1: Identifying the steps of the research process
- Step 2: Determining study strengths and weaknesses
- Step 3: Evaluating the credibility and meaning of study findings

Nursing students and practicing nurses usually conduct critical appraisals that are focused on identifying the steps of the research process in a study. This type of critical appraisal may be written in outline format, with headings identifying the steps of the research process. A more in-depth critical appraisal includes not only this step but also determines study strengths and weaknesses and evaluates the study findings' credibility and meaning. We encourage you to read the Shipowick and associates' (2009) study, and conduct a comprehensive critical appraisal using the guidelines presented earlier in this chapter. Compare your ideas with the critical appraisal presented in this section.

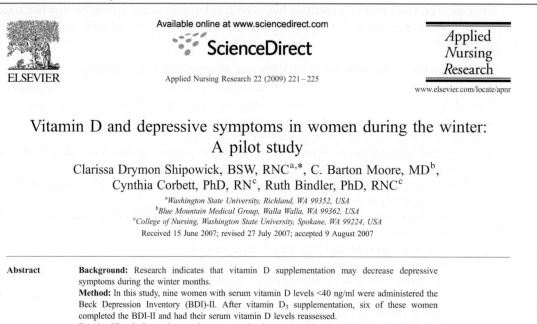

Available online at www.sciencedirect.com

ScienceDirect

ELSEVIER

Applied Nursing Research 22 (2009) 221–225

Applied
Nursing
Research

www.elsevier.com/locate/apnr

Vitamin D and depressive symptoms in women during the winter: A pilot study

Clarissa Drymon Shipowick, BSW, RNC[a],*, C. Barton Moore, MD[b],
Cynthia Corbett, PhD, RN[c], Ruth Bindler, PhD, RNC[c]

[a]*Washington State University, Richland, WA 99352, USA*
[b]*Blue Mountain Medical Group, Walla Walla, WA 99362, USA*
[c]*College of Nursing, Washington State University, Spokane, WA 99224, USA*

Received 15 June 2007; revised 27 July 2007; accepted 9 August 2007

Abstract

Background: Research indicates that vitamin D supplementation may decrease depressive symptoms during the winter months.

Method: In this study, nine women with serum vitamin D levels <40 ng/ml were administered the Beck Depression Inventory (BDI)-II. After vitamin D_3 supplementation, six of these women completed the BDI-II and had their serum vitamin D levels reassessed.

Results: Vitamin D supplementation was associated not only with an increase in the serum D levels by an average of 27 ng/ml but also with a decline in the BDI-II scores of an average of 10 points.

Discussion: This study suggests that supplemental vitamin D_3 reduces depressive symptoms.
© 2009 Elsevier Inc. All rights reserved.

1. Vitamin D and depressive symptoms in women during the winter

It has been hypothesized that low vitamin D levels in the winter account for exacerbation of melancholia (Vasquez, Manso, & Cannell, 2004). Vitamin D can be obtained through food consumption or synthesized by the body from sun exposure. For people living in northern climates (above 37° latitude), the oblique angle of the sun's rays during the autumn and winter precludes vitamin D synthesis, and vitamin D deficiency or insufficiency is common (Rucker, Allen, Fick, & Hanley, 2002).

In the United States, laboratories use a different version of the metric system (nanograms per milliliter) to measure 25-OH serum vitamin D levels, whereas the International System of Units is used worldwide (nanomoles per liter). The following 25-OH serum vitamin D levels are used as criteria for this study. Vitamin D deficiency is defined as serum levels <20 ng/ml or <50 nmol/L. The prefix *nano* is one billionth of a unit of measurement (Pickett, 2000). Vitamin D insufficiency is defined as serum vitamin D levels >20 but <40 ng/ml or >50 but <100 nmol/L. Optimal vitamin D levels are defined as between 40 and 65 ng/ml or between 100 and 160 nmol/L (Vasquez et al., 2004). Toxic levels do not occur until circulating levels are greater than 125 ng/ml or 312 nmol/L (Holick & Jenkins, 2003).

Research shows that women are more susceptible to depression than men (Kornstein & Sloan, 2003). Women under 40 years of age are four times more likely to have seasonal affective disorder than men (Gaines, 2005). According to the World Health Organization (WHO), by 2020, depression will be the leading cause of disability worldwide (WHO, 2000).

Studies indicate that vitamin D deficiency is associated with increased depressive symptoms (Armstrong et al., 2006; Jorde, Waterloo, Haug, & Svartberg, 2005). Thus, vitamin D supplementation may provide a natural, inexpensive, and accessible remedy for seasonal mood fluctuations and an adjunct for individuals with depressive symptoms.

2. Purpose of the study

The following research questions guided the study: (a) Is there a significant relationship between serum vitamin D

* Corresponding author. Tel.: +1 509 522 2747.
E-mail address: cshipowick@charter.net (C.D. Shipowick).

222   *C.D. Shipowick et al. / Applied Nursing Research 22 (2009) 221–225*

levels and depressive symptoms? and (b) Do depressive symptoms in women with low serum vitamin D levels improve 8 weeks after initiation of vitamin D_3 supplementation (5,000 IU daily) during the fall and winter?

3. Conceptual model

Vitamin D_3 is hydoxylated in the liver to become 25-OH vitamin D, the major circulating form of vitamin D. It is activated in the kidneys to become the hormone 1,25-OH vitamin D where it is tightly regulated. Certain organs including the brain also have the capacity to activate vitamin D (Holick & Jenkins, 2003). Both unactivated and activated vitamin D can cross the blood–brain barrier (Kiraly, Kiraly, Hawe, & Makhani, 2006). Based on these data, a biopsychological framework of vitamin D as a hormone that influences depressive symptoms served as an emerging model (Fig. 1). Three physiologic pathways between vitamin D and depressive symptoms were identified: (a) Vitamin D in its active form in the body has been shown to stimulate serotonin (Gaines, 2005), a neurotransmitter that is associated with mood elevation; (b) Vitamin D has been

associated with down-regulation of glucocorticoid receptor gene activation, which is found to be up-regulated in depression; and (c) Vitamin D has also been found to be neuroprotective, shielding neurons from toxins such as glucocorticoids and other excitotoxic insults (Obradovic, Gronemeyer, Lutz, & Rein, 2006).

4. Literature review

In a descriptive study of patients with fibromyalgia ($N = 75$; 70 females and 5 males) at a clinic in Belfast, Ireland, during the winter season, 10% were found to be vitamin D deficient, 42% had levels that were labeled inadequate, and only 23% had levels considered to be adequate (Armstrong et al., 2006). The Hospital Anxiety and Depression Scale (HADS), a tool used to measure mood disorders, was completed by these patients. Using a Kruskal–Wallis analysis of variance (ANOVA), a statistically significant difference ($p \le .05$) between the HADS scores of the group with the lowest vitamin D levels and the other two groups was found, suggesting a link between anxious and depressive symptoms and vitamin D deficiency.

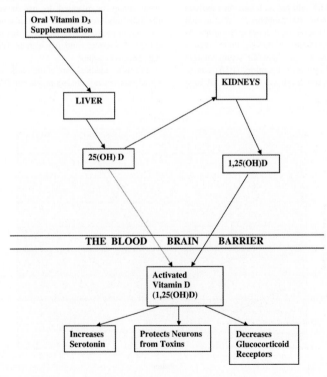

Fig. 1. The biopsychological model of vitamin D: hormone that elevates mood. From *The UV Advantage* (Fig. 1.3: New understanding of how vitamin D benefits health), by M. Holick & M. Jenkins, 2003, New York, NY: Ibooks Inc. Adapted with permission.

Continued

C.D. Shipowick et al. / Applied Nursing Research 22 (2009) 221–225   223

Table 1
Paired samples statistics and tests ($n = 6$)

Paired samples	M	Difference in means	SD	Average SD	t	p
BDI-II (1)	31.8333	10.66667	4.79236	7.7616	3.366	.020
BDI-II (2)	21.1667		11.07098			
25-OH-D (1)	21.8333	−26.33333	8.32867	15.68014	−4.114	.009
25-OH-D (2)	48.1667		20.01416			

In an Australian study during the summer, serum vitamin D levels were collected from patients with unipolar and bipolar depression ($N = 17$). Only 3 of the 17 participants had adequate vitamin D levels. The mean serum vitamin D level among the general population in the same geographic area was found to be 34 nmol/L higher. This study suggests that a higher proportion of depressed patients are vitamin D deficient (Berk et al., 2007).

The Tromso study, conducted in northern Norway, measured serum calcium and parathyroid hormone levels in 7,950 participants. Subsequently, a secondary analysis of 21 participants who had been experiencing secondary hyperparathyroidism without renal failure was conducted. The 21 participants with altered calcium metabolism demonstrated neuropsychological problems. A relationship between serum vitamin D levels and depressive symptoms was also documented. Using ANOVA, there was a statistically significant association between serum vitamin D levels and the Beck Depression Inventory (BDI) scores, indicating that a low serum level was indicative of high

depressive symptoms. This association did not appear to be the result of covariation with any other variables. Low serum vitamin D levels correlated with higher BDI scores, identifying a negative correlation between vitamin D levels and depressive symptoms (Jorde et al., 2005).

5. Methods and procedure

Following university institutional review board approval and the approval of the clinical agency where the study was carried out, a quasi-experimental pretest–posttest design was implemented with female participants acting as their own pre-post control. Female patients ($N = 9$) being treated at a medical clinic in southeastern Washington for vitamin D deficiency or insufficiency voluntarily participated in this study. Initial evaluations took place between January and March. During these months, vitamin D stores are typically low and the impact of vitamin D supplementation should be most visible in participants. The following were excluded from the study: (a) those with mental impairments such as dementia or language barriers that may have inhibited answering written questions; (b) women who were using or planned to use tanning beds or other phototherapy; (c) women who planned on traveling to sunnier, more tropical areas (e.g., Mexico, Hawaii, Arizona) during the winter; and (d) women taking or planning to take antidepressants.

Per usual medical care at the clinic, participants who had blood tests that indicated serum vitamin D levels below 40 ng/ml

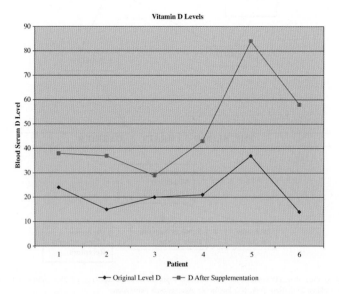

Fig. 2. Comparing vitamin D levels before and after supplementation. This graph shows that vitamin D_3 supplementation is associated with an increase in serum 25-OH vitamin D levels by an average of 27 ng/ml after 8 weeks.

were advised to initiate vitamin D_3 supplementation (5,000 IU) by their physician. Before vitamin D_3 supplementation, women were informed of the research opportunity. Women agreeing to participate completed the BDI-II survey prior to initiating vitamin D_3 supplementation. The BDI-II is a commonly used depression screening tool with demonstrated reliability and validity. The following criteria are used universally in the scoring of the BDI-II and for this study. Potential scores range from 0 to 63 with normal (0–13), mild depression (14–19), moderate depression (20–28), and severe depression (29–63) as designated. After the 8 weeks of D_3 supplementation, participants returned to the clinic to have their vitamin D level rechecked per usual clinic protocol and once again completed the BDI-II survey. Participants gave permission for their medical records to be accessed to document serum vitamin D levels for the study. Of the nine participants, six provided BDI-II and serum vitamin D levels 8 weeks after vitamin D_3 supplementation.

6. Data analysis and results

SPSS 14.0 was used to perform statistical analysis. The participants who did not complete the postsupplement measurements were not included in the correlational and inferential analyses. Cronbach's alpha for the BDI-II was .81 at baseline and .95 at follow-up.

Six participants completed the study. This subsample had a mean age of 42.2 years ($SD = 13.17$, range = 23–55). Their

baseline and follow-up mean serum vitamin D levels were 21.8 ($SD = 8.33$, range = 14–37) and 48.2 ($SD = 20.01$, range = 29–84), respectively ($t = -4.11$, $p = .009$). The baseline and follow-up mean BDI-II scores were 31.8 ($SD = 4.79$, range = 26–40) and 21.2 ($SD = 11.07$, range = 8–37), respectively ($t = 3.37$, $p = .02$; Table 1). Normal serum vitamin D levels (>40 ng/ml) were achieved after supplementation for three participants (Fig. 2). These same three participants had BDI-II scores of 14 or below after supplementation (Fig. 3).

7. Discussion

Following supplementation, serum vitamin D levels increased in all participants with an average increase of 27 ng/ml. At the prescribed intake of 5,000 IU daily, a significant reduction in depressive symptoms was realized after supplementation. Further, among the three women with a postsupplementation serum vitamin D level greater than 40, all had BDI-II scores of 14 or less, suggestive of normal mood with minimal depressive symptoms.

The Armstrong study statistically associated depressive and anxious symptoms with low serum vitamin D levels. The Berk study found low vitamin D levels prevalent in patients diagnosed with unipolar or bipolar depression, and the Tromso study associated low vitamin D levels with higher scores on the BDI, indicative of depressive symptoms. The current study associated higher vitamin D levels with lower BDI-II scores, indicating less depressive

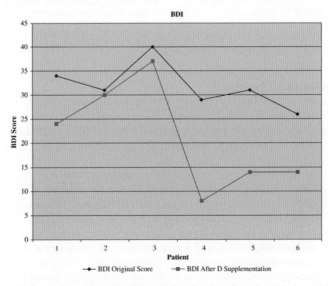

Fig. 3. Comparing BDI-II scores before and after supplementation. This graph shows that vitamin D supplementation is associated with a decline (improved mood: a negative correlation) in BDI-II scores of an average of about 10 points.

Continued

RESEARCH EXAMPLE—cont'd

C.D. Shipowick et al. / Applied Nursing Research 22 (2009) 221–225 225

symptoms with more optimal vitamin D levels. Further research with a larger sample size and stronger design is warranted to continue to investigate the clinical utility of vitamin D₃ supplementation.

8. Limitations and conclusions

Replication of this study with a larger, adequately powered sample is needed to provide a more definitive understanding of the relationship between vitamin D supplementation and seasonal depressive symptoms. Additionally, further research to determine factors related to vitamin D₃ dosing is needed. The reasons for three of the women not achieving serum vitamin D₃ levels above 40 ng/ml are unclear. It may be that these women were not consistently taking vitamin D₃, that they required longer than 8 weeks of supplementation to achieve optimal vitamin D levels, or that a higher vitamin D₃ dose was needed to achieve optimal vitamin D levels. More frequent analyses of serum vitamin D levels and measuring adherence to supplementation are warranted in future studies. Future studies should be conducted with a randomized and blinded design to account for placebo effect.

In summary, this pilot study provides evidence to suggest that women who suffer from seasonal depressive symptoms may benefit from vitamin D₃ supplementation if serum vitamin D levels are low (<40 ng/ml). These findings are consistent with other studies that indicate that higher vitamin D levels improve sense of well-being (Armstrong et al., 2006; Berk et al., 2007; Jorde et al., 2005).

Acknowledgments

We are grateful to Robert Bendall for his statistical expertise and to Mary DeRose for her work behind the scenes and her troubleshooting expertise.

References

Armstrong, D. J., et al. (2006). Vitamin D deficiency is associated with anxiety and depression in fibromyalgia. *Clinical Rheumatology, 26*(4), 348–355.
Berk, M., et al. (2007). Vitamin D deficiency may play a role in depression. *Medical Hypotheses, 4*(1), 1–4.
Gaines, S. (2005). The saddest season. *Minnesota Medicine, 88*, 25–32.
Holick, M., & Jenkins, M. (2003). *The UV advantage.* New York, NY: Ibooks Inc.
Jorde, R., Waterloo, K., Saleh, F., Haug, E., & Svartberg, J. (2005). The Tromso study. *Journal of Neurology, 10*, 27–32.
Kiraly, S., Kiraly, M., Hawe, R., & Makhani, N. (2006, January). Vitamin D as a neuroactive substance: Review. *Scientific World Journal, 6*, 125–139.
Kornstein, S., & Sloan, D. (2003). Gender differences in depression and response to antidepressant treatment. *Psychiatric Clinics North America, 26*, 581–594.
Obradovic, D., Gronemeyer, H., Lutz, B., & Rein, T. (2006). Cross-talk of vitamin D and glucocorticoids in hippocampal cells. *Journal of Neurochemistry, 96*, 500–509.
Pickett J, (Ed.) (2000). *The American heritage dictionary of the English language.* 4th ed. Boston: Houghton Mifflin Company, p. 1167.
Rucker, D., Allen, J., Fick, G., & Hanley, D. (2002). Vitamin D insufficiency in a population of healthy western Canadians. *Canadian Medical Association Journal, 166*, 1517–1524.
Vasquez, A., Manso G., & Cannell, J. (2004). The clinical importance of vitamin D: A paradigm shift with implications for all healthcare providers. *Alternative Therapies in Health and Medicine, 10*, 28–36.
World Health Organization. (2000). Setting the WHO agenda for mental health. *Bulletin of the World Health Organization,* (Vol. 78, p. 500).

(From Shipowick, C. D., Moore, C. B., Corbett, C., & Bindler, R. [2009]. Vitamin D and depressive symptoms in women during the winter: A pilot study. *Applied Nursing Research, 22*[3], 221-225.)

Critical Appraisal
Step 1: Steps of the Research Process

1. *Abstract:* The study abstract included the problem, sample of women with serum vitamin D levels less than 40 ng/mL, sample size of nine, with six completing the study, treatment of vitamin D₃ supplementation, dependent variable of depressive symptoms measured with the Beck Depression Inventory II (BDI-II), key results, and conclusions. The study purpose and design were not included in the abstract.

2. *Problem:*
"Research shows that women are more susceptible to depression than men (Sloan & Kornstein, 2003). Women under 40 years of age are four times more likely to have seasonal affective disorder than men (Gaines, 2005). According to the World Health Organization (WHO), by 2020, depression will be the leading cause of disability worldwide (WHO, 2000). Studies indicate that vitamin D deficiency is associated with increased depressive symptoms (Armstrong et al., 2007; Jorde et al., 2006). Thus, vitamin D supplementation may provide a natural, inexpensive, and accessible remedy for seasonal mood fluctuations and an adjunct for individuals with depressive symptoms." (Shipowick et al., 2009, p. 221)

3. *Purpose:* The purpose is not clearly stated in the study, but it is evident from the title and problem that the purpose of this quasi-experimental study was to examine the effect of vitamin D₃ supplementation on depressive symptoms of women during the winter months.

4. *Literature review:* A minimal review of literature is presented in this research report. Shipowick and associates (2009) identified three studies that linked vitamin D to depression. Armstrong and co-workers (2007) found that patients with the lowest vitamin D levels had the highest anxiety and depression scores. This suggested a link between anxious and depressive symptoms and vitamin D deficiency. Berk and colleagues (2007) found that a higher proportion of depressed patients were vitamin D–deficient, supporting the link between depression and vitamin D level. Jorde and associates (2005) found a "statistically significant association between serum vitamin D levels and the Beck Depression Inventory (BDI) scores, indicating that a low serum level was indicative of high depressive symptoms" (Shipowick et al., 2009; p. 223).

5. *Framework:* A biopsychological model is appropriate and clearly presented as the framework for this study. Shipowick and co-workers (2009) described their model in the following way:
   "Vitamin D_3 is hydroxylated in the liver to become 25-OH vitamin D, the major circulating form of vitamin D. It is activated in the kidneys to become the hormone 1,25-OH vitamin D where it is tightly regulated. Certain organs including the brain also have the capacity to activate vitamin D (Holick & Jenkins, 2003). Both unactivated and activated vitamin D can cross the blood-brain barrier (Kiraly et al., 2006). Based on these data, a biopsychological framework of vitamin D as a hormone that influences depressive symptoms served as an emerging model (see Figure 12-1 of this study as follows). Three physiological pathways between vitamin D and depressive symptoms were identified: (a) vitamin D in its active form in the body has been shown to stimulate serotonin (Gaines, 2005), a neurotransmitter that is associated with mood elevation; (b) vitamin D has been associated with down-regulation of glucocorticoid receptor gene activation, which is found to be unregulated in depression; and (c) vitamin D has also been found to be neuroprotective, shielding neurons from toxins such as glucocorticoids and other excitotoxic insults (Obradovic, Gronemeyer, Lutz, & Rein, 2006)." (Shipowick et al., 2009, p. 222)

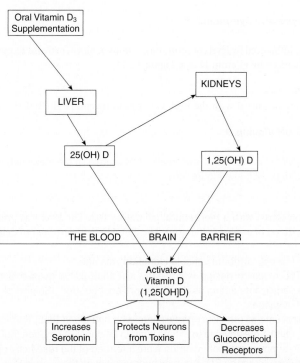

FIG 12-1 The biopsychological model of vitamin D, a hormone that elevates mood. (Adapted from Holick, M., & Jenkins, M. (2003). The UV advantage. New York: Ibooks; and Shipowick, C. D., Moore, C. B., Corbett, C., & Bindler, R. [2009]. Vitamin D and depressive symptoms in women during the winter: A pilot study. *Applied Nursing Research, 22*[3], 222.)

Continued

6. *Research questions and hypothesis*
   "The following research questions guided the study: (a) Is there a significant relationship between serum vitamin D levels and depressive symptoms? and (b) Do depressive symptoms in women with low serum vitamin D levels improve 8 weeks after initiation of vitamin D_3 supplementation (5000 IU [International Units] daily) during the fall and winter?" (Shipowick et al., 2009, pp. 221-222)
7. *Variables:* Shipowick and co-workers (2009) clearly presented the conceptual and operational definitions for the independent variable (vitamin D_3 supplementation) and dependent variables (depression symptoms and 25-OH vitamin D). The conceptual definitions are linked to the study framework, and the operational definitions are linked to the study methodology. The conceptual and operational definitions for these variables are provided in the following excerpt.

Independent Variable: Vitamin D_3 Supplementation
Conceptual Definition
Vitamin D_3 improves depressive symptoms through:
   "...three physiological pathways: (a) its active form in the body stimulates serotonin, a neurotransmitter associated with mood elevations; (b) it is associated with down-regulation of glucocorticoid receptor gene activation, which is up-regulated in depression; and (c) it is neuroprotective, shielding neurons from toxins such as glucocorticoids and other excitotoxic insults." (Shipowick et al., 2009, p. 222; see Figure 12-1)

Operational Definition
The treatment of vitamin D_3 supplementation was implemented by providing the subjects with 5000 IU of vitamin D_3 daily for 8 weeks.

Dependent Variable: Depressive Symptoms
Conceptual Definition
Depressive symptoms are influenced by levels of serotonin, actions of glucocorticoid receptors, and neurons exposed to toxins, which are influenced by vitamin D (see Figure 12-1).

Operational Definition
Depressive symptoms were measured with the Beck Depression Inventory II (BDI-II), a Likert scale.

Dependent Variable: 25-OH Vitamin D
Conceptual Definition
   "Vitamin D_3 is hydroxylated in the liver to become 25-OH vitamin D, the major circulating form of vitamin D." (Shipowick et al., 2009, p. 222; see Figure 12-1)

Operational Definition
25-OH vitamin D was measured with a biochemical laboratory test. The level was pretested to determine if the women met the sample criteria of a value < 40 ng/ml. The 25-OH was post-tested to determine if the participants' value was > 40 ng/ml.

8. *Attribute variables:* The only attribute variable identified was age.
9. *Research design:* The research design was clearly identified as "a quasi-experimental pretest-posttest design with female participants acting as their own pre-post control" (Shipowick et al., 2009, p. 223).
   a. *Treatment or intervention:*
      "Per usual medical care at the clinic, participants who had blood tests that indicated serum vitamin D levels below 40 ng/ml were advised to initiate vitamin D_3 supplementation (5000 IU) by their physicians. Before vitamin D_3 supplementation, women were informed of the research opportunity. Women agreeing to participate completed the BDI-II survey prior to initiating the vitamin D_3 supplementation." (Shipowick, 2009, pp. 223-224)
      The women participants took the 5000 IU vitamin D_3 supplement daily for 8 weeks.
   b. *Group assignment:* The study has only one group of 9 women who served as their own control. This means they completed BDI-II scale as the pretest and then took the 5000 IU of vitamin D_3 supplement

treatment for 8 weeks and then were post-tested for depressed symptoms with the BDI-II. Thus, the pretest is considered the control and the post-test is conducted to determine the effect of the treatment. The pretest scores are compared with the post-test scores to determine the effect of the vitamin D_3 treatment (Grove et al., 2013).

10. *Sample*
    a. *Sample criteria:* Sample inclusion criteria were females being treated for vitamin D deficiency or insufficiency with vitamin D level below 40 ng/mL as measured by the serum level of 25-OH vitamin D. "The following were excluded from the study: (a) those with mental impairments such as dementia or language barriers that may have inhibited answering written questions; (b) women who were using or planned to use tanning beds or other phototherapy; (c) women who planned on traveling to sunnier, more tropical areas (e.g., Mexico, Hawaii, Arizona) during the winter; and (d) women taking or planning to take antidepressants." (Shipowick et al., 2009, p. 223)
    b. *Sampling method:* Nonprobability sample of convenience is indicated by the women being asked to take part in the study, and then they voluntarily participated.
    c. Sample size and attrition: The sample size was $N=9$. Three participants were lost from the study, indicating a 33% attrition rate, and six (67%) completed the study. This study included no mention of power analysis or acceptance rate for study participation.
11. *Institutional review board and type of consent:*
    "Following university institutional review board approval and the approval of the clinical agency where the study was carried out..." (Shipowick et al., p. 223). "Before vitamin D_3 supplementation, women were informed of the research opportunity. Women agreeing to participate completed the BDI-II." (Shipowick et al., 2009, p. 224)
12. *Study setting:* The setting was a medical clinic in southeastern Washington state. The women took the vitamin D_3 supplements daily in their homes.
13. *Measurement methods:* The study included the dependent variable depressive symptoms that was measured with one measurement method, the BDI-II Likert scale. However, the sample inclusion criteria required that the women have a serum 25-OH vitamin D level prior to the study, and this level was also post-tested so it might be considered a second dependent variable. Therefore both measurement methods are included in the following table.

Name of Measurement Method	Author	Type of Measurement Method	Level of Measurement	Reliability or Precision	Validity or Accuracy
Beck Depression Inventory II (BDI-II)	Beck	Likert Scale	Interval	BDI-II, commonly used depression screening tool with demonstrated reliability; for this study, the BDI-II had Cronbach alphas of 0.81 at baseline and 0.95 at follow-up.	BDI-II had demonstrated validity in previous studies and was used in Jorde and associates' (2005) study cited in the literature review; successive use validity because scale is used in previous studies and current study

Continued

RESEARCH EXAMPLE—cont'd

Name of Measurement Method	Author	Type of Measurement Method	Level of Measurement	Reliability or Precision	Validity or Accuracy
25-OH vitamin D level	Biochemical measure	Physiological measurement method—laboratory test of serum vitamin D level	Ratio	Precision of laboratory test not addressed in the study; no discussion of the collection and analysis of the serum for the vitamin D levels; serum collection done in same clinic for pre- and post-tests	Vitamin D is hydroxylated in the liver to become 25-OH vitamin D, the major circulating form of vitamin D; thus, 25-OH vitamin D is the most accurate measure of vitamin D in the body to identify deficiencies.

14. *Data collection procedures:* The women were screened for their 25-OH vitamin D level in January to March. If the vitamin D level was less than 40 ng/mL, the women were informed of the study and asked to participate. Those volunteering to participate in the study then were asked to complete the BDI-II and then started on the 5000 IU of vitamin D_3 every day for 8 weeks. At the end of the eighth week, the women again were asked to complete the BDI-II to document their depression symptoms. The 25-OH vitamin D level was also determined. Those involved in treatment implementation and data collection were not identified. The training of individuals for data collection and implementation of the treatment was not described.

15. *Statistical analyses:* The Statistical Package for the Social Sciences (SPSS) 14.0 was used to perform the statistical analyses. Only the six participants completing the study were included in the analyses. The analyses conducted are summarized in the following table.

Purpose of Analysis	Analysis Technique	Statistic	Result	Probability (*p*)
Description of subjects' age	Mean	$\bar{x}$	42.2	
	Standard deviation	SD	13.17	
	Range	Range	23-55	
Description of depression symptoms measured with the BDI-II			Pretest Post-test	
	Mean	$\bar{x}$	31.8333 21.1667	
	Standard deviation	SD	4.79236 11.07098	
		Average SD	7.7616	
	Differences in means	Mean difference	10.66667	
	Line graph		Figure 12-3	

Purpose of Analysis	Analysis Technique	Statistic	Result	Probability (p)
Description of 25-OH vitamin D levels			Pretest Post-test	
	Mean	$\bar{x}$	21.8333 48.1667	
	Standard deviation	SD Average SD	8.32867 15.68014	
	Differences in means	Mean difference	−26.33333	
	Line graph		Figure 12-2	
Difference between pretest and post-test on depressive symptoms	Dependent or paired t-test	t	3.366	p=0.020
Difference between pretest and post-test for 25-OH vitamin D level	Dependent or paired t-test	t	−4.114	p=0.009

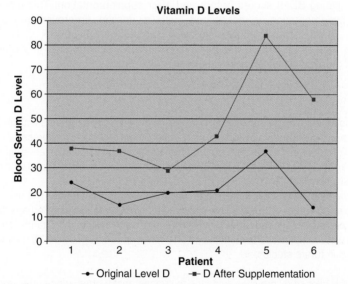

FIG 12-2 Comparing vitamin D levels before and after supplementation. This graph shows that vitamin D_3 supplementation is associated with an increase in serum 25-OH vitamin D levels by an average of 27 ng/mL after 8 weeks. (From Shipowick, C. D., Moore, C. B., Corbett, C., & Bindler, R. (2009). Vitamin D and depressive symptoms in women during the winter: A pilot study. *Applied Nursing Research, 22*[3], 223.)

Continued

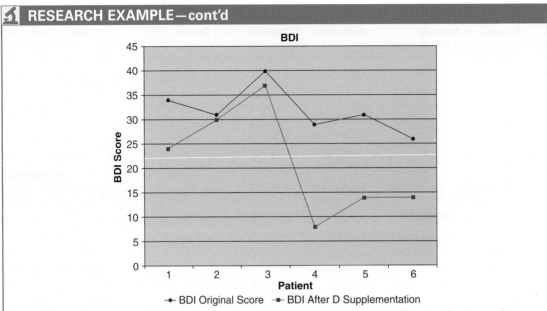

FIG 12-3 Comparing BDI-II scores before and after supplementation. This graph shows that vitamin D supplementation is associated with a decline (improved mood: a negative correlations) in BDI-II scores of an average of 10 points. (From Shipowick, C. D., Moore, C. B., Corbett, C., & Bindler, R. [2009]. Vitamin D and depressive symptoms in women during the winter: A pilot study. *Applied Nursing Research, 22*[3], 223.)

16. *Interpretation of findings:*
    "Following supplementation, serum vitamin D levels increased in all participants with an average increase of 27 ng/ml. At the prescribed intake of 5000 IU daily, a significant reduction in depressive symptoms was realized after supplementation. Further, among the three women with a postsupplementation serum vitamin D level greater than 40, all had BDI-II scores of 14 or less, suggestive of normal mood with minimal depressive symptoms." (Shipowick et al., 2009, p. 224)

17. *Limitations of the study:* The small sample size was identified as a limitation. The reasons for three of the women not achieving serum vitamin D_3 levels above 40 ng/mL were unclear. Perhaps they were not taking the vitamin D_3 consistently or needed longer than 8 weeks to achieve optimal vitamin D levels of 40 to 65 ng/mL. The design was identified as a limitation, and Shipowick and colleagues (2009) recommended the use of stronger designs in future studies.

18. *Conclusions:*
    "In summary, this pilot study provides evidence to suggest that women who suffer from seasonal depressive symptoms may benefit from vitamin D_3 supplementation if serum vitamin D levels are low (<40 ng/ml). These findings are consistent with other studies that indicate that higher vitamin D levels improve sense of well-being (Armstrong et al., 2007; Berk et al., 2007; Jorde et al., 2005)." (Shipowick et al., 2009, p. 225)

19. *Implications for nursing:* The researchers provide no specific implications for nursing practice.

20. *Suggestions for further research:*
    "Further research with a larger sample size and stronger design is warranted to continue to investigate the clinical utility of vitamin D_3 supplementation.... Replication of this study with a larger, adequately powered sample is needed to provide a more definitive understanding of the relationship between vitamin D supplementation and seasonal depressive symptoms. Additionally, further research to determine factors related to vitamin D_3 dosing is needed.... More frequent analyses of serum vitamin D levels and measuring adherence to supplementation are warranted in future studies. Future studies should be conducted with a randomized and blinded design to account for placebo effect." (Shipowick et al., 2009, p. 225)

Step 2: Study Strengths and Weaknesses

This section discusses the strengths and weaknesses of the steps of the research process and the logical links among these steps. The abstract, problem, purpose, literature review, framework, methodology, results, and discussion elements of the Shipowick and associates' (2009) article are critically appraised.

Abstract

The abstract is very brief and includes the study problem, sample size, significant results, and conclusions. The abstract would have been strengthened by including the study purpose and design (APA, 2010).

Problem and Purpose

The research problem is clearly identified in the abstract and in the first few paragraphs of the article. This is a significant clinical problem that could be detected, managed, and monitored by nurses in collaboration with physicians. Vitamin D insufficiency is a very common problem in healthcare today, as is depression. Additional research is needed to determine the impact of vitamin D supplementation on depression symptoms (Brown, 2014; O'Mathuna et al., 2011). The purpose is not clearly stated in the study, but is inferred from the study title and research questions (Creswell, 2014).

Literature Review

The literature review is brief, including only three studies, and would have been strengthened by the addition of more correlational and quasi-experimental studies focused on the impact of vitamin D supplementation on mood. However, the three studies cited provide a basis for conducting this study. The references cited in the study and the reference list included some errors, such as the Armstrong and co-workers' study having a 2006 date in the research report, but the source is actually a 2007 publication. The Kornstein and Sloan (2003) article is really Sloan and Kornstein (2003), and the pages for the Gaines (2005) article are pages 30 to 33. In addition, a final summary of what is known and not known about the problem studied would have added clarity to the literature review (Grove et al., 2013).

Framework

The framework section is a major strength of this study. Shipowick and colleagues (2009) provided a clear, concise, appropriate physiological framework for their study (Smith & Liehr, 2008). The biopsychological model presented in the study provides a clear link of how vitamin D as a hormone elevates mood and decreases depressive symptoms (Figure 12-1). The study framework also provided clear conceptual definitions of the independent and dependent variables, and these conceptual definitions provided a basis for operationalizing these variables in this study (Grove et al., 2013).

Methods

The study design is a single group pretest and post-test, with subjects serving as their own control. This is a weak design because there is only a treatment group and no comparison group to determine if the treatment is effective or if the change from pretest to post-test is caused by extraneous variables (Creswell, 2014; Shadish et al., 2002). However, the design does provide a means to examine the two research questions. The sample size was small, $N = 9$, and no power analysis was conducted to determine an adequate sample size for the study (Aberson, 2010). In addition, the study has a high attrition rate (33.3%), with three subjects dropping out of the study before the 8 weeks of the treatment were completed. No rationale is provided for why the subjects did not complete the study. However, the study results were significant, indicating that the sample was adequately powered, and no type II error occurred (Aberson, 2010; Grove et al., 2013).

The sampling method was one of convenience, and there is greater potential for sampling error with a nonprobability sample than a random sample. However, the researchers provide very strong sample inclusion and exclusion criteria that limit the potential effects of extraneous variables and improve the representativeness of the sample. Only the age of the participants is given, and it would have been helpful to include the ethnicity and history of depression when describing the sample. The study seemed ethical because it was approved for conduct by the IRBs of the university and clinic and informed consent was obtained from the study participants (Hoe & Hoare, 2012).

The study included a strong treatment of vitamin D_3 supplementation, 5000 IU daily for 8 weeks. However, the researchers needed to provide more detail about how the treatment was implemented. If the treatment was implemented by more than one person, the training to promote consistency in the administration of treatment needed to be addressed (Santacroce et al., 2004).

Continued

> ### RESEARCH EXAMPLE—cont'd
>
> The BDI-II is a strong measurement strategy for depression and has been used in many other studies over the years. In addition, the Cronbach alphas were strong and supported the reliability of the BDI-II in this study. However, the measurement section would have been strengthened by a more detailed discussion of the reliability and validity of the BDI-II based on previous research (DeVon et al., 2007; Hoe & Hoare, 2012; Roberts & Stone, 2003; Waltz et al., 2010). The researchers discussed the scoring for the BDI-II and indicated that the scores could range from 0 to 63. They also indicated the meaning for the different scores, with normal scores from 0 to 13, mild depression scores from 14 to 19, moderate depression scores from 20 to 28, and severe depression scores from 29 to 63.
>
> The 25-OH vitamin D level is the strongest measurement of vitamin D levels in the body and is the most effective way to identify women with insufficient vitamin D levels. Additional discussion was needed, however, of the precision and accuracy of the laboratory in determining the 25-OH vitamin D levels in this study (DeKeyser & Pugh, 1990). Shipowick and colleagues (2009) did not indicate who collected the data. If more than one person collected data, the reliability or consistency of the data collection process needs to be addressed (Grove et al., 20013; Santacroce et al., 2004).
>
> #### Results
>
> The statistical techniques used to analyze data from the BDI-II and the 25-OH vitamin D levels were clearly identified and appropriate. The analysis techniques (descriptive and inferential) are appropriate for the level of measurement of the variables (Grove, 2007; Plichta & Kelvin, 2013). The results are clearly and concisely presented in narrative form, table, and graphs to facilitate understanding. The sample size was small but adequate to detect significant differences between the pretests and post-tests for depression symptoms and vitamin D levels. This section would have been strengthened by linking the results to the two research questions (Hoare & Hoe, 2013).
>
> #### Discussion
>
> The findings were as expected, and the statistical and clinical significance of the findings are clearly addressed (Brown, 2014; Hoare & Hoe, 2013). The findings were supportive of the study framework and consistent with previous research, which was documented in the article. The conclusions were clearly expressed and appropriate based on the study results and findings. The researchers identified the study limitations and provided specific appropriate ideas for future studies to overcome the limitations of this study. A randomized clinical trial design was recommended, which would greatly strengthen the quality of the study and credibility of the findings (Mittlbock, 2008). The researchers did not make recommendations for nursing practice but focused on the need for additional research before making changes in practice.
>
> #### Step 3: Credibility and Meaning of the Study Findings
>
> The Shipowick and associates' (2009) study examined significant clinical problems (seasonal depression and vitamin D deficiencies in women) and examined the effectiveness of vitamin D_3 supplementation for these problems. This study has many strengths and few weaknesses, which leads one to conclude that the findings are credible and an accurate reflection of reality. The findings—women who suffer from seasonal depressive symptoms may benefit from vitamin D_3 supplementation if their vitamin D levels are low—are supportive of the study framework (Figure 12-1 of this example). In addition, these findings are consistent with those of previous researchers (Armstrong et al., 2007; Berk et al., 2007; Jorde et al., 2006).
>
> The findings of the Shipowick and co-workers' (2009) study increase our understanding of the link between vitamin D and depressive symptoms in women and provide direction for future studies. Vitamin D_3 has potential to be an effective treatment for seasonal depression in women with low vitamin D levels. Because of the small sample size and limitations of the study design, however, the researchers do not recommend generalizing these findings from the sample to the population. Shipowick and colleagues provided excellent, detailed directions for future studies. They did not recommend using the findings in practice at this time. Clinically, patients are currently being tested for deficiencies in vitamin D levels and treated with 5000 IU of vitamin D_3, even though research is still inadequate to recommend treatment of depressive symptoms with vitamin D. This is an important area for further research.

UNDERSTANDING THE QUALITATIVE RESEARCH CRITICAL APPRAISAL PROCESS

Nurses in every phase and field of practice need experience in critically appraising qualitative and quantitative studies. Although qualitative studies require a different approach to critical appraisal than quantitative studies (Sandelowski, 2008), appraisal in both cases has a common purpose—determining the rigor with which the methods were applied and the extent to which the conclusions of the study were trustworthy. Critical appraisal of qualitative studies focuses on how the integrity of the design and methods will affect the credibility and meaningfulness of the findings and their usefulness in clinical practice (Pickler, 2007). Different criteria have been used to appraise qualitative studies critically (Burns, 1989; Clissett, 2008; Cohen & Crabtree, 2008; Morse, 1991; Schoe, Høstrop, Lyngsø, Larsen, & Poulsen, 2011). We include a set of criteria synthesized from these published criteria and have organized them into three broad steps similar to those used for critical appraisal of quantitative studies. Therefore the qualitative research critical appraisal process consists of (1) identifying the components of the qualitative research process in studies, (2) determining study strengths and weaknesses, and (3) evaluating the trustworthiness and meaning of study findings. Each step includes the questions to be addressed to reflect the philosophical orientation of qualitative research.

Step 1: Identifying the Components of the Qualitative Research Process in Studies

The first step of the critical appraisal process is similar to looking at a map of an entire country and observing the boundaries and key topographical features, such as mountains and lakes. You might find the cities to which you want to travel and identify the best route to travel from one to the other. At this point, you are not identifying the quality of the roads or unique aspects of the various cities you want to visit. This type of overview allows you to orient yourself to the country. In the same way, the first step of the critical appraisal process provides you with an overview of the study.

Guidelines for Identifying the Components of the Research Process in Qualitative Studies

Begin your appraisal by looking at the entire article, beginning with the title and abstract (review the principles presented in Box 12-1). What is the title? Is the abstract descriptive of the study? Continue your review and find the major headings of the article to determine if the major components of a research report are present.

Were the following parts of the research report plainly identified (APA, 2010)?

- Introduction section, with the problem, purpose, literature review, framework (if applicable), and objectives and questions
- Methods section, with the qualitative approach, sample, and data collection methods
- Results section, with the specific results presented as themes and supported by direct quotes from participants
- Discussion section, with the findings, conclusions, limitations, transferability to other groups, implications for practice, and suggestions for future research (Brown, 2014; Grove et al., 2013)

As you read the study report in more depth, identify and describe each of the following aspects of the study and its report.

Guidelines for Identifying the Components of a Qualitative Study

1. Introduction
   a. Describe the qualifications of the authors to conduct the study. Did the authors acknowledge any potential bias or personal connection related to the study topic and steps taken to reduce bias?
   b. Discuss the clarity of the article title. Is the title clearly focused and does it include the focus and population of the study? Does the title indicate the type of study conducted—phenomenology, grounded theory, ethnography, exploratory-descriptive qualitative, or historical research (Creswell, 2013, 2014; Fawcett & Garity, 2009; Hoe & Hoare, 2012)?
   c. Discuss the quality of the abstract (includes purpose, qualitative approach, sample, and key results; APA, 2010).
2. State the problem.
   a. Significance of the problem
   b. Background of the problem
   c. Problem statement
3. State the purpose.
4. Examine the literature review.
   a. Is the literature review identified as such? In some research articles, the literature review will be identified clearly as a review of the literature; some authors may incorporate the review into the background and significance.
   b. Did the author cite quantitative and qualitative studies relevant to the focus of the study? What other types of literature did the author include?
   c. Identify the disciplines of the authors of studies cited in this paper and the journals in which they published their studies. Does it appear that the author searched databases outside of the *Cumulative Index to Nursing and Allied Health Literature* (CINAHL) for relevant studies?
   d. Are the references current? Are classic or groundbreaking studies included, which may be older?
   e. Did the author evaluate or indicate the weaknesses of the available studies (Grove et al., 2013; Hart, 2009)?
5. Identify the study framework or philosophical orientation of the study.
   a. Did the authors cite primary sources to support the framework or philosophical orientation of the study?
   b. If the study was a grounded theory study, did the researcher develop a theoretical description or diagram as part of the study findings (Creswell, 2013)?
6. List the research objectives (aims) or questions, if identified.
7. Identify the qualitative approach used to answer the research questions (phenomenology, grounded theory, ethnography, exploratory-descriptive, historical, or other approach). If the specific qualitative approach was not identified, what aspects of the method, such as natural settings or coding, indicate that a qualitative approach was used (Creswell, 2013; Munhall, 2012)?
8. Describe the sample and setting.
   a. Identify inclusion and exclusion criteria.
   b. What methods did the researchers use to recruit participants?
   c. Identify the sample size.
   d. Identify the characteristics of the sample.

3. Study framework or philosophical orientation
   a. If a framework was used, are its major concepts reflected in the questions asked during data collection and in the findings?
   b. If a framework was developed from the findings (grounded theory study), is it clearly linked to the study findings?
4. Was the philosophical orientation of the qualitative approach identified? Was a primary source for the philosophy cited (Grove et al., 2013; Munhall, 2012)?
5. Research objectives or questions
   a. Are the objectives or questions presented clearly?
   b. Are the objectives or questions linked to the research purpose?
6. Qualitative approach
   a. Did the researchers select a qualitative approach that produced data to meet the objectives or answer the research questions?
   b. For a study with no identified qualitative approach, did the researcher provide a rationale for why a qualitative study was conducted (Creswell, 2014; Grove et al., 2013)?
7. Sample and setting
   a. Did the sampling method yield participants who had experience with the topic of the study and could provide data to address the research questions?
   b. Were participants excluded from the study because of age, socioeconomic status, or ethnicity without a sound rationale?
   c. Were the rights of human subjects protected?
   d. If potential participants refused to participate or participants did not complete the study, did the researcher acknowledge these issues as limitations?
   e. Did the setting in which data were collected protect the confidentiality and promote the comfort of the participants?
   f. If participants became upset during data collection, describe the measures taken to provide them with emotional support (Cowles, 1988).
8. Data collection
   a. Were questions used during the interview or focus group relevant to the study's research objectives or questions (Grove et al., 2013; Maxwell, 2013)?
   b. Did the interviews last long enough for the researcher to gather robust, thorough descriptions of the participants' perspectives?
   c. If focus groups were conducted, were the size, composition, and length adequate to promote group interaction and to produce robust data?
   d. Were observations conducted at times and for long enough periods to collect rich data that allows for a thorough description of the culture, setting, or process of interest (Wolf, 2012)?
9. Data analysis
   a. Were the data analysis processes described thoroughly enough to be able to evaluate the logic of the researcher's decisions and support the rigor of the study?
   b. Were the measures to increase the trustworthiness of the study adequate to give the reader confidence in the findings (Cohen & Crabtree, 2008; Mackey, 2012; Wolf, 2012)?
10. Interpretation of findings
    a. Were the findings linked to quotes or specific observations?
    b. Did the researcher address variations in the findings by relevant sample characteristics?

    c. If the findings were unexpected, what explanations were given for why this may have occurred?

11. Limitations
    a. Did the researchers acknowledge the limitations and their potential effects on the findings? Were there limitations that the researchers did not acknowledge?
    b. Were the limitations the result of factors under the researcher's control or external factors over which the researcher had no control?

12. Conclusions
    a. Did the conclusions logically flow out of the findings?
    b. Did the recommendations for future studies flow out of the findings?
    c. Did the researchers identify other settings or participants to whom the findings might be applicable?

Step 3: Evaluating the Trustworthiness and Meaning of Study Findings

The final step in the critical appraisal of qualitative studies is based on the information that you have identified and the conclusions that can be made from the first two steps of the process. Evaluating the trustworthiness of a study involves determining the credibility, transferability, dependability, and confirmability of the study findings. Although these terms can be defined individually, strategies used by the researchers to enhance the dependability of the findings directly affects the credibility and confirmability of the findings. Similarly, the findings are transferable (applicable) when the sample is described thoroughly, and the reader has confidence in the credibility, dependability, and confirmability of the findings.

Guidelines for Evaluating the Trustworthiness and Meaning of Study Findings

1. Could the limitations of the study have been prevented?
2. Do the findings provide a credible reflection of reality?
3. Does the study expand nurses' understanding of the phenomenon studied? If so, how can the findings be used in nursing practice and education?
4. What do the findings add to the current body of knowledge related to theory and education?
5. How does this study support future knowledge development?
6. Did the overall presentation of the study fit its purpose, method, and findings?
7. Was the presentation logical and clearly written (Cohen & Crabtree, 2008)?
8. Did the researchers provide ideas for further research?
9. State the conclusion or summary of the critical appraisal of the study (Grove et al., 2013).

EXAMPLE OF A CRITICAL APPRAISAL OF A QUALITATIVE STUDY

Bultas (2012) conducted a qualitative study about the experiences of preschool children with autism when they visit healthcare providers. A critical appraisal of the study was done to demonstrate the application of the critical appraisal guidelines to a published qualitative study. A copy of the study is provided here so that you may read it and work through the critical appraisal yourself. The study is followed by the three steps of critical appraisal.

Journal of Pediatric Nursing (2012) **27**, 460–470

ELSEVIER

The Health Care Experiences of the Preschool Child With Autism

Margaret W. Bultas PhD, RN, CPNP-PC*

St. Louis University, School of Nursing, St. Louis, MO

Key words:
Autism;
Health care;
Preschool child;
Mother

It is known that children with autism spectrum disorder (ASD) visit health care providers (HCPs) more frequently than typically developing peers, and mothers experience barriers in this process. The purpose of this interpretive phenomenological study was to gain a better understanding of a mother's experiences of taking her child with ASD to the HCP. Two themes related to the health care experience of the child surfaced from the study. These themes included feelings that HCPs do not "get" the complexity of caring for the child and marginalization of mothers by the HCP. The need for creation of child-specific profiles emerged from this study.
© 2012 Elsevier Inc. All rights reserved.

Background

THE PREVALENCE OF autism spectrum disorder (ASD) in the population has increased significantly since it was first described in the 1940s. The complex health care needs of children with ASD, along with their unique developmental characteristics, require an innovative approach to health care. Because of this, it is important to study and understand more about the health care experiences of children with ASD, as it can reveal concerns, feelings, resources, and barriers in the delivery of their health care.

There is little nursing literature that identifies specifics regarding the needs of mothers during health care visits for their child with ASD. Certainly, the literature indicates that mothers are dissatisfied with the lack of information received and their difficulty in accessing health care for their child (Minnes & Steiner, 2008; Ruble, Heflinger, Renfrew, & Saunders, 2005). However, there is a lack of information regarding these mothers' specific needs and concerns related to their children's health care experiences.

What does exist in the literature is evidence that mothers of children with autism have a keen sense and understanding of their child (Caronna, Augustyn, & Zuckerman, 2007;

Inglese, 2009; Nadel & Poss, 2007). Researchers also know that empowering the mother of a child with ASD leads to an overall better outcome for the child (Kuhn & Carter, 2006). Mothers are most frequently the caregiver that interacts with their child's health care provider (HCP). This is especially true in the early ages of a child's life. Therefore, mothers are uniquely situated to provide important information regarding their child with ASD's health care experiences.

Review of Literature

Increasing Prevalence of Autism

Autism was first described in the 1940s by Dr. Leo Kanner, a psychiatrist. Dr. Kanner presented several case studies of children who demonstrated "fascinating peculiarities" and a condition that differed "markedly and uniquely from anything reported so far" (Kanner, 1943, p. 217). The children showed little affection toward their parents, preferred to be alone, and were able to master skills such as patterning and counting at a very early age (Kanner, 1943). Since then, the definition and diagnostic criteria for ASD has been refined.

The prevalence of ASD in 2002 was estimated to be approximately 1 per 150 children in North America as noted

* Corresponding author: Margaret W. Bultas, PhD, RN, CPNP-PC.
E-mail address: mbultas@juno.com.

0882-5963/$ – see front matter © 2012 Elsevier Inc. All rights reserved.
doi:10.1016/j.pedn.2011.05.005

Continued

by the Centers for Disease Control and Prevention and The Council on Children with Disabilities (Centers for Disease Control and Prevention, 2007; Johnson, Myers, & The Council on Children with Disabilities, 2007). Most recent epidemiological studies now estimate this prevalence to be 1 in 110 children, an increase in prevalence of approximately 57% (Centers for Disease Control and Prevention, 2009). Data show that since 1980, these rates have continued to climb at alarming rates (Blaxill, 2004; Fombonne, 2003; Newschaffer, Falb, & Gurney, 2005).

As these numbers have continued to rise over the last four decades, HCPs continue to try to understand more about the cause of this disorder. What is known is that evidence shows that males are four times more likely than females to be diagnosed with an ASD (Centers for Disease Control and Prevention, 2009). In addition, there is sufficient evidence suggesting an underlying genetic cause of autism (Pickler & Elias, 2009). A sibling predisposition to developing ASD provides more supporting evidence of this genetic link (Nadel & Poss, 2007). Biological and environmental triggers, although what these triggers may be is not known, are also reported to play a role in the increased prevalence of this disorder (Waldman, Nicholson, Adilov, & Williams, 2008). Reasons for the increased prevalence in ASD rates still has not been agreed upon by researchers. Changes in diagnostic criteria, variations in methods of assessing population characteristics, greater awareness among HCPs and parents, or even a true increase in the incidence of ASD are among the possible explanations of the causes of this increase in prevalence (Coo et al., 2008; Waldman et al., 2008).

The statistics for ASDs is frightening to all parents, affected or not by this disorder. Of an even bigger concern is that there continues to be no validated medical treatment for ASDs. Without a determined cause of ASD and no preventative strategies or cures, the increase in children diagnosed with ASD is not expected to diminish.

Health Care for a Child With ASD

A diagnosis of ASD frequently starts with the child's primary HCP. The HCP administers screening tools and developmental questionnaires along with addressing concerns from parents. Neurologists and psychiatrists are just some of the specialists that, along with the child's primary provider, become regular HCPs for a child with ASD. It comes as no surprise that the child with ASD interfaces with the health care field many times in the early years (Myers, 2009).

The Complex Health Care Needs of a Child With Autism

Children with ASD often have coexisting health care needs (Department of Health and Human Services [DHHS],

2008; Liptak, Stuart, & Auigner, 2006). These conditions include seizures, environmental allergies, gastrointestinal complaints, psychiatric diagnoses, behavioral difficulties, and sometimes intellectual disabilities. These conditions lead to a greater number of HCP interactions and complicate the child's treatment. Evidence reveals that children with ASD see their HCPs with more frequency than typically developing children (Liptak, Stuart, et al., 2006); they present with ongoing needs and require ongoing medical management (Myers, 2009).

One of the difficulties in treating comorbidities, in children with autism, is that the child's biological response to usual medical treatments and therapies for these conditions is frequently unpredictable (Volkmar, Wiesner, & Westphal, 2006). The primary reason for these atypical responses may be due to the wide range of behaviors displayed by children with ASD, further evidence that they have increasingly complex medical needs (Volkmar et al., 2006). Children with ASD have reactions in the environment that are not typical and neither are their reactions to medical treatments.

Several studies document the health care expenditures of children with disabilities and specifically children with ASD. Estimates of health care expenditures for this population have been between 3 and 10 times greater for children with autism than that of typically developing children (Croen, Najjar, Ray, Lotspeich, & Bernal, 2006). These increased health care expenditures are another indication that children with ASD are frequent consumers of health care services. Several studies also support the claim that a diagnosis of autism places a significant financial health care burden on the family (Croen et al., 2006; Liptak, Stuart, et al., 2006; Shimabukuro, Grosse, & Rice, 2008).

Meeting the Unique Health Care Needs of the Child and Family

The HCP of children with ASD and their families admit that they have concerns when caring for this population. These concerns include feelings of inadequacy and a lack of confidence in treating and providing service for the child with an ASD (Minnes & Steiner, 2008; Rhoades, Scarpa, & Salley, 2007). Certainly, the increasing prevalence of ASDs has led to increased awareness of the need to screen for the disorder. However, HCPs have difficulty understanding how to manage the health and comorbidities and providing the resources necessary for families with a child with autism (Johnson et al., 2007).

The family of a child who has a disability has significant needs. Those needs include increased amounts of health information, increased amounts of health education related to their child's specific disabilities, and increased time from the HCP to provide this information (Guralnick, 2004). It has been shown that when mothers of children with autism have increased amounts of information and resources available, stress and anxiety are decreased for the mother (Pelchat & Lefebvre, 2004; Tsai, Tsai, & Shyu, 2008). The complexity of ASD also necessitates a multifaceted, but individualized, approach to the child's medical needs. This approach must take into account the child's individuality, strengths, and limitations along with the family's unique characteristics (Johnson, Kastner, & The Committee/Section on Children With Disabilities, 2005).

One of the concerns that mothers have with their HCPs is the perception that providers are not always listening or taking their concerns seriously. A traditional approach in providing pediatric care includes the use of techniques such as reassurance or even allowing more time for a child to achieve a developmental milestone (Caronna et al., 2007). Professional experience often demonstrates to HCPs that simple reassurance to parents is often all that is necessary. However, parents frequently have important concerns and even a "sixth sense" that something may not be right. Parents who are simply reassured and sent on their way may not feel respected or feel that their concerns are important. Several studies have demonstrated that families consider their HCPs to be aware and "up to date" on the new aspects of care related to autism. However, families feel that providers lack an understanding of the impact that the disorder has on the family (Liptak, Orlando, et al., 2006). Families also desire more information that is specific and individual to their child's condition, which can be difficult given the wide range of associated behaviors and the range of disability inherent in a diagnosis of autism.

Medical Homes

A medical home is a primary care provider that serves as a central case coordinator for the child. The American Academy of Pediatrics (2002) defines a *medical home* as family-centered, accessible, and providing all aspects of pediatric care to include direct care, management, and facilitation of that care. Although children with ASD see multiple specialists for comorbidities, there is evidence that children with ASDs frequently lack a medical home (Mandell, Cao, Ittenbach, & Pinto-Martin, 2006). This lack of a medical home can adversely affect the child's delivery of health care, leading to a less than holistic approach. The American Psychological Association recently developed a policy statement supporting the need for research related to family-centered medical homes in addressing the needs of children (Stille et al., 2010).

Collaboration and Partnerships

Collaboration between mother and provider is an important part of any health care visit, but it becomes even more essential when the patient is a child with ASD. With parents' increased access to health information, there is a need to ask more questions and develop a deeper partnership with HCPs. A typical visit to the HCP is anything but typical when it is for a child who has a diagnosis of autism.

Parents are frequently good predictors of their child's unique reactions to new or unusual surroundings; however, there have been only a few studies that have looked at interventions focused on this type of planning and parent involvement for the child with ASD. The importance of planning and collaborating with parents when a child with ASD has the need for health care is supported by two studies examining surgical outcomes in children with ASD (Van Der Walt & Moran, 2001; Seid, Sherman, & Seid, 1997). Both of these studies looked at surgical outcomes for children with ASD whose parents were contacted prior to their child's surgical date. This prior contact with the parent allowed HCPs an opportunity to gather important information to plan for the child's anticipated surgery. Van Der Walt and Moran found that early communication with parents of children with autism, to individualize the anesthetic plan for the child's surgery, led to decreased patient and parent stress and a smoother postoperative phase for the child. Similarly, Seid et al. also found that early involvement and communication with parents of children with autism undergoing ENT surgery led to quicker discharges and less-complicated postoperative courses. Both of these studies support the importance of listening, communicating, and collaborating with a parent of a child with ASD to improve the health care experience for the child with ASD.

Significance of the Study

Although fathers are involved in childcare, mothers often fulfill a greater role related to childrearing in the typical American family (Tehee, Honan, & Hevey, 2009). Frequently, health care visits become the responsibility of the mother in the early years (Liptak, Stuart, et al., 2006). Therefore, mothers both arrange and take the child to the health care visit. Because preschool children frequently visit the HCP and the child with ASD has difficulty with changes in routine and social interactions, the mother of a child with ASD is uniquely situated to describe these health care experiences.

Purpose and Aims of the Study

The purpose of this interpretive phenomenological study was to gain a better understanding of mothers' experiences when they take their preschool-age child with ASD to the HCP. Specific aims of this study included the following:

1. Revealing the mothers' concerns and feelings related to the health care experiences and needs of their preschool-age child with ASD.
2. Examining resources and barriers that mothers experience when taking their child to the HCP and how these affect the visit and the outcome of the visit.

Continued

3. Describing, from the mothers' perspective, the behaviors of the preschool child with ASD during health care visits.

Exploring and understanding more about the mothers' experiences of their child's health care visits are critical. Their perspective provides important insights. In the ever changing face of health care for the child with ASD, understanding the concerns, feelings, resources, and roadblocks that occur in the delivery of health care enables HCPs to better meet the needs of this growing population of health care consumers.

Methods

Interpretive Phenomenology

Interpretive phenomenology was chosen as the methodology for this study. Interpretive phenomenology provides an opportunity for the researcher to explore the meanings and experiences of people and their lives. It is derived from Heidegger's philosophy that the concept and meaning of "being" cannot be separated from the person's world because the person's "world" shapes who they are (Leonard, 1994). Using a phenomenological approach allows the researcher to derive meanings within the context of the participant's surroundings and environment. Heidegger also stresses that traditional science can limit one's ability to understand the human experience and further restrict the ability to generate answers to important questions (Leonard, 1994). Therefore, the benefit of using a phenomenological approach is that it can help uncover and discover experiences in the context of the person's world. More specifically, Heidiggerian phenomenology focuses on a viewpoint that the experiences center on the relationship of the person within their world (Leonard, 1994).

Specific goals of interpretive phenomenology include hearing and understanding the voice of the participant, accurately presenting this voice, seeking a greater understanding of a phenomena, and uncovering differences and commonalities of events (Benner, 1994; Collingridge & Gantt, 2008). Understanding the experiences of caring for and living with a child with ASD requires an approach that allows for situated understanding. There is a uniqueness with which autism affects a child and a mother. Everyday life for the parent and a child with ASD is not ordinary when compared with other families. Even usual events, such as meeting health care needs, can become extraordinary. Therefore, studying and understanding the meaning of these events should be done in context. Describing experiences, as they are, is a goal of interpretive phenomenology, and the purpose and specific aims of this study fit well with these overall goals.

Sample

The study enrolled 11 mothers who had a preschool child with ASD. Inclusion criteria for the study required that mothers have primary caregiving responsibilities for their child, the child had received a diagnosis of ASD from a medical provider, the child was between the ages of 36 and 72 months and not enrolled in kindergarten, and the mothers were English speaking. All mothers enrolled in this study were at least 18 years of age.

Source

Institutional review board approval was received prior to recruitment. Participants for this study were recruited through a parent resource and advocacy group for families with a child with ASD. This resource group included a list-serve. A recruitment flyer for this study was e-mailed through their list-serve and communication alerts.

Procedure

Participants who contacted the researcher had the study explained to them and were screened over the telephone. Participants were then provided with written and informed consent at the first face-to-face meeting prior to being interviewed. Study participants were interviewed three times over a 2- to 4-week period. Each interview lasted between 1 and 2 hours. Interviews were semistructured and used interview guides both adapted and developed by the researcher. Information gathered focused on experiences during the child's health care visit and information about the child. In addition to the interview guides, participants also completed a demographic questionnaire and the Auchenbach Child Behavior Checklist (CBC; Auchenbach & Rescorla, 2000), a child behavior rating tool. Interviews took place in a location of the participants choosing. Two participants requested meeting at a local coffee house, whereas the other 9 participants preferred to meet in their home. All interviews were digitally recorded and transcribed by a transcriptionist.

Data Analysis and Interpretation

Transcribed interviews were analyzed by the researcher using a paradigm case and thematic analysis. The interpretation process started with analysis of one particular participant that stood out as rich in content and meaningful. This became the paradigm case that was used to compare, contrast, and explore the other cases as they were read and evaluated for common themes (Spichiger, 2009). All of the interviews were read, several times each, and highlighted for significant information as they were compared and contrasted to each other. The process of moving back and forth between the transcripts and the themes helped further develop the themes and subthemes (Spichiger, 2009). Identifying the common themes was done through the construction of a blank table that outlined the specific aims of the study. During the process of reading and rereading the transcripts, key information was transferred to the large table under the appropriate specific aim heading. After the table was completed and all interviews had been read and analyzed, the table was reviewed, which further highlighted and made apparent the themes and subthemes. The use of these strategies was helpful in understanding the embedded knowledge and information that occurred within the text of the interview (Benner, 1994). The researcher's forestructure, meaning the background, experiences, and prior knowledge that one brings to the situation at hand, is part of the interpretive process; however, there were no predetermined or defined themes that the researcher began with.

Interpretive sessions were then held to review the paradigm case, themes, and subthemes. There were three interpretive sessions that included two other doctoral students who were also using interpretive and qualitative methodologies for their studies and an experienced qualitative researcher whose background is in interpretive phenomenology. Large portions of raw transcript were provided ahead of time to the session participants for their review. During the sessions, the raw data and researcher-identified themes were reviewed and discussed with the group. The use of these sessions verified the results of the thematic analysis, clarified the subthemes, and also strengthened the study design.

Demographic questionnaires and the Auchenbach CBC were also used as part of the data in this study. Demographic questionnaires were helpful in the construction of the interpretive summaries that were used as background information on the participants. The Auchenbach CBC was scored as well. Information from this tool identified and verified the presence of behavioral concerns in the participants' children. Children's behaviors were rated in the borderline or clinical range for pervasive developmental problems; this means that their parents' ratings of their behaviors were consistent with behaviors that could be considered a pervasive developmental delay, such as ASD (Auchenbach & Rescorla, 2000).

Validity and Trustworthiness of the Data

Evaluating the trustworthiness of a study is crucial to evaluating its merit and value (Lincoln & Guba, 1985). Lincoln and Guba focus on four criteria to establish reliability of a study: credibility, confirmability, transferability, and dependability. These four criteria were met in the analysis of the data in this study.

Credibility refers to the truthfulness of the findings, whereas *confirmability* refers to the degree of bias in the results (Lincoln & Guba, 1985). Both of these were met through the member check during the interpretive sessions. The engagement of the researcher with parents over a 2- to 4-week period of 3- to 6-hour-long interviews supported the credibility and confirmability of the findings. To reduce bias, the forestructure of the researcher was clearly stated up front. It should also be noted, however, that forestructure is considered an important aspect and strength of interpretive phenomenological work as it enhances the richness and deepness of the analysis (Benner, 1994). Lastly, there is evidence of triangulation as the data were analyzed through the use of a paradigm case, thematic analysis, and interpretive sessions.

Transferability and dependability were also met. *Transferability* refers to the degree that those findings can be applied in other contexts, whereas *dependability* refers to the consistency of the findings (Lincoln & Guba, 1985). The use of three separate interviews that probed for rich descriptions supports the transferability of the findings. Dependability and accuracy of the findings were verified through the interpretive sessions. In addition, interpretive methodology relies on the adequacy, length, and depths of the interviews to achieve those consistent findings (Angen, 2000). Interviews in this study averaged 1 to 2 hours in length, and all participants were interviewed three separate times.

Results

Demographic results of the study revealed that the 11 mothers ranged in age from 28 to 44 years. Nine mothers described themselves as Caucasian, whereas the other 2 described themselves as either African American or Hispanic. All of the mothers were married to the child's father and living as a family at the time of the interviews. Seven of the mothers reported an income of $20,000–$60,000 per year, whereas 4 mothers reported a family income of greater than $100,000 per year. Ten of the children were male, with only one of the mother's having a daughter with ASD.

The data from these mothers' interviews related to the health care experiences of the mother and child, which centered around two main themes. First, mothers expressed concern that their child's HCP and their office staff "just didn't get it." They felt that their HCPs and the office staff simply did not understand the complexity of ASD and how the diagnosis of ASD affects every decision, task, and every moment of the day. Second, HCPs marginalized and ignored the mothers' concerns, especially those that are related to their child's cognitive and social development. In addition, there were general barriers to care that became apparent during the interviews. It should be noted that the actual HCPs' names were not collected so the researcher was unable to determine if the providers practiced in a medical home model.

Continued

RESEARCH EXAMPLE—cont'd

Theme 1: They Just Don't "Get It"

An overwhelming concern expressed by mothers was a feeling that HCPs did not really understand the effects of ASD on every aspect of the child and family and how difficult it was to make accommodations for a child with ASD. The mothers felt that the HCP did understand the definition and diagnosis of ASD but that they did not understand the deep impact of ASD on the family or were unable to use that knowledge to accommodate the child's needs. It was not always evident, to the mothers, that the provider and office staff recognized the importance of tailoring the approach to the child's care leading to a positive health care encounter and outcome for the child and mother.

Several subthemes related to this feeling of not grasping the holistic effects and complexity that ASD has on the child and family surfaced. These subthemes included a need to acknowledge the expertise of the mother in working with and caring for the child, a need to recognize the emotional and physical toll of autism on the entire family, and a need to understand the mother's need to seek out alternative therapies and treatments in an effort to help her child. The phrase "they just don't get it" summed up the feelings of these mothers.

Acknowledging the Expertise of the Mother...Moms Know Best

Some mothers felt that their HCP did not understand that the actual approach and delivery of health care services must be adjusted to accommodate the child with ASD. Providers did not always recognize that examining a child with ASD would not ensue in the same manner that it would for a typically developing child. For example, many children with ASD have exaggerated fears or anxieties that cause them to behave in a less than positive manner. One mother felt as if she had just one small request that could really reduce her son's anxieties and fears and improve the overall outcome of the health care visit; however, her awareness of her son's fears was ignored. The following is what she said:

> Marie: ...But, ever since that time, if he sees a person with a white coat, I mean if we go to the pediatrician for just a well visit or if he's sick or something, I have to ask them before they go in the room "can you please remove your coat?" If they don't and they're like "no, he'll be all right," it's hold down, it's scream, "no, no mommy, no, no mommy!"

> Int: Are people receptive to that request to remove a white lab coat?

> Marie: No, doctors are not. And I have actually switched doctors because of that reason. I've called around. It's very hard because I know that they are doctors and they are versed in lots of different things, but when their specialty is not in autism they don't realize how [much it affects him].

Not Recognizing the Emotional Toll of Autism on the Family

Another concern that became apparent was that HCPs did not understand or could not appreciate how deeply ASD affected all aspects of these mothers' lives. The day-to-day difficulty that ASD imparts in their lives takes an emotional toll on them and their family. Kristy is a 28-year-old mother who is currently enrolled in nursing school. Her past medical experiences influenced her decision to pursue this career. Kristy's experience was that her son's HCP's office had not taken the time to really consider or understand her situation and how her son's ASD impacted not only his health but also her ability to care for him. Her disappointment with this aspect of health care influenced her decision to become a nurse.

> Kristy: They [health care providers] don't understand. If they knew half of what my life was like and what my son goes through every day, then they would understand. And actually, I have to credit a lot of that to nursing because one of the things that we're learning in nursing... you can't judge somebody by their cover because you have no idea who they are, where they are, how they got where they are, and one of the things that we've been taught [in nursing school] is that it really helps to prevent judgment when you actually sit down and you talk to someone and you find out why they are the way they are or how they got there.

Kristy also describes how difficulties related to her son's ASD, such as his disrupted sleep pattern, affect her ability to cope with day-to-day tasks. Several mothers also expressed a similar concern. Many of the HCPs were focused solely on the medical aspect of the child's health and often ignored the developmental needs of both the child and the family. However, a child's developmental needs and the family situation are also important to the child's health and the delivery of health care. Kristy felt as if the HCP did not understand that she needed help with her son's other concerns—the concerns that were not clearly a medical problem, such as an infection or illness. She felt that if there was not a medication to prescribe to solve or cure the problem, then her primary HCP was not interested in addressing the problem.

Understanding the Need to Seek Out Alternate Therapies and Treatment

The last subtheme of "not getting it" involved a need for HCPs to better understand the mothers' need to consider alternative therapies or treatments for their children. There was an expressed desire that the HCP have an open mind to the mothers' consideration of alternative treatments. Mothers wanted the HCP to understand and recognize the reasons why they felt compelled to consider all possible treatments; it was a way for them to do something to help their child. Although resources exist to help parents evaluate and consider alternative therapies, such as the "Checklist for Considering Nonstandard or Controversial Practices" provided by Prelock (2006, p. 375), mothers desired to have these conversations with their HCPs.

One mother desired that her HCP discuss the treatments that she had investigated and was considering for her son. She wanted the provider to talk about these with her with an open mind and wanted the provider's expertise in discussing the benefits and possible consequences of these treatments. She needed this openness so that she could make an informed decision related to the use of these treatments for her son.

> Nancy: And that is why when I told you that I experienced two different doctors approach in the same office it was because of their willingness to discuss alternative treatments. Both of them are really committed and good doctors, I cannot say a bad thing at all. But one of them was more open minded....if you [a parent] want to have an alternative approach to treating autism or try different approaches, some doctors can be a little more resistant to discussing this.

Theme 2: Marginalized by Those Who Should Care

The second major theme that surfaced from the participants' transcripts was a marginalization or silencing of the mothers' concerns by the HCP. Mothers experienced a lack of support when they reported concerns of delayed development to their child's HCP. HCPs did not always see these parent concerns as important. Several mothers were told by the provider not to worry about delays in development since their child was a boy and boys do not mature as quickly as girls. Unfortunately, it has been shown that gender may play an important role in an HCP's decision to refer a child with a developmental delay with girls being more readily referred for follow-up than boys (Sices, Feudtner, McLaughlin, Drotar, & Williams, 2004). These concerns were sometimes deferred at more than one well care visit, thereby delaying their child's diagnosis by several months.

> Mary: Between 6 and 9 months...[that's when] I started wondering. My parents as teachers person, she said, "he's just delayed because he was late with all of his gross motor skills" and I started worrying...and I worked with kids who had autism so I knew all the signs....Then after his 9 month shots, between 9 12 months, we lost him [to autism]. And when we went back for his 12 month shots...I just wish I hadn't done those I said, "doctor, there is something wrong. He's not making eye contact, he's not trying to say mama, dada, he wasn't walking, and he wasn't pulling up on furniture." I said, "everything is delayed, everything is delayed, there's something wrong." She goes, "oh some kids just blossom later." I heard the same thing at 15 months [when] she said, "let's wait three more months."

Despite reassurances such as this, several mothers were so convinced that something was wrong they sought outside evaluations and help without the knowledge of their child's HCP. Eventually, these mothers returned to their child's provider with a diagnosis of ASD. This became a basis of distrust between HCP and mother in many cases. Some relationships between mother and provider never healed, and the mothers eventually found a new HCP for their child.

Barriers to Care

Through the interviews, mothers' identified both child and environmental barriers as obstacles in the delivery of the child's health care services. Child behaviors often complicated both the flow of the visit and the mothers' abilities to remember instructions provided by the HCP regarding the child's needs. In addition, environmental barriers such as wait times and waiting room setup affected visit outcomes.

Boredom was a prevalent behavior that the mothers described in their children. This boredom was seen in both the waiting and the examination room. Mothers often identified both of these areas as having little available to do while the child waited. This translated into the child partaking in inappropriate activities, such as getting into the trash can and into cabinets, or even negative physical behaviors, such as screaming or running. The consequences to these behaviors were often the need to discipline the child and receiving judgmental looks and stares from other parents or office staff.

Many of the health care offices that mothers visited lacked toys or developmentally appropriate manipulative toys available for the children. In addition, excessive wait times exacerbated the children's boredom, anxiety, and fears. Mothers' ability to be patient and to calm their children became difficult and added to the mothers' stress. This stress also affected the mothers' ability to concentrate on the providers' instructions and to fully remember the concerns, questions, and reasons for the health care visit. Many mothers felt as if their HCP's office did not provide an adequate environment or the physical resources necessary to meet not only their child's needs but also the needs of typically developing children.

Discussion

Early Referral for Developmental Concerns

All mothers enrolled in the study voiced that they had concerns of developmental delays in their children and that their providers were either slow to respond with referrals or delayed attention to these concerns. Delays were sometimes several months. Several factors may be responsible for a provider's reluctance to refer a child for evaluation of ASD. These factors include the limited time that providers spend

Continued

with patients, limited training in identifying red flags indicative of ASD, and a reluctance to raise concerns of ASD due to uncomfortable feelings related to upsetting parents, and possible emotional reactions from parents (Rhoades et al., 2007). There is a need for providers to not only listen and give credibility to parent concerns but also act early on them. Early screening and identification of ASD provide a child with the opportunity for early enrollment into educational programs, the only established method for treating autism (Nadel & Poss, 2007).

Creating a Child–Family Profile

Overwhelmingly, mothers in this study suggested creating some type of profile that explained more about their child and the child's needs to create a positive health care experience. Development of this profile, with input from the mother or family, would provide staff and HCPs a reference that would identify information necessary to work effectively with their child. This profile would not be a medical history but rather a reference that included important information about routine and behaviors that could negatively impact the child's experience. A profile such as this would help HCPs have a better understanding of the child and family.

Developing the Profile

Many mothers in the study felt stress and anxiety over their need to "drive" the health care visit by repeating child-specific instructions and information on every visit. Using the parent as a consultant in developing a profile for care was recommended by Seid et al. (1997) in their study on perioperative interventions for children with ASD. The authors found that fostering that collaborative relationship and using the parent as a resource minimized negative outcomes for the child with ASD (Seid et al., 1997). In addition, the accuracy of the parent's predictions regarding the behaviors of a child with autism in a health care setting was supported in a study conducted by Marshall, Sheller, Mancl, and Williams (2008). This study used parents to predict their child's ability to cooperate during dental procedures. It concluded that parents not only preferred being involved in decisions regarding their child's ability to behave and cooperate during these procedures but also were accurate in predicting how their child would respond to and behave to specific interventions (Marshall et al., 2008). Recognizing the value of the mother's knowledge and experience with her own child and then using it as an asset in providing care is important. Incorporating suggestions from parents reflects a true family-centered approach that involves the parent and the provider discussing how to achieve the best outcomes for the child (Inglese, 2009).

Several aspects should be addressed when developing this patient profile. First, the mother or primary caregiver for the child should be interviewed and actively involved in the development of the profile. Although this seems obvious, ample time and care should be taken in interviewing them.

Mothers also expressed a desire for their HCP to understand more about their child and the unique needs and abilities of the child. It would be important to address the child's developmental level and clearly note that on the profile. Because autism is a spectrum disorder, there is a wide range of physical and psychosocial abilities. Some children are verbal, whereas others are not. It is also important to recognize and note any specific alterations in activities of daily living for the child. For example, many children with ASD have alterations in sleep, diet, or other issues that affect the ability of the mother to provide their care.

Identifying and noting child anxieties, fears, and antecedents to these feelings is critical to provide a more positive health care experience. The child's behavior, as a result of these feelings, should be clearly noted so that staff and providers in the office working with the child on the day of the visit are aware of them. Many children with ASD have sensory difficulties to sound, light, or touch. They may need an adapted approach to being weighed or having their temperature taken, for example.

Another important piece in developing the patient profile is identifying office-related physical barriers to care. Some children are less anxious in an open waiting room, whereas others may benefit from being in a smaller area, such as the examination room. Wait times for office visits may also need to be decreased to optimize the child's behavior. Several mothers tried contacting their child's HCP's office prior to leaving for their appointment to find out if the provider was behind schedule. However, several offices would not provide them with information on the length of the wait for their HCP. Having a plan for these issues should be discussed early. If the office is unable to provide parents with information on wait times, then having the office provide an appropriate environment for the child to wait, to decrease anxieties and fears, would be an option.

In addition, the patient profile should address a process for completing necessary paperwork for the health care visit. Some parents expressed that it was beneficial for them to complete and read any necessary paperwork, such as immunization information and checkout paperwork, as soon as they arrived at the office or to have it sent to them prior to the visit. Completing paperwork either during or after the visit was difficult especially when their child was upset from the visit. This was especially evident for the mothers that had to bring more than one child with them to the visit.

Discussing and understanding more about the use of any complementary and alternative treatments and medicine (CAM) that mothers may be using are also important to note on the patient profile. Many parents have investigated these types of treatments in an effort to enhance their child's development or bridge gaps in their delays. HCPs need to maintain an open line of communication regarding the use of CAM in their patients. It is important that parents and providers have the opportunity to discuss the treatment's safety and efficacy and the implications of a parent's desire to withhold a medically tested intervention that there may be a misunderstanding about, such as immunizations. Mothers said they desire this open communication even when the provider does not recommend the use of CAM.

Lastly, the length of time needed or allowed for the appointment should also be addressed. Often, the parents of a child with ASD need an extended length of visit either due to child behavior or other factors that complicate the delivery of their health care. Mothers understand the busy nature of the health care office but often can predict when they have issues that may require more time. Mothers in this study clearly did not want to extend the length of time spent in the health care office on a regular basis but recognized that there were times when they need additional time to discuss their child's health concerns.

Mothers' Pearls

Environmental barriers and child behaviors during the health care visit clearly became obstacles in experiencing a positive outcome with the health care visit. Although mothers packed toys and snacks for their child, having additional items in the waiting or examination rooms was one of the recommendations from study participants. Some offices may not have toys readily available due to concerns related to infection control. However, many mothers felt that offices should provide hand sanitizer and wipes or clean the toys on a regular basis because it was important to have developmentally appropriate manipulatives for their children to play with while they waited. Mothers felt this was as important for the typically developing child as it was for their child with autism. One mother remarked that her HCP's office used to have a large fish tank in the waiting area and that it really held her son's attention. She noted that typically developing children were also intrigued and interested in the fish tank.

Mothers also recommended that the HCP provide them with written instructions specific to their child's care addressed at that visit. The overwhelming nature of a visit, which was often complicated with negative child behaviors due to anxiety and waiting, made it difficult for many mothers to remember the HCP's instructions. Mothers that were provided with written instructions appreciated them and used them as a reference when they returned home and had questions. Several mothers noted that having this written information saved them from calling the office to ask about information they had forgotten.

Of special note, all offices visited by the participants provided some type of reinforcement or reward at the completion of the health care visit. This was often in the form of a sticker, piece of candy, or a small toy. All mothers remarked that this was beneficial and a practice that should continue.

Limitations of the Study

There were several limitations of this study. Traditionally, sample sizes for interpretive phenomenology are small (Collingridge & Gantt, 2008) due to the nature of the work. The use of multiple interviews with each mother, however, helped to both strengthen and verify the data (Pohlman, 2005). With this type of work, even small sample sizes can provide understandings that are transferable. The second potential limitation was that participants were being asked to recall situations and stories. The nature of the interviews asked mothers to recall and provide stories that were retrospective and that could have led to inaccuracies. In an effort to minimize some of these effects, the researcher tried to meet with participants over several weeks in anticipation of an interview capturing a recent health care visit. However, only five participants had health care encounters while enrolled in the study. A third possible limitation of the study was related to the participants' possibly not fully disclosing or sharing information. In an effort to minimize this effect, the researcher planned several interviews with each mother to establish a relationship with the mothers to increase their level of comfort with the researcher.

Conclusion

In conclusion, it is clear that HCPs will be interfacing and caring for an increased number of children with ASD. The unique needs and approach necessary in caring for children with ASD can complicate the delivery of health care services. Mothers are an important resource for their child's HCP. Taking the time to understand the effects of ASD on the entire family, acknowledging the mother's expertise regarding her child, and acting on her concerns can reduce barriers to quality care. A child-specific profile can be used to identify environmental, psychological, and physical barriers to care. A profile such as this also provides opportunities for increased collaboration that facilitates good parent–provider communication, increased confidence levels for the HCPs, reduction of negative health care outcomes for this growing population, and reduced costs in health care encounters over the long term. Research focused on evaluating the use of a profile, similar to what is described here, along with evaluating the experiences of mothers whose HCPs practice within a medical home model is recommended to further enhance the delivery of health care to this population of children.

Acknowledgments

This research was funded by the Goldfarb School of Nursing at Barnes Jewish College and the Tao Iota Chapter of Sigma Theta Tau. I would like to acknowledge the

Continued

following people for their support of this project: Jean Bachman, DSN, RN; Dawn Garzon, PhD, RN, PNP-BC, CPNP-PC, FAANP; Shawn Pohlman, PhD, RN; and Rebecca McCathren, PhD. Study results were disseminated at the 21st Annual Convention of the Society of Pediatric Nurses, April 2011, Las Vegas, NV.

References

American Academy of Pediatrics, & Medical home initiatives for children with special health care needs advisory committee. (2002). The medical home. *Pediatrics, 110,* 184–186.

Angen, M. J. (2000). Evaluating interpretive inquiry: Reviewing the validity debate and opening the dialogue. *Qualitative Health Research, 10,* 378–395.

Auchenbach, T. M., & Rescorla, L. A. (2000). *Manual for ASEBA preschool forms & profiles.* Burlington, VT: University of Vermont, Research Center for Children, Youth & Families.

Benner, P. (1994). *Interpretive phenomenology: Embodiment, caring, and ethics in health and illness.* Thousand Oaks, CA: Sage Publications, Inc.

Blaxill, M. F. (2004). What's going on? The question of time trends in autism. *Public Health Reports, 119,* 536–551.

Caronna, E. B., Augustyn, M., & Zuckerman, B. (2007). Revisiting parental concerns in the age of autism spectrum disorders. *Archives of Pediatric and Adolescent Medicine, 161,* 406–408.

Centers for Disease Control and Prevention. (2009). Prevalence of autism spectrum disorders—Autism and developmental disabilities monitoring network, United States, 2006. *MMWR Surveillance Summaries, 58*(SS 10), 1–20.

Centers for Disease Control and Prevention. (2007). Prevalence of autism spectrum disorders—Autism and developmental disabilities monitoring network, 14 sites, United States 2002. *MMWR Surveillance Summaries, 56,* 12–28.

Collingridge, D. S., & Gantt, E. E. (2008). The quality of qualitative research. *American Journal of Medical Quality, 23,* 389–395.

Coo, H., Ouellette-Kuntz, H., Lloyd, J. E., Kasmara, L., Holden, J. J., & Lewis, M. E. (2008). Trends in autism prevalence: Diagnostic substitution revisited. *Journal of Autism and Developmental Disorders, 38,* 1036–1046.

Croen, L. A., Najjar, D. V., Ray, T., Lotspeich, L., & Bernal, P. (2006). A comparison of health care utilization and costs of children with and without autism spectrum disorders in a large group-model health plan. *Pediatrics, 118,* e1203–e1211.

Department of Health and Human Services [DHHS]. (2008). *Autism spectrum disorders: Pervasive developmental disorders.* Retrieved from http://www.nimh.nih.gov/health/publications/autism/nimhautism spectrum.pdf.

Fombonne, E. (2003). Epidemiological surveys of autism and other pervasive developmental disorders: An update. *Journal of Autism and Developmental Disorders, 33,* 365–382.

Guralnick, M. J. (2004). Family investments in response to the developmental challenges of young children with disabilities. In A. Kalil, & T. DeLeire (Eds.), *Family investments in children's potential* (pp. 119–136). Mahwah, NJ: Lawrence Erlbaum Associates, Publishers.

Inglese, M. D. (2009). Caring for children with autism spectrum disorder, part II: Screening, diagnosis, and management. *Journal of Pediatric Nursing, 24,* 49–59.

Johnson, C., Kastner, T., & The Committee/Section on Children With Disabilities. (2005). Helping families raise children with special health care needs at home. *Pediatrics, 115,* 507–511.

Johnson, C. P., Myers, S. M., & The Council on Children with Disabilities. (2007). Identification and evaluation of children with autism spectrum disorders. *Pediatrics, 120,* 1183–1215.

Kanner, L. (1943). Autistic disturbances of affective contact. *Nervous Child, 2,* 217–250.

Kuhn, J. C., & Carter, A. S. (2006). Maternal self-efficacy and associated parenting cognitions among mothers of children with autism. *American Journal of Orthopsychiatry, 76,* 564–575.

Leonard, V. W. (1994). A Heideggerian phenomenological perspective on the concept of person. In *Interpretive phenomenology: Embodiment, caring, and ethics in health and illness.* Thousand Oaks: Sage Publications, Inc.

Lincoln, Y. S., & Guba, E. G. (1985). *Naturalistic inquiry.* Newbury Park, CA: Sage Publications.

Liptak, G. S., Orlando, M., Yingling, J. T., Theurer-Kaufman, K. L., Malay, D. P., Tompkins, L. A., et al. (2006). Satisfaction with primary health care received by families of children with developmental disabilities. *Journal of Pediatric Health Care, 20,* 245–252.

Liptak, G. S., Stuart, T., & Auigner, P. (2006). Health care utilization and expenditures for children with autism: Data from U. S. national samples. *Journal of Autism and Developmental Disorders, 36,* 871–879.

Mandell, D. S., Cao, J., Ittenbach, R., & Pinto-Martin, J. (2006). Medicaid expenditures for children with autistic spectrum disorders: 1994–1999. *Journal of Autism and Developmental Disorders, 36,* 475–485.

Marshall, J., Sheller, B., Mancl, L., & Williams, B. (2008). Parental attitudes regarding behavior guidance of dental patients with autism. *Pediatric Dentistry, 30,* 400–407.

Minnes, P., & Steiner, K. (2008). Parent views on enhancing the quality of health care for their children with fragile X syndrome, autism or Down syndrome. *Child Care, Health and Development, 35,* 250–256.

Myers, S. (2009). Management of autism spectrum disorders in primary care. *Pediatric Annals, 38,* 42–49.

Nadel, S., & Poss, J. E. (2007). Early detection of autism spectrum disorders: Screening between 12 and 24 months of age. *Journal of the American Academy of Nurse Practitioners, 19,* 408–417.

Newschaffer, C. J., Falb, M. D., & Gurney, J. G. (2005). National autism prevalence trends from United States special education data. *Pediatrics, 115,* e277–e282.

Pelchat, D., & Lefebvre, H. (2004). A holistic intervention program for families with a child with a disability. *Journal of Advanced Nursing, 48,* 124–131.

Pickler, L., & Elias, E. (2009). Genetic evaluation of the child with an autism spectrum disorder. *Pediatric Annals, 38,* 26–29.

Pohlman, S. (2005). The primacy of work and fathering preterm infants: Findings from an interpretive phenomenological study. *Advances in Neonatal Care, 5,* 204–216.

Prelock, P. (2006). *Autism Spectrum Disorders: Issues in Assessment and Intervention.* Austin, TX: Pro-Ed, Inc.

Rhoades, R. A., Scarpa, A., & Salley, B. (2007). The importance of physician knowledge of autism spectrum disorder: Results of a parent survey. *BMC Pediatrics, 7.* Retrieved from http://www.biomedcentral.com/content/pdf/1471-2431-7-37.pdf.

Ruble, L. A., Heflinger, C. A., Renfrew, J. W., & Saunders, R. C. (2005). Access and service use by children with autism spectrum disorders in Medicaid managed care. *Journal of Autism and Developmental Disorders, 35,* 3–13.

Seid, M., Sherman, M., & Seid, A. B. (1997). Perioperative psychosocial interventions for autistic children undergoing ENT surgery. *International Journal of Pediatric Otorhinolaryngology, 40,* 107–113.

Shimabukuro, T. T., Grosse, S. D., & Rice, C. (2008). Medical expenditures for children with an autism spectrum disorder in a privately insured population. *Journal of Autism and Developmental Disorders, 38,* 546–552.

Sices, L., Feudtner, C., McLaughlin, J., Drotar, D., & Williams, M. (2004). How do primary care physicians manage children with possible developmental delays? A national survey with an experimental design. *Pediatrics, 113,* 274–282.

Spichiger, E. (2009). Family experiences of hospital end-of-life care in Switzerland: An interpretive phenomenological study. *International Journal of Palliative Nursing, 15,* 332–337.

Stille, C., Turchi, R. M., Antonelli, R., Cabana, M. D., Cheng, T. L., Laraque, D., et al. The Academic Pediatric Association task Force on the Family-Centered Medical Home. (2010). The family-centered medical home: Specific considerations for child health research and policy. *Academic Pediatrics, 10,* 211–217.

Tehee, E., Honan, R., & Hevey, D. (2009). Factors contributing to stress in parents of individuals with autistic spectrum disorders. *Journal of Applied Research in Intellectual Disabilities, 22,* 34–42.

Tsai, W., Tsai, J., & Shyu, Y. L. (2008). Integrating the nurturer–trainer roles: Parental and behavior/symptom management processes for mothers of children with autism. *Social Science & Medicine, 67,* 1798–1806.

Van Der Walt, J. H., & Moran, C. (2001). An audit of perioperative management of autistic children. *Paediatric Anesthesia, 11,* 401–408.

Volkmar, F. R., Wiesner, L. A., & Westphal, A. (2006). Healthcare issues for children on the autism spectrum. *Current Opinion in Psychiatry, 19,* 361–366.

Waldman, M., Nicholson, S., Adilov, N., & Williams, J. (2008). Autism prevalence and precipitation rates in California, Oregon, and Washington Counties. *Archives of Pediatric and Adolescent Medicine, 162,* 1026–1034.

(From Bultas, M. W. (2012). The health care experiences of the preschool child with autism. *Journal of Pediatric Nursing, 27*(5), 460–470.)

Critical Appraisal

Step 1: Identifying the Components of the Qualitative Research Process

1. Introduction

- *Qualifications of the researcher:* Dr. Bultas is a certified pediatric nurse practitioner. Her PhD degree was earned in 2010, and her dissertation was called "The Mother's Perspective: Understanding More About the Healthcare Experiences of the Preschool Child with Autism" (Bultas, 2010). She did not indicate in this article any potential bias or personal connection to the topic of autism. The St. Louis University website has a record of her scholarly work, which includes seven peer-reviewed publications on topics related to pediatric nursing (http://www.slu.edu/Documents/nursing/Bultas13.pdf).

- *Article title:* The title indicates that the article is about the healthcare experiences of younger children with autism, but does not indicate the type of qualitative approach that was used. The title does not indicate that data were collected from the mothers of autistic children and not the children themselves. Because collecting data from parents and other caregivers was probably the only feasible means of exploring the healthcare needs of autistic children, a more appropriate title would be "Mothers' Perspectives on Healthcare Visits of Their Preschool Children with Autism: An Interpretive Phenomenological Study."

- *Abstract:* The abstract did include the qualitative approach in the purpose statement. The sample size and data collection methods were not identified. The two major themes and primary conclusion of the study comprised the remainder of the five-sentence abstract.

2. Problem

- *Significance:* The section of the article called "Significance" included the justification for obtaining data from the mothers instead of the fathers or both parents. Mothers were identified as the parent who most frequently take children to healthcare visits. These preschool children frequently needed to see a healthcare provider (HCP). The actual significance of the study was found in the review of the literature section.

  "Most recent epidemiological studies now estimate the prevalence [autism] to be 1 in 110 children, an increase in prevalence of approximately 57% (Centers for Disease Control and Prevention, 2009)....The statistics for ASDs [autism spectrum disorders] is frightening to all parents, affected or not by this disorder. Of an even bigger concern is that there continues to be no validated medical treatment for ASDs." (Bultas, 2012, p. 461)

- *Background:* The background of the problem included the history of when autism was first described and how autism is typically diagnosed via screening tools administered by the child's primary healthcare provider. Autism is more prevalent in boys. Genes and unknown biological and environmental triggers were mentioned as possible causes of autism. Additional background information was provided on the complex and unique healthcare needs of children and families affected by autism (Bultas, 2012).

Continued

RESEARCH EXAMPLE—cont'd

"One of the difficulties in treating comorbidities, in children with autism, is that the child's biological response to usual medical treatments and therapies for these conditions is frequently unpredictable (Volkmar, Wiesnar, & Westphal, 2006)....Children with ASD have reactions in the environment that are not typical and neither are their reactions to medical treatments....The family of a child who has a disability has significant needs." (Bultas, 2012, p. 461)

"One of the concerns that mothers have with their HCPs is the perception that providers are not always listening or taking their concerns seriously....Professional experience often demonstrates to HCPs that simple reassurance to parents is often all that is necessary. However, parents frequently have important concerns and even a 'sixth sense' that something may not be right....Families often desire more information that is specific and individual to their child's condition, which can be difficult given the wide range of associated behaviors and the range of disability inherent in the diagnosis of autism." (Bultas, 2012, p. 462)

- *Problem statement:*

  "There is a lack of information regarding these mothers' specific needs and concerns related to their children's healthcare experiences" (Bultas, 2012, p. 460).

3. Purpose

"The purpose of this interpretive phenomenological study was to gain a better understanding of mothers' experiences when they take their preschool-age child with ASD to the HCP." (Bultas, 2012, p. 462)

4. Literature Review

The literature review was clearly marked with a major heading. Of the 45 sources cited in the paper, Bultas (2012) cited 15 of them to support statements that provided information and background on autism. Five references were cited related to the method of interpretive phenomenology. Four government sources were cited with prevalence rates, documenting the significance of the ASDs. Ten research papers reported analyses conducted with large databases created by insurance companies or government entities. Researchers who collected original data related to the healthcare of autistic and developmentally challenged children were cited 11 times. The studies were predominantly quantitative, although a few qualitative studies were referenced. Bultas (2012) reviewed literature from government, pediatrics, psychiatry, social science, and child development sources. Bultas (2012) cited the first professional publication identifying autism (Kanner, 1943), an example of a classic article that was appropriate to include, despite its age. Four other sources were older than 1995. The remaining references included five from 2000 to 2004 and 35 references published in or since 2005. The article reports part of the data collected by Bultas for her dissertation, which she completed in 2010. It does not appear that she updated her literature review between completing her dissertation and publishing the article. She did not note strengths or weaknesses of the studies that she reviewed.

5. Study Framework or Philosophical Orientation of the Study

The philosophical orientation of the study was interpretive phenomenology. As support for this qualitative approach, Bultas (2012) cited a book by Benner (1994) on interpretive phenomenology and a chapter in the book by Leonard (1994). Although Dr. Benner is the nurse expert on interpretative phenomenology, Bultas (2012) did not cite Heidegger, the originator of interpretive phenomenology.

6. Objectives (Aims) or Research Questions

"Specific aims of this study included the following:

1. Revealing the mothers' concerns and feelings related to the healthcare experiences and needs of their preschool-age child with ASD.
2. Examining resources and barriers that mothers experience when taking their child to the HCP and how these affect the visit and the outcome of the visit.
3. Describing, from the mothers' perspective, the behaviors of the preschool child with ASD during healthcare visits." (Bultas, 2012, pp. 461-462)

7. Qualitative Approach
Interpretive phenomenology was the philosophical orientation and qualitative approach for the study.

8. Sample and Setting
- *Inclusion and exclusion criteria:* The inclusion criteria for the study "required that mothers have primary caregiving responsibilities for their child, their child had received a diagnosis of ASD from a medical provider, the child was between the ages of 36 months and 72 months and not enrolled in kindergarten, and the mothers were English speaking." (Bultas, 2012, p. 463).
  Exclusion criteria were not mentioned in the article.
- *Sample:* Eleven mothers who participated were 28 to 44 years old. Racial-ethnic diversity of the group was limited with nine whites and two participants who reported being African American or Hispanic. Four mothers had household incomes more than $100,000, with the rest reporting that their income was between $20,000 and $60,000 per year. The children were primarily sons ($n = 10$). The mothers were all "married to the child's father and living as a family at the time" (Bultas, 2012. P. 464).
- *Recruitment and human subjects protection:* Bultas (2012, p. 463) recruited participants through a "parent resource and advocacy group for families with a child with ASD" by sending a recruitment flyer through an electronic "list-serve and communication alerts." The study and its recruitment plans and data collection procedures were approved by an IRB prior to recruitment. Initial contact was made by telephone to screen potential participants and ensure that they met the inclusion criteria. The researcher met the mothers for interviews in a local coffee shop or the participants' homes, with the participants selecting their preferred location. The settings were appropriate because the mothers were comfortable in their chosen location. Informed consent was obtained and documented during the first meeting. No information was provided about whether any mothers refused to participate or about response plans in case mothers became upset during the interviews. Bultas (2012) conducted three interviews with each mother and made no mention of any mothers who did not participate in all three interviews.

9. Data Collection Procedures
Semistructured interviews were the method of data collection and followed a researcher-developed interview guide. The interview guide was not included in the article, so the interview questions cannot be compared to the study aims. With each of the 33 interviews (three per each participant) lasting from 1 to 2 hours, the researcher collected a substantial amount of data. To understand the mothers' experiences better, Bultas (2012) requested that each mother complete a child behavior checklist as well as the demographic questionnaire. "All interviews were digitally recorded and transcribed by a transcriptionist" (Bultas, 2012, p. 463). No mention was made of field notes or journal entries.

10. Data Analysis Process
Digital recordings were professionally transcribed prior to analysis by Bultas (2012). Immersion in the data was accomplished by reading the transcripts "several times each, and highlighted for significant information as they were compared and contrasted to each other" (Bultas, 2012, p. 463). An audit trail was created by entering themes into a table based on the researcher's "background, previous experience, and prior knowledge" (Bultas, 2012, p. 464). A paradigm case, defined as a participant with a particularly rich experience, was identified and analyzed first. A researcher experienced in interpretive phenomenology and two other doctoral students analyzed significant portions of the transcripts independently prior to meeting for three interpretive sessions. Using the methods described, the interpretation of the data was verified.
- *Trustworthiness of the findings:* Bultas (2012) included a section in the article in which she described measures taken to evaluate the trustworthiness of the study. She identified aspects of the data collection and analysis that supported credibility, confirmability, transferability, and dependability, which are the four criteria of quality proposed by Lincoln and Guba (1985). Repeated interviews allowed the participants to verify previous data that were collected and provided them with the opportunity to add information to previous interview data, an example of member checking. The number and length of interviews, use of a paradigm case, identification of the researcher's perspectives on the topic, and interpretive sessions were described as measures taken to ensure the trustworthiness of the study and its findings.

Continued

11. Interpretation of Findings

In the review of the literature, Bultas (2012) described parental concerns that providers were unaware of the impact of autism on the family and failed to acknowledge or address the concerns of parents in a respectful way. The same concerns were revealed in the data analysis, as indicated by the themes of "they just don't 'get it'" and "marginalized by those who should care" (Bultas, 2012, pp. 465-466). Providers did not recognize the extensive knowledge that mothers of children with autism have of their children. They also did not recognize the "emotional toll of autism on the family" (p. 465). If they chose to seek alternative treatments, mothers indicated that they wanted support and information from providers. The findings were consistent with the limited findings that had been previously published. One unexpected finding was the mothers' desire for healthcare providers to be supportive and informative about the use of complementary and alternative therapies.

12. Limitations

Bultas (2012) acknowledged the limitations of a small sample size, participants being asked to recall previous experiences, and participants not disclosing pertinent information. With each limitation, she reiterated the strategies used to minimize the limitations, such as conducting multiple interviews with each mother, meeting with participants over several weeks, and developing a relationship with the mothers.

13. Conclusions

Bultas (2012) emphasized in the conclusions the importance of the findings in light of the increased prevalence of autism and unique needs of families affected by autism.

> "HCPs will be interfacing and caring for an increased number of children with ASD. The unique needs and approach necessary in caring for children with ASD can complicate the delivery of healthcare services. Mothers are an important resource for their child's HCP. Taking the time to understand the effects of ASD on the entire family, acknowledging the mother's expertise regarding her child, and acting on her concerns can reduce barriers to quality care." (Bultas, 2012, p. 468)

14. Transferability of the Findings

The mothers identified the need for waiting and examination rooms to have developmentally appropriate toys, along with sanitizing wipes or hand cleanser to minimize the risk of infection. "Mothers felt this was as important for the typically developing child as it was for their child with autism" (Bultas, 2012, p. 468). Although not stated by Bultas (2012), the recommendation to develop a child profile is transferable to any child with special needs seeking care in an HCP's office. The child profile will contain information to remind HCPs of ways to remove barriers for care and increase the effectiveness of the communication between the HCPs and mothers.

15. Implications for Nursing Practice

In addition to the mothers' recommendation related to a child profile and having toys available, they also identified that written instructions needed to be sent home with the mothers to provide information they need to care for their children at home (Bultas, 2012). The mothers also recommended that a reinforcement given at the end of the visit by many HCPs, such as a sticker or small toy, should be continued. The overall nursing implication of the study finding is to listen to mothers and other caregivers, because they know their family members better than HCPs can know them (Bultas, 2012). HCPs can meet the patient's unique needs by partnering with and learning from mothers and others who provide routine care to the patient at home.

16. Future studies

Bultas (2012) noted that research is needed to test the use of a child profile and evaluate the care that families affected by autism receive in the context of the medical home model.

Step 2: Determining Study Strengths and Weaknesses

Research Problem, Purpose, and Objectives

The problem of providing effective care for children with autism is a significant problem because of the prevalence of the condition and the challenges of meeting the unique healthcare needs of the families affected by autism.

The purpose was clear and stated the study's focus. The research objectives were clear and linked to the study purpose (Fawcett & Garity, 2009; Maxwell, 2013).

Review of the Literature

The multidisciplinary review was well organized. The references cited supported the need for the study and appropriateness of the study's methods. Although little information was provided about the quality of the studies reviewed, the findings of previous studies and information from other references were synthesized and compared to each other. The gap in knowledge addressed by the study was clearly identified.

Philosophical Orientation and Qualitative Approach

Interpretive phenomenology was the philosophical basis for the study. No primary source was provided; however, Dr. Benner (1994) was cited as the authority who developed the specific type of phenomenology used by Bultas (2012). Providing information from Heidegger and citing a primary source would have strengthened the description of the qualitative approach. The qualitative approach was congruent with the study purpose and objectives.

Sample and Setting

The participants had experience with the research topic and were valuable sources of data. The inclusion criterion that mothers had to speak English may have limited participation of some mothers. The rights of human subjects were protected through the recruiting and data collection phases of the study. Informed consent was obtained prior to data collection. The protection of the participants was also enhanced by allowing them to select the setting for the interviews. Bultas (2012) did not provide information about potential participants who were approached about the study but did not participate. She also did not note whether arrangements were made in advance to address the emotional needs of the participants in case the topic was upsetting to them (Cowles, 1988).

Data Collection

Repeated interviews were conducted to address the research objectives. The interviews lasted between 1 and 2 hours, and each participant was interviewed three times. The total time spent with each participant, a strength of the study, was more than enough to develop robust responses to the research questions. The specific questions used during the interview were not included in the article. The findings produced from the interviews related to the objectives of the study, so one can infer that the interview questions were relevant (Maxwell, 2013).

Data Analysis

Bultas (2012) provided a thorough description of the data analysis, beginning with immersion in the data following transcription of the interviews. She used several strategies to structure the review process, including identifying a paradigm case for comparison to each subsequent interview and completing a table of themes related to each study aim.

> "During the process of reading and rereading the transcripts, key information was transferred to the large table under the appropriate specific aim heading. After the table was completed and all interviews had been read and analyzed, the table was reviewed, which further highlighted and made apparent the themes and subthemes." (Bultas, 2012, p. 464)

She also provided a thorough description of the interpretive sessions that were part of the data analysis. These sessions were valuable to the researcher at the time but also to the reader, because using them supported the trustworthiness of the study. In addition, the trustworthiness of the study was directly addressed in a section of the paper titled "Validity and Trustworthiness of the Data" (Bultas, 2012, p. 464). The use of multiple strategies to enhance trustworthiness increases the reader's confidence in the findings (Cohen & Crabtree, 2008; Murphy & Yielder, 2010). The support provided for the trustworthiness of the study is a major strength of the article.

Interpretation of Findings

Bultas (2012) provided quotes to support each theme and subtheme. She did not address variations in findings based on sample characteristics. The sample was homogeneous because of limiting the study to a particular age group of children and narrowly defining the research problem as the lack of knowledge related to the healthcare

Continued

RESEARCH EXAMPLE—cont'd

visit. The unexpected findings related to wanting to discuss complementary and alternative therapies were not explained and were not mentioned in the literature review.

Limitations

The acknowledged limitations of the study were minimized to the extent possible by the researcher's well-designed study. One limitation—the few children who had healthcare visits during the study—was not under the control of the researcher.

Conclusions

The conclusions and recommendations for future studies were logically congruent with the findings. Bultas (2012) recommended conducting a study to evaluate the use of a child profile, a potential intervention that was identified in the data.

Step 3: Evaluating the Trustworthiness and Meaning of Study Findings

Bultas (2012) conducted a well-designed study that minimized the limitations to a great degree. As a result, the findings provide a credible view of the healthcare needs of children with autism from the perspective of their mothers. The findings can be used in nursing practice as support for creating a child profile that the provider and mother of a child with autism can develop collaboratively. Mothers' suggestions related to the toys needed in the waiting room and scheduling of visits would be appropriate for children with autism, as well as for other children with developmental needs. In nursing education, these strategies can be shared as part of a pediatric nursing course. Including the findings in an update for pediatric nurses would be appropriate for continuing nursing education. The findings of this study expand current EBP knowledge and can be used to provide patient-centered care to mothers and their children with autism. This type of knowledge promotes the accomplishment of the QSEN (2013) competencies for prelicensure nursing students. Bultas (2012) noted that the findings could be used to support testing a child profile as an intervention for children with developmental needs.

The congruence of the purpose, method, and findings was clearly demonstrated throughout the presentation of the study. The article was organized and clearly written. The study's strengths exceed its few weaknesses, and it can serve as a strong example of interpretive phenomenology.

KEY CONCEPTS

- An intellectual critical appraisal of research requires careful examination of all aspects of a study to judge its strengths, weaknesses, credibility, meaning, and significance.
- Research is critically appraised to broaden understanding, improve practice, and provide a background for conducting a study.
- All nurses, including students, practicing nurses, nurse educators, and nurse researchers, need expertise in the critical appraisal of research.
- The research critical appraisal process includes identifying the steps of the research process in studies, determining study strengths and weaknesses, and evaluating the credibility and meaning of study findings.
- Strong quantitative study is guided by a clear, concise problem and purpose and appropriate objectives, questions, or hypotheses. The study framework is appropriate; the design is relevant, with limited threats to validity; data analyses address the study objective, questions, or hypotheses; and the study findings are credible and an accurate reflection of reality.
- Critical appraisals of qualitative studies include identifying the components of the qualitative research process, determining study strengths and weaknesses, and evaluating the trustworthiness and meaning of the study findings.

- Strong qualitative studies are based on a philosophical orientation and qualitative approach that are specified. Building on that foundation, the researcher implements data collection and analysis methods that enhance the study's trustworthiness.
- Detailed guidelines are provided for conducting critical appraisals of quantitative and qualitative studies.
- Example critical appraisals are provided for a quantitative study and a qualitative study.

REFERENCES

Aberson, C. L. (2010). *Applied power analysis for the behavioral sciences.* New York: Routledge Taylor & Francis.

Agency for Healthcare Research and Quality (AHRQ). (2013). *AHRQ home.* Retrieved February 19, 2013 from, http://www.ahrq.gov.

Alligood, M. R. (2010). *Nursing theory: Utilization & application.* Maryland Heights, MO: Mosby Elsevier.

American Nurses Credentialing Center (ANCC). (2013). *Magnet program overview.* Retrieved February 18, 2013 from, http://www.nursecredentialing.org/Magnet/ProgramOverview.aspx.

American Psychological Association (APA). (2010). *Publication manual of the American Psychological Association* (6th ed.). Washington, DC: Author.

Armstrong, D. J., Meenagh, G. K., Bickle, I., Lee, A. S. H., Curran, S., & Finch, M. B. (2007). Vitamin D deficiency is associated with anxiety and depression in fibromyalgia. *Clinical Rheumatology, 26*(4), 551–554.

Benner, P. (1994). *Interpretive phenomenology: Embodiment, caring, and ethics in health and illness.* Thousand Oaks, CA: Sage Publications.

Berk, M., Sanders, K. M., Pasco, J. A., Jacka, F. N., Williams, L. J., Hayles, A. L., et al. (2007). Vitamin D deficiency may play a role in depression. *Medical Hypotheses, 69*(6), 1316–1319.

Bialocerkowski, A., Klupp, N., & Bragge, P. (2010). Research methodology series: How to read and critically appraise a reliability article. *International Journal of Therapy and Rehabilitation, 17*(3), 114–120.

Brown, S. J. (2002). Focus on research methods. Nursing intervention studies: A descriptive analysis of issues important to clinicians. *Research in Nursing & Health, 25*(4), 317–327.

Brown, S. J. (2014). *Evidence-based nursing: The research-practice connection* (3rd ed.). Sudbury, MA: Jones & Bartlett.

Bultas, M. W. (2010). *The mother's perspective: Understanding more about health care experiences of the preschool child with autism.* University of Missouri—St. Louis, ProQuest, UMI Dissertations Publishing, 3427619.

Bultas, M. W. (2012). The health care experiences of the preschool child with autism. *Journal of Pediatric Nursing, 27*(5), 460–470.

Burns, N. (1989). Standards for qualitative research. *Nursing Science Quarterly, 2*(1), 44–52.

Centers for Disease Control and Prevention. (2009). Prevalence of autism spectrum disorders—Autism and developmental disabilities monitoring network, United States, 2006. *MMWR Surveillance Summaries, 58*(SS 10), 1–20.

Chinn, P. L., & Kramer, M. K. (2011). *Integrated theory and knowledge development in nursing* (8th ed.). St. Louis: Elsevier Mosby.

Clissett, P. (2008). Evaluating qualitative research. *Journal of Orthopaedic Nursing, 12*(2), 99–105.

Cohen, D. J., & Crabtree, B. F. (2008). Evaluative criteria for qualitative research in health care: Controversies and recommendations. *Annals of Family Medicine, 6*(4), 331–339.

Cowles, K. (1988). Issues in qualitative research on sensitive topics. *Western Journal of Nursing Research, 10*(2), 163–179.

Craig, J., & Smyth, R. (2012). *The evidence-based practice manual for nurses* (3rd ed.). Edinburgh: Churchill Livingstone Elsevier.

Creswell, J. W. (2013). *Qualitative inquiry & research design: Choosing among five approaches* (3rd ed.). Thousand Oaks, CA: Sage.

Creswell, J. W. (2014). *Research design: Qualitative, quantitative and mixed methods approaches* (3rd ed.). Thousand Oaks, CA: Sage.

DeKeyser, F. G., & Pugh, L. C. (1990). Assessment of reliability and validity of biochemical measures. *Nursing Research, 39*(5), 314–317.

DeVon, H. A., Block, M. E., Moyle-Wright, P., Ernst, D. M., Hayden, S. J., et al. (2007). A psychometric toolbox for testing validity and reliability. *Journal of Nursing Scholarship, 39*(2), 155–164.

Doran, D. M. (2011). *Nursing outcomes: The state of the science* (2nd ed.). Canada: Jones & Bartlett Learning.

Fawcett, J., & Garity, J. (2009). *Evaluating research for evidence-based nursing practice.* Philadelphia: F. A. Davis.

Gaines, S. (2005). The saddest season. *Minnesota Medicine, 88*(11), 30–33.

Gloeckner, M. B., & Robinson, C. B. (2010). A nursing journal club thrives through shared governance. *Journal for Nurses in Staff Development, 26*(6), 267–270.

Grove, S. K. (2007). *Statistics for health care research: A practical workbook.* St. Louis: Saunders Elsevier.

Grove, S. K., Burns, N., & Gray, J. R. (2013). *The practice of nursing research: Appraisal, synthesis, and generation of evidence* (7th ed.). St. Louis: Elsevier Saunders.

Hart, C. (2009). *Doing a literature review: Releasing the social science imagination.* Thousand Oaks, CA: Sage Publications.

Hoare, Z., & Hoe, J. (2013). Understanding quantitative research: Part 2. *Nursing Standard (Royal College of Nursing [Great Britain]), 27*(18), 48–55.

Hoe, J., & Hoare, Z. (2012). Understanding quantitative research: Part 1. *Nursing Standard (Royal College of Nursing [Great Britain]), 27*(15-17), 52–57.

Holick, M., & Jenkins, M. (2003). *The UV advantage.* New York: Ibooks.

Jorde, R., Waterloo, K., Salech, F., Haug, E., & Svartberg, J. (2006). Neuropsychological function in relation to serum parathyroid hormone and serum 25-hydroxyvitamin D levels: The Tromso study. *Journal of Neurology, 253*(4), 464–470.

Kanner, L. (1943). Autistic disturbances of affective contact. *Nervous Child, 2,* 217–250.

Kiraly, S., Kiraly, M., Hawe, R., & Makhami, N. (2006, January). Vitamin D as a neuroactive substance: Review. *Scientific World Journal, 6,* 125–139.

Leonard, V. W. (1994). A Heideggerian phenomenological perspective on the concept of person. In P. Benner (Ed.), *Interpretive phenomenology: Embodiment, caring, and ethics in health and illness* (pp. 43–64). Thousand Oaks, CA: Sage Publications.

Lincoln, Y. S., & Guba, E. G. (1985). *Naturalistic inquiry.* Thousand Oaks, CA: Sage Publications.

Mackey, M. (2012). Evaluation of qualitative research. In P. L. Munhall (Ed.), *Nursing research: A qualitative perspective* (pp. 517–531). (5th ed.). Sudbury, MA: Jones & Bartlett.

Maxwell, J. (2013). *Qualitative research design: An interactive approach* (3rd ed.). Thousand Oaks, CA: Sage Publications.

Melnyk, B. M., & Fineout-Overholt, E. (Eds.). (2011). *Evidence-based practice in nursing & healthcare: A guide to best practice.* (2nd ed.). Philadelphia: Lippincott, Williams, & Wilkins.

Miles, M., Huberman, A., & Saldana, J. (2014). *Qualitative data analysis: A methods sourcebook* (3rd ed.). Thousand Oaks, CA: Sage Publications.

Mittlbock, M. (2008). Critical appraisal of randomized clinical trials: Can we have faith in the conclusions? *Breast Care, 3*(5), 341–346.

Morrison, D. M., Hoppe, M. J., Gillmore, M. R., Kluver, C., Higa, D., & Wells, E. A. (2009). Replicating an intervention: The tension between fidelity and adaptation. *AIDS Education and Prevention, 21*(2), 128–140.

Morse, J. M. (1991). Evaluating qualitative research. *Qualitative Health Research, 1*(3), 283–286.

Munhall, P. L. (2012). *Nursing research: A qualitative perspective* (5th ed.). Sudbury, MA: Jones & Bartlett.

Murphy, F., & Yielder, J. (2010). Establishing rigor in qualitative radiography. *Radiography, 16*(1), 62–67.

National Institute of Nursing Research (NINR). (2013). *What is nursing research?* Retrieved February 18, 2013 from, https://www.ninr.nih.gov.

O'Mathuna, D. P., Fineout-Overholt, E., & Johnston, L. (2011). Critically appraising quantitative evidence for clinical decision making. In B. M. Melnyk, & E. Fineout-Overholt (Eds.), *Evidence-based practice in nursing & healthcare: A guide to best practice* (pp. 81–134) (2nd ed.). Philadelphia: Lippincott Williams & Wilkins.

Obradovic, D., Gronemeyer, H., Lutz, B., & Rein, T. (2006). Cross-talk of vitamin D and glucocorticoids in hippocampal cells. *Journal of Neurochemistry, 96*(2), 500–509.

Petty, N., Thomson, O., & Stew, G. (2012). Ready for a paradigm shift? Part 2: Introducing qualitative research methodologies and methods. *Manual Therapy, 17*(5), 378–384.

Pickler, R. H. (2007). Evaluating qualitative research studies. *Journal of Pediatric Health Care, 21*(3), 195–197.

Plichta, S. B., & Kelvin, E. (2013). *Munro's statistical methods for health care research* (6th ed.). Philadelphia: Lippincott Williams & Wilkins.

Pyrczak, F. (2008). *Evaluating research in academic journals: A practical guide to realistic evaluation* (4th ed.). Los Angeles: Pyrczak.

Quality and Safety Education for Nurses (QSEN). (2013). *Pre-licensure knowledge, skills, and attitudes (KSAs).* Retrieved February 11, 2013 from, http://qsen.org/competencies/pre-licensure-ksas.

Roberts, W. D., & Stone, P. W. (2003). Ask an expert: How to choose and evaluate a research instrument. *Applied Nursing Research, 16*(1), 70–72.

Ryan-Wenger, N. A. (2010). Evaluation of measurement precision, accuracy, and error in biophysical data for clinical research and practice. In C. F. Waltz, O. L. Strickland, & E. R. Lenz (Eds.), *Measurement in nursing and health research* (pp. 371–383). (4th ed.). New York: Springer.

Sandelowski, M. (2008). Justifiying qualitative research. *Research in Nursing & Health, 31*(3), 193–195.

Sandelowski, M., & Barroso, J. (2007). *Handbook for synthesizing qualitative research.* New York: Springer.

Santacroce, S. J., Maccarelli, L. M., & Grey, M. (2004). Methods: Intervention fidelity. *Nursing Research, 53*(1), 63–66.

Schoe, L., Høstrup, H., Lyngsø, E., Larsen, S., & Poulsen, I. (2011). Validation of a new assessment tool for qualitative research articles. *Journal of Advanced Nursing, 68*(9), 2086–2094.

Shadish, W. R., Cook, T. D., & Campbell, D. T. (2002). *Experimental and quasi-experimental designs for generalized causal inference.* Chicago: Rand McNally.

Sherwood, G., & Barnsteiner, J. (2012). *Quality and safety in nursing: A competency approach to improving outcomes.* Ames, IA: Wiley-Blackwell.

Shipowick, C. D., Moore, C. B., Corbett, C., & Bindler, R. (2009). Vitamin D and depressive symptoms in women during the winter: A pilot study. *Applied Nursing Research, 22*(3), 221–225.

Sloan, D. M., & Kornstein, S. G. (2003). Gender differences in depression and response to antidepressant treatment. *Psychiatric Clinics of North America, 26*(3), 581–594.

Smith, M. J., & Liehr, P. R. (2008). *Middle range theory for nursing* (2nd ed.). New York: Springer.

Volkmar, F. R., Wiesner, L. A., & Westphal, A. (2006). Healthcare issues for children on the autism spectrum. *Current Opinion in Psychiatry, 19*(4), 361–366.

Waltz, C. F., Strickland, O. L., & Lenz, E. R. (2010). *Measurement in nursing and health research* (4th ed.). New York: Springer.

Wolf, M. (2012). Ethnography: The method. In P. L. Munhall (Ed.), *Nursing research: A qualitative perspective* (pp. 285–338) (5th ed.). Sudbury, MA: Jones & Bartlett.

World Health Organization. (2000). Setting the WHO agenda for mental health. *Bulletin of the World Health Organization, 78*(4), 500.

CHAPTER OVERVIEW

LEARNING OUTCOMES

After completing this chapter, you should be able to:

1. Identify the benefits and barriers related to evidence-based practice in nursing.
2. Critically appraise systematic reviews, meta-analyses, meta-syntheses, and mixed-methods systematic reviews of current research evidence.
3. Use the PICOS format to formulate clinical questions to identify evidence for use in practice.
4. Describe the models used to promote evidence-based practice in nursing.

5. Apply the Iowa Model of Evidence-Based Practice for implementing evidence-based changes in your practice.
6. Implement research-based protocols, algorithms, and policies in your practice.
7. Apply the Grove Model to implement national evidence-based guidelines in your practice.
8. Describe the significance of evidence-based practice centers and translational research in developing evidence-based health care.

KEY TERMS

Ancestry searches, p. 432
Best research evidence, p. 415
Citation bias, p. 433
Duplicate publication
  bias, p. 433
Evidence-based
  guidelines, p. 453
Evidence-based practice
  (EBP), p. 415
Evidence-based practice centers
  (EPCs), p. 460
Forest plot, p. 436
Funnel plot, p. 433
Grey literature, p. 424
Grove Model for Implementing
  Evidence-Based Guidelines
  in Practice, p. 456
Heterogeneity, p. 430
Iowa Model of Evidence-Based
  Practice, p. 450

Language bias, p. 433
Location bias of studies, p. 433
Mean difference, p. 435
Meta-analysis, p. 430
Metasummary, p. 437
Meta-synthesis, p. 437
Methodological bias, p. 433
Mixed-methods systematic
  review, p. 441
  Multilevel synthesis, p. 441
  Parallel synthesis, p. 441
Odds ratio *(OR)*, p. 435
Outcome reporting bias, p. 433
PICO format, p. 443
PICOS format, p. 423
Publication bias, p. 433
Research-based protocols, p. 450
Risk difference *(RD)*, p. 436
Risk ratio *(RR)* or relative
  risk, p. 435

Standardized mean difference
  (SMD), p. 435
Stetler Model of Research
  Utilization to Facilitate
  Evidence-Based
  Practice, p. 447
Phase I: Preparation, p. 448
Phase II: Validation, p. 448
Phase III: Comparative
  Evaluation/Decision
  Making, p. 448
Phase IV: Translation/
  Application, p. 449
Phase V: Evaluation, p. 449
Systematic review, p. 421
Time lag bias of studies, p. 433
Translational research, p. 461

Research evidence has greatly expanded over the last 30 years as numerous quality studies in nursing, medicine, and other healthcare disciplines have been conducted and disseminated. These studies are commonly communicated via conferences, journals, and the Internet. The expectations of society and the goals of healthcare systems are the delivery of quality, safe, cost-effective health care to patients, families, and communities, nationally and internationally. To ensure the delivery of quality health care, the care must be based on the current best research evidence available. Healthcare agencies are emphasizing the delivery of evidence-based health care, and nurses and physicians are focused on evidence-based practice (EBP). With the emphasis on EBP over the last 2 decades, outcomes have improved for patients, healthcare providers, and healthcare agencies (Brown, 2014; Craig & Smyth, 2012; Doran, 2011; Higgins & Green, 2008; Melnyk & Fineout-Overholt, 2011).

Evidence-based practice (EBP) is an important theme in this text that was defined in Chapter 1 as the conscientious integration of best research evidence with clinical expertise and patient values and needs in the delivery of quality, safe, cost-effective health care (Craig & Smyth, 2012; Institute of Medicine, 2001; Sackett, Straus, Richardson, Rosenberg, & Haynes, 2000). Best research evidence is produced by the conduct and synthesis of numerous high-quality studies in a selected health-related area. The concept of best research evidence was described in Chapter 1, and the processes for synthesizing research evidence (systematic review, meta-analysis, meta-synthesis, and mixed-methods systematic review) were defined.

This chapter builds on previous EBP discussions in this text to provide you with strategies for implementing the best research evidence in your practice and moving the profession of nursing toward EBP. This chapter examines the benefits and barriers related to implementing evidence-based care in nursing. Guidelines are provided for critically appraising research syntheses (systematic reviews, meta-analyses, meta-syntheses, and mixed-methods systematic reviews) to determine the knowledge that is ready for use in practice. Two nursing models developed to facilitate EBP in healthcare agencies are introduced. Expert researchers, clinicians, and consumers—through government agencies, professional organizations, and healthcare agencies—have developed an extensive number of evidence-based guidelines. A framework for reviewing the quality of these evidence-based guidelines and for using them in practice is provided. This chapter concludes with a discussion of the nationally designated EBP centers and translational research implemented to promote evidence-based health care.

BENEFITS AND BARRIERS RELATED TO EVIDENCE-BASED NURSING PRACTICE

EBP is a goal for the profession of nursing and each practicing nurse. At the present time, some nursing interventions are evidence-based, or supported by the best research knowledge available from systematic reviews, meta-analyses, meta-syntheses, and mixed-methods systematic reviews. However, many nursing interventions require additional research to generate essential knowledge for making changes in practice. Some nurses readily use research-based interventions, and others are slower to make changes in their practice based on research. Some clinical agencies are supportive of EBP and provide resources to facilitate this process, but other agencies have limited support for the EBP process. This section identifies some of the benefits and barriers related to EBP to assist you in delivering evidence-based care to your patients.

Benefits of Evidence-Based Nursing Practice

The greatest benefits of EBP are improved outcomes for patients, providers, and healthcare agencies. Organizations and agencies nationally and internationally have promoted the synthesis of the best research evidence in thousands of healthcare areas by teams of expert researchers and clinicians. These research syntheses, such as systematic reviews and meta-analyses, have provided the basis for developing strong evidence-based guidelines for practice. These guidelines identify the best treatment plan, or gold standard, for patient care in a selected area to promote quality health outcomes. Students and clinical nurses have easy access to numerous evidence-based guidelines to assist them in making the best clinical decisions for their patients. These evidence-based syntheses and guidelines are found in presentations and publications and can be easily accessed online through the National Guideline Clearinghouse (NGC, 2014a) in the United States (http://www.guideline.gov/browse/by-topic.aspx), the Cochrane Collaboration (2014) in England (http://www.cochrane.org/cochrane-reviews), and the Joanna Briggs Institute (2014) in Australia (http://www.joannabriggs.org/index.html). Additional EBP resources are presented later in this chapter.

Healthcare agencies are highly supportive of EBP because it promotes quality, cost-effective care for patients and families and meets accreditation requirements. The Joint Commission (2014) revised their accreditation criteria to emphasize patient care quality achieved through EBP. Approximately 25% of chief nursing officers (CNOs) identified the movement toward evidence-based nursing practice as their number one priority (Nurse Executive Center, 2005).

Many CNOs and healthcare agencies are trying to obtain or maintain Magnet status, which documents the excellence of nursing care in an agency. Approval for Magnet status is obtained through the American Nurses Credentialing Center (ANCC). The national and international healthcare agencies that currently have Magnet status can be viewed online at the ANCC (2014) website (http://www.nursecredentialing.org/Magnet/FindaMagnetFacility.aspx). The Magnet Recognition

Program recognizes EBP as a way to improve the quality of patient care and revitalize the nursing environment. Selection criteria for Magnet status that require healthcare agencies to promote the conduct of research and use of research evidence in practice follow.

Force 6: Quality Care

"Research and Evidence-Based Practice

22. Describe how current literature, appropriate to the practice setting, is available, disseminated, and used to change administrative and clinical practices.

23. Discuss the institution's policies and procedures that protect the rights of participants in research protocols. Include evidence of consistent nursing involvement in the governing body responsible for protection of human subjects in research.

24. Provide evidence that research consultants are actively involved in shaping nursing research infrastructure, capacity, and mentorship.

25. Provide a copy of the nursing budget or other sources of funding for the past year, the current year-to-date, and the future projection, highlighting the allocation and utilization of resources for nursing research.

26. Supply documentation of all nursing research activities that are ongoing, including internal validation studies, internal and external research, and participation in surveys completed within the past twelve (12) month period.

27. Provide evidence of education and mentoring activities that have effectively engaged staff nurses in research- and/or evidence-based practice activities.

28. Describe resources available to nursing staff to support participating in nursing research and nursing research utilization activities."

Nursing Executive Center, 2005, p. 15

These selection criteria include critical elements for EBP, especially financial support for and outcomes related to research activities. Important research-related outcomes to be documented by agencies for Magnet status include nursing studies conducted and professional publications and presentations by nurses. For each study, the title of the study, principal investigator or investigators, role of nurses in the study, and study status need to be documented (Horstman & Fanning, 2010).

The Quality and Safety Education for Nurses (QSEN, 2013) project was implemented to improve prelicensure nurses' "knowledge, skills, and attitudes (KSAs) that are necessary to continuously improve the quality and safety of the healthcare systems within which they work." QSEN competencies were developed in six areas essential for students and registered nurses' (RNs) practice—patient-centered care, teamwork and collaboration, EBP, quality improvement (QI), safety, and informatics. QSEN competencies were introduced in Chapter 1 and are linked to study findings in all chapters in this text. You can view the competencies on the QSEN Institute website (http://qsen.org/competencies/pre-licensure-ksas). EBP is an important area in your prelicensure education, and educators and students need to work toward achieving the following EBP competencies:

"Participate effectively in appropriate data collection and other research activities.
Adhere to Institutional Review Board (IRB) guidelines.
Base individualized care plan on patient values, clinical expertise, and evidence.
Read original research and evidence reports related to area of practice.
Locate evidence reports related to clinical practice topics and guidelines.

Participate in structuring the work environment to facilitate integration of new evidence into standards of practice.

Question rationale for routine approaches to care that result in less-than-desired outcomes or adverse events.

Consult with clinical experts before deciding to deviate from evidence-based protocols."

QSEN, 2013

Students and RNs demonstrating these EBP competencies are able to provide quality, safe care to patients and to accomplish the goals outlined for Magnet status. Sherwood and Barnsteiner (2012) provide details on the QSEN competencies and educational experiences to promote the KSAs of prelicensure and graduate nurses. In working toward EBP, students and practicing nurses are encouraged to embrace the benefits of EBP; critically appraise current research evidence; refine agency protocols, algorithms or clinical decision trees, and policies based on current research; use the evidence-based guidelines available; and collect data as needed for research projects.

Barriers to Evidence-Based Nursing Practice

Barriers to the EBP movement have been practical and conceptual. One of the most serious barriers is the lack of research evidence available regarding the effectiveness of many nursing interventions. EBP requires synthesizing research evidence from randomized controlled trials (RCTs) and other types of intervention studies, and these types of studies are still limited in nursing. Mantzoukas (2009) reviewed the research evidence in 10 high-impact nursing journals, including *Nursing Research, Research in Nursing & Health, Western Journal of Nursing Research, Journal of Nursing Scholarship,* and *Advances in Nursing Science,* between 2000 and 2006 and found that the studies were 7% experimental, 6% quasi-experimental, and 39% nonexperimental. However, RCTs and quasi-experimental studies conducted to determine the effectiveness of nursing interventions did increase during that time period.

Systematic reviews and meta-analyses conducted in nursing are limited when compared with other disciplines, such as medicine and psychology. In addition, nurse authors of these research syntheses have sometimes indicated that there is inadequate research evidence to support using certain nursing interventions in practice (Craig & Smyth, 2012; Mantzoukas, 2009). Bolton, Donaldson, Rutledge, Bennett, and Brown (2007, p. 123S) conducted a review of "systematic/integrative reviews and meta-analyses on nursing interventions and patient outcomes in acute care settings." Their literature search covered 1999 to 2005 and identified 4000 systematic-integrative reviews and 500 meta-analyses covering the following seven topics selected by the authors—staffing, caregivers, incontinence, care of older adults, symptom management, pressure ulcer prevention and treatment, and developmental care of neonates and infants. The authors found a limited association between nursing interventions and processes and patient outcomes in acute care settings, as indicated by the following:

"The strongest evidence was for the use of patient risk-assessment tools and interventions implemented by nurses to prevent patient harm. We observed significant variation in the methods to measure the effect of independent variables (nursing interventions) on patient outcomes. Results indicate the need for more research measuring the effect of specific nursing interventions that may impact acute care patient outcomes."

Bolton et al., 2007, p. 123S

Extensive evidence has been generated through nursing research, but additional studies are needed that focus on determining the effectiveness of nursing interventions on patient outcomes

(Bolton et al., 2007; Doran, 2011; Mantzoukas, 2009). Identifying the areas in which research evidence is lacking is an important first step in developing the evidence needed for practice. Well-designed experimental and quasi-experimental studies are needed to test selected nursing interventions and to use that understanding to generate sound evidence for practice. Nurses also need to be more active in conducting quality syntheses (systematic reviews, meta-analyses, and meta-syntheses) of research evidence in selected areas (Finfgeld-Connett, 2010; Higgins & Green, 2008; Moore, 2012; Rew, 2011).

Another concern is that the research evidence is generated based on population data and then is applied in practice to individual patients. Sometimes it is difficult to transfer research knowledge to individual patients, who respond in unique ways or have unique needs. More work is needed to promote the use of evidence-based guidelines with individual patients. The National Institutes of Health (NIH, 2012) is supporting translational research to improve the use of research evidence with different patient populations in various settings. Patients who have poor outcomes when managed according to an evidence-based guideline need to be reported and, if possible, their circumstances should be published as a case study. Electronic health records (EHRs) now make it possible to determine patient outcomes of care that have been delivered using EBP guidelines.

Another serious barrier is that some healthcare agencies and administrators do not provide the resources necessary for nurses to implement EBP. Their lack of support might include the following: (1) inadequate access to research journals and other sources of synthesized research findings and evidence-based guidelines; (2) inadequate knowledge on how to implement evidence-based changes in practice; (3) heavy workload, with limited time to make research-based changes in practice; (4) limited authority to change patient care based on research findings; (5) limited support from nursing administrators or medical staff to make evidence-based changes in practice; (6) limited funds to support research projects and research-based changes in practice; and (7) minimal rewards for providing evidence-based care to patients and families (Butler, 2011; Eizenberg, 2010; Straka, Brandt, & Brytus, 2013). The success of EBP is determined by all involved, including healthcare agencies, administrators, nurses, physicians, and other healthcare professionals. We all need to take an active role in ensuring that the health care provided to patients and families is based on the best research available.

SEARCHING FOR EVIDENCE-BASED SOURCES

EBP requires searching a variety of databases and websites for the best research evidence for use in practice. You can identify research syntheses such as systematic reviews, meta-analyses, meta-syntheses, and mixed-methods systematic reviews through searches of electronic databases, national library sites, EBP organizations, and professional organizations. Some of the key resources for EBP are identified in Table 13-1. At least 2500 new systematic reviews are reported in English and indexed in MEDLINE each year (Liberati, Altman, Tetzlaff, Mulrow, Gotzsche, Ioannidis, et al., 2009). The Cochrane Collaboration library of systematic reviews is an excellent resource, with more than 11,000 entries relevant to nursing and health care (http://www.cochrane.org/cochrane-reviews). In 2009, the Cochrane Nursing Care Field (CNCF) was developed to support the conduct, dissemination, and use of systematic reviews in nursing. The Joanna Briggs Institute also provides resources for locating and conducting research syntheses in nursing (see Table 13-1). Chapter 6 provides additional direction for searching electronic databases for individual studies and research syntheses. Once you have identified research syntheses of interest, you need to appraise these sources critically for relevant research evidence for use in your practice.

TABLE 13-1 EVIDENCE-BASED PRACTICE RESOURCES

RESOURCE	DESCRIPTION
Electronic Databases	
CINAHL *(Cumulative Index to Nursing and Allied Health Literature)*	CINAHL is an authoritative resource covering the English-language journal literature for nursing and allied health. The database was developed in the United States and includes sources published from 1982 to the present.
MEDLINE (PubMed, National Library of Medicine)	MEDLINE was developed by the National Library of Medicine in the United States; it provides access to more than 11 million MEDLINE citations back to the mid-1960s and to additional life science journals.
MEDLINE with MeSH	Also developed by the National Library of Medicine, MEDLINE with MeSH provides authoritative medical information on medicine, nursing, dentistry, veterinary medicine, the healthcare system, preclinical services, and more.
PsychINFO	The American Psychological Association developed this database that includes professional and academic literature for psychology and related disciplines from 1887 to the present.
CANCERLIT	CANCERLIT, containing information on cancer, was developed by the U.S. National Cancer Institute.
National Library Sites	
Cochrane Library	The Cochrane Library provides high-quality evidence for those providing and receiving health care and those involved in research, teaching, funding, and administration of health care at all levels. Included is the Cochrane Collaboration, which has many systematic reviews of research (http://www.cochrane.org/ reviews).
National Library of Health (NLH)	NLH, located in the United Kingdom, provides searchable evidence-based sources at http://www.evidence.nhs.uk.
Evidence-Based Practice Organizations and Collections	
National Guideline Clearinghouse (NGC)	The Agency for Healthcare Research and Quality (AHRQ) developed NGC to house the thousands of evidence-based guidelines that have been developed for use in clinical practice; these can be accessed online at http://www.guidelines.gov.
Cochrane Nursing Care Field (CNCF)	Cochrane Collaboration includes over 7000 reviews in 11 different fields; one is the CNCF, which supports the conduct, dissemination, and use of systematic reviews in nursing. Most libraries subscribe to the Cochrane Collaboration but free access to abstracts and reviews can be found at http://cncf.cochrane.org.
National Institute for Health and Clinical Excellence (NICE)	The NICE was organized in the United Kingdom to provide access to current evidence-based guidelines, similar to NGC (http://nice.org.uk).
Joanna Briggs Institute (JBI)	JBI, an international evidence-based organization originating in Australia, has a search website that includes evidence summaries, systematic reviews, systematic review protocols, evidence-based recommendations for practice, best practice information sheets, consumer information sheets, and technical reports; see "Search the Joanna Briggs Institute" (http://www.joannabriggs.edu.au/Search. aspx).
Nursing Reference Center (NRC)	The NRC includes a collection of rigorously reviewed, evidence-based care sheets that provide current best practice for over 700 interventions and clinical conditions. This source requires a subscription, so check with your librarian. You can access this resource at http://www.ebscohost.com/pointOfCare/nrc-about.

CRITICALLY APPRAISING RESEARCH SYNTHESES

Research evidence is usually synthesized using the following processes: systematic review, meta-analysis, meta-synthesis, and mixed-method systematic review. These synthesis processes were introduced in Chapter 1, and the following section provides guidelines for critically appraising these synthesis processes to determine the status of knowledge for use in practice.

Critically Appraising Systematic Reviews

A systematic review is a structured, comprehensive synthesis of the research literature to determine the best research evidence available to address a healthcare question. A systematic review involves identifying, locating, appraising, and synthesizing quality research evidence for clinicians to use in practice (Bettany-Saltikov, 2010a; Craig & Smyth, 2012; Higgins & Green, 2008; Liberati et al., 2009; Rew, 2011). Systematic reviews are often conducted by two or more researchers and/or clinicians in a selected area of interest to determine the best research knowledge in that area (see Grove, Burns, & Gray [2013] for the process of conducting a systematic review).

Systematic reviews need to be conducted with rigorous research methodology to promote the accuracy of the findings and minimize the reviewers' bias. Table 13-2 provides a checklist for

TABLE 13-2	CHECKLIST FOR CRITICALLY APPRAISING PUBLISHED SYSTEMATIC REVIEWS AND META-ANALYSES		
SYSTEMATIC REVIEW STEPS		**STEP COMPLETE (YES OR NO)**	**COMMENTS: QUALITY AND RATIONALE**
1. Did the title indicate that a systematic review, meta-analysis, or both were conducted?			
2. Was an abstract included that provided a structured summary of purpose, data sources, study eligibility criteria, participants, interventions, outcomes, study appraisal and synthesis methods, results, key findings, conclusions, and implications for practice?			
3. Was the clinical question clearly expressed and significant? Was the PICOS (**p**articipants, **i**ntervention, **c**omparative interventions, **o**utcomes, and **s**tudy design) format used to develop the question and focus the systematic review or meta-analysis?			
4. Were the purpose and objectives or aims of the research synthesis clearly expressed and used to direct it?			
5. Were the search criteria clearly identified? Was the PICOS format used to identify the search criteria, and were the years covered, language, and publication status of sources identified in the search criteria?			
6. Was a comprehensive, systematic search of the literature conducted using explicit criteria identified in step 3? Were the search strategies clearly reported with examples? Did the search include published studies, grey literature, and unpublished studies?			

Continued

SYSTEMATIC REVIEW STEPS	STEP COMPLETE (YES OR NO)	COMMENTS: QUALITY AND RATIONALE
TABLE 13-2 **CHECKLIST FOR CRITICALLY APPRAISING PUBLISHED SYSTEMATIC REVIEWS AND META-ANALYSES—cont'd**		
7. Was publication bias addressed, including any time lag bias, location bias, duplicate publication bias, citation bias, and language bias?		
8. Was the process for the selection of studies for the review clearly identified and consistently implemented? Was the selection process expressed in a flow diagram such as Figure **13-1**?		
9. Were key elements (population, sampling process, design, intervention, outcomes, and results) of each study clearly identified and presented in a table?		
10. Was a quality critical appraisal of the studies conducted? Were the results related to participants, types of interventions, outcomes, and outcome measurement methods? Were possible methodological and reporting biases clearly discussed related to each study (i.e., in table and narrative format)?		
11. Was a meta-analysis conducted as part of the systematic review? Was a rationale provided for conducting the meta-analysis? Were the details of the meta-analysis process and results clearly described?		
12. Were the results of the systematic review or meta-analysis clearly described (i.e., in narrative and table)? Were details of the study interventions compared and contrasted in a table? Were the outcome variables clearly identified and the quality of the measurement methods addressed?		
13. Did the report conclude with a clear discussion section? a. Were the review findings summarized to identify the current best research evidence? b. Were the limitations of the review and how they might have affected the findings addressed? c. Were the recommendations for further research, practice, and policy development addressed?		
14. Did the authors of the review develop a clear, concise, quality report for publication? Was the report inclusive of the items identified in the PRISMA statement, which are included in this table (Liberati et al., 2009; Moher et al., 2009)?		

critically appraising the steps of systematic reviews and meta-analyses. These steps are based on the Preferred Reporting Items for Systematic Reviews and Meta-Analyses (PRISMA; Liberati et al., 2009) statement and other relevant sources to guide nurses in conducting systematic reviews (Bettany-Saltikov, 2010a, 2010b; Higgins & Green, 2008; Moore, 2012; Rew, 2011). The PRISMA statement was developed in 2009 by an international group of expert researchers and clinicians to improve the quality of reporting for systematic reviews and meta-analyses. It includes 27 items, which can be found at http://prisma-statement.org and are detailed in the article by Liberati and colleagues (2009). If the review process is clearly detailed in the report, others can replicate the process and verify the findings.

A systematic review conducted by Choi and Hector (2012) is presented here as an example, with the application of the critical appraisal steps outlined in Table 13-2. They conducted a systematic review that included a meta-analysis to determine the effectiveness of fall prevention programs in reducing the number and rate of falls in hospital and community agencies. You can find the publication by Choi and Hector (2012) in the CINAHL database of your closest library (see Table 13-1 for a description of CINAHL). We recommend that you read this article and use the guidelines in Table 13-2 to critically appraise this systematic review and compare your findings with the following discussion.

Step 1

Did the title indicate if a systematic review or meta-analysis was conducted? Choi and Hector (2012, p. 188.e21) titled their research synthesis as "Effectiveness of Intervention Programs in Preventing Falls: A Systematic Review of Recent 10 Years and Meta-Analysis." The authors clearly indicated the types of research syntheses (systematic review and meta-analysis) included in their publication.

Step 2

Did the abstract include a structured summary of the research synthesis? Choi and Hector (2012) provided a clear, concise abstract that identified the purpose of the systematic review, data sources, study eligibility criteria, studies selected for review (17 RCTs), types of fall prevention programs, primary outcomes of number of falls and fall rates, critical appraisal of studies, results, conclusions, and implications for practice.

Step 3

Was a significant, clear clinical question developed to direct the research synthesis? A systemic review or meta-analysis is best directed by a relevant clinical question that focuses the review process and promotes the development of a quality synthesis of research evidence. One of the most common formats used to develop a relevant clinical question to guide a systematic review is the PICO or PICOS format described in the *Cochrane Handbook for Systematic Reviews of Interventions* (Higgins & Green, 2008). The PICOS format includes the following elements:

P—Population or participants of interest (see Chapter 9 on sampling)

I—Intervention needed for practice (see Chapter 8 on nursing interventions)

C—Comparisons of the intervention with control, placebo, standard care, variations of the same intervention, or different therapies (see Chapter 8)

O—Outcomes needed for practice (see Chapter 10 on measurement methods and Chapter 14 on outcomes research)

S—Study design (see Chapter 8 on types of study designs)

Choi and Hector (2012) noted that falls were the leading cause of injury and deaths among older adults, with the direct medical costs estimated to be over $19.2 billion in 2000. Research syntheses had been conducted on fall prevention programs from the 1990s to 2000, but not for the last decade. What was not known was the effectiveness of the fall prevention interventions studied from 2000 to 2009. The population was older adults, and the intervention was fall prevention programs. The studies reviewed included different types of interventions, with most of the fall prevention programs including multiple approaches, such as individualized exercises for strength, coordination and balance, occupational therapy, home environmental and behavioral assessments, cognition assessment, medical examination, gait stability, and medication review. The intervention group was compared with groups receiving standard care, no treatment, or a variation of the treatment. The primary outcomes measured were number of falls and fall rate. The study design included synthesis of only RCTs using guidelines from the Cochrane Collaboration handbook (Higgins & Green, 2008; see Chapter 8 for a description of RCTs). The study design (RCTs) clearly focused the literature review but might have eliminated some important studies that could have expanded the knowledge related to the intervention, fall prevention programs.

Step 4

Were the purpose and objectives or aims of the review expressed? Systematic reviews of research include a purpose and sometimes specific aims or objects to guide the synthesis process (Bettany-Saltikov, 2010a; Rew, 2011). The purpose identifies the major goal or focus of the review. Choi and Hector (2012, p. 188.e13) identified their purpose as follows: "To examine the reported effectiveness of fall-prevention programs for older adults by reviewing randomized controlled trials from 2000 to 2009." This clearly focused purpose was used to direct their systematic review and meta-analysis, and no additional objectives were identified.

Step 5

Was the literature search criteria clearly identified? Research reports of systematic reviews or meta-analyses need to identify the inclusion and exclusion criteria used to direct the literature search (see Table 13-2). The PICOS format might be used to develop the search criteria with more detail being developed for each of the elements. These search criteria might focus on the following: (1) type of research methods, such as quantitative, qualitative, or outcomes research; (2) population or type of study participants; (3) study designs, such as description, correlational, quasi-experimental, experimental, qualitative, or mixed methods; (4) sampling processes, such as probability or nonprobability sampling methods; (5) intervention and comparison interventions; and (6) specific outcomes to be measured. The search criteria also need to indicate the years for the review, language, and publication status (Bettany-Saltikov, 2010b; Higgins & Green, 2008; Rew, 2011).

Often searches have been limited to published sources in common databases, which excludes the grey literature from the research synthesis. Grey literature refers to studies that have limited distributions, such as theses and dissertations, unpublished research reports, articles in obscure journals, articles in some online journals, conference papers and abstracts, conference proceedings, research reports to funding agencies, and technical reports (Benzies, Premji, Hayden, & Serrett, 2006; Conn, Valentine, Cooper, & Rantz, 2003). Most grey literature is difficult to access through database searches and is often not peer-reviewed, with limited referencing information. These are some of the main reasons why grey literature is not included in systematic reviews and meta-analyses. However, excluding grey literature might result in misleading, biased results. Studies with significant findings are more likely to be published than studies with nonsignificant findings and are usually published in more high-impact, widely distributed journals that are indexed in computerized databases (Conn et al., 2003). Studies with significant findings are more likely to have duplicate publications, which should not be included in the systematic review or meta-analysis. More details on identifying publication bias are provided in the next section on critically apprais-ing meta-analyses.

Choi and Hector (2012) designed their literature search strategies and their protocol for con-ducting their systematic review using sources such as the Cochrane Collaboration handbook (Higgins & Green, 2008) and the PRISMA statement (Liberati et al., 2009; Moher, Liberati, Tetzlaff, Altman, & PRISMA Group, 2009). PICOS format was also implemented with the litera-ture search being directed by population of older adults, intervention of fall prevention programs, comparison of intervention groups with standard care and control groups, outcomes of number of falls and fall rates, and study designs limited to RCTs. The date restriction for the search was 2000 to 2009 based on the lack of research syntheses conducted in the last decade. The search was limited to published studies reported in English, which could result in important studies being omitted from the systematic review.

Step 6

Was a comprehensive, systematic search of the research literature conducted? The key search terms, different databases searched, and search results need to be recorded in the systematic review and meta-analysis publications. Sometimes authors provide a table that identifies the search terms and criteria. The PRISMA statement recommends presenting the full electronic search strat-egy used for at least one major database, such as CINAHL or MEDLINE (Liberati et al., 2009). The search strategies used to identify grey literature and other unpublished studies need to be identified.

Choi and Hector (2012, p. 188.e14) described their search of the literature in the following:

"A thorough search of the scientific and medical literature was conducted using major biomed-ical electronic databases: Medline, PubMed, PsycINFO, CINAHL, and RefWorks. This rigorous literature examination selected articles in peer-reviewed journals published in the English lan-guage, with full-text availability, targeting both men and women, in RCTs, with primary out-comes measures as either the number of falls or the fall rate, with fall-intervention follow-up of a minimum of 5 months, and published from 2000 to 2009. We excluded articles with unidentified study design. . . . Key words used were the combination of falls, recurrent falls, fall-prevention programs, interventions, programs, injuries, older adults, RCTs, and/or long-term care facilities. A total of 17,325 studies were generated from the 5 electronic data bases."

Step 7

Was publication bias addressed? Choi and Hector (2012) recognized the publication bias that occurs with using only published sources and not including grey literature. They also limited their search to the English language, resulting in a language bias. They noted that 33 studies were duplicated across the databases, and these were excluded, thus reducing the potential for duplication bias.

Step 8

Was the process for selecting the studies for review detailed? The selection of studies for inclusion in a systematic review or meta-analysis is a complex process that initially involves the review and removal of duplicate sources. The abstracts of the remaining studies are reviewed by two or more authors and sometimes by an external reviewer to ensure that they meet the criteria identified in step 5 (see Table 13-2). The abstracts might be excluded based on the study participants, interventions, outcomes, or design not meeting the search criteria (Bettany-Saltikov, 2010b; Higgins & Green, 2008; Liberati et al., 2009). After the abstracts meeting the designated criteria are identified, the next step is to retrieve the full-text citation for each study. If studies do not meet criteria, they need to be removed, with a rationale provided. The study selection process is best demonstrated by a flow diagram that was developed by the PRISMA Group (Liberati et al., 2009). Figure 13-1 shows this diagram, which has four phases: (1) identification of the sources; (2) screening of the sources based on set criteria; (3) determining if the sources meet eligibility requirements; and (4) identifying the studies included in the review.

Choi and Hector (2012) provided a description of their selection of sources and a flow diagram that documented the final results of the 17 RCTs included in their systematic review, with a

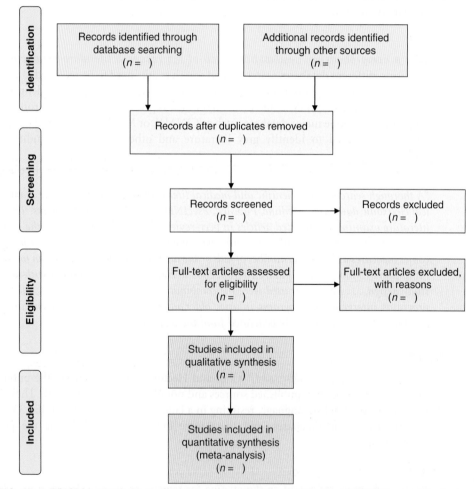

FIG 13-1 PRISMA 2009 Flow Diagram. Identification, screening, eligibility, and inclusion of research sources in systematic reviews and meta-analyses. (From Moher, D., Liberati, A., Tetzlaff, J., Altman, D. G., & PRISMA Group. (2009). *Preferred reporting items for systematic reviews and meta-analyses: The PRISMA statement.* Retrieved July 17, 2013, from http://www.prisma-statement.org.)

meta-analysis. The following excerpt identifies the steps that they took to select their studies for inclusion in their research synthesis:

"There were 33 studies duplicated across databases that were excluded.... Studies with titles and abstracts unlikely to be relevant were excluded (n = 15,419) followed by exclusion of studies that did not identify an RCT (n = 1619). A total of 287 potentially relevant studies were reviewed by the primary author (M. C.). We excluded studies of fall-prevention programs for children (n = 27). The primary search (completed from July 2009 to March 2010) generated a total of 227 studies.... Of the 227 publications that met the criteria for meta-analysis, 17 studies remained [Figure 13-2]."

Choi and Hector, 2012, p. 188.e14

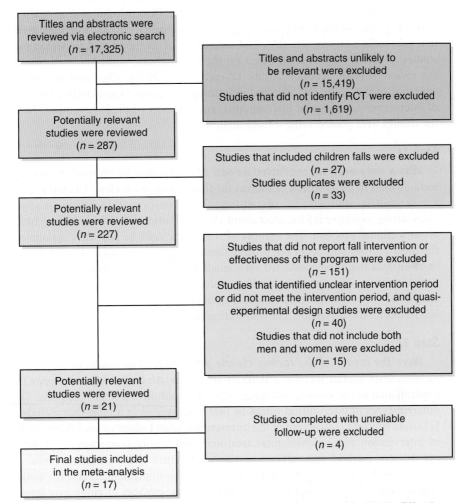

FIG 13-2 Flow chart of study selection. (From Choi, M., & Hector, M. (2012). Effectiveness of intervention programs in preventing falls: A systematic review of recent 10 years and meta-analysis. *Journal of the American Medical Directors Association, 13*(2), 188.e15. Figure 1.)

Step 9

Were key elements of the studies presented? Critical appraisals of studies for systematic reviews and meta-analyses are best done by constructing a table describing the characteristics of the included studies, such as the purposes of the studies, populations, sampling processes, interventions, outcomes, and results (Bettany-Saltikov, 2010b; Higgins & Green, 2008; Liberati et al., 2009). Choi and Hector (2012) detailed the key elements of the 17 studies in a table. The table included authors of the study, year, sample size of control and intervention groups, intervention and follow-up period, intervention model, setting, mean age of subjects, and brief description of the intervention programs. The table would have been stronger if the sampling methods, outcomes measured, and key results for the 17 studies had been included in a table format.

Step 10

Were the studies critically appraised? Two or more experts need to review the studies independently and make judgments about their quality. The critical appraisal of the studies is often difficult because of the differences in types of participants, designs, sampling methods, intervention protocols, outcome variables and measurement methods, and presentation of results. The studies are often rank-ordered based on their quality and contribution to the development of the review (Bettany-Saltikov 2010b; Liberati et al., 2009). Choi and Hector's (2012) critical appraisal of the 17 studies involved examining the sample characteristics in the studies, types of interventions, settings of interventions, and intensity of the intervention. The final results of the studies were pooled using a meta-analysis.

Step 11

Was a meta-analysis conducted as part of the systematic review? Some authors conduct a meta-analysis in the synthesis of sources for their systematic review (Liberati et al., 2009). Because a meta-analysis involves the use of statistics to summarize results of different studies, it usually provides strong, objective information about the effectiveness of an intervention or solid knowledge about a clinical problem. The authors of the review need to provide a rationale for conducting the meta-analysis and detail the process that they used to conduct this analysis. For example, a meta-analysis might be conducted on a small group of similar studies to determine the effect of an intervention. The systematic review conducted by Choi and Hector (2012) included a meta-analysis of the 17 studies and provided a detailed discussion of the rationale for the meta-analysis and results for this procedure. The next section provides more details on conducting a meta-analysis.

Step 12

Were the results of the review clearly presented? The results of a systematic review and meta-analysis should include a description of the study participants, types of interventions implemented in the studies, outcomes measured, and measurement methods. The results of the different types of intervention might be best summarized in a table that includes the following: (1) study source; (2) structure of the intervention (stand-alone or multifaceted); (3) specific type of intervention (e.g., physiological treatment, education, counseling, or behavioral therapy); (4) delivery method (e.g., demonstration and return demonstration, verbal, video, or self-administered); (5) length of time the intervention is implemented; and (6) statistical difference between the intervention and control, standard care, placebo, or alternative intervention groups (Liberati et al., 2009).

The specific outcomes, including primary and secondary outcomes, of the studies might also be best summarized in a table. This table might include (1) the study source, (2) outcome variable(s), with an indication as to whether it was a primary or secondary outcome in the study, (3) measurement method used for each study outcome variable, and (4) quality of the measurement methods, such as the reliability and validity of a scale or the precision and accuracy of a physiological measure.

Choi and Hector (2012) included a description of the 17 fall prevention interventions in a table indicating that most of the interventions were multifactorial rather than an individual action. The interventions and their follow-up period had to be at least 5 months. The authors indicated that the primary outcomes of number of falls and fall rates were measured in different ways in the studies, which limited the quality of the results and findings of the systematic review and meta-analysis. The following excerpt presents the key results from the systematic review and meta-analysis:

> *"Overall, a significant 14% fall reduction was found in the number of falls and fall rate during the follow-up along with an even more significant fall reduction in multifactorial interventions studies (n= 15, 14%) and nursing homes (n= 3, 55%). The significant fall-prevention effect in multifactorial intervention program in our analysis was consistent with results of several prior studies and inconsistent with 2 earlier meta-analysis efforts that reported that a single intervention specifically focusing on exercise alone was more effective in reducing falls.... The intensity of the intervention did not demonstrate any significant fall reduction rate."*
>
> *Choi & Hector, 2012, p. 188.e19*

Step 13

Did the report conclude with a clear discussion section?   In a systematic review or meta-analysis, the discussion of the findings includes an overall evaluation of the types of interventions implemented and the outcomes measured. You can also expect the methodological issues or limitations of the review to be addressed. A quality discussion section explicitly connects the findings to the study's framework to identify the theoretical implications of the findings. Finally, the discussion section needs to provide recommendations for further research, practice, and policy development (Bettany-Saltikov, 2010b; Higgins & Green, 2008; Liberati et al., 2009).

Choi and Hector (2012) provided a discussion of their findings, limitations, and recommendations for research and practice. The report would have been strengthened by including a framework and linking the findings back to the framework to indicate current knowledge regarding the effect of fall prevention programs on number of falls and fall rates. The following excerpt summarizes the key aspects of the discussion section of their report:

> *"We conclude that interventions to prevent falls in older adults were modestly effective, in multifactorial intervention with a 10% reduction in fall rates, 9% in community settings, and 12% on Model 1 intervention types (initial intervention and subsequent follow-up)"* (Choi & Hector, 202 p 188.e20).

The limitations included studies with small sample sizes, varying types of fall prevention interventions, and measurements of outcomes of number of falls and fall rate in various ways. Several of the 17 studies concluded that the intervention made no significant difference. They also noted that the search of the literature might have been more rigorous in identifying additional studies.

> *"We found a few observations that might be valuable for future research. Studies need to be carefully designed to examine their results over an extended period of time (at least 6 months) if they are to be meaningful. Excluding observational studies with significant variations of outcome measures would help to reduce confounders. Eliminating quasi-experimental studies would help to yield an unbiased estimate of the effect size. Including only studies of RCTs*

may reduce publication bias. . . . We certainly would encourage the inclusion of more random-ized controlled studies to reduce sampling error variation, even if the results turned out not to be positive."

Choi and Hector, 2012, p. 188.e20

Implications for practice

"Implementing intervention programs to prevent falls by older adults seems to be plausible and highly desirable, but the overall effectiveness of intervention programs are not supported strongly by significant statistical results. The following are recommendations for healthcare providers to attempt to reduce fall rates in clinical practice: (1) identify an individual's risk factors for falls; (2) determine predisposing and precipitating factors if the patient has a history of falls, and intervene accordingly; (3) provide intervention programs and management focusing on lower-extremity balance and strengthening; (4) consider psychological factors such as fear of fall-ing and self-imposed restriction of activity; and (5) classify injuries when they do occur based on the International Classification of Diseases."

Choi & Hector, 2012, p. 188.e20

Systematic reviews and meta-analyses provide important, evidence-based knowledge for use in practice. Choi and Hector's (2012) recommendations provide clear evidence-based interventions that students and RNs might use to reduce the falls in their agencies and institutions. The QSEN (2013) implication is that critically appraising systematic reviews and using relevant evidence in practice is essential for achieving EBP.

Step 14

Was a clear concise report developed for publication? The systematic review or meta-analysis report needs to include the content discussed in the previous 13 steps. You can use Table 13-2 when critically appraising a systematic review, indicate if the step is present, and comment about its qual-ity with, supporting rationale. In summary, Choi and Hector (2012) developed a strong systematic review and meta-analysis for publication. The title clearly indicates the types of syntheses con-ducted. The clinical question addressed followed the PICOS format, and the purpose of the syn-thesis is clearly focused. The search of the literature might have been more rigorous and included additional studies, especially grey literature. The selection of studies for the synthesis was clearly presented in a flow chart and documented with rationale. The studies selected for the systematic review and meta-analysis were critically appraised, and the results from these syntheses were clearly presented in tables and narrative. The publication concluded with relevant findings, limitations, and recommendations for research and practice.

Critically Appraising Meta-Analyses

A meta-analysis is conducted to pool or combine statistically the results from previous studies into a single quantitative analysis that provides one of the highest levels of evidence about the effective-ness of an intervention (Andrel, Keith, & Leiby, 2009; Craig & Smyth, 2012; Higgins & Green, 2008; Liberati et al., 2009). This approach has objectivity because it includes analysis techniques to deter-mine the effect of an intervention while examining the influences of variations in the studies included in the meta-analysis. The studies included in a meta-analysis need to be examined for variations or heterogeneity in areas such as sample characteristics, sample size, design, types of interventions, and outcome variables and measurement methods (Higgins & Green, 2008).

Heterogeneity in the studies included in a meta-analysis can lead to different types of biases (see later). Meta-analyses that include more homogeneous (similar) studies have less bias and usually provide more valid findings (Moore, 2012).

Statistically combining data from several studies results in a large sample size, with increased power to determine the true effect of a specific intervention on a particular outcome (see Chapter 9 for a discussion of power). The ultimate goal of a meta-analysis is to determine if an intervention (1) significantly improves outcomes, (2) has minimal or no effect on outcomes, or (3) increases the risk of adverse events. Meta-analysis is also an effective way to resolve conflicting study findings and controversies that have arisen related to a selected intervention (Higgins & Green, 2008).

Strong evidence for using an intervention in practice can be generated from a meta-analysis of multiple, quality studies such as RCTs and quasi-experimental studies. However, the conduct of a meta-analysis depends on the accuracy, clarity, and completeness of information presented in studies. Box 13-1 provides a list of information that needs to be included in a research report

---

BOX 13-1 RECOMMENDED REPORTING FOR AUTHORS TO FACILITATE META-ANALYSIS

Demographic Variables Relevant to Population Studied
Age
Gender
Marital status
Ethnicity
Education
Socioeconomic status

Methodological Characteristics
Sample size (experimental and control groups)
Type of sampling method
Sampling refusal rate and attrition rate
Sample characteristics
Research design
Groups included in study—experimental, control, comparison, placebo groups
Intervention protocol and fidelity discussion
Data collection techniques
Outcome measurements
- Reliability and validity of instruments
- Precision and accuracy of physiological measures

Data Analysis
Names of statistical tests
Sample size for each statistical test
Degrees of freedom for each statistical test
Exact value of each statistical test
Exact p value for each test statistic
One-tailed or two-tailed statistical test
Measures of central tendency (mean, median, and mode)
Measures of dispersion (range, standard deviation)
Post hoc test values for ANOVA (analysis of variance) test of three or more groups

to facilitate the conduct of a meta-analysis. You might use the information in Box 13-1 as a checklist to determine if the reports of RCTs and quasi-experimental studies are complete.

The steps for critically appraising a meta-analysis are similar to those for critically appraising a systematic review that were detailed earlier (see Table 13-2). The following information is provided to increase your ability to appraise critically meta-analysis studies. The PRISMA statement, Cochrane Collaboration guidelines for meta-analysis (Higgins & Green, 2008), and other resources (Andrel et al., 2009; Conn & Rantz, 2003; Moore, 2012; Turlik, 2010) were used to provide details for critically appraising a meta-analysis. Conn's (2010) meta-analysis to determine the effect of physical activity interventions on depressive symptom outcomes in healthy adults is presented as an example.

Clinical Question for a Meta-Analysis

The clinical question developed for a meta-analysis is usually clearly focused: "What is the effectiveness of a selected intervention?" The PICOS (*p*articipants or population, *i*ntervention, *c*omparative interventions, *o*utcomes, and *s*tudy design) format discussed earlier might be used to generate the clinical question (Higgins & Green, 2008; Liberati et al., 2009; Moher et al., 2009). Conn (2010) indicated that only one previous meta-analysis had examined the effect of physical activities (PAs) on depressive symptoms among subjects without clinical depression. Therefore, Conn wanted to address the following clinical question: "What is the effect of PA on depressive symptoms in healthy adults?"

Purpose and Questions to Direct a Meta-Analysis

Researchers need to identify the purpose of their meta-analysis and the questions or objectives that guide the analysis. Conn clearly identified the following relevant purpose and research questions to guide her meta-analysis:

> *"This meta-analysis synthesized depressive symptom outcomes of supervised and unsupervised PA interventions among healthy adults. . . . This meta-analysis addressed the following research questions:*
>
> *(1) What are the overall effects of supervised PA and unsupervised PA interventions on depressive symptoms in healthy adults without clinical depression?*
>
> *(2) Do interventions' effects on depressive symptom outcomes vary depending on intervention, sample, and research design characteristics?*
>
> *(3) What are the effects of interventions on depressive symptoms among studies comparing treatment subjects with before versus after interventions?"*
>
> **Conn, 2010, pp. 128-129**

Search Criteria and Strategies for Meta-Analyses

The methods for identifying search criteria and selecting search strategies are similar for meta-analyses and systematic reviews. The search criteria are usually narrowly focused for a meta-analysis to identify the specific studies examining the effect of a particular intervention. The search needs to be rigorous and should include published sources identified through varied databases and unpublished studies identified through other types of searches (see earlier). Conn (2010) clearly identified her detailed search strategies in the following excerpt. She used ancestry searches, which involves the use of citations from relevant studies to identify additional studies.

Primary Study Search Strategies

"Multiple search strategies were used to ensure a comprehensive search and thus limit bias while moving beyond previous reviews. An expert reference librarian searched 11 computerized databases (e.g., MEDLINE, PsychINFO, EMBASE) using broad search terms (sample MEDLINE intervention terms: adherence, behavior therapy.... PA terms: exercise, physical activity, physical fitness). ... Search terms for depressive symptoms were not used to narrow the search because many PA intervention studies report depressive symptom outcomes but do not consider these the main outcomes of the study and thus papers are not indexed by these terms. Several research registers were examined including Computer Retrieval of Information on Scientific Projects and RCT, which contains 14 active registers and 16 archived registers. Computerized author searches were completed for project principal investigators located from research registers and for the first three authors on eligible studies. Author searches were completed for dissertation authors to locate published papers. Ancestry searches were conducted on eligible and review papers. Hand searches were completed for 114 journals which frequently report PA intervention research."

Conn, 2010, p. 129

Possible Biases for Meta-Analyses and Systematic Reviews

Even with rigorous literature searches, authors of meta-analyses and systematic reviews are often limited to mainly published studies. The nature of the sources can lead to biases and flawed or inaccurate conclusions in the research syntheses. The common biases that can occur in conducting and reporting research syntheses include publication bias (e.g., time lag bias, location bias, duplicate publication bias, citation bias, and language bias); bias from poor study methodology; and outcome reporting bias (see Table 13-2). Publication bias occurs because studies with positive results are more likely to be published than studies with negative or inconclusive results. Higgins and Green (2008) found that the odds were four times greater that positive study results would be published versus negative results. Time lag bias of studies, a type of publication bias, occurs because studies with negative results are usually published later, sometimes 2 to 3 years later, than studies with positive results. Sometimes studies with negative results are not published at all, whereas studies with positive results might be published more than once (duplicate publication bias). Location bias of studies can occur if studies are published in lower impact journals and indexed in less searched databases. A citation bias occurs when certain studies are cited more often than others and are more likely to be identified in database searches. Language bias can occur if searches focus just on studies in English, and important studies exist in other languages.

Methodological bias is often related to design and data analysis problems in studies. For example, studies might have limitations related to the sample, intervention, outcome measurements, and analysis techniques that result in methodological bias. Outcome reporting bias occurs when study results are not reported clearly and with complete accuracy. For example, reporting bias occurs when researchers selectively report positive results and not negative results, or positive results might be addressed in detail, with limited discussion of negative results. Higgins and Green (2008) provided a much more comprehensive discussion of potential biases in systematic reviews and meta-analyses.

Publication, methodological, and outcome reporting biases can weaken the validity of the findings from meta-analyses and systematic reviews. An analysis method termed the *funnel plot* can be used to assess for biases in a group of studies. Funnel plots provide graphic representations of possible effect sizes (*ESs*) for interventions in selected studies (see Chapter 9 for the calculation of *ES*). The *ES*, or strength of an intervention in a study, can be calculated by determining the difference between the experimental and control groups for the outcome variable. The mean difference between the experimental and control groups for several studies is easier to determine if the outcome variable is measured by the same scale or instrument in each study. However, the standardized mean difference *(SMD)* must be calculated in a meta-analysis when the same outcome, such as depression, is measured by different scales or methods. More details are provided on *SMD* later in this section.

Figure 13-3 shows a funnel plot of the *SMDs* from 13 individual studies. The *SMDs* from the studies are fairly symmetrical or are equally divided by the line through the middle of the funnel in the graph. A symmetrical funnel plot indicates limited publication bias. Asymmetry of the funnel plot is mainly the result of publication bias but also of methodological bias, reporting bias, heterogeneity in the studies' sample sizes and interventions, and chance. In Figure 13-3, the studies with small sample sizes are toward the bottom of the graph, and the studies with larger samples are toward the top. Figure 13-3 is presented to help you understand the funnel plot diagrams included in systematic reviews and meta-analyses.

Conn (2010) provided a quality discussion of her literature search results and the risk of publication bias in her meta-analysis. The following includes key content related to the search results and the possible biases:

"Comprehensive searches yielded 70 reports.. . . The supervised PA [physical activity] two-group comparison included 1,598 subjects. The unsupervised PA two-group comparison included 1,081 subjects. The treatment single-group comparisons included 1,639 supervised PA and 3,420 unsupervised PA subjects.. . . Most primary studies were published articles (s = 54), and the remainder were dissertations (s = 14), book chapter (s = 1), and conference presentation materials (s = 1; s indicates the number of reports). Publication bias was evident in the funnel plots for supervised and unsupervised PA two-group outcome comparisons and for treatment group, pre- vs. post-intervention supervised PA and unsupervised PA comparisons. The control group pre- and post-comparison distributions on the funnel plots suggested less publication bias than plots of treatment groups. Unless otherwise specified, all results are from the treatment vs. control comparisons."

Conn, 2010, p. 131

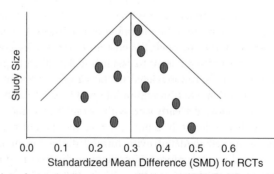

FIG 13-3 Funnel plot of standardized mean differences (*SMDs*) for randomized controlled trials (RCTs) with limited bias. (From Grove, S. K., Burns, N., & Gray, J. R. (2013). *The practice of nursing research: Appraisal, synthesis, and generation of evidence* (7th ed.). St. Louis: Elsevier Saunders.)

Results of Meta-Analysis for Continuous Outcomes

Many nursing studies examine continuous outcomes or outcomes that are measured by methods that produced interval- or ratio-level data. Physiological measures to examine blood pressure produce ratio-level data. Likert scales, such as the Center for Epidemiologic Studies Depression Scale (CES-D), produce interval-level data (see Chapter 10 for a copy of the CES-D). Therefore, blood pressure and depression are continuous outcomes. The effect of an intervention on a continuous outcome in a meta-analysis is determined by the mean difference between two groups. The mean difference is a standard statistic that identifies the absolute difference between two groups. It is an estimate of the amount of change caused by the intervention (e.g., physical activity) on the outcome (e.g., depression), on average, compared with the control group. The mean difference is reported in a meta-analysis to identify the effect of an intervention but is appropriate only if the outcome is measured by the same scale in all the studies (Higgins & Green, 2008).

A standardized mean difference (SMD), or *d*, is a summary statistic that is reported in a meta-analysis when the same outcome is measured by different scales or methods. The *SMD* is also sometimes referred to as the standardized mean effect size. For example, in the meta-analysis by Conn (2010), depression was commonly measured with three different scales—Profile of Mood States, Beck Depression Inventory, and CES-D. Studies that have differences in means in the same proportion to the standard deviations have the same *SMD (d)*, regardless of the scales used to measure the outcome variable. The differences in the means and standard deviations in the studies are assumed to be the result of the measurement scales and not variability in the outcome (Higgins & Green, 2008, p. 256).

Conn's (2010) meta-analysis result identified a standardized mean effect size of 0.372 (moderate *ES*) between the treatment and control groups for the 38 supervised PA studies and *SMD* of 0.522 (strong *ES*) among the 22 unsupervised PA studies. (Chapter 9 provides values for determining small, moderate, and strong *ESs*.) This meta-analysis documented that supervised and unsupervised PA reduced symptoms of depression in healthy adults or adults without clinical depression. Therefore, a decrease in depression is another important reason for encouraging patients to be involved in structured and unstructured physical activities. The results of this meta-analysis support the QSEN (2013) competencies of locating, reading, and integrating research evidence in practice.

Results of Meta-Analysis for Dichotomous Outcomes

If the outcome data examined in a meta-analysis are dichotomous, risk ratios, odds ratios, and risk differences are usually reported to indicate the effect of the intervention on the measured outcome. These terms are introduced in this chapter, but more information is available in Craig and Smyth (2012), Higgins and Green (2008), and Sackett and associates (2000). With dichotomous data, every participant fits into one of two categories, such as clinically improved or no clinical improvement, effective screening device or ineffective screening device, or alive or dead. The risk ratio, also called the relative risk (*RR*), is the ratio of the risk of subjects in the intervention group to the risk of subjects in the control group for having a particular health outcome. The health outcome is usually adverse, such as the risk of a disease (e.g., cancer) or the risk of complications or death (Higgins & Green, 2008).

The odds ratio (*OR*) is defined as the ratio of the odds of an event occurring in one group, such as the treatment group, to the odds of it occurring in another group, such as the standard care group. The *OR* is a way of comparing whether the odds of a certain event is the same for two groups. An example is the odds of medication adherence or nonadherence for an experimental group receiving education and specialized medication packaging intervention versus a group receiving standard practice or care.

The risk difference (*RD*), also called the *absolute risk reduction,* is the risk of an event in the experimental group minus the risk of the event in the control or standard care group. Higgins and Green (2008), Fernandez and Tran (2009), and Grove and co-workers (2013) provide more details on the results from meta-analyses with dichotomous data.

Magnus, Ping, Shen, Bourgeois, and Magnus (2011) conducted a meta-analysis of the effectiveness of mammography screening in reducing breast cancer mortality in women 39 to 49 years old. Because mammography screening is significant in reducing breast cancer mortality in women older than 50 years, and early detection of breast cancer increases survival, annual routine mammography screening has been recommended for all women 40 to 47 years old in the United States. Thus, "the primary aim of the current study was, after a quality assessment of identified randomized controlled trials (RCTs), to conduct a meta-analysis of the effectiveness of mammography screening [*intervention*] in women aged 39-49 [*population*] in reducing breast cancer mortality [*dichotomous outcome*]. The second aim was to compare and discuss the results of previously published meta-analyses" (Magnus et al., 2011, p. 845). The following describes the methods, results, and conclusions of this meta-analysis:

> "*Methods:* PubMed/MEDLINE, OVID, COCHRANE, and Educational Resources Information Center (ERIC) databases were searched, and extracted references were reviewed. Dissertation abstracts and clinical trials databases available online were assessed to identify unpublished works. All assessments were independently done by two reviewers. All trials included were RCTs, published in English, included data on women aged 39-49, and reported relative risk (RR)/odds ratio (OR) or frequency data.
>
>   *Results:* Nine studies were identified.... The individual trials were quality assessed, and the data were extracted using predefined forms.... Seven RCTs with the highest quality score were combined, and a significant pooled RR estimate of 0.83 (95% confidence interval [CI] 0.72-0.97) was calculated."
>
>

Magnus et al., 2011, p. 845

The results of the study are graphically represented in Figure 13-4 using a forest plot. A forest plot is a type of diagram used to present the meta-analysis results of studies with dichotomous outcomes (Grove et al., 2013; Fernandez & Tran, 2009). The plot clearly identifies the names of the seven studies included in the meta-analysis on the left side of the figure. The *RR* and *CI* for each study are identified with a block and horizontal line. The numerical *RR* and 95% *CI* values are identified on the right side of the plot, with the percentage of weight given to each study in the meta-analysis. Most of the studies show homogeneity with odds ratios left of the vertical line, except for the Stockholm study. Magnus and colleagues (2011, p. 845) concluded that "Mammography screenings were effective and generate a 17% reduction in breast cancer mortality in women 39-49 years of age. The quality of the trials varied, and providers should inform women in this age group about the positive and negative aspects of mammography screenings."

Critically Appraising Meta-Syntheses

Qualitative research synthesis is the process and product of systematically reviewing and formally integrating the findings from qualitative studies (Sandelowski & Barroso, 2007). The process for conducting a synthesis of qualitative research is still evolving. Various synthesis methods have appeared in the literature, such as meta-synthesis, meta-ethnography, meta-study, meta-narrative, qualitative metasummary, qualitative meta-analysis, and aggregated analysis (Barnett-Page & Thomas, 2009; Kent & Fineout-Overholt, 2008; Sandelowski & Barroso, 2007; Walsh & Downe, 2005). Despite Sandelowski and Barroso receiving NIH funding to develop meta-synthesis processes, qualitative

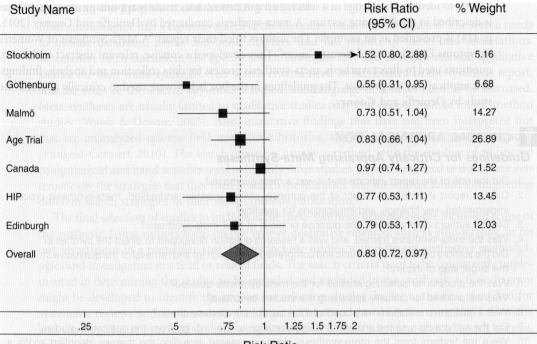

Study Name		Risk Ratio (95% CI)	% Weight
Stockhoim		1.52 (0.80, 2.88)	5.16
Gothenburg		0.55 (0.31, 0.95)	6.68
Malmö		0.73 (0.51, 1.04)	14.27
Age Trial		0.83 (0.66, 1.04)	26.89
Canada		0.97 (0.74, 1.27)	21.52
HIP		0.77 (0.53, 1.11)	13.45
Edinburgh		0.79 (0.53, 1.17)	12.03
Overall		0.83 (0.72, 0.97)	

Risk Ratio

FIG 13-4 Forest Plot. This shows the individual randomized controlled trials and overall pooled estimate from the seven original randomized controlled trials, with a high-quality score addressing the impact of mammography screening on breast cancer mortality in women 39 to 49 years old. *CI,* Confidence interval. (From Magnus, M. C., Ping, M., Shen, M. M., Bourgeois, J., & Magnus, J. H. (2011). Effectiveness of mammography screening in reducing breast cancer mortality in women aged 39-49 years: A meta-analysis. *Journal of Women's Health, 20*(6), 848.)

researchers are currently not in agreement that it is possible to meta-synthesize qualitative studies or, if it is, what is the appropriate method to use to accomplish this process. Despite the lack of consensus on the process for meta-syntheses, qualitative researchers recognize the importance of summarizing qualitative findings to determine the knowledge that might be used in practice and for policy development (Barnett-Page & Thomas, 2009; Finfgeld-Connett, 2010; Sandelowski & Barroso, 2007). The Cochrane Collaboration recognizes the importance of synthesizing qualitative research, and the Cochrane Qualitative Methods Group was developed as a forum for the discussion and development of methodology in this area (Higgins & Green, 2008).

The qualitative research synthesis method that seems to be gaining momentum in the nursing literature is meta-synthesis. Methodological articles have been published to describe meta-synthesis, but this method is still evolving (Finfgeld-Connett, 2010; Kent & Fineout-Overholt, 2008; Walsh & Downe, 2005). A meta-synthesis is defined as the systematic compilation and integration of qualitative study results to expand understanding and develop a unique interpretation of study findings in a selected area. The focus is on interpretation rather than on combining study results, as with quantitative research synthesis. A meta-synthesis involves the breaking down of findings from different studies to discover essential features and then combining these ideas into a unique, transformed whole. Sandelowski and Barroso (2007) identified metasummary as a step in conducting meta-synthesis. A metasummary is the summarizing of findings across qualitative

Guidelines for Critically Appraising Mixed-Methods Systematic Reviews

1. Did the title identify the type of research synthesis that was conducted?
2. Was a clear, concise abstract presented that included the purpose, clinical question addressed, data sources, review methodology, results, findings, and recommendations for practice?
3. Were the purpose and questions guiding the mixed-methods systematic review identified?
4. What were the search criteria for quantitative, qualitative, and mixed-methods studies?
5. Were the search strategies identified for locating relevant quantitative, qualitative, and mixed-methods studies?
6. Was a rigorous search of the literature conducted and detailed in the final report?
7. Was the process for selecting relevant quantitative, qualitative, and mixed-methods studies for the synthesis detailed?
8. Was a table of information of studies included that demonstrated a comparative appraisal of the studies?
9. Were critical appraisals of the studies summarized in the final report?
10. Was a clear synthesis of study findings presented? Did this synthesis integrate the findings from quantitative, qualitative, and mixed-method studies? (Bettany-Saltikov, 2010a, 2010b; Creswell, 2014; Higgins & Green, 2008)

Wulff, Cummings, Marck, and Yurtseven (2011) conducted a mixed-methods systematic review to examine the association of medication administration technologies and patient safety. The title indicated that a mixed-method systematic review was conducted. The abstract clearly and concisely covered the aim of the review, search process, review methods, results, and conclusions. Wolff and associates (2011, p. 2080) noted that "the aim of the study was to evaluate the research evidence on relationships between the use of medication administration technologies and incidence of medication administration incidents and preventable adverse drug events to inform decision-making about existing technology options." The authors systematically searched 13 databases with keywords such as medication, drugs, pharm system, medication errors, and safety. A total of 37,705 titles and abstracts were screened, and 108 full-text manuscripts were retrieved and reviewed.

Wulff and co-workers (2011) presented a flow chart to document the selection of the 12 manuscripts included in the mixed-methods systematic review. These 12 studies included the following designs: five preintervention and postintervention studies, five correlational studies, and two qualitative studies. The elements of the 12 studies were compared in two different tables. The tables included the study source, medication technology intervention studied, setting, sample size, study design, outcomes measured, and results. Most of the healthcare agencies measured short-term outcomes focused on medication errors, with less focus on adverse drug events and patient safety outcomes. The authors recognized the publication bias of only reviewing titles and abstracts in English. The studies reviewed mainly reported positive findings, with less coverage of negative and nonsignificant findings, which is another publication bias.

The major focus of this review was the synthesis of the 10 quantitative studies that identified the benefits of implementing medication administration technologies to improve patient safety. However, the problem identified by the quantitative and qualitative studies was that nurses develop workarounds when implementing different types of medication administration technologies, which could compromise patient safety. Wulff and colleagues (2011) recommended that additional intervention studies be conducted with a framework, hypotheses, and experimental or RCT designs to produce stronger, evidence-based knowledge for practice. This knowledge is essential to guide the selection and use of medication administration technologies in healthcare agencies to promote patient safety, which is a QSEN (2013) competency area.

DEVELOPING CLINICAL QUESTIONS TO IDENTIFY EXISTING RESEARCH-BASED EVIDENCE FOR USE IN PRACTICE

EBP requires using the most current research evidence in practice. Many research-based protocols, algorithms, and guidelines have been published for nurses to use in their practice. Thousands of research syntheses (systematic reviews, meta-analyses, meta-syntheses, and mixed-methods systematic reviews) are available through libraries and national and international organizations and collections. Many individual studies in selected areas require identification, review, and summarizing for use in practice (see Chapter 6). Students and practicing nurses need to use this current research evidence in practice (see Table 13-1 for resources that include current research evidence). Use of current best research evidence in practice is usually organized by a relevant clinical question formulated using the PICO format. The PICO format is very similar to the PICOS format introduced earlier to guide systematic reviews and meta-analyses. However, the PICO format is also implemented to organize research evidence to address a clinical problem.

P—Population or participants of interest in your clinical setting

I—Intervention needed for practice

C—Comparisons of interventions to determine the best intervention for your practice

O—Outcomes needed for practice and ways to measure the outcomes in your practice

You can use the PICO format to identify relevant studies, meta-analyses, and integrative reviews needed to develop evidence-based protocols, algorithms, guidelines, and policies for practice. Some publications include a systematic review and guidelines for practice. For example, Nicoll and Hesby (2002) developed a systematic review of the research literature focused on intramuscular (IM) injection techniques. This review provided the basis for their development of a clinical practice guideline entitled "Intramuscular Injection: Guidelines for Evidence-Based Technique." The goal of their systematic review and evidence-based guidelines was the "elimination of complications from IM injections" (Nicoll & Hesby, 2002, p. 152). The researchers summarized the medications routinely administered by the IM route with site recommendations in Table 13-3. This table includes the medication class, generic and brand names of the medication, and recommended site and needle size for selected IM injections. The recommendations for sites and needle size (length and gauge) were for infants, toddlers, and adults. This is valuable research evidence for you to use when giving an IM injection of a particular medication to patients of all ages in your practice (Cocoman & Murray, 2008; Greenway, 2004). Table 13-4 presents the clinical practice guideline for giving IM injections using an evidence-based technique.

You can use the PICO format to determine the evidence-based delivery of an IM injection.

P—Population is adults needing influenza virus vaccine by IM injection. Confirm that the vaccine must be given by IM injection.

I—Intervention to deliver the right medication by the right route at the right site using the appropriate needle size (length and gauge; Cocoman & Murray, 2008; Greenway, 2004).

C—Comparison of interventions reveals that influenza virus vaccine should be given to adults in the deltoid site with 25- to 38-mm, 22- to 25-gauge needles (see Table 13-3). The evidence-based technique for giving the IM injection is given in Table 13-4.

O—Outcome desired is an IM injection of vaccine without complications.

TABLE 13-3   MEDICATIONS ROUTINELY ADMINISTERED BY THE INTRAMUSCULAR ROUTE WITH SITE RECOMMENDATIONS

MEDICATION CLASS	GENERIC NAME	BRAND NAMES (SELECTED)*	RECOMMEND SITES AND NEEDLE SIZE†
Antibiotics	Streptomycin sulfate	Streptomycin sulfate injection	Adults—ventrogluteal (VG) with 38-mm, 18- to 25-gauge needle
	Penicillin G benzathine, penicillin G procaine	Bicillin, Wycillin, Pfizerpen	Infants and young children—vastus lateralis with 16- to 25-mm, 22- to 25-gauge needle
Biologicals, including immune globulins, vaccines, and toxoids	Diphtheria and tetanus toxoids adsorbed	DT (pediatric), Td (adult)	Adults—deltoid with 25- to 38-mm, 22- to 25-gauge needle Hepatitis
	Diphtheria, tetanus, and acellular pertussis	Acel-Immune, Infanrix, Tripedia, Certiva	B and rabies must be given in the deltoid site. Immune globulin may be given in the deltoid (volumes of 2 mL or less) or VG site (volumes
	Haemophilus influenzae type b conjugate	ActHIB	of >2 mL).
	Haemophilus influenzae type b conjugate and hepatitis B (recombinant)	Comvax	Toddlers and older children— deltoid, if the muscle mass is adequate, with 16- to 32-mm, 22- to 25-gauge needle
	Hepatitis A vaccine, inactivated	Havrix, Vaqta	Infants, young children, and those with inadequate muscle mass at the deltoid site—vastus lateralis with
	Hepatitis B vaccine (recombinant)	Engerix-B, Recombivax HB	22- to 25-mm, 22- to 27-gauge needle
	Hepatitis B immune globulin (human)	BayHep B, Nabi-HB	
	Hepatitis A inactivated and hepatitis B (recombinant)	Twinrix	
	Immune globulin for pre- and postexposure prophylaxis for hepatitis A infection		
	Influenza virus vaccine	Fluogen, FluShield, Fluvirin, Fluzone	
	Lyme disease vaccine	LYMErix	
	Pneumococcal vaccine, polyvalent	Prevnar	
	Rabies vaccine, adsorbed	RabAvert	
	Rabies immune globulin (human)		
	Rho(D) immune globulin (human)	BayRho-D, MICRhoGAM, RhoGAM, WinRho SDF	

TABLE 13-3	MEDICATIONS ROUTINELY ADMINISTERED BY THE INTRAMUSCULAR ROUTE WITH SITE RECOMMENDATIONS—cont'd		
MEDICATION CLASS	**GENERIC NAME**	**BRAND NAMES (SELECTED)**	**RECOMMEND SITES AND NEEDLE SIZE**
	Tetanus immune globulin (human)	BayTet	
	Tetanus toxoid, adsorbed	Tetanus Toxoid, Adsorbed, Purogenated	
Hormonal agents	Medroxyprogesterone acetate	Depo-Provera	Adults—VG with 38- mm, 18- to 25-gauge needle (these
	Chorionic gonadotropin	Novarel, Pregnyl	medications typically not indicated
	Menotropin	Humegon, Repronex	for infants and young children)
	Testosterone enanthate	Delatestryl	

*Selected brand names are included to be illustrative of products widely used in the United States; in other countries in which the generic products are available (this is particularly true in the case of vaccines), they may go by different names. All brand names are copyrighted trademarks of their respective companies.

†Needle sizes are provided in metric lengths to conform to the international standard; for U.S. readers, corresponding needle sizes in inches are as follows: 16 mm $= ^5/_8$"; 22 mm $= ^7/_8$"; 25 mm $= 1$"; 32 mm $= 1\,^1/_4$"; 38 mm $= 1\,^1/_2$".

(From Nicoll, L. H., & Hesby, A. (2002). Intramuscular injection: An integrative research review and guideline for evidence-based practice. *Applied Nursing Research, 16*(2), 150.)

TABLE 13-4	CLINICAL PRACTICE GUIDELINE

Intramuscular Injection Guidelines for Evidence-Based Technique

Patient Population
Infants, toddlers, children, and adults receiving medication by the IM route for curative or prophylactic purposes

Objective
Administration of medication to maximize its therapeutic effect for the patient and minimize or eliminate patient injury and discomfort associated with the procedure

Key Points
"An injection should only be given if it is necessary—and each injection that is given must be safe" (WHO, 1998).
Justification for IM injection. Consider:
- Medication characteristics, including formulation, onset and intensity of effect, and duration of effect*
- Patient characteristics, including compliance, uncooperativeness, reluctance, or inability to take medication via another route*

Site selection. Site is the single most consistent factor associated with complications and injury. Consider: Age of patient:
- Infants—vastus lateralis is the preferred site.*
- Toddlers and children—vastus lateralis or deltoid*
- Adults—ventrogluteal or deltoid*

Medication type
- Biologicals (including immune globulins, vaccines, and toxoids)—vastus lateralis (infants and young children); deltoid in older children and adults*

Continued

TABLE 13-4 **CLINICAL PRACTICE GUIDELINE**—cont'd

- Hepatitis B and rabies must be given in the deltoid; injection in other sites decreases the immunogenicity of the medication.
- Depot formulations—ventrogluteal site*
- Medications that are known to be irritating, viscous or in oily solutions should be administered at the ventrogluteal site.*

Medication volume
- Small volumes of medication (≤2 mL) may be given in the deltoid site.*
- Large volumes of medication (2-5 mL) should be given in the ventrogluteal site.

Always use bony landmarks to identify the site properly *

Preparation of the medication. Consider:

Equipment

Needle length corresponds to the site of injection and age of patient according to the following guidelines:
- Vastus lateralis—16 mm to 25 mm*
- Deltoid (children)—16 mm to 32 mm*
- Deltoid (adults)—25 mm to 38 mm*
- Ventrogluteal (adults)—38 mm*

Needle gauge—often dependent on needle length. In general, most biologicals and medications in aqueous solutions can be administered with a 20- to 25-gauge needle; medications in oil-based solutions require 18- to 25-gauge needles[†]

Always use a new, sterile syringe and needle for every injection. *

Use a filter needle to withdraw medication from a glass ampule* or rubber-topped vial.[§]

With a filter needle, change needle before injection.*

Use the markings on the syringe barrel to determine the correct dose.*

Do not include an air bubble in the syringe *

Patient preparation and positioning. Consider site of injection:
- Deltoid—patient may sit or stand.[†] A child may be held in an adult's lap.*
- Ventrogluteal—patient may stand, sit, or lay laterally or supine.*
- Vastus lateralis—infants and young children may lay supine or be held in an adult's lap.*
- Remove clothing at the site for adequate visualization and palpation of bony landmarks.[†]
- Position patient to relax the muscle.*

Injection procedure
- Cleanse the site with alcohol and allow to dry.[†]
- Insert needle into the muscle using a smooth, steady motion.[†]
- Research on two alternate techniques to reduce pain at the moment of injection is inconclusive at this time, but warrants further study.[‡,§]
- Aspirate for 5 to 10 seconds.*
- Inject slowly at a rate of 10 sec/mL.[†]
- After injection, wait 10 seconds before withdrawing the needle.[†]
- Withdraw needle slowly; apply gentle pressure with a dry sponge.[†]

Postinjection
- Assess site for complications, immediately and 2 to 4 hours later, if possible.
- Instruct patient regarding assessment, self-management of minor reactions, and when to report more serious problems.*
- Properly and promptly dispose of all equipment.*

Note. Needle sizes are provided in metric lengths to conform to international standard; for U.S. readers, corresponding needle sizes in inches are as follows: 16 mm = $^5/_8$"; 22 mm = $^7/_8$"; 25 mm = 1"; 32 mm = $1^1/_4$"; 38 mm = $1^1/_2$".

Criteria for grading of the evidence:

*Empirical data from published research reports, recommendations of established advisory panels, and generally accepted scientific principles.

[†]Surveys, reviews, consensus among clinicians, and expert opinion.

[‡]Published case reports.

[§]Anecdotal evidence and letters.

From Nicoll, L. H., & Hesby, A. (2002). Intramuscular injection: An integrative research review and guideline for evidence-based practice. *Applied Nursing Research, 16*(2), 159.

You can use Tables 13-3 and 13-4 to ensure that you give IM injections using the best research evidence available. You can then share this evidence with others in clinics, hospitals, or rehabilitation centers to promote EBP for the delivery of IM injections (QSEN, 2013).

MODELS TO PROMOTE EVIDENCE-BASED PRACTICE IN NURSING

EBP is a complex phenomenon that requires integration of the best research evidence with clinical expertise and patient values and needs in the delivery of quality, cost-effective care. The two models most commonly used to implement research evidence in practice are the Stetler Model of Research Utilization to Facilitate Evidence-Based Practice (Stetler, 2001) and the Iowa Model of Evidence-Based Practice to Promote Quality of Care (Titler et al., 2001). These two models are discussed in this section.

Stetler Model of Research Utilization to Facilitate Evidence-Based Practice

An initial model for research utilization in nursing was developed by Stetler and Marram in 1976 and expanded and refined by Stetler in 2001 to promote EBP for nursing. The Stetler Model of Research Utilization to Facilitate Evidence-Based Practice (Figure 13-6) provides a comprehensive framework to enhance the use of research evidence by nurses to facilitate an EBP. The research evidence can be used at the institutional or individual level. At the institutional level, study findings

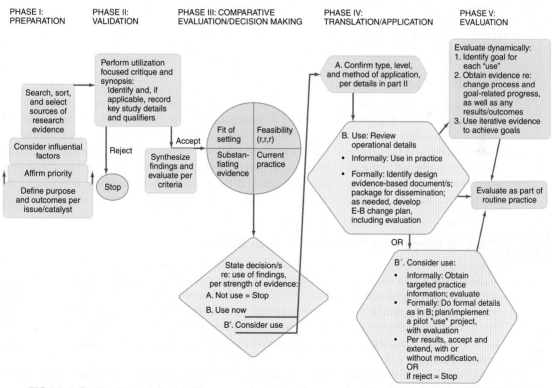

FIG 13-6 Stetler Model, Part I. Shown are the steps of research utilization to facilitate EBP. (From Stetler, C. B. (2001). Updating the Stetler model of research utilization to facilitate evidence-based practice. *Nursing Outlook, 49*(6), 276.)

are synthesized and the knowledge generated is used to develop or refine policies, algorithms, procedures, protocols, or other formal programs implemented in the institution. Individual nurses, such as RNs, educators, and policymakers, summarize research and use the knowledge to make practice decisions, influence educational programs, and guide political decision making. For example, the evidence-based guidelines for giving IM injections discussed in the previous section can be implemented at the individual level to promote quality outcomes for IM injections given by nurses.

Stetler's model is included in this text to encourage the use of research evidence by individual nurses and healthcare institutions to facilitate the development of EBP. The five phases of the Stetler (2001) model are briefly described in the following sections: (1) preparation, (2) validation, (3) comparative evaluation and decision making, (4) translation and application, and (5) evaluation.

Phase I: Preparation

The intent of Stetler's (2001) model is to make using research evidence in practice a conscious, critical thinking process that is initiated by the user. Thus, Phase I: Preparation, involves determining the purpose, focus, and potential outcomes of making an evidence-based change in a clinical agency. Agency priorities and other external and internal factors that could be influenced by or could influence the proposed practice change need to be examined. Once the agency, individuals, or committee identify and approve the purpose of the evidence-based project, a detailed search of the literature is conducted to determine the strength of the evidence available for use in practice (see Chapter 6 for directions in searching the literature). The research literature might be reviewed to solve a difficult clinical, managerial, or educational problem; provide the basis for a policy, algorithm, or protocol; or prepare for an in-service program or other type of professional presentation.

Phase II: Validation

In Phase II: Validation, the research reports are critically appraised to determine their scientific soundness (Fawcett & Garity, 2009; Hoare & Hoe, 2013; Hoe & Hoare, 2012). If the studies are limited in number, weak, or both, the findings and conclusions are considered inadequate for use in practice and the process stops. If a systematic review, meta-analysis, and/or meta-synthesis have been conducted in the area in which you want to make an evidence-based change, this greatly strengthens the quality of the research evidence. If the research knowledge base is strong in the selected area, the clinical agency must make a decision regarding the priority of using the evidence in practice.

Phase III: Comparative Evaluation/Decision Making

Phase III: Comparative Evaluation includes four parts: (1) substantiation of the evidence; (2) fit of the evidence with the healthcare setting; (3) feasibility of using research findings; and (4) concerns with current practice (see Figure 13-6). Substantiating evidence is produced by replication, in which consistent, credible findings are obtained from several studies in similar practice settings. The studies generating the strongest research evidence are systematic reviews and meta-analyses of RCTs. However, quasi-experimental studies also provide extremely strong evidence for making a change in an agency. To determine the fit of the evidence in the clinical agency, examine the characteristics of the setting to determine the forces that will facilitate or inhibit implementation of the evidence-based change, such as a policy, protocol, or algorithm, for nursing practice. Stetler (2001) believes that the feasibility of using research evidence in practice involves examining the three Rs related to making changes in practice: (1) potential risks, (2) resources needed, and (3) readiness of those involved. The final comparison involves determining whether the research information provides credible, empirical evidence for making changes in the current practice. The research evidence needs to document that an intervention increased the quality in current practice by solving practice problems and improving patient outcomes. By conducting phase III, you can assess the overall benefits and risks of using the research evidence in a practice setting. If the benefits are much greater than the risks for the organization, individual nurse, or both, using the research-based intervention in practice is feasible.

During the decision-making aspect of phase III, three decisions are possible: (1) to use the research evidence; (2) to consider using the evidence; and (3) not to use the research evidence (see Figure 13-6). The decision to use research knowledge in practice depends mainly on the strength of the evidence. Depending on the research knowledge to be used in practice, the individual RN, hospital unit, or agency might make this decision. Another decision might be to consider use of the available research evidence in practice. When a change is complex and involves multiple disciplines, additional time is often needed to determine how the evidence might be used and what measures will be taken to coordinate the involvement of different healthcare professionals in the change. A final option might be not to use the research evidence in practice because the current evidence is not strong, or the risks or costs of change in current practice are too high in comparison with the benefits (Stetler, 2001).

Phase IV: Translation/Application

Phase IV: Translation/Application involves planning for and actual use of the research evidence in practice. The translation phase involves determining exactly what knowledge will be used and how that knowledge will be applied to practice. The use of the research evidence can be cognitive, instrumental, or symbolic. With cognitive application, the research base is a means of modifying a way of thinking or one's appreciation of an issue (Stetler, 2001). For example, cognitive application may improve the nurse's understanding of a situation, allow analysis of practice dynamics, or improve problem-solving skills for clinical problems. Instrumental application involves using research evidence to support the need for change in nursing interventions or practice protocols. Symbolic or political utilization occurs when information is used to support or change a current policy. The application phase includes the following steps for planned change: (1) assess the situation to be changed; (2) develop a plan for change; and (3) implement the plan. During the application phase, the protocols, policies, or algorithms developed with research knowledge are implemented in practice (Stetler, 2001). An agency may conduct a pilot project on a single hospital unit to implement the change in practice. The agency would then evaluate the results of this project to determine if the change should be extended throughout the healthcare agency.

Phase V: Evaluation

The final stage, Phase V: Evaluation, is to evaluate the impact of the research-based change on the healthcare agency, personnel, and patients. The evaluation process can include formal and informal activities conducted by administrators, nurse clinicians, and other health professionals. Informal evaluations might include self-monitoring or discussions with patients, families, peers, and other professionals. Formal evaluations can include case studies, audits, quality improvement, and translational or outcomes research projects. The goal of Stetler's (2001) model is to increase the use of research evidence in nursing to facilitate EBP. This model provides detailed steps to encourage nurses to become change agents to make the necessary improvements in practice based on research evidence.

Iowa Model of Evidence-Based Practice

Nurses have been actively involved in conducting research, synthesizing research evidence, and developing evidence-based guidelines for practice. These activities support their strong commitment to EBP, which could be facilitated by the Iowa model. The Iowa Model of Evidence-Based Practice provides direction for the development of EBP in a clinical agency. This EBP model was initially developed by Titler and associates in 1994 and revised in 2001 (Figure 13-7). In a healthcare agency, there are triggers that initiate the need for change, and the focus should always be to make changes based on the best research evidence. These triggers can be problem-focused and evolve from risk management data, process improvement data, benchmarking data, financial data, and clinical problems. The triggers can also be knowledge-focused, such as new research findings, change in national agencies or organizational standards and guidelines, expanded philosophy of care, or questions from the institutional standards' committee. The triggers are evaluated and prioritized based on the needs of the clinical agency. If a trigger is considered an agency priority, a group is formed to search for the best evidence to manage the clinical concern (Titler et al., 2001).

In some situations, the research evidence is inadequate to make changes in practice, and additional studies are needed to strengthen the knowledge base. Sometimes the research evidence can be combined with other sources of knowledge (e.g., theories, scientific principles, expert opinion, and case reports) to provide fairly strong evidence for use in developing research-based protocols for practice. Research-based protocols are structured guidelines for implementing nursing interventions in practice that are based on current research evidence. The strongest evidence comes from systematic reviews that include meta-analyses of RCTs. However, meta-syntheses, mix-methods systematic reviews, and individual studies also provide important evidence for changing practice. The levels of research evidence are described in Chapter 1 (see Figure 1-3) and also presented inside the front cover of this text.

The research-based protocols or evidence-based guidelines developed could be pilot-tested on a particular unit and then evaluated to determine the impact on patient care. If the outcomes are favorable from the pilot test, the change would be made in practice and monitored over time to determine its impact on the agency environment, staff, costs, and patient and family (Titler et al., 2001). If an agency strongly supports the use of the Iowa model, implements patient care based on the best research evidence, and monitors changes in practice to ensure quality care, the agency is promoting EBP.

Application of the Iowa Model of Evidence-Based Practice

Preparing to use research evidence in practice raises some important questions. Which research findings are ready for use in clinical practice? What are the most effective strategies for implementing research-based protocols or evidence-based guidelines in a clinical agency? What are the outcomes from using the research evidence in practice? Do the risk management data, process improvement data, benchmarking data, or financial data support making the change in practice based on the research evidence? Is the research-based change proposed an agency priority? We suggest that effective strategies for using research evidence in practice will require a multifaceted approach that takes into consideration the evidence available, attitudes of the practicing nurses, the organization's philosophy, and national organizational standards and guidelines (ANCC, 2014; Brown, 2014; Melnyk & Fineout-Overholt, 2011; The Joint Commission, 2014). In this section, the steps of the Iowa model (Titler et al., 2001) guide the use of a research-based intervention in a hospital to facilitate EBP.

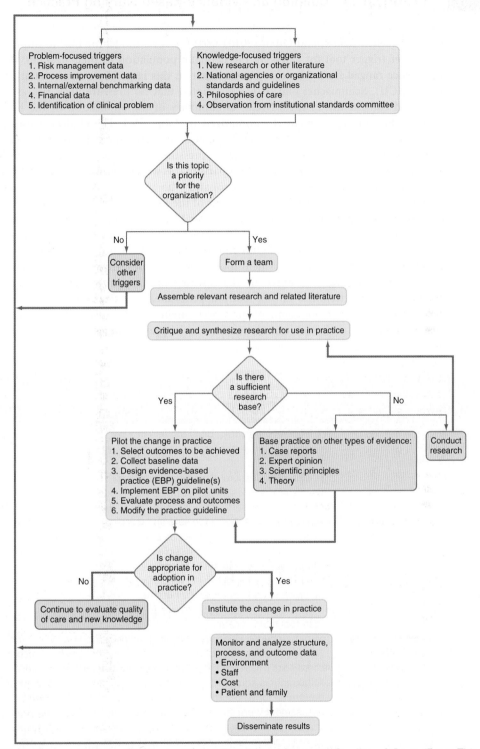

FIG 13-7 Iowa Model of Evidence-Based Practice to Promote Quality of Care. (From Titler, M. G., Kleiber, C., Steelman, V. J., Rakel, B. A., Budreau, G., Everett, L. Q., et al. (2001). The iowa model of evidence-based practice to promote quality care. *Critical Care Nursing Clinics of North America, 13*(4), 497–509.)

Schumacher, Askew, and Otten (2013) used the Iowa model for EBP to implement a pressure ulcer trigger tool for assessing the neonatal population in their hospital. Pressure ulcer prevalence ranged from 0% to 1% per quarter in this large Midwest neonatal intensive care unit (NICU). Schumacher and co-workers noted that no pressure ulcer risk assessment tool was used consistently in their NICU. A summary of the application of the Iowa model of EBP to this clinical problem is summarized in Table 13-5. The clinical question addressed was generated using the PICO format. Population was the infants in the NICU. The intervention to be implemented was a three-question pressure ulcer trigger tool to assess if the neonates were at risk for skin breakdown. The comparison was with the Braden Q tool, the standard care or usual practice of determining the neonates who were at risk for pressure ulcers (PUs). The outcome measured was the effectiveness of the PU trigger tool as compared to the Braden Q tool in assessing neonates who are at risk for PU. The studies that had examined the effectiveness of different neonatal PU assessment tools were critically appraised. The tools in these studies were judged to be too long for routine clinical use. Schumacher and colleagues (2013) developed a shorter trigger assessment tool based on the research evidence: "Trigger Questions for Pressure Ulcer Risk Proposed by the Institute for Clinical Systems Improvement: Is the infant: Moving extremities and/or body appropriately for developmental age? Responding to discomfort in a developmentally appropriate manner? Demonstrating adequate tissue perfusion based on the clinical formula (mean arterial pressure = gestational age and/or capillary refill <3 s)?" (Schumacher et al., 2013, p. 48).

TABLE 13-5   **USE OF THE IOWA MODEL FOR EVIDENCE-BASED PRACTICE PROJECTS TO ESTABLISH A CLINICAL TOOL FOR EVALUATION OF PRESSURE ULCER RISK IN AN NICU**

1. Generate the question from either a problem or new knowledge.	For infants in the NICU, does the use of a pressure ulcer trigger tool perform equally as well as the Braden Q to identify an infant at risk? **P**—Infant in the NICU **I**—Use of a pressure ulcer trigger tool **C**—Usual practices of assessing all with Braden Q **O**—Trigger tool performs equally as well as the Braden Q for risk identification
2. Determine relevance to organizational priorities.	Our hospital is committed to safe and reliable care and ensuring a flawless patient experience. This includes preventing hospital-acquired pressure ulcers—a "never event." Possible impact/outcomes may include: • Potential increase in WOC referrals • Correct triggering of infants requiring further pressure ulcer risk assessment and prevention strategies by nursing • Preservation of nursing time because the trigger tool is a shorter and easier to use tool that indicates for whom full assessment is needed.
3. Develop a team to gather and appraise evidence.	Team members included a clinical nurse specialist, two WOC nurses, NICU Nursing Practice Council members, and electronic medical records experts. According to IHI, all premature infants are at risk for pressure ulcer development. Although this statement is visionary, it does not assist the bedside nurse to determine for whom to provide interventions. Referrals to the WOC nurse for assessment were based on clinical judgment, and no assessment tools were in place. Risk assessment tools are available for the neonatal population but were judged to be lengthy and time-consuming for every nurse, every shift. A trigger tool was developed, based on IHI pediatric trigger questions to help the nurse determine whom to refer for full assessment.

TABLE 13-5	USE OF THE IOWA MODEL FOR EVIDENCE-BASED PRACTICE PROJECTS TO ESTABLISH A CLINICAL TOOL FOR EVALUATION OF PRESSURE ULCER RISK IN AN NICU—cont'd
4. Determine if the evidence answers the question.	Reasonable evidence is present to warrant implementation of this practice. The three IHI trigger questions are based on the concepts of the Braden Q and could trigger those at risk and requiring further assessment and intervention.
5. If there is sufficient evidence, pilot the change in practice.	Prior to implementation, 10 patients were randomly selected to test the feasibility of implementing trigger questions. The three trigger questions were asked of the nurses caring for each patient, and results were compared to a Braden Q score generated by a WOC nurse. We noted that patients with high risk, as defined by the Braden Q, were also identified as at-risk based on the three trigger questions. The three trigger questions were embedded into the electronic medical record. Pressure ulcer data were collected through the surveillance provided by skin team nurses as part of their usual duties.
6. Evaluate structure, process, and outcome data.	The HAPU rate for the NICU remains low and has not changed since the implementation of the trigger tool. The number of WOC nurse consultations has remained stable since implementation of the three trigger questions into NICU nurse practice.
7. Disseminate results.	Results and appropriate feedbacks have been shared with the NICU nurses via the NICU practice

HAPU, Hospital-acquired pressure ulcer; *IHI,* Institute for Healthcare Improvement; *NICU,* neonatal intensive care unit; *WOC,* Wound, ostomy, and continence.
From Schumacher, B., Askew, M., & Otten, K. (2013). Development of a pressure ulcer trigger tool for the neonatal population. *Journal of Wound, Ostomy, and Continence Nursing, 40*(1), Table 1, p. 47.

Schumacher and associates (2013) found that their three-question PU trigger assessment tool was as effective as the Braden Q tool in determining neonatal risk for pressure ulcers. Their findings are summarized in the following study excerpt:

> *"Following implementation of the trigger questions in 2009, we observed no net increase in the number of WOC [wound, ostomy, and continence] referrals per 1000 patients. Nevertheless, our PU [pressure ulcer] prevalence in the NICU remains low at 0.01 per 1000 patient days. Comparison of results from the 3 trigger questions and the Braden Q scoring by the WOC nurse demonstrated that most infants are correctly identified by the tool, with the exception of those very immature infants who may be at risk for medical device-related ulcers. . . .*
>
> *We implemented a 3-item trigger tool to aid NICU nurses identifying neonates at risk for PU development. While these questions do not quantify risk, we have found that they are an efficient initial screening tool when combined with additional assessment and management in consultation with a WOC nurse."*
>
> **Schumacher et al., 2013, p. 50**

IMPLEMENTING EVIDENCE-BASED GUIDELINES IN PRACTICE

EBP in nursing and medicine has expanded extensively since the 1990s. Research knowledge is generated every day that needs to be critically appraised and synthesized to determine the best evidence for use in practice (Brown, 2104; Craig & Smyth, 2012; Melnyk, Fineout-Overholt, Stillwell, & Williams, 2010). This section discusses the evidence-based guidelines developed based on the current, best research evidence available by expert researchers and clinicians for use in practice. For example, Chobanian and co-workers (2003) conducted an excellent systematic review to determine the best research evidence available for assessing, diagnosing, and managing hypertension (HTN). This systematic review, which included several meta-analyses, was used to develop the "Seventh Report of the Joint National Committee on Prevention, Detection, and Treatment of High Blood Pressure" (JNC 7; National Heart, Lung, and Blood Institute [NHLBI], 2003). The JNC 7 guideline for the management of HTN, introduced in Chapter 1, is the currently recognized guideline by the NHLBI. James and colleagues (2014; panel members appointed to the Eighth Joint National Committee [JNC 8]) released 2014 Evidence-Based Guideline for the Management of High Blood Pressure in Adults, but the guideline is not affiliated with NHLBI or any other organization. In January of 2014, the American Society of Hypertension and the International Society of Hypertension released clinical practice guidelines for the management of hypertension in the community (Weber et al., 2014). The JNC 7 and the most recent guidelines by the American and International Societies of Hypertension (Weber et al., 2014) are presented as an example later in this section.

History of the Development of Evidence-Based Guidelines

Since the 1980s, the Agency for Healthcare Research and Quality (AHRQ) has had a major role in identifying health topics and developing evidence-based guidelines for these topics (http://www.ahrq.gov). In the late 1980s and early 1990s, panels or teams of experts were often charged with developing clinical guidelines for the AHRQ. The AHRQ solicited the members of the panel, who usually included nationally recognized researchers in the topic area, expert clinicians (such as physicians, nurses, pharmacists, and social workers), healthcare administrators, policy developers, economists, government representatives, and consumers. The group designated the scope of the guideline and conducted extensive reviews of the literature, including relevant systematic reviews, meta-analyses, meta-syntheses, mixed-methods systematic reviews, individual studies, and theories.

The best research evidence available was synthesized to develop recommendations for practice. The guidelines were examined for their usefulness in clinical practice, impact on health policy, and cost-effectiveness. Consultants, other researchers, and additional expert clinicians often were asked to review the guidelines and provide input. Based on the experts' critique, the AHRQ revised and packaged the guidelines for distribution to healthcare professionals. Some of the first guidelines focused on the following healthcare problems: (1) acute pain management in infants, children, and adolescents; (2) prediction and prevention of pressure ulcers in adults; (3) urinary incontinence in adults; (4) management of functional impairments with cataracts; (5) detection, diagnosis, and treatment of depression; (6) screening, diagnosis, management, and counseling about sickle cell disease; (7) management of cancer pain; (8) diagnosis and treatment of heart failure; (9) low back problems; and (10) otitis media diagnosis and management in children.

National Guideline Clearinghouse Resources

At the present time, standardized guideline development ranges from a structured process such as the one just discussed to a less structured process in which a guideline might be developed by a healthcare organization, healthcare plan, or professional organization. The AHRQ initiated the National Guideline Clearinghouse (NGC; 2014b) in 1998 to store the evidence-based practice guidelines. Initially, the NGC had 200 guidelines, but now the collection has expanded to thousands of clinical practice guidelines. The NGC is a publicly available database of evidence-based clinical practice guidelines and related documents. Free Internet access to these guidelines is available at http://www.guideline.gov. The NGC is updated weekly with new content that the AHRQ produces in partnership with the American Medical Association and America's Health Insurance Plans. The key components of the NGC and its user-friendly resources can be found on the AHRQ website (http://www.guideline.gov/index.aspx). Some of the critical information on the NGC is provided here to show you what is available and how to access the NGC resources:

- Structured abstracts (summaries) about the guideline and its development
- Links to full-text guidelines, where available, and/or ordering information for print copies
- Downloads of the complete NGC summary for all guidelines represented in the database
- A guideline comparison utility that gives users the ability to generate side-by-side comparisons for any combination of two or more guidelines
- Unique guideline comparisons, called *Guideline Syntheses*

These are prepared by NGC staff and compare guidelines covering similar topics, highlighting areas of similarities and differences. NGC Guideline Syntheses often provide a comparison of guidelines developed in different countries, providing insight into commonalities and differences in international health practices.

- An electronic forum, NGC-L, for exchanging information on clinical practice guidelines, their development, implementation, and use
- An annotated bibliography database in which users can search for citations for publications and resources about guidelines, including guideline development and methodology, structure, evaluation, and implementation

Other features include the following (NGC, 2014a; http://www.guideline.gov/browse/by-topic.aspx):

- *What's New* enables users to see what guidelines have been added each week and includes an index of all guidelines in NGC.
- *NGC Update Service* is a weekly electronic mailing of new and updated guidelines posted to the NGC website.
- *Detailed Search* enables users to create very specific search queries based on the various attributes found in the *NGC Classification Scheme.*
- *NGC Browse* permits users to scan for guidelines available on the NGC site by disease or condition, treatment or intervention, or developing organization.
- Full-text guidelines and/or companion documents are available through the guideline developer and can be downloaded.
- The *Glossary* provides definitions of terms used in the standardized abstracts (summaries).

The NGC provides varied audiences with an easy to use mechanism for obtaining objective, detailed information on clinical practice guidelines. The NGC (2014a) also provides a list of the guidelines that are in the process of being developed. In addition to the evidence-based guidelines, the AHRQ has developed many tools to assess the quality of care provided by the evidence-based guidelines. You can search the AHRQ (2013) website (http://www.qualitymeasures.ahrq.gov) for an appropriate tool to measure a variable in a research project or evaluate outcomes of care in a clinical agency.

Numerous professional organizations, healthcare agencies, universities, and other groups provide evidence-based guidelines for practice, which can be found on the following websites:

- Academic Center for Evidence-Based Nursing—http://www.acestar.uthscsa.edu
- Association of Women's Health, Obstetric, and Neonatal Nurse—http://awhonn.org
- Centers for Health Evidence—http://www.cche.net
- Guidelines Advisory Committee—http://www.gacguidelines.ca
- Guidelines International Network—http://www.g-i-n.net

- HerbMed, Evidence-Based Herbal Database, 1998, Alternative Medicine Foundation—http://www.herbmed.org
- MD Consult—http://www.mdconsult.com/php/286943359-1063/homepage
- National Association of Neonatal Nurses—http://www.nann.org
- National Institute for Clinical Excellence (NICE)—http://www.nice.org.uk/catcg2.asp?c=20034
- Oncology Nursing Society—http://www.ons.org
- U.S. Preventive Services Task Force—http://www.uspreventiveservicestaskforce.org/about.htm

Implementing Evidence-Based Guidelines for Management of Hypertension in Practice

Evidence-based guidelines have become the standards for providing care to patients in the United States and other countries. A few nurses have participated in committees that have developed these evidence-based guidelines, and many nurses are using these guidelines in their practices. An evidence-based guideline for the assessment, diagnosis, and management of high blood pressure is provided as an example. This guideline was developed from the JNC 7 report that was published in the *Journal of the American Medical Association* (Chobanian et al., 2003). The NIH, Department of Health and Human Services, and National Heart, Lung, and Blood Institute (NHLBI) developed educational materials to present the specifics of this guideline to promote its use by healthcare providers. This guideline is presented in Figure 13-8; it provides clinicians with direction for the following: (1) classification of blood pressure as normal, prehypertension, and HTN stages 1 and 2; (2) conduct of a diagnostic workup of HTN; (3) assessment of the major cardiovascular disease risk factors; (4) assessment of the identification of causes of HTN; and (5) treatment of HTN. The American Society of Hypertension and the International Society of Hypertension guidelines include the same classification of HTN—prehypertension, stage 1 hypertension, and stage 2 hypertension (Weber et al., 2014).

Algorithms or clinical decision trees provide direction for the selection of the most appropriate treatment methods for each patient with an illness or disease. Figure 13-8 includes an algorithm for managing patients diagnosed with HTN (NHLBI, 2003). In their international HTN guidelines, Weber and colleagues (2014) provided a more detailed algorithm for the management of HTN (Figure 13-9). This algorithm includes starting with lifestyle changes like the JNC 7 algorithm. However, Weber and colleagues provide direction for management of HTN in both Black and non-Black patients. Starting drug therapy for special cases (patients with kidney disease, diabetes, coronary disease, stroke history, and heart failure) are presented in the algorithm and detailed in the discussion of the guidelines. This algorithm can assist nurses and physicians in implementing the best treatment plans for patients of different cultures, ages, and chronic illnesses (see Figure 13-9).

RNs and students need to assess the usefulness and quality of each evidence-based guideline before they implement it in their practice. Figure 13-10 presents the Grove Model for Implementing Evidence-Based Guidelines in Practice. In this model, nurses identify a practice problem, search for the best research evidence to manage the problem in their practice, and note that an evidence-based guideline has been developed. The quality and usefulness of the guideline must be assessed by the nurse before it is used in practice, which involves examining the following: (1) authors of the guideline; (2) significance of the healthcare problem; (3) strength of the research evidence; (4) link to national standards; and (5) cost-effectiveness of using the guideline in practice. The quality of the JNC 7 guideline is examined as an example using the four criteria identified in the Grove model (see Figure 13-10). The authors of the JNC 7 guideline were expert researchers,

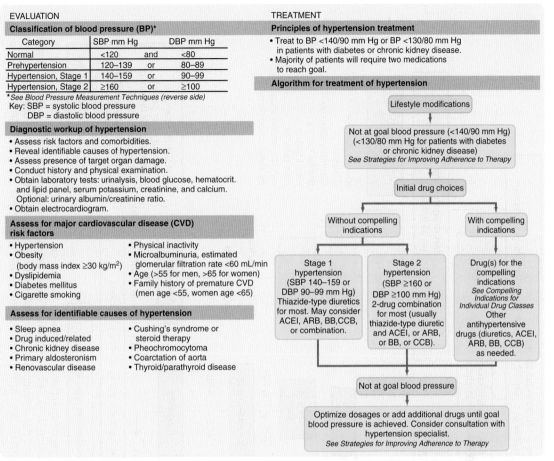

EVALUATION

Classification of blood pressure (BP)*

Category	SBP mm Hg		DBP mm Hg
Normal	<120	and	<80
Prehypertension	120–139	or	80–89
Hypertension, Stage 1	140–159	or	90–99
Hypertension, Stage 2	≥160	or	≥100

*See Blood Pressure Measurement Techniques (reverse side)
Key: SBP = systolic blood pressure
DBP = diastolic blood pressure

Diagnostic workup of hypertension

- Assess risk factors and comorbidities.
- Reveal identifiable causes of hypertension.
- Assess presence of target organ damage.
- Conduct history and physical examination.
- Obtain laboratory tests: urinalysis, blood glucose, hematocrit. and lipid panel, serum potassium, creatinine, and calcium. Optional: urinary albumin/creatinine ratio.
- Obtain electrocardiogram.

Assess for major cardiovascular disease (CVD) risk factors

- Hypertension
- Obesity (body mass index ≥30 kg/m²)
- Dyslipidemia
- Diabetes mellitus
- Cigarette smoking
- Physical inactivity
- Microalbuminuria, estimated glomerular filtration rate <60 mL/min
- Age (>55 for men, >65 for women)
- Family history of premature CVD (men age <55, women age <65)

Assess for identifiable causes of hypertension

- Sleep apnea
- Drug induced/related
- Chronic kidney disease
- Primary aldosteronism
- Renovascular disease
- Cushing's syndrome or steroid therapy
- Pheochromocytoma
- Coarctation of aorta
- Thyroid/parathyroid disease

TREATMENT

Principles of hypertension treatment

- Treat to BP <140/90 mm Hg or BP <130/80 mm Hg in patients with diabetes or chronic kidney disease.
- Majority of patients will require two medications to reach goal.

Algorithm for treatment of hypertension

Lifestyle modifications

Not at goal blood pressure (<140/90 mm Hg) (<130/80 mm Hg for patients with diabetes or chronic kidney disease) *See Strategies for Improving Adherence to Therapy*

Initial drug choices

Without compelling indications

With compelling indications

Stage 1 hypertension (SBP 140–159 or DBP 90–99 mm Hg) Thiazide-type diuretics for most. May consider ACEI, ARB, BB,CCB, or combination.

Stage 2 hypertension (SBP ≥160 or DBP ≥100 mm Hg) 2-drug combination for most (usually thiazide-type diuretic and ACEI, or ARB, or BB, or CCB).

Drug(s) for the compelling indications *See Compelling Indications for Individual Drug Classes* Other antihypertensive drugs (diuretics, ACEI, ARB, BB, CCB) as needed.

Not at goal blood pressure

Optimize dosages or add additional drugs until goal blood pressure is achieved. Consider consultation with hypertension specialist. *See Strategies for Improving Adherence to Therapy*

FIG 13-8 Reference card from the Seventh Report of the Joint National Committee on Prevention, Detection, Evaluation, and Treatment of High Blood Pressure [JNC 7]. (From U.S. Department of Health and Human Services, National Institutes of Health, National Heart, Lung, and Blood Institute. (2003). *Reference card from the Seventh Report of the Joint National Committee on Prevention, Detection, Evaluation, and Treatment of High Blood Pressure.* Bethesda, MD: NIH Publication No. 03-5231. Retrieved August 3, 2009, from www.nhlbi.nih.gov/guidelines/hypertension/jnc7card.htm.)

clinicians (physicians), policy developers, healthcare administrators, and the National High Blood Pressure Education Program Coordinating Committee. These authors have the expertise to develop an evidence-based guideline for HTN.

> "Hypertension is a significant healthcare problem because it affects approximately 50 million individuals in the United States and approximately 1 billion individuals worldwide. . . . Hypertension is the most common primary diagnosis in the United States with 35 million office visits as the primary diagnosis. . . . Recent clinical trials have demonstrated that effective BP [blood pressure] control can be achieved in most patients with hypertension, but the majority will require 2 or more antihypertensive drugs."

> *Chobanian et al., 2003, p. 2562*

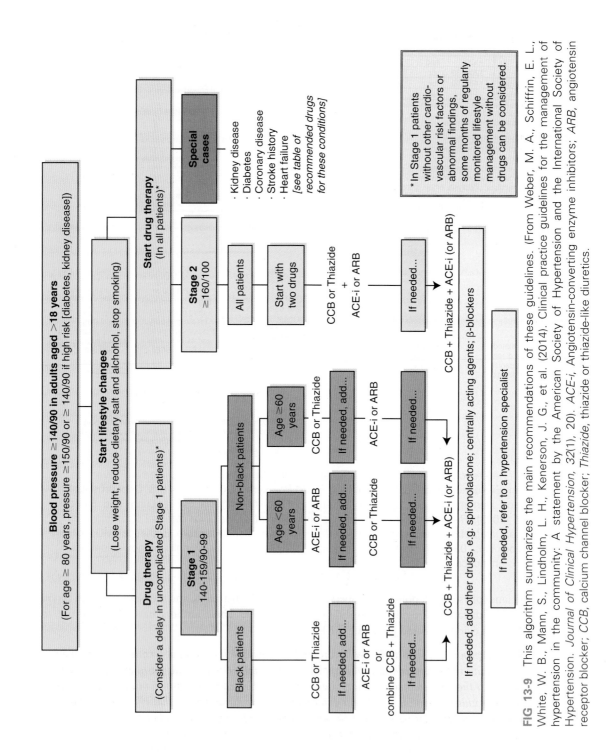

FIG 13-9 This algorithm summarizes the main recommendations of these guidelines. (From Weber, M. A., Schiffrin, E. L., White, W. B., Mann, S., Lindholm, L. H., Kenerson, J. G., et al. (2014). Clinical practice guidelines for the management of hypertension in the community: A statement by the American Society of Hypertension and the International Society of Hypertension. *Journal of Clinical Hypertension, 32*(1), 20). *ACE-i,* Angiotensin-converting enzyme inhibitors; *ARB,* angiotensin receptor blocker; *CCB,* calcium channel blocker; *Thiazide,* thiazide or thiazide-like diuretics.

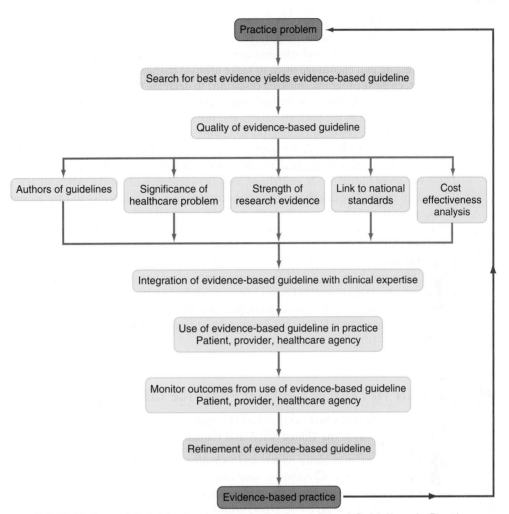

FIG 13-10 Grove Model for Implementing Evidence-Based Guidelines in Practice.

The research evidence for the development of the JNC 7 guideline was extremely strong. The JNC 7 report included 81 references; 9 (11%) of the references were meta-analyses and 35 (43%) were RCTs; 44 (54%) sources are considered extremely strong research evidence. The other references were strong and included retrospective analyses or case-controlled studies, prospective or cohort studies, cross-sectional surveys or prevalence studies, and clinical intervention studies (Nonrandom; Chobanian et al., 2003). The JNC 7 provides the national standard for the assessment, diagnosis, and treatment of HTN. The recommendations from the JNC 7 are supported by the U.S. Department of Health and Human Services and disseminated through NIH publication No. 03-5231. Use of the JNC 7 guideline in practice is cost-effective because the clinical trials have shown that "antihypertensive therapy has been associated with 35% to 40% mean reductions in stroke incidence; 20% to 25% in myocardial infarction [MI]; and more than 50% in HF [heart failure]" (Chobanian et al., 2003, p. 2562).

The next step is for nurses and physicians to use the JNC 7 guideline in their practice to classify patients' blood pressures and assess their major cardiovascular disease (CVD) risk factors (see Figure 13-8). Nurses and students can use this information to educate patients about their blood pressure and encourage them to make lifestyle changes (e.g., weight loss, no added salt in their diet, exercise program, smoking cessation) to decrease their CVD risks. Nurses also need to examine the outcomes for the patient, nurse, physician, and healthcare agency. The outcomes would be recorded in the patients' charts and possibly in a database (because of the implementation of EHRs) and would include the following: (1) blood pressure readings for patients; (2) incidence of diagnosis of HTN based on the JNC 7 or international HTN guidelines (Weber et al., 2014); (3) appropriateness of the treatments implemented to manage HTN based on JNC7 or international HTN guidelines; and (4) incidence of stroke, MI, and HF over 5, 10, 15, and 20 years. The healthcare agency outcomes include the access to care by patients with HTN, patient satisfaction with care, and the cost related to diagnosis and treatment of HTN and the complications of stroke, MI, and HF. EBP guidelines are refined in the future based on clinical outcomes, outcome studies, and new RCTs and meta-analyses. The JNC 7 guidelines are currently under revision but the guidelines proposed by James and colleagues (2014) have not been approved by government or professional organizations. Currently the JNC 7 and the international HTN guidelines published by Weber and colleagues (2014) provide the most relevant evidence-based guidelines for the management of HTN in adults. The use of these evidence-based HTN guidelines and additional guidelines promote an EBP for nurses (see Figure 13-10).

INTRODUCTION TO EVIDENCE-BASED PRACTICE CENTERS

In 1997, the AHRQ launched its initiative to promote EBP by establishing 12 evidence-based practice centers (EPCs) in the United States and Canada.

> *"The EPCs develop evidence reports and technology assessments on topics relevant to clinical, social science/behavioral, economic, and other healthcare organization and delivery issues—specifically those that are common, expensive, and/or significant for the Medicare and Medicaid populations. With this program, AHRQ became a 'science partner' with private and public organizations in their efforts to improve the quality, effectiveness, and appropriateness of health care by synthesizing the evidence and facilitating the translation of evidence-based research findings. Topics are nominated by non-federal partners such as professional societies, health plans, insurers, employers, and patient groups."*
>
> *AHRQ, 2012; http://www.ahrq.gov/clinic/epc*

Under the EPC program, the AHRQ awards 5-year contracts to institutions to serve as EPCs. EPCs review all relevant scientific literature on clinical, behavioral, organizational, and financial topics to produce evidence reports and technology assessments. These reports are used to inform and develop coverage decisions, quality measures, educational materials, tools, guidelines, and research agendas. The EPCs also conduct research on the methodology of systematic reviews.

The AHRQ (2012) website (http://www.ahrq.gov/clinic/epc) provides the names of the EPCs and the focus of each center. This site also provides a link to the evidence-based reports produced by these centers. These EPCs have had an important role in the development of evidence-based guidelines since the 1990s and will continue to make significant contributions to EBP in the future.

INTRODUCTION TO TRANSLATIONAL RESEARCH

Some barriers to EBP have resulted in the development of a new type of research to improve the translation of research knowledge to practice. This new research methodology, termed *transitional research,* is being supported by the NIH (2012). Translational research is an evolving concept defined by the NIH as the translation of basic scientific discoveries into practical applications. Basic research discoveries from the laboratory setting need to be tested in human studies. Also, the outcomes from human clinical trials need to be adopted and maintained in clinical practice. Translational research is being encouraged by medicine and nursing to increase the implementation of evidence-based interventions in practice and determine if these interventions are effective in producing the outcomes desired in clinical practice (Chesla, 2008; NIH, 2012). Translational research was originally part of the National Center for Research Resources. However, in December 2011, the National Center for Advancing Translation Sciences (NCATS) was developed as part of the NIH institutes and centers (NIH, 2012).

The NIH wanted to encourage researchers to conduct translational research and developed the Clinical and Translational Science Awards (CTSA) consortium in October 2006. The consortium started with 12 centers located throughout the United States and expanded to 39 centers in April 2009. The program was fully implemented in 2012, with about 60 institutions involved in clinical and translational science.

The CTSA consortium is mainly focused on expanding the translation of medical research to practice. Titler (2004, p. S1) defined transitional research for the nursing profession as the "Scientific investigation of methods, interventions, and variables that influence adoption of evidence-based practices (EBPs) by individuals and organizations to improve clinical and operational decision making in health care. This includes testing the effect of interventions on promoting and sustaining the adoption of EBPs." Baumbusch and colleagues (2008) provided an agenda for translational research and developed a collaborative model for knowledge translation between research and practice in clinical settings. Callard, Rose, and Wykes (2012) identified four different phases of translational research and stressed the importance of including service users in these types of studies. As you search the literature for relevant research syntheses and studies, you will note that translation studies are being published in nursing. Whittemore and colleagues (2009) conducted a translation study to promote the transfer of a diabetic prevention program to primary care. These types of studies will assist you in translating research findings to your practice and determining the impact of EBP on patients' health. However, federal funding is needed to expand the conduct of transitional research in nursing.

We hope that the content in this chapter increases your understanding of EBP, critical appraisal of research syntheses, application of EBP models, and implementation of EBP guidelines. We encourage you to take an active role in moving nursing toward EBP that improves outcomes for patients, nurses, and healthcare agencies.

KEY CONCEPTS

- Evidence-based practice (EBP) is the conscientious integration of best research evidence with clinical expertise and patient values and needs in the delivery of quality, safe, cost-effective health care.
- Best research evidence is produced by the conduct and synthesis of numerous high-quality studies in a health-related area.

- There are benefits and barriers associated with EBP. The benefits of EBP are that the standards for hospital accreditation by The Joint Commission support EBP, as does the Magnet Hospital Program managed by the American Nurses' Credentialing Center.
- The Quality and Safety Education for Nurses (QSEN) Institute has identified competencies for prelicensure nurses to promote the use of evidence-based knowledge in practice.
- Guidelines are provided for critically appraising the research synthesis processes of systematic review, meta-analysis, meta-synthesis, and mixed-methods systematic review. These synthesis processes are used to determine the best research evidence in a selected area and quality of the research evidence available for practice.
- A systematic review is a structured, comprehensive synthesis of the research literature to determine the best research evidence available to address a healthcare question. A systematic review involves identifying, locating, appraising, and synthesizing quality research evidence for expert clinicians to use to promote EBP.
- A meta-analysis is conducted to pool the results from previous studies statistically into a single quantitative analysis that provides one of the highest levels of evidence about the effectiveness of an intervention.
- Meta-synthesis is defined as the systematic compilation and integration of qualitative study results to expand understanding and develop a unique interpretation of study findings in a selected area. The focus is on interpretation rather than on combining study results, as with quantitative research synthesis.
- Reviews that include syntheses of various quantitative, qualitative, and mixed-methods studies are referred to as mixed-methods systematic reviews in this text.
- The PICO format is described for generating a clinical question to guide the use of current research evidence in practice. Evidence-based guidelines are provided for administering IM injections to children, adolescents, and adults.
- Two models have been developed to promote EBP in nursing, the Stetler Model of Research Utilization to Facilitate EBP (Stetler, 2001) and the Iowa Model of EBP to Promote Quality of Care (Titler et al., 2001).
- The phases of the revised Stetler model are (I) preparation, (II) validation, (III) comparative evaluation/decision making, (IV) translation/application, and (V) evaluation.
- The Iowa model provides guidelines for implementing patient care based on the best research evidence and monitoring changes in practice to ensure quality care.
- The process for developing evidence-based guidelines is described, and an example of the guideline for assessment, diagnosis, and treatment of hypertension is provided.
- The Grove Model for Implementing Evidence-Based Guidelines in Practice is provided to assist nurses in determining the quality of evidence-based guidelines and the steps for using these guidelines in practice.
- An excellent source for evidence-based guidelines is the National Guideline Clearinghouse, initiated by the AHRQ in 1998.
- Evidence-based practice centers (EPCs), created by the AHRQ in 1997, have had an important role in the conduct of research, development of systematic reviews, and formulation of evidence-based guidelines in selected practice areas.
- Translational research is an evolving concept defined by the NIH as the translation of basic scientific discoveries into practical applications.

REFERENCES

Agency for Healthcare Research and Quality (AHRQ). (2012). *Evidence-based practice centers: Synthesizing scientific evidence to improve quality and effectiveness in health care.* Retrieved July 15, 2013, from, http://www.ahrq.gov/clinic/epc.

Agency for Healthcare Research and Quality (AHRQ). (2013). *National Quality Measures Clearinghouse (NQMC).* Retrieved July 15, 2013, from, http://qualitymeasures.ahrq.gov.

American Nurses Credentialing Center. (2014). *Find a magnet organization.* Silver Springs, MD: Author. Retrieved February 11, 2014, from, http://www.nursecredentialing.org/Magnet/FindaMagnetFacility.aspx.

Andrel, J. A., Keith, S. W., & Leiby, B. E. (2009). Meta-analysis: A brief introduction. *Clinical and Translational Science, 2*(5), 374–378.

Barnett-Page, E., & Thomas, J. (2009). Methods for the synthesis of qualitative research: A critical review. *BMC Medical Research Methodology, 9*(59). http://dx.doi.org/10.1186/147-2288-9-59.

Baumbusch, J. L., Kirkham, S. R., Khan, K. B., McDonald, H., Semeniuk, P., Tan, E., et al. (2008). Pursuing common agendas: A collaborative model for knowledge translation between research and practice in clinical settings. *Research in Nursing & Health, 31*(2), 130–140.

Benzies, K. M., Premji, S., Hayden, K. A., & Serrett, K. (2006). State-of-the-evidence reviews: Advantages and challenges of including grey literature. *Worldviews on Evidence-Based Nursing, 3*(2), 55–61.

Bettany-Saltikov, J. (2010a). Learning how to undertake a systematic review: Part 1. *Nursing Standard, 24*(50), 47–56.

Bettany-Saltikov, J. (2010b). Learning how to undertake a systematic review: Part 2. *Nursing Standard, 24*(51), 47–58.

Bolton, L. B., Donaldson, N. E., Rutledge, D. N., Bennett, C., & Brown, D. S. (2007). The impact of nursing interventions: Overview of effective interventions, outcomes, measures, and priorities for future research. *Medical Care Research and Review, 64*(Suppl. 2), 123S–143S.

Brown, S. J. (2014). *Evidence-based nursing: The research-practice connection* (3rd ed.). Sudbury, MA: Jones & Bartlett.

Butler, K. D. (2011). Nurse practitioners and evidence-based nursing practice. *Clinical Scholars Review, 4*(1), 53–57.

Callard, F., Rose, D., & Wykes, T. (2012). Close to the bench as well as the bedside: Involving service users in all phases of translational research. *Health Expectations, 15*(4), 389–400.

Chesla, C. A. (2008). Translational research: Essential contributions from interpretive nursing science. *Research in Nursing & Health, 31*(4), 381–390.

Chobanian, A. V., Bakris, G. L., Black, H. R., Cushman, W. C., Green, L. A., Izzo, J. L., et al. (2003). The Seventh Report of the Joint National Committee on Prevention, Detection, Evaluation, and Treatment of High Blood Pressure: The JNC 7 Report. *Journal of the American Medical Association, 289*(19), 2560–2572.

Choi, M., & Hector, M. (2012). Effectiveness of intervention programs in preventing falls: A systematic review of recent 10 years and meta-analysis. *Journal of the American Medical Directors Association, 13*(2), 188.e13–188.e21. http://dx.doi.org/10.1016/j.jamda.2011.04.022.

Cochrane Collaboration. (2014). *Cochrane reviews.* Retrieved February 11, 2014, from, http://www.cochrane.org/cochrane-reviews.

Cocoman, A., & Murray, J. (2008). Intramuscular injections: A review of best practice for mental health nurses. *Journal of Psychiatric and Mental Health Nursing, 15*(5), 424–434.

Conn, V. S. (2010). Depressive symptom outcomes of physical activity interventions: Meta-analysis findings. *Annals of Behavioral Medicine, 39*(2), 128–138.

Conn, V. S., & Rantz, M. J. (2003). Research methods: Managing primary study quality in meta-analyses. *Research in Nursing & Health, 26*(4), 322–333.

Conn, V. S., Valentine, J. C., Cooper, H. M., & Rantz, M. J. (2003). Methods: Grey literature in meta-analyses. *Nursing Research, 52*(4), 256–261.

Craig, J., & Smyth, R. (2012). *The evidence-based practice manual for nurses* (3rd ed.). Edinburgh, Scotland: Churchill Livingstone Elsevier.

Creswell, J. W. (2014). *Research design: Qualitative, quantitative and mixed methods approaches* (4th ed.). Thousand Oaks, CA: Sage.

Denieffe, S., & Gooney, M. (2011). A meta-synthesis of women's symptoms experience and breast cancer. *European Journal of Cancer Care, 20*(4), 424–435.

Doran, D. M. (2011). *Nursing sensitive outcomes: The state of the science* (2nd ed.). Sudbury, MA: Jones & Bartlett.

Eizenberg, M. M. (2010). Implementation of evidence-based nursing practice: Nurses' personal and professional factors? *Journal of Advanced Nursing, 67*(1), 33–42.

Fawcett, J., & Garity, J. (2009). *Evaluating research for evidence-based nursing practice.* Philadelphia: F. A. Davis.

Fernandez, R. S., & Tran, D. T. (2009). The meta-analysis graph: Clearing the haze. *Clinical Nurse Specialist CNS, 23*(2), 57–60.

Finfgeld-Connett, D. (2010). Generalizability and transferability of meta-synthesis research findings. *Journal of Advanced Nursing, 66*(2), 246–254.

Greenway, K. (2004). Using the ventrologluteal site for intramuscular injection. *Nursing Standard, 18*(25), 39–42.

Grove, S. K., Burns, N., & Gray, J. R. (2013). *The practice of nursing research: Appraisal, synthesis, and generation of evidence* (7th ed.). Philadelphia: Elsevier Saunders.

Harden, A., & Thomas, J. (2005). Methodological issues in combining diverse study types in systematic reviews. *International Journal of Social Research Methodology, 8*(3), 257–271.

Higgins, J. P., & Green, S. (2008). *Cochrane handbook for systematic reviews of interventions: Cochrane book series.* West Sussex, UK: The Cochrane Collaboration and John Wiley & Sons.

Hoare, Z., & Hoe, J. (2013). Understanding quantitative research: Part 2. *Nursing Standard, 27*(18), 48–55.

Hoe, J., & Hoare, Z. (2012). Understanding quantitative research: Part 1. *Nursing Standards, 27*(15–17), 52–57.

Horstman, P., & Fanning, M. (2010). Tips for writing magnet evidence. *Journal of Nursing Administration, 40*(1), 4–6.

Institute of Medicine. (2001). *Crossing the quality chasm: A new health system for the 21st century.* Washington, DC: National Academy Press.

James, P. A., Opari, S., Carter, B. L., Cushman, W. C., Dennison-Himmelfarb, C., Handler, J., et al. (2014). 2014 Evidence-based guideline for the management of high blood pressure in adults: Report from the panel members appointed to the Eighth Joint National Committee (JNC 8). *JAMA, 311*(5), 507–520.

Joanna Briggs Institute. (2014). *Welcome to the Joanna Briggs Institute: Home.* Retrieved February 11, 2014, from, http://www.joannabriggs.org/index.html.

Kent, B., & Fineout-Overholt, E. (2008). Using meta-synthesis to facilitate evidence-based practice. *Worldviews on Evidence-Based Nursing, 5*(3), 160–162.

Liberati, A., Altman, D. G., Tetzlaff, J., Mulrow, C., Gotzsche, P. C., Ioannidis, J. P., et al. (2009). The PRISMA Statement for reporting systematic reviews and meta-analyses of studies that evaluate healthcare interventions: Explanation and elaboration. *Annals of Internal Medicine, 151*(4), W-65–W-94.

Magnus, M. C., Ping, M., Shen, M. M., Bourgeois, J., & Magnus, J. H. (2011). Effectiveness of mammography screening in reducing breast cancer mortality in women aged 39-49 years: A meta-analysis. *Journal of Women's Health, 20*(6), 845–852.

Mantzoukas, S. (2009). The research evidence published in high impact nursing journals between 2000 and 2006: A quantitative content analysis. *International Journal of Nursing Studies, 46*(4), 479–489.

Melnyk, B. M., & Fineout-Overholt, E. (2011). *Evidence-based practice in nursing & healthcare: A guide to best practice* (2nd ed.). Philadelphia: Lippincott, Williams, & Wilkins.

Melnyk, B. M., Fineout-Overholt, E., Stillwell, S. B., & Williamson, K. M. (2010). The seven steps of evidence-based practice. *American Journal of Nursing, 110*(1), 51–53.

Moher, D., Liberati, A., Tetzlaff, J., Altman, D. G., & PRISMA Group. (2009). *Preferred Reporting Items for Systematic Reviews and Meta-Analyses: The PRISMA Statement.* Retrieved July 9, 2013 from, http://www.prisma-statement.org.

Moore, Z. (2012). Meta-analysis in context. *Journal of Clinical Nursing, 21*(19/20), 2798–2807.

National Guideline Clearinghouse (NGC). (2014a). *National Guideline Clearinghouse: Guidelines by topics.* Retrieved February 11, 2014, from, http://www.guideline.gov/browse/by-topic.aspx.

National Guideline Clearinghouse (NGC). (2014b). *National Guideline Clearinghouse: Home.* Retrieved February 11, 2014, from, http://www.guideline.gov/.

National Heart, Lung, and Blood Institute. (2003). *The Seventh Report of the Joint National Committee on Prevention, Detection, Evaluation, and Treatment of High Blood Pressure (JNC 7).* Bethesda, MD: National Institutes of Health. Retrieved July 9, 2013 from, www.nhlbi.nih.gov/guidelines/hypertension.

National Institutes of Health (NIH). (2012). *NIH: National Center for Translational Science.* Retrieved July 9, 2013 from, http://www.ncrr.nih.gov/clinical_research_resources/clinical_and_translational_science_awards/index.asp.

Nicoll, L. H., & Hesby, A. (2002). Intramuscular injection: An integrative research review and guideline for evidence-based practice. *Applied Nursing Research, 16*(2), 149–162.

Nurse Executive Center. (2005). *Evidence-based nursing practice: Instilling rigor into clinical practice.* Washington, DC: Advisory Board Company.

Quality and Safety Education for Nurses (QSEN). (2013). *Pre-licensure knowledge, skills, and attitudes (KSAs).* Retrieved February 11, 2014, from, http://qsen.org/competencies/pre-licensure-ksas.

Rew, L. (2011). The systematic review of literature: Synthesizing evidence for practice. *Journal for Specialists in Pediatric Nursing, 16*(1), 64–69.

Sackett, D. L., Straus, S. E., Richardson, W. S., Rosenberg, W., & Haynes, R. B. (2000). *Evidence-based medicine: How to practice & teach EBM* (2nd ed.). London: Churchill Livingstone.

Sandelowski, M., & Barroso, J. (2007). *Handbook for synthesizing qualitative research.* New York: Springer.

Schumacher, B., Askew, M., & Otten, K. (2013). Development of a pressure ulcer trigger tool for the neonatal population. *Journal of Wound, Ostomy, and Continence Nursing, 40*(1), 46–50.

Sherwood, G., & Barnsteiner, J. (2012). *Quality and safety in nursing: A competency approach to improving outcomes.* Ames, IA: Wiley-Blackwell.

Stetler, C. B. (2001). Updating the Stetler Model of Research Utilization to facilitate evidence-based practice. *Nursing Outlook, 49*(6), 272–279.

Stetler, C. B., & Marram, G. (1976). Evaluating research findings for applicability in practice. *Nursing Outlook, 24*(9), 559–563.

Straka, K. L., Brandt, P., & Brytus, J. (2013). Brief report: Creating a culture of evidence-based practice and nursing research in a pediatric hospital. *Journal of Pediatric Nursing, 28*(4), 374–378.

The Joint Commission. (2014). *About our standards.* Retrieved February 11, 2014, from, http://www. jointcommission.org/standards_information/standards.aspx.

Titler, M. G. (2004). Overview of the U.S. invitational conference "Advancing Quality Care Through Translation Research." *Worldviews on Evidence-Based Nursing, 1*(1), S1–S5.

Titler, M. G., Kleiber, C., Steelman, V. J., Rakel, B. A., Budreau, G., Everett, L. Q., et al. (1994). Research-based practice to promote the quality of care. *Nursing Research, 43*(5), 307–313.

Titler, M. G., Kleiber, C., Steelman, V. J., Rakel, B. A., Budreau, G., Everett, L. Q., et al. (2001). The Iowa Model of Evidence-Based Practice to promote quality care. *Critical Care Nursing Clinics of North America, 13*(4), 497–509.

Turlik, M. (2010). Evaluating the results of a systematic review/meta-analysis. *Podiatry Management,* Retrieved from, www.podiatrym.com.

Walsh, D., & Downe, S. (2005). Meta-synthesis method for qualitative research: A literature review. *Journal of Advanced Nursing, 50*(2), 204–211.

Weber, M. A., Schiffrin, E. L., White, W. B., Mann, S., Lindholm, L. H., Kenerson, J. G., et al. (2014). Clinical practice guidelines for the management of hypertension in the community: A statement by the American Society of Hypertension and the International Society of Hypertension. *Journal of Clinical Hypertension, 16*(1), 14–26.

Whittemore, R., Melkus, G., Wagner, J., Dziura, J., Northrup, V., & Grey, M. (2009). Translating the diabetes prevention program to primary care: A pilot study. *Nursing Research, 58*(1), 2–12.

Wulff, K., Cummings, G. G., Marck, P., & Yurtseven, O. (2011). Medication administration technologies and patient safety: A mixed-method systematic review. *Journal of Advanced Nursing, 67*(10), 2080–2085.

CHAPTER 14

Outcomes Research

Diane Doran, RN, PhD, FCAHS

CHAPTER OVERVIEW

LEARNING OUTCOMES

After completing this chapter, you should be able to:

1. Explain the theoretical basis of outcomes research.
2. Discuss the history of outcomes research in nursing.
3. Describe the role of outcomes research in determining the effect of nursing on health outcomes.
4. Differentiate outcomes research from other types of research conducted by nurses.
5. Identify the methodologies used in published outcomes studies.
6. Critically appraise published outcomes studies.

KEY TERMS

Outcomes research, now an established field of health research, focuses on the end results of patient care. More specifically, outcomes research is concerned with the effectiveness of healthcare interventions and health services (Doran, 2011; Jefford, Stockler, & Tattersall, 2003). In the context of nursing, it focuses on how a patient's health status changes as a result of the nursing care received or the nursing services delivered. The Agency for Healthcare Research and Quality (AHRQ) suggests that "outcomes research seeks to understand the end results of particular healthcare practices and interventions. End results include effects that people experience and care about, such as change in the ability to function. In particular, for individuals with chronic conditions, where cure is not always possible, end results include quality of life as well as mortality. By linking the care people receive to the outcomes they experience, outcomes research has become the key to developing better ways to monitor and improve quality of care" (AHRQ, 2013).

The momentum propelling outcomes research comes primarily from policy makers, insurers, and the public. In these times of economic efficiency in the public health sector, there is a growing demand for data that justify the interventions and the costs of care and for systems of care that demonstrate improved patient outcomes. In that regard, nursing-sensitive outcomes have become an issue of increasing interest because of national concerns related to the quality of patient care. The interest in research on outcomes is clearly relevant to the nursing profession. Because nurses are at the forefront of care delivery, the demand for professional accountability regarding patient outcomes dictates that we can identify and document outcomes influenced by our care.

This chapter addresses the theoretical basis of outcomes research, provides a brief history of the emerging endeavors to examine outcomes, explains the importance of outcomes research designed to examine nursing practice, and highlights methodologies used in outcomes research. The chapter concludes with an introduction to guidelines that might be used to critically appraise outcomes studies. The movement to outcomes research and the approaches described in this chapter are a worldwide phenomenon.

Outcomes research differs significantly from the other types of research addressed in this text. It is a more complex study. Its designs are different, and the researchers engaged in it are often from a mix of disciplines, such as economics and public health, as well as from nursing. The studies use a unique theoretical framework to focus on health outcomes. In keeping with the interprofessional perspective of outcomes research, a broad base of literature from a variety of disciplines was used to develop the content for this chapter.

THEORETICAL BASIS OF OUTCOMES RESEARCH

The theorist Avedis Donabedian (1976, 1978, 1980, 1982, 1987) proposed a theory of quality health care and provided a process for evaluating it. Donabedian's theory still dominates outcomes research. Other theories of outcomes have since been developed, but we will limit our discussion to Donabedian's theory. Although quality is the overriding construct of Donabedian's theory, he never actually defined this concept himself (Mark, 1995). The World Health Organization (WHO; 2009, p. 13) defined quality of care as the "degree to which health services for individuals and populations increase the likelihood of desired health outcomes and are consistent with current professional knowledge."

Donabedian (1987) represented the key concepts and relationships in his theory using a cube. The cube shown in Figure 14-1 helps explain the elements of quality health care. The three dimensions of the cube are health, the subjects of care, and the providers of care. The cube also incorporates three of the many aspects of health—physical-psychological function, psychological function, and social function. Donabedian (1987, p. 4) proposed that "the manner in which we conceive of health, and of our responsibility for it, makes a fundamental difference to the concept of quality and, as a result, to the methods that we use to assess and assure the quality of care."

Loegering, Reiter, and Gambone (1994) modified Donabedian's levels to include the patient, patient's family, and community as providers as well as recipients of care. They suggest that access to care is one dimension of the provision of care by the community. Figure 14-2 illustrates their modifications.

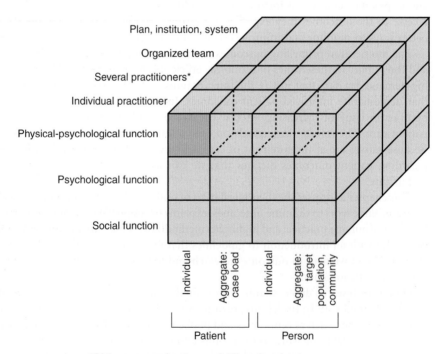

*Of the same profession or of different professions

FIG 14-1 Level and scope of concern as factors in the definition of quality. (From Donabedian, A. (1987). Some basic issues in evaluating the quality of health care. In L. T. Rinke (Ed.), *Outcome measures in home care: Vol. 1* (pp. 3–28). New York: National League of Nursing.)

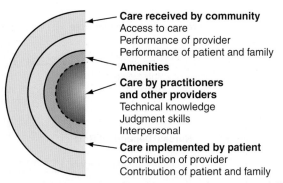

Care received by community
Access to care
Performance of provider
Performance of patient and family
Amenities
Care by practitioners
and other providers
Technical knowledge
Judgment skills
Interpersonal
Care implemented by patient
Contribution of provider
Contribution of patient and family

FIG 14-2 Various levels at which the quality of health care can be assessed. (From Donabedian, A. (1988). The quality of care: How can it be assessed? *Journal of the American Medical Association, 260*(12), 1744–1748.)

Donabedian (1987, 2005) identified three foci of evaluation in appraising quality—structure (e.g., nursing units, hospitals, home health agencies), process (of how care is provided, such as a practice style or standard of care), and outcomes (end results of care). Each of these constructs is addressed in this chapter. A complete quality assessment program requires the simultaneous inclusion of all three and an examination of the relationships among them. However, researchers have had little success in accomplishing this theoretical goal. Studies designed to examine all three constructs would require sufficiently large samples of various structures, each with the various processes being compared and large samples of subjects who have experienced the outcomes of those processes. The funding required and cooperation necessary to accomplish this goal have not yet been realized; however, there are examples of nursing research in which two or more aspects have been evaluated. Numerous studies conducted by nurses in the United States (Aiken, Clarke, Sloane, Lake, & Cheney, 2008; Kutney-Lee, Sloane, & Aiken, 2013; Stone, Mooney-Kane, Larson, Horan, Glance, Zwanziger, et al., 2007; Yoder, Xin, Norris, & Yan, 2013), Canada (Doran et al., 2006a, 2006b; Doran, Sidani, Keatings, & Doidge, 2002; McGillis Hall et al., 2003; Tourangeau, 2003; Tourangeau et al., 2007), and internationally (Bakker et al., 2011; Oh, Park, Jin, Piao, & Lee, 2013; Van den Heede, et al., 2009) have explored the relationships among nursing interventions, nursing services, and patient outcomes. Nursing interventions reflect the care delivered by nurses. A falls risk assessment or pressure ulcer risk assessment are examples of nursing interventions. Nursing services is a general concept referring to the organization and administration of nursing activities. Nursing service variables that have been studied include the skill mix and configuration of nursing personnel; staffing levels; assignment patterns (primary, functional, or team); shift patterns; levels of nursing education, experience, and expertise; ratios of full-time to part-time nurses; level and type of nursing leadership available centrally and on units; cohesion and communication among the nursing staff and between nurses and physicians; implementation of clinical care maps for patients with selected diagnoses; and the interrelationships of these factors.

NURSING-SENSITIVE OUTCOMES

Irvine, Sidani, and McGillis Hall (1998) adapted Donabedian's (1987) theory of quality in their development of the Nursing Role Effectiveness Model. The Nursing Role Effectiveness Model,

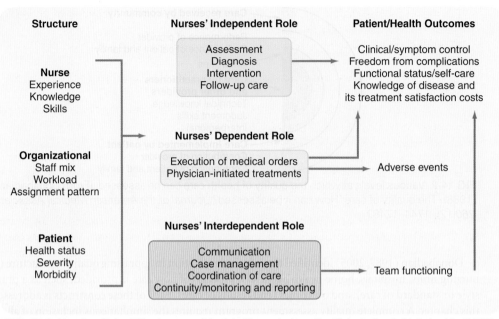

FIG 14-3 Nursing Role Effectiveness Model. (From Irvine, D., Sidani, S., & Hall, L. M. (1998). Linking outcomes to nurses' roles in health care. *Nursing Economics, 16*(2), 58–64.)

presented in Figure 14-3, was developed to guide conceptualization and research related to nursing-sensitive outcomes. It also provided the theoretical basis for a systematic review of the "state of the science on nursing-sensitive outcomes measurement" (Doran, 2011). The Nursing Role Effectiveness Model is based on Donabedian's (1987) quality framework and has three major components—structure, the nurses' role, and patient and health outcomes. Structure in outcomes has three subcomponents—nurse, organization, and patient. Nurse variables that influence the quality of nursing care include factors such as experience level, knowledge, and skill level. Organizational components that can affect the quality of nursing care include staff mix, workload, and assignment patterns. Patient characteristics that can affect the quality of care and outcomes include health status, severity, and morbidity. The nurse's role in outcomes has three subcomponents—nurse's independent role, nurse's dependent role, and nurse's interdependent role. Independent role functions include assessment, diagnosis, nurse-initiated interventions, and follow-up care. The patient and health outcomes of the independent role are clinical and symptom control, freedom from complications, functional status and self-care, knowledge of disease and its treatment, satisfaction, and costs. The dependent role functions include execution of medical orders and physician-initiated treatments. It is the dependent role functions that can lead to patient and health outcomes of adverse events. Interdependent role functions include communication, case management, coordination of care, and continuity, monitoring, and reporting. The interdependent role results in team functioning and affects the patient and health outcomes of the independent role. Patient and health outcomes are clearly interwoven into the entire care context. The propositions of the Nursing Role Effectiveness Model are as follows (Irvine et al., 1998, p. 62):

• Nursing's capacity to engage effectively in the independent, dependent, and interdependent role functions is influenced by individual nurse variables, patient variables, and organizational structure variables.

- The nurse's interdependent role function depends on the ability to communicate and articulate her or his opinion to other members of the healthcare team.
- Nurse, patient, and system structural variables have a direct effect on clinical, functional, satisfaction, and cost outcomes.
- The nurse's independent role function can have a direct effect on clinical, functional, satisfaction, and cost outcomes.
- Medication errors and other adverse events associated with the nurse's dependent role function can ultimately affect all categories of patient outcome.
- Nursing's interdependent role function can affect the quality of interprofessional communication and coordination, with the recognition that the nature of interprofessional communication and coordination can influence other important patient outcomes and costs, such as risk-adjusted length of stay, risk-adjusted mortality rates, excess home care costs following discharge, unplanned visits to the physician or emergency department, and unplanned rehospitalization.

The Nursing Role Effectiveness Model (see Figure 14-3) provided a framework for conceptualizing nursing-sensitive outcomes (Doran, 2011) and directed the selection of keywords that were used in the systematic review of the state of the science on nursing-sensitive outcomes measurement. The methodology and results of this systematic review are discussed next.

Conceptual and empirical research articles were included in the systematic review. Conceptual papers were included if they discussed the definition and domains of a patient outcome concept, or if they presented the results of a concept analysis designed to explicate the conceptual definition and dimensions of the outcome concept. Empirical papers were included if they described the development of an instrument to measure the outcome concept or evaluated the psychometric properties of the instrument. Papers that reported results of studies that examined the relationship among nursing structural variables, nursing interventions, and outcomes were included. The review focused on studies that were conducted in acute care, home care, primary care, and long-term care settings. For each empirical paper, the authors made note of the date of publication, study design (e.g., randomized controlled trial [RCT], case control, prospective cohort, or descriptive), setting, sample, response rate, and study limitations. This information was important for determining the generalizability of the study results to specific clinical contexts (i.e., external validity) and for determining threats to internal validity, such as response bias or the influence of confounding variables (see Chapter 8 for a discussion of types of design validity). A confounding variable is an extraneous variable whose presence affects the variables being studied so that the findings might not be an accurate reflection of reality. Researchers select study designs to reduce the effect of extraneous variables. The review also included information about the specific structural or nursing intervention variables and their relationships with the outcome variables examined.

One of the results of this systematic review was the identification of nurse-sensitive patient outcomes (Doran, 2011). A **nursing-sensitive patient outcome** (NSPO) is sensitive because it is influenced by nursing care decisions and actions. It may not be caused by nursing but is associated with nursing. In various situations, "nursing" might be the individual nurse, nurses as a working group, approach to nursing practice, nursing unit, or institution that determines the numbers of nurses, their salaries, educational levels of nurses, assignments of nurses, workload of nurses, management of nurses, and policies related to nurses and nursing practice. It might even include the architecture of the nursing unit. In whatever form, nursing actions have a role in the outcome, even though acts of other professionals, organizational acts, and patient characteristics and behaviors often are involved in the outcome. What patient outcomes can you think of that might be nursing-sensitive? Examples of nursing-sensitive outcomes from Doran and colleagues' review and their definitions are summarized in Table 14-1.

TABLE 14-1	NURSING-SENSITIVE PATIENT OUTCOMES AND DEFINITIONS
OUTCOME CONCEPT	**DEFINITION**
Functional status	Functional status is a multidimensional construct that consists of, at least, behavioral (e.g., performance of activities of daily living), psychological (e.g., mood), cognitive (e.g., attention, concentration), and social (e.g., activities associated with roles) components (Knight, 2000; Doran, 2011).
Self-care	Self-care behavior entails the practice of actions or activities that individuals initiate and perform, within time frames, on their own behalf in the interest of maintaining life, healthy functioning, continued personal development, and well-being (Jenerette & Murdaugh, 2008; Orem, 2001; Sidani, 2011a).
Symptoms	"Symptoms refer to (a) sensations or experiences reflecting changes in a person's biopsychosocial functions, (b) a patient's perception of an abnormal physical, emotional, or cognitive state, (c) the perceived indicators of change in normal functioning, as experienced by patients, or (d) subjective experience reflecting changes in the biopsychosocial functioning, sensations, or cognition of an individual" (Sidani, 2011b, p. 132).
Pain	Pain has been defined as "an unpleasant sensory and emotional experience associated with actual or potential tissue damage, or described in terms of such damage" (Merskey & Bogduk, 1994, p. 210).
Adverse outcome	An adverse outcome is defined as consequence of injury caused by medical management or complication rather than by the underlying disease itself, and generally includes prolonged health care, a resulting disability, or death at the time of discharge (WHO, 2009).
Psychological distress	Psychological distress has been defined as "the emotional condition that one feels in response to having to cope with situations that are unsettling, frustrating, or perceived as harmful or threatening" (Lazarus & Folman's work as cited in Howell, 2011, p. 289).
Patient satisfaction	"Patient satisfaction is frequently defined as the extent to which patients' expectations of care match the actual care received" (Spence Laschinger, Gilbert, & Smith, 2011, p. 362).
Mortality rate	Mortality, in its simplest meaning, reflects death. "When examining death as a quality-of-care outcome, rates of death are examined for specific patient samples or populations" (Tourangeau, 2011, p. 411).
Healthcare utilization	"Healthcare utilization can be thought of as the sum or aggregate of services consumed by patients in their attempts to maintain or regain a level of health status, along with the costs of these services" (Clarke, 2011, p. 441).

ORIGINS OF OUTCOMES AND PERFORMANCE MONITORING

Florence Nightingale has been credited as being the first nurse to collect data to identify nursing's contribution to quality care and conduct research into patient outcomes (Magnello, 2010; Montalvo, 2007). However, efforts to collect data systematically to assess outcomes in more modern times did not gain widespread attention in the United States until the late 1970s. At that time, concerns about quality of care prompted the development of the *Universal Minimum Health Data Set*, which was followed shortly thereafter by the *Uniform Hospital Discharge Data Set* (Kleib, Sales, Doran, Mallette, & White, 2011). These data sets facilitated consistency in data collection among healthcare organizations by prescribing the data elements to be gathered. The aggregated data were then used to perform an assessment of quality of care in hospitals and provide information on patients discharged from hospitals.

Over time, other countries developed similar data sets. In Canada, "Standards for Management Information Systems" (MIS) were developed in the 1980s. With the establishment of the Canadian Institute for Health Information (CIHI) in 1994, the MIS became a set of national standards used to collect and report financial and statistical data from health service organizations' daily operations (CIHI, 2012). Simultaneously, CIHI implemented a national Discharge Abstract Database (DAD), which has become a key resource in outcomes research. However, those data sets did not include information about nursing care delivered to patients in the hospital (Kleib et al., 2011). Without that information, the contribution of nursing care to patient, organizational, and system outcomes was rendered invisible. This major gap in information was addressed by the development of nursing minimum data sets in the United States, Canada, and other countries worldwide.

FEDERAL GOVERNMENT INVOLVEMENT IN OUTCOMES RESEARCH

There are now several national outcomes' initiatives in the United States and other countries focused on the development of methods for measuring and reporting patient health outcomes. We provide an overview on some of the national outcome initiatives in the United States, starting with the work of the AHRQ, and then focus specifically on examples of national nursing outcome initiatives. These initiatives are paving the way for outcomes research by building tools and methodologies for measuring patient outcomes and building large secondary databases that are sources for outcomes research.

Agency for Healthcare Research and Quality (AHRQ)

The AHRQ, as a part of the U.S. Department of Health and Human Services (DHHS), supports research designed to improve the outcomes and quality of health care, reduce healthcare costs, address patient safety and medical errors, and broaden access to effective services. The AHRQ website (http://www.ahrq.gov) is a valuable source of information about outcomes research, funding opportunities, and results of recently completed research, including nursing research. In 2010, the AHRQ was awarded $25 million in funding to support efforts by states and health systems to implement and evaluate patient safety approaches and medical liability reform models. In addition, AHRQ invested $17 million to expand projects to help prevent health care–associated infections (HAIs), the most common complication of hospital care. The AHRQ initiated several major research efforts to examine medical outcomes and improve quality of care. One of the most current initiatives is comparative effectiveness research, which is described in the next section.

American Recovery and Reinvestment Act

Funding from the American Recovery and Reinvestment Act (Recovery Act), signed into law in 2009, allowed AHRQ to expand its work in support of comparative effectiveness research, including enhancing the Effective Health Care Program. A total of $473 million was designated for funding patient-centered outcomes research (AHRQ, 2010). The AHRQ program provides patients, clinicians, and others with evidence-based information to make informed decisions about health care through activities such as comparative effectiveness reviews conducted through AHRQ's Evidence-Based Practice Center (EPC). The AHRQ has a broad research portfolio that involves almost every aspect of health care, including:
- Clinical practice
- Outcomes and effectiveness of care
- Evidence-based practice
- Primary care and care for priority populations
- Healthcare quality

- Patient safety and medical errors
- Organization and delivery of care and use of healthcare resources
- Healthcare costs and financing
- Health information technology
- Knowledge transfer

National Quality Forum

The National Quality Forum (NQF) was created in 1999 as a national standard-setting organization for healthcare performance measures (NQF, 2013a). The NQF portfolio of voluntary consensus standards includes performance measures, serious reportable events, and preferred practices (i.e., safe practices). A complete list of measures included in the NQF portfolio can be found online (http://www.qualityforum.org/Measures_Reports_Tools.aspx). Approximately one third of the measures in NQF's portfolio are measures of patient outcomes, such as mortality, readmissions, health functioning, depression, and experience of care. The NQF includes several nursing-sensitive measures in its performance measurement portfolio. Those that were submitted by the American Nurses Association (ANA) under the National Database of Nursing Quality Indicators (see later) include the following:

- Nursing staff skill mix
- Nursing hours per patient day
- Catheter-associated urinary tract infection (UTI) rate
- Central line–associated bloodstream infection rate
- Fall and injury rates
- Hospital- and unit-acquired pressure ulcer rates
- Nurse turnover rate
- RN practice environment scale
- Ventilator-associated pneumonia rate

These indicators are the first nationally standardized performance measures of nursing-sensitive outcomes in acute care hospitals and are designed to assess healthcare quality, patient safety, and a professional and safe work environment. Although most of the measures in use focus on the failure to meet expected standards, the NQF believes that quality is as much about influencing positive outcomes as about avoiding negative outcomes. Therefore, the NQF is currently developing national standards to evaluate the quality of health care based on how patients feel. It notes that "national quality assessment programs usually measure and reward practices based on improving clinical processes such as re-hospitalization or infection rates. While this type of information is important and useful to clinicians, it doesn't always take into account what is most important to the patient and families of the patient receiving care, such as the management of long-term symptoms or ability to conduct daily activities" (NQF, 2013b).

National Database of Nursing Quality Indicators

In 1994, the ANA, in collaboration with the American Academy of Nursing Expert Panel on Quality Health Care, launched a plan to identify indicators of quality nursing practice and collect and analyze data using these indicators throughout the United States (Mitchell, Ferketich, & Jennings, 1998). The goal was to identify and/or develop nursing-sensitive quality measures. Donabedian's theory was used as the framework for the project. Together, these indicators were referred to as the ANA Nursing Care Report Card, which could facilitate benchmarking or setting a desired standard that would allow comparisons of hospitals in terms of their nursing care quality.

In 1998, the ANA provided funding to develop a national database to house data collected using nursing-sensitive quality indicators. This became the National Database of Nursing Quality Indicators (NDNQI; Montalvo, 2007). Participation in NDNQI meets requirements for the Magnet Recognition Program, and 20% of database members participate for that reason (see Chapters 1 and 13 for a discussion of Magnet status). Detailed guidelines for data collection, including definitions and decision guides, are provided by the NDNQI (2013). The NDNQI nursing-sensitive indicators are summarized in Table 14-2.

TABLE 14-2 AMERICAN NURSES ASSOCIATION NATIONAL DATABASE OF NURSING QUALITY INDICATORS

INDICATOR	SUBINDICATOR	MEASURE
1. Nursing hours per patient day*,[†]	a. Registered nurse (RN) b. Licensed practical nurse, licensed vocational nurse (LPN, LVN) c. Unlicensed assistive personnel UAP)	Structure
2. Patient falls*,[†]		Process and outcome
3. Patient falls with injury*,[†]	a. Injury level	Process and outcome
4. Pediatric pain assessment, intervention, reassessment (AIR) cycle		Process
5. Pediatric peripheral intravenous infiltration rate		Outcome
6. Pressure ulcer prevalence	a. Community-acquired b. Hospital-acquired c. Unit-acquired	Process and outcome
7. Psychiatric physical and sexual assault rate		Outcome
8. Restraint prevalence[†]		Outcome
9. RN education/certification		Structure
10. RN satisfaction survey options*,[‡]	a. Job satisfaction scales b. Job satisfaction scales short form c. Practice environment scale (PES)[†]	Process and outcome
11. Skill mix: Percentage of total nursing hours supplied by ANA and NQF*,[†]	a. RN b. LPN, LVN c. UAP d. No. of total nursing hours supplied by agency staff (%)	Structure
12. Voluntary nurse turnover[†]		Structure
13. Nurse vacancy rate		Structure

14. Nosocomial infections
  a. Urinary catheter–associated urinary tract infection (UTI)[†]
  b. Central line catheter–associated bloodstream infection (CABSI)*,[†]
  c. Ventilator-associated pneumonia (VAP)[†]
		Outcome

*Original ANA nursing-sensitive indicator.
[†]NQF-endorsed nursing-sensitive indicator.
[‡]The RN survey is annual, whereas the other indicators are quarterly.

Other organizations currently involved in efforts to study nursing-sensitive outcomes include the Collaborative Alliance for Nursing Outcomes California Database (CALNOC, 2013a), Center for Medicare & Medicaid Services (CMS) Hospital Quality Initiative, American Hospital Association, the Federation of American Hospitals, The Joint Commission and, in Canada, the Canadian Nurses Association National Nursing Quality Report. For further information on these outcome initiatives, you can review Doran, Mildon, and Clarke's (2011) knowledge synthesis of the state of science on nursing outcomes measurement and international nursing report card initiatives. This knowledge synthesis was a review of nursing-sensitive outcome and report card initiatives in the United States, Canada, United Kingdom, and Belgium.

Oncology Nursing Society

The Oncology Nursing Society (ONS, 2012) is a professional organization of more than 35,000 RNs and other healthcare providers dedicated to excellence in patient care, education, research, and administration in oncology nursing. The ONS has taken a leadership role among specialty nursing organizations in developing an evidence-based practice (EBP) resource area on its website (http://www.ons.org/ClinicalResources). The site provides nurses with a guide to identify, critically appraise, and use evidence to solve clinical problems. The ONS website also assists nurses, in particular advanced practice nurses, who are helping others develop EBP protocols. The outcomes resource area is helpful to nurses for achieving desired outcomes for people with cancer by providing outcome measures, resource cards, and evidence tables.

ADVANCED PRACTICE NURSING OUTCOMES RESEARCH

Demonstrating the value of advanced practice nurses' (APNs) roles within the healthcare system has been the focus of much of the outcomes research in nursing, probably because advance practice roles are often under threat when healthcare organizations restructure under cost constraints or when new advanced practice roles are first introduced, as was the case with the nurse practitioner role. Therefore, we review some of the outcomes research related to advanced practice nursing in this next section.

The ANA recognizes four types of APNs—certified registered nurse anesthetists (CRNAs), certified nurse-midwives (CNMs), clinical nurse specialists (CNSs), and nurse practitioners (NPs). Studying APNs requires a determination of what happens during the process of APN care. This care involves a set of activities within, among, and between practitioners and patients and includes technical and interpersonal elements. The process of care is complex and somewhat mysterious. However, clearly describing what occurs during the process is essential to developing a comprehensive understanding of how APNs affect outcomes.

There is abundant research demonstrating the safety and effectiveness of APNs. DiCenso and colleagues (2010) conducted a search of all RCTs ever published, comparing APNs to usual care in terms of patient, provider, and/or health system outcomes. They found a total of 78 trials—28 of primary care NPs, 17 of acute care NPs, 32 of CNSs, and one of a combined CNS-NP role. Findings consistently showed that care by APNs resulted in equivalent or improved outcomes. Moore and McQuestion (2012) conducted a systematic review of the outcomes of the CNS role, focusing on chronic disease patient populations. Many of the studies showed that CNSs had a positive impact on patients living with chronic illnesses. Key outcomes included an improvement in quality of life, patient and health provider satisfaction, fewer and shorter rehospitalizations, and lower costs of care. Examples of outcomes that have been found to be sensitive to APN processes of care are summarized in Table 14-3.

TABLE 14-3   OUTCOMES ASSOCIATED WITH ADVANCED PRACTICE NURSES' PROCESSES OF CARE

OUTCOMES	EXAMPLES
Patient outcomes	Disease- or condition-specific outcomes, such as changes in signs of disease: • Physical symptoms • Psychosocial outcomes • Prevention of complications of treatment • Self-management • Patient satisfaction
Organizational outcomes Nursing outcomes	Unit or hospital length of stay—total healthcare costs Improvement in nursing knowledge and skills Enhancing nursing participation in continuing professional development Increasing nursing job satisfaction

From Doran, D. M., Sidani, S., & Di Pietro, T. (2010). Nursing-sensitive outcomes. In J. S. Fulton, B. Lyon, & K. Goudreau (Eds.), *Foundations of clinical nurse specialist practice* (pp. 35-37). New York: Springer.

OUTCOMES RESEARCH AND NURSING PRACTICE

Outcome studies provide rich opportunities to build a stronger scientific underpinning for nursing practice. Nurse researchers have been actively involved in the effort to examine the outcomes of patient care. Ideally, we would like to understand the outcomes of nursing practice within a one to one nurse-patient relationship; however, in most cases, the nursing effect is shared because more than one nurse cares for a patient. In addition, nurse managers and nurse administrators have control over the nursing staff and the environment of nursing practice, and this control affects the autonomy of the nurse to implement practice. Consequently, outcomes research must first focus on how nursing care is organized, rather than on what nurses do. When that occurs, we may begin to determine how what nurses do influences patient outcomes (Lake, 2006). In the next section of this chapter, we provide a description of approaches to evaluating outcomes, structural variables, and processes of care.

Evaluating Outcomes of Care

The goal of outcomes research is the evaluation of outcomes as defined by Donabedian; however, this goal is not as easily realized. Donabedian's (1987) theory requires that identified outcomes be clearly linked with the process that caused the outcome. Researchers need to define the process and justify the causal links with the selected outcomes. The identification of desirable outcomes of care requires dialogue between the recipients and providers of care. Although the providers of care may delineate what is achievable, the recipients of care must clarify what is desirable. A desirable outcome would address issues of specific concern to patients, such as long-term symptoms or ability to conduct activities of daily living. The outcomes must also be relevant to the goals of the health professionals, healthcare system of which the professionals are a part, and society.

Outcomes are time-dependent. Some outcomes may not be apparent for a long period after the process that is purported to have caused them, whereas others may be identified immediately. Some outcomes are temporary, and others are permanent. Therefore, an appropriate time frame must be established for determining the selected outcomes.

The second step is to evaluate the impact of various structural elements on the process of care and on outcomes. This evaluation requires a comparison of different structures that provide the same processes of care. In evaluating structures, the unit of measure is the structure. The evaluation requires access to a sufficiently large sample of "like" structures, with similar processes and outcomes, which can then be compared with a sample of another structure providing the same processes and examining the same outcomes. For example, in nursing research, nurses might want to compare various structures providing primary health care, such as the private physician office, health maintenance organization (HMO), rural health clinic, community-oriented primary care clinic, and nurse-managed center. Alternatively, nurse researchers might examine nursing care provided within the structures of a private outpatient surgical clinic, private hospital, county hospital, and teaching hospital associated with a health science center. In each of these examples, the focus of research would be the impact of structure on the processes and outcomes of care. Table 14-4 lists some current outcomes studies that have examined the impact of structure of care on patient outcomes.

In the United States, nursing homes, home healthcare agencies, and hospitals are required to collect specifically measured quality variables and to report them to the federal government. This mandate was established because of considerable variation in the quality of care in these structures. Various government agencies analyze the quality of these structures so that they can adequately oversee the quality of care provided to the U.S. public. These data are made available to the general public so that individuals can make their own determination of the quality of care provided by various nursing homes, home healthcare agencies, and hospitals. Researchers can also access these data for studies of the quality of various structures. To access these data on the Internet, you can search using the phrases "nursing home compare," "home health compare," and "hospital compare." In addition to being able to select a specific hospital, nursing home, or home healthcare agency, you can access considerable general information about quality related to each of these structures of health care.

Evaluating Process of Care

Clinical management has been an art rather than a science for most health professionals. Understanding the process sufficiently to study it must begin with careful reflection, dialogue, and observation. There are multiple components of clinical management, many of which have not yet been clearly defined or tested. Three components of process that are of particular interest to Donabedian (1982, 1987) are standards of care, practice styles, and costs of care. Standards of care and practice styles are included in the following sections but costs of care are discussed later in this chapter, with the methodologies of evaluation.

Standards of Care

A standard of care is a norm on which quality of care is judged. Clinical guidelines, critical paths, and care maps define standards of care for particular situations. In that regard, Donabedian (1987) recommended the development of specific criteria to be used as a basis for judging the quality of care. These criteria may take the form of clinical guidelines or care maps based on prior validation that the care contributed to the desired outcomes. The clinical guidelines published by the AHRQ (2011) established norms or standards against which the validity of clinical management can be judged. These norms are now established through clinical practice guidelines available through the National Guideline Clearinghouse (NGC) within the AHRQ (see http://www.guideline.gov). Chapter 13 provides a detailed discussion of the NGC and its resources.

Practice Styles, Practice Pattern, and Evidence-Based Practice

The style of a practitioner's practice is another dimension of the process of care that influences quality; however, it is problematic to judge what constitutes goodness in style and to justify the decisions made regarding it. Practice pattern is a concept closely related to practice style. Practice style represents variation in how care is provided, whereas practice pattern represents variation in what care is provided.

EBP is another dimension of the process of care that is considered a critical aspect of professional practice (Stetler & Caramanica, 2007). The ultimate goals of EBP are improved patient health status and quality of care (Graham, Bick, Tetroe, Strause, & Harrison, 2011). Therefore, the impact of EBP should be assessed through the measurement of patient outcomes. Very few empirical studies have assessed the impact of evidence-based nursing practice on patient outcomes. One of them, a study by Davies, Edwards, Ploeg, and Virani (2008), found that implementation of best practice guidelines in nursing resulted in improved outcomes in diverse settings, but there was considerable variability in the indicators evaluated, suggesting the need for more research in this area. Table 14-5 lists some outcomes studies that have examined the impact of process of care on patient outcomes.

METHODOLOGIES FOR OUTCOMES STUDIES

Outcomes research methodologies have been developed to link the care that people receive with the results they experience, thereby providing better ways to monitor and improve the quality of care (Clancy & Eisenberg. 1998). This section describes some of the current methodologies used in conducting outcomes research, including sampling methods, research strategies or designs, measurement processes, and statistical approaches. These descriptions are not sufficient to guide you in using the approaches described; rather, they provide a broad overview of the variety of methodologies you will see in outcomes studies. This knowledge will help you understand and critically appraise the methodologies used in published outcomes studies. For additional information, you can refer to the citations in each section and to other sources of outcomes research (Doran, 2011; Grove, Burns, & Gray, 2013). Outcomes studies cross a variety of disciplines; therefore, the emerging methodologies are being enriched by a cross-pollination of ideas, some of which are new to nursing research.

Samples and Sampling

The preferred methods of obtaining samples are different in outcomes studies. Random sampling is seldom used, with the exception of an RCT, when a specific intervention or healthcare service is being evaluated. Usually, heterogeneous samples (with varied types of patients), rather than homogeneous (with similar patients) samples, are obtained in outcomes research. Rather than using sampling criteria, which restrict subjects included in the study to decrease possible biases, reduce the variance, and increase the possibility of identifying a statistically significant difference, outcomes researchers seek large heterogeneous samples that reflect, as much as possible, all patients who would be receiving care in a real healthcare context. For example, samples need to include patients with various comorbidities and patients with varying levels of health status. In addition, individuals should be identified who do not receive treatment for their condition.

Devising ways to evaluate the representativeness of such samples is problematic. For a sample to be representative, it must be as much like the target population as possible, particularly in relation to the variables being studied. Because the target population in outcomes research is often heterogeneous, there are a large number of variables for which sample representativeness

TABLE 14-5	STUDIES INVESTIGATING THE RELATIONSHIP BETWEEN PROCESS VARIABLES AND OUTCOMES
YEAR	**STUDY**
2013	Effken, J.A., Gephart, S.M., Brewer, B.B., & Carley, K.M. (2013). Using ORA, a network analysis tool, to assess the relationship of handoffs to quality and safety outcomes. *CIN: Computers, Informatics, Nursing, 31*(1), 36-44.
2012	Rosted, E., Wagner, L, Hendriksen, C., & Poulsen, I. (2012). Geriatric nursing assessment and intervention in an emergency department: A pilot study. *International Journal of Older People Nursing, 7*(2), 141-151.
2012	Cossette, S., Frasure-Smith, N., Dupuis, J., Juneau, M., & Guertin, M.C. (2012). Randomized controlled trial of tailored nursing interventions to improve cardiac rehabilitation enrollment. *Nursing Research, 61*(2), 111-120.
2012	Sermeus, M.J., Park, J.S., & Park, H. (2012). Effect of sleep-inducing music on sleep in persons with percutaneous transluminal coronary angiography in the cardiac care unit. *Journal of Clinical Nursing, 21*(5-6), 728-735.
2012	Yuenyong, S., O'Brien, B., & Jirapeet, V. (2012). Effects of labour support from close female relative on labor and maternal satisfaction in a Thai setting. *Journal of Obstetric, Gynecologic, & Neonatal Nursing, 41*(1), 45-56.
2012	Ruesch, C., Mossakowski, J., Forrest, J., Hayes, M., Jahrsdoerfer, M., Comeau, E., & Singleton, M. (2012). Using nursing expertise and telemedicine to increase nursing collaboration and improve patient outcomes. *Telemedicine Journal & E-Health, 18*(8), 591-595.
2010	Sidani S., & Doran, D. (2010). Relationships between processes and outcomes of nurse practitioners in acute care: An exploration. *Journal of Nursing Care Quality, 25*(1), 31-38.
2010	Poochikian-Sarkissian, S., Sidani, S., Ferguson-Paré, M., & Doran, D. (2010). Examining the relationship between patient-centred care and outcomes. *Canadian Journal of Neuroscience Nursing 32*(4), 14-21.
2006	Kutzleb, J., & Reiner, D. The impact of nurse-directed patient education on quality of life and functional capacity in people with heart failure. *Journal of the American Academy of Nurse Practitioners, 18*(3), 116-123.
2006	Sidani, S., Doran, D.M., Porter, H., LeFort, S., O'Brien-Pallas, L., Zahn, C., Laschinger, H., & Sarkissian, S. (2006). Processes of care: Comparison between nurse practitioners and physician residents in acute care. *Canadian Journal of Nursing Leadership 19*(1), 69-85.
2006	Doran, D.M., Harrison, M., Spence-Laschinger, H., Hirdes, J., Rukholm, E., Sidani, S., McGillis Hall, L., & Tourangeau, A. (2006a). Nursing-sensitive outcomes data collection in acute care and long-term care settings. *Nursing Research, 55*(2S), S75-S81.
2006	Doran, D.M., Harrison, M., Spence-Laschinger, H., Hirdes, J., Rukholm, E., Sidani, S., McGillis Hall, L., & Tourangeau, A., & Cranley, L. (2006b). Relationship between nursing interventions and outcome achievement in acute care settings. *Research in Nursing & Health, 29*(1), 61-70.
2003	Doran, D.M., O'Brien-Pallas, L., Sidani, S., McGillis Hall, L., Petryshen, P., Hawkins, J., Watt-Watson, J., & Thompson, D. (2003). An evaluation of nursing sensitive outcomes for quality care. *Journal of International Nursing Perspectives, 3*(3), 109-125.

needs to be determined. Another challenge in outcomes research is to develop strategies for locating untreated individuals and including them in follow-up studies. The intent is to determine whether outcomes differ between those treated and those untreated. To address some of these challenges, outcomes researchers have used large databases as sample sources in observational research designs.

Large Databases as Sample Sources

One source of samples for outcomes studies is large databases. As illustrated in Figure 14-4, two broad categories of databases emerge from patient care encounters, clinical databases and administrative databases (Waltz, Strickland, & Lenz, 2010).

Clinical databases are created by providers such as hospitals, HMOs, accountable care organizations, and healthcare professionals. The clinical data are generated as a result of routine documentation of care or in relation to a research protocol. Some databases are data registries that have been developed to gather data related to a particular disease, such as heart disease or cancer (Lee & Goldman, 1989). With a clinical database, you can link observations made by many practitioners over long periods of time. Links can be made between the process of care and outcomes (Mitchell et al., 1994; Moses, 1995).

Administrative databases are created by insurance companies, government agencies, and others not directly involved in providing patient care. Administrative databases have standardized sets of data for enormous numbers of patients and providers (McDonald & Hui, 1991). An example is the Medicare database managed by the CMS. The administrative databases can be used to determine the incidence or prevalence of disease, geographic variations in medical care use, characteristics of medical care, and outcomes of care. Examples of large database indicators used to assess the quality of care are provided in Table 14-6. Initiatives such as CALNOC (2013b) and NDNQI (2013; Montalvo, 2007) are making nursing data more accessible for large database research.

Study Designs

Although RCTs are considered the gold standard for clinical research, most outcomes studies use quasi-experimental or observational research designs, which are suitable for addressing questions of effectiveness and efficiency. Like RCTs, outcomes research sometimes seeks to provide evidence about which interventions work best for which types of patients and under what circumstances. However, the "intervention" being evaluated is not limited to medications or new clinical procedures, but may also include the provision of particular services or resources, or even the enforcing of specific policies and regulations, by legislative and financial bodies. Outcomes research often considers additional parameters such as cost, timeliness, convenience, geographic accessibility,

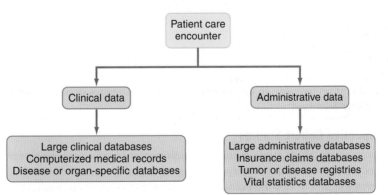

FIG 14-4 Types of databases emanating from patient care encounters. (From Grove, S. K., Burns, N., & Gray, J. R. (2013). *The practice of nursing research: Appraisal, synthesis, and generation of evidence* (7th ed.). St. Louis: Elsevier Saunders.)

TABLE 14-6	SOME LARGE DATABASE INDICATORS USED TO MONITOR NURSING STRUCTURAL, PROCESS, AND OUTCOME INDICATORS	
TYPE OF INDICATOR	**INDICATOR**	**SOURCE**
Structural	Nursing (e.g., RN, LPN, UAP) hours per patient day	National Database Nursing Quality Indicators (NDNQI, 2013) Collaborative Alliance for Nursing Outcomes (CALNOC, 2013a) National Quality Forum (NQF, 2013b)
	Staff mix (RN, LPN, LVN, UAP)	NDNQI (2013) CALNOC (2013a) NQF (2013)
	Nurse turnover	NDNQI (2013) CALNOC (2013a) NQF (2013)
	RN practice environment	NDNQI (2013) NQF (2013b)
Process	Risk assessment for pressure ulcers	CALNOC (2013a)
	Physical restraints	NDNQI (2013) CALNOC (2013a)
	Prevention protocols in place	CALNOC (2013a) B-NMDS (Belgian nursing minimum data set; Sermeus et al., 2008; Van den Heede, et al., 2009)
	Medication administration accuracy	CALNOC (2013a)
Outcome	Patient falls, injury falls	NDNQI (2013) CALNOC (2013a) NQF (2013b)
	Catheter-associated urinary tract infection rate	NDNQI (2013) NQF (2013)
	Hospital-acquired pressure ulcer	NDNQI (2013) CALNOC (2013a) NQF (2013b)
	Central line–associated bloodstream infection rate	NDNQI (2013) CALNOC (2013a) NQF (2013b)

LPN, Licensed practical nurse; *LVN*, licensed vocational nurse; *RN*, registered nurse; *UAP*, unlicensed assistive personnel.

and patient preferences. In the next section, common types of designs used in outcomes research are briefly discussed.

Prospective Cohort Studies

A prospective cohort study is an epidemiological study in which the researcher identifies a group of people who are at risk for experiencing a particular event and then follows them over time to observe whether or not the event occurs. Sample sizes for these studies often must be very large, particularly if only a small portion of the at-risk group will experience the event. The entire group is followed over time to determine the point at which the event occurs, variables associated with the event, and outcomes for those who experienced the event in comparison with those who did not.

The Harvard Nurses' Health Study is an example of a prospective cohort study. This study recruited 100,000 nurses to determine the long-term consequences of the use of birth control pills. Every 2 years, or more often, nurses complete a questionnaire about their health and health behaviors. The study has now been in progress for more than 20 years. Multiple studies reported in the literature have used the large data set yielded by the study. The following summary describes a prospective cohort study on smoking and the risk of psoriasis in women. It uses the Nurses' Health Study II, a second study using a younger population than that in the Harvard study (Setty, Curhan, & Choi, 2007). The researchers were able to obtain an extremely large heterogeneous sample for their study by using data from the Nurses' Health Study:

> "Background: *Psoriasis is a common, chronic, inflammatory skin disorder. Smoking may increase the risk of psoriasis.*
>
> Methods: *Over a 14-year time period from 1991 to 2005, the relation between smoking status, duration, intensity, cessation, exposure to second-hand smoke, and incident of psoriasis was prospectively examined in 78,532 women from the Nurses' Health Study II. The primary outcome was incident, self-reported, physician-diagnosed psoriasis.*
>
> Results: *Eight-hundred-eighty-seven incident cases of psoriasis were documented. The multivariate relative risk (RR) of psoriasis was 1.78 (95% confidence interval [CI], 1.46 to 2.16) for current smokers and 1.37 (95% CI, 1.17 to 1.59) for past smokers in comparison with persons who had never smoked. The multivariate RR of psoriasis was 1.60 (95% CI, 1.31 to 1.97) for those who had smoked 11 to 20 pack-years and 2.05 (95% CI, 1.66 to 2.53) for those who had smoked 21 or more pack-years in comparison with nonsmokers. The multivariate RR of psoriasis was 1.61 (95% CI, 1.30 to 2.00) for those who quit smoking less than 10 years ago, 1.31 (95% CI, 1.05 to 1.64) for those who had quit 10 to 19 years ago, and 1.15 (95% CI, 0.88 to 1.51) for those who had quit 20 or more years ago in comparison with persons who had never smoked. An increased risk of psoriasis was associated with prenatal and childhood exposure to passive smoke.*
>
> Conclusions: *The prospective analysis suggests that current and past smoking, and cumulative measures of smoking, were associated with the incidence of psoriasis. After 20 years of smoking cessation, the risk of the incident psoriasis among ex-smokers decreases nearly to that of persons who have never smoked."*
>
> **Setty et al., 2007, p. 953**

Retrospective Cohort Studies

A retrospective cohort study is an epidemiological study in which the researcher identifies a group of people who have experienced a particular event. This is a common research technique used in the field of epidemiology to study occupational exposure to chemicals. Events of interest to nursing that could be studied in this manner include a procedure, episode of care, nursing intervention, or diagnosis. Nurses might use a retrospective cohort study to follow a cohort of women who had undergone mastectomy for breast cancer or of patients in whom a urinary bladder catheter was placed during and after surgery. The cohort is evaluated after the event to determine the occurrence of changes in health status, usually the development of a particular disease or death. Nurses might be interested in the pattern of recovery after an event or, in the case of catheterization, the incidence of bladder infections in the months after surgery.

On the basis of the study findings, epidemiologists calculate the relative risk of the identified change in health for the group. Relative risk is the probability of the outcome occurring in the exposed group versus that in the nonexposed group. For example, if death were the occurrence of interest, the expected number of deaths would be determined. The observed number of deaths divided by the expected number of deaths and multiplied by 100 yields a standardized mortality ratio (SMR), which is regarded as a measure of the relative risk of the studied group to die of a particular condition. In nursing studies, patients might be followed over time after discharge from a healthcare facility to determine complication rates and the SMR (Swaen & Meijers, 1988).

In retrospective studies, researchers commonly ask patients to recall information relevant to their previous health status. This information is often used to determine the amount of change occurring before and after an intervention. Recall can easily be distorted, thereby misleading researchers in determining outcomes. Therefore, recall should be used with caution. Herrmann (1995) identified three sources of distortion in recall: (1) the question posed to the subject may be conceived or expressed incorrectly; (2) the recall process may be in error; and (3) the research design used to measure recall may result in the recall's appearing to be different from what actually occurred. Herrmann (1995, p. AS90) also identified four bases of recall:

Direct recall: The subject "accesses the memory without having to think or search memory," resulting in correct information.

Indirect recall: The subject "accesses the memory after thinking or searching memory," resulting in correct information.

Limited recall: "Access to the memory does not occur but information that suggests the contents of the memory is accessed," resulting in an educated guess.

No recall: "Neither the memory nor information relevant to the memory may be accessed," resulting in a wild guess.

The following abstract, developed by Doran and associates (2013), in their study of adverse events and outcomes in the Canadian home care population, is presented as an example of a retrospective cohort study. It is also an example of a study that used large secondary databases as data sources.

"Background: *Home care (HC) is a critical component of the ongoing restructuring of health care in Canada. It impacts three dimensions of healthcare delivery: primary health care, chronic disease management, and aging at home strategies. The purpose of our study is to investigate a significant safety dimension of HC, the occurrence of adverse events and their related outcomes. The study reports on the incidence of HC adverse events, the magnitude of the events, the types of events that occur, and the consequences experienced by HC clients in the province of Ontario.*

Methods: *A retrospective cohort design was used, utilizing comprehensive secondary databases available for Ontario HC clients from the years 2008 and 2009. The data were derived from the Canadian Home Care Reporting System, the Hospital Discharge Abstract Database, the National Ambulatory Care Reporting System, the Ontario Mental Health Reporting System, and the Continuing Care Reporting System. Descriptive analysis was used to identify the type and frequency of the adverse events recorded and the consequences of the events. Logistic regression analysis was used to examine the association between the events and their consequences.*

Results: *The study found that the incident rate for adverse events for the HC clients included in the cohort was 13%. The most frequent adverse events identified in the databases were injurious falls, injuries from other than a fall, and medication-related incidents. With respect to outcomes, we determined that an injurious fall was associated with a significant increase in the odds of a client requiring long-term-care facility admission and of client death. We further determined that three types of events, delirium, sepsis, and medication-related incidents were associated directly with an increase in the odds of client death.*

Conclusions: *Our study concludes that 13% of clients in home care experience an adverse event annually. We also determined that an injurious fall was the most frequent of the adverse events and was associated with increased admission to long-term care or death. We recommend the use of tools that are presently available in Canada, such as the Resident Assessment Instrument and its Clinical Assessment Protocols, for assessing and mitigating the risk of an adverse event occurring."*

Doran et al., 2013, p. 227

Population-Based Studies

Population-based studies are conducted within the context of the patient's community rather than the context of the medical system. With this method, all cases of a condition occurring in the defined population are included, not just the cases treated at a particular healthcare facility. The latter could introduce a selection bias. The researcher might make efforts to include individuals with the condition who had not received treatment.

Community-based norms of tests and survey instruments obtained in this manner provide a clearer picture of the range of values than the limited spectrum of patients seen in specialty clinics. Estimates of instrument sensitivity and specificity are more accurate (see Chapter 10). This method enables researchers to understand the natural history of a condition or the long-term risks and benefits of a particular intervention (Guess et al., 1995). Bakker and co-workers (2011) conducted a study examining the differences in birth outcomes related to maternal age. The following is an abstract of their study:

"Background: *Previous studies have shown that birth weight and preterm birth are strong predictors of neonatal morbidity and mortality. Maternal age might be a modifiable determinant of weight and gestational age at birth. In most Western countries, the age of mothers having their first child is increasing due to prolonged education, professional commitment, delayed marriage, and other personal reasons. It has been suggested that older maternal age is associated with increased risks of pregnancy complications, such as gestational hypertension or diabetes, preterm delivery, fetal malformations, and fetal death.*

Methods: *This is a population-based prospective cohort study with 8,568 mothers and their children based in Rotterdam, Netherlands. Maternal age, sociodemographic, lifestyle-related determinants, and birth outcomes were obtained from questionnaires and hospital records. The main outcome measures were birth weight, preterm delivery, small-for-gestational-age, and large-for-gestational-age babies. Multivariate linear and logistic regression analyses were used to analyze study data.*

Results: *In this study, mothers aged 30-34.9 years had no differences in risk of preterm delivery. Mothers <20 years had the highest risk of delivering small-for-gestational-age babies (OR 1.6, 95% CI: 1.1-2.5); however, after adjustment for sociodemographic and lifestyle-related determinants this increased risk was not present. Mothers >40 years had the highest risk of delivering large-for-gestational-age babies (OR 1.3, 95% CI: 0.8-2.4); however no associations of maternal age with the risks of delivering large-for-gestational-age babies could be explained by sociodemographic and lifestyle-related determinants.*

Conclusions: *Younger mothers have an increased risk of small-for-gestational age babies, whereas older mothers have an increased risk of large-for-gestational-age babies when compared with mothers aged 30-34.9 years. Sociodemographic and lifestyle-related determinants cannot entirely explain these differences."*

Bakker et al., 2011, p. 500

be described in the research report. This step requires that the study design include baseline measures of patient status, such as demographic characteristics, functional status, and disease severity measures. An analysis of improvement allows for better judgments to be made about the appropriate use of various treatments (Fasting & Gisvold, 2003).

CRITICAL APPRAISAL OF OUTCOMES STUDIES

This section discusses approaches for critically appraising outcomes studies. Guyatt and colleagues (2008) published the *Users' Guides to the Medical Literature,* which outlines the methodology for critically appraising study designs, including those typically used in outcomes research. This guide provides worksheets used to summarize the results of a critical appraisal. The worksheets that are most relevant to outcomes research are those that address studies of economic analysis, retrospective cohort design, health-related quality of life, and prospective cohort design. An example of the types of questions to consider in critically appraising outcome studies of health-related quality of life are provided in the following section.

Questions Guiding the Critical Appraisal of Outcomes Studies

This section provides questions to assist you in critically appraising outcomes studies. These questions are organized by three broad questions: "Are the results valid?", "What are the results?", and "How can I apply the results to patient care?"

Are the results valid?

- In a prospective cohort study, did the exposed and control groups start and finish with the same risk of outcome?
- In nursing outcome studies, exposure could refer to a particular nursing intervention, staffing model or staff mix, or even healthcare policy.
- Three subquestions need to be considered in addressing the original question about the validity of the study results:
  - Were patients similar for factors or variables known to be associated with the outcome (or was statistical adjustment used to control for differences between the exposed and control groups)?
  - Were the circumstances and methods for detecting the outcome similar? Did the researchers use the same method for measuring the outcome in the exposed and control groups?
  - Was the follow-up sufficiently complete? Ideally, we would like to see approximately 80% follow-up in both control and exposed groups.

In a retrospective cohort study, did the exposed and control groups have the same chance of being exposed in the past? In a retrospective cohort study, the researcher would be interested in determining whether outcomes differ for individuals exposed in the past to a particular health risk, health condition, or health service by following individuals longitudinally after the particular exposure. The following questions need to be addressed in retrospective cohort studies:

- Were cases and controls similar with respect to the indication or circumstances that would lead to exposure? For example, were they all equally eligible to receive the particular nursing intervention or receive care under the particular staffing model?
- Were the circumstances and methods for determining exposure similar for cases and controls? In a retrospective cohort study, investigators look back in time to determine exposure to a particular intervention or determine the existence of a particular condition. To answer this question, you would need to determine if the study used the same approach for determining exposure in the control and intervention groups.

What are the results?

- How strong is the association between exposure and outcome? Were the results statistically significant?
- How precise was the estimate of effect? Were the confidence intervals for the effect large or small? Small confidence intervals reflect greater precision in the estimate of effect.

In a study of an outcome such as health-related quality of life (HRQL):

- Did the investigators measure aspects of patients' lives that patients consider important? To answer this question, you would need to consider whether the authors described the content of their measure of health-related quality of life (HRQL) in sufficient detail so that it is possible to make a judgment about the relevance of the measure for the particular patient population, and/or whether the authors provided direct evidence from their study or indirect evidence from previous studies that the HRQL measure is important to the patient population being investigated.
- Did the HRQL instrument work in the intended way? This question requires an appraisal of the psychometric properties of the HRQL instrument with regard to reliability and validity.
- Were important aspects of HRQL omitted from measurement? This question requires an appraisal of the content validity of the instrument with regard to whether the instrument was complete in its measurement of HRQL.

How can I apply the results to patient care?

- Were the study patients similar to the patient in my practice setting?
- Was follow-up sufficiently long to assess an impact on outcome?
- Is the exposure (e.g., intervention, staffing model, healthcare policy) similar to what might occur in my practice setting?
- What is the magnitude of effect? This question requires you to consider whether the effect was clinically important to make it worthwhile to change practice?
- Are there any benefits that are known to be associated with exposure? This question asks you to consider whether the benefits for patients and/or practice settings are sufficiently worthwhile to suggest that you would want to act on the results.

Example Critical Appraisal of an Outcomes Study

An example of a critical appraisal of a quality of life outcome study is provided below.

RESEARCH EXAMPLE

Critical Appraisal of an Outcomes Study

Research Study Excerpt

Orwelius and colleagues (2013, p. 229) investigated long-term health-related quality of life (HRQoL or HRQL) after burns. Their study abstract is as follows:

"Background: Health-related quality of life (HRQoL) is reduced after a burn, and is affected by coexisting conditions. The aims of the investigation were to examine and describe effects of coexisting disease on HRQoL, and to quantify the proportion of burned people whose HRQoL was below that of a reference group matched for age, gender, and coexisting conditions.

Method: A nationwide study covering 9 years...examined HRQoL 12 and 24 months after the burn with the SF-36 questionnaire. The reference group was from the referral area of one of the hospitals.

Continued

RESEARCH EXAMPLE—cont'd

Results: The HRQoL of the burned patients was below that of the reference group mainly in the mental dimensions, and only single patients were affected in the physical dimensions. The factor that significantly affected most HRQoL dimensions ($n=6$) after the burn was unemployment, whereas only smaller effects could be attributed directly to the burn.

Conclusion: Poor HRQoL was recorded for only a small number of patients, and the declines were mostly in the mental dimensions when compared with a group adjusted for age, gender, and coexisting conditions. Factors other than the burn itself, such as mainly unemployment and pre-existing disease, were most important for the long-term HRQoL experience in these patients."

Critical Appraisal

The study used a retrospective cohort design. Individuals who experienced a burn were followed for 24 months to determine the impact of the burn, along with other factors, on changes in HRQoL. The exposed group consisted of all Swedish-speaking patients 18 years or older admitted with burns of 10% or more of total body surface area or duration of stay in the burn unit of 7 days or more in 2000 to 2009 (hereafter referred to as the burn cohort). The unexposed cohort was identified from a public health survey of one county in Sweden, which was completed in 1999 (hereafter referred to as the healthy reference cohort). The two cohorts were not similar for all factors known to be associated with HRQoL. For example, the burn cohort had more males, fewer individuals with higher education, more single individuals, and fewer individuals not employed or retired than the healthy reference cohort. These differences could have influenced HRQoL and, in this study, the investigators accounted for the differences statistically in their analysis. Although the circumstances for detecting the outcome were different for both cohorts, the method of assessment—namely, the SF-36 (Ware & Sherbourne, 1992)—was the same. The SF-36 is a well-recognized HRQoL measure, with high reliability and validity established in a representative Swedish population and burn population (Edgar, Dawson, Hankey, Phillips, & Wood, 2010).

Follow-up in the burn cohort was 24 months, a duration that is considered sufficiently long for detecting change in HRQoL. Of the eligible burn patients, 61% were recruited into the cohort and follow-up of these individuals at 24 months was 48%. Response after two reminders in the healthy reference cohort was 61%. Incomplete follow-up of both cohorts could mean that there are systematic differences (i.e., response bias) between individuals who responded to the survey from those who did not, thus influencing the generalizability of the study findings. There were statistically significant differences in HRQoL between the burn and healthy reference cohorts, primarily in the mental dimension, and the authors reported clinically significant improvements in physical function and role function scores among the burn cohort. The factor that most significantly affected HRQoL after the burn was unemployment, whereas only small effects could be attributed directly to the burn. In conclusion, there were some threats to the validity of the study findings, particularly with regard to differences between the burn and healthy reference cohorts and incomplete follow-up. Some of these differences were accounted for statistically in the analysis. Strengths of the study included use of a reliable and valid measure of HRQoL and statistically and clinically significant effects. Translations of these findings to a North American population would depend on how similar the Swedish population is to the North American population and how similar health care of burn patients is between them.

KEY CONCEPTS

- Outcomes research examines the end results of patient care.
- The scientific approaches used in outcomes studies differ in some important ways from those used in traditional research.
- Donabedian (1987, 2005) developed the theory on which outcomes research is based.
- Quality is the overriding construct of the theory, although Donabedian never defined this term.
- The three major concepts of the theory are health, subjects of care, and providers of care.
- Donabedian identified three objects of evaluation in appraising quality—structure, process, and outcome.

- The goal of outcomes research is to evaluate outcomes as defined by Donabedian, whose theory requires that identified outcomes be clearly linked with the process that caused the outcome.
- Clinical guideline panels are established to incorporate available evidence on health outcomes.
- Outcomes studies provide rich opportunities to build a stronger scientific underpinning for nursing practice.
- A nursing-sensitive patient outcome is "sensitive" because it is influenced by nursing.
- Organizations currently involved in efforts to study nursing-sensitive outcomes include the American Nurses Association, National Quality Forum, Collaborative Alliance for Nursing Outcomes, Veterans Affairs Nursing Outcomes Database, Center for Medicare & Medicaid Services Hospital Quality Initiative, American Hospital Association, Federation of American Hospitals, The Joint Commission, and Agency of Healthcare Research and Quality.
- An area of interest is the process of care delivered by APNs (nurse practitioners, nurse midwives, nurse anesthetists, and clinical nurse specialists).
- Outcome design strategies tend to have less control than traditional research designs discussed in this text, except for randomized controlled trials (RCTs).
- Some of the common outcomes studies' methodologies include prospective cohort studies, retrospective cohort studies, population-based studies, economic analysis, and ethical studies.
- Outcomes studies generally use large representative, heterogeneous samples rather than random samples.
- Statistical approaches used in outcomes studies include new approaches to examining measurement reliability, strategies to analyze change, and the analysis of improvement.
- Dissemination is an important aspect of the outcomes research process because it ensures that the study results will have an impact on patients, providers, and healthcare organizations.
- Critical appraisal of outcomes studies focuses on similarity of exposed and unexposed cohorts, adequacy and completeness of follow-up, reliability and validity of the outcome measure(s), and statistical and clinical significance of the study findings.
- An example critical appraisal of a current outcomes study is provided.

REFERENCES

Agency for Healthcare Research and Quality (AHRQ). (2013). *Outcomes research: Fact Sheet.* Retrieved July 30, 2013 from, http://www.ahrq.gov/research/findings/factsheets/outcomes/outfact/index.html.

Agency for Healthcare Research and Quality (AHRQ). (2011). *National Guideline Clearinghouse.* Retrieved July 30, 2013 from, http://www.guideline.gov.

Agency for Healthcare Research and Quality (AHRQ). (2010). *HHS awards $437 million in patient-centered outcomes research funding.* Retrieved July 30, 2013 from, http://www.ahrq.gov/health-care-information/topics/topic-arra.html.

Aiken, L. H., Clarke, S. P., Sloane, D. M., Lake, E. T., & Cheney, T. (2008). Effects of hospital care environment on patient mortality and nurse outcomes. *Journal of Nursing Administration,* 38(5), 223–229.

Bakker, R., Steegers, E., Biharie, A., Mackenbach, J., Hofman, A., & Jaddoe, V. (2011). Explaining differences in birth outcomes in relation to maternal age: The Generation R Study. *BJOG: An International Journal of Obstetrics and Gynaecology,* 118(4), 500–509.

Bettger, J. A., Coster, W. J., Latham, N. K., & Keysor, J. J. (2008). Analyzing change in recovery patterns in the year after acute hospitalization. *Archives of Physical Medicine & Rehabilitation,* 89(7), 1267–1275.

Bombardier, C., & Tugwell, P. (1987). Methodological considerations in functional assessment. *Journal of Rheumatology,* 14(Suppl. 15), 7–10.

Boz, C., Ozmenoglu, M., Alioglu, Z., Velioglu, S., Altunayoglu, V., & Gazioglu, S. (2004). Local cold effect on the excitability recovery curve of the sympathetic skin response. *Electromyography & Clinical Neurophysiology,* 44(8), 497–501.

Brenner, M. H., Curbow, B., & Legro, M. W. (1995). The proximal-distal continuum of multiple health outcome measures: The case of cataract surgery. *Medical Care, 33*(4 Suppl.), AS236–AS244.

Canadian Institute for Health Information (CIHI). (2012). *Frequently asked questions about the MIS Standards.* Retrieved July 30, 2013 from, http://www.cihi.ca/cihi-ext-portal/internet/en/document/standards+and+data+submission/standards/mis+standards/mis_faq.

Clancy, C. M., & Eisenberg, J. M. (1998). Outcomes research: Measuring the end results of health care. *Science, 282*(5387), 245–246.

Clarke, S. P. (2011). Health care utilization. In D. M. Doran (Ed.), *Nursing outcomes: The state of the science* (pp. 439–485) (2nd ed.). Sudbury, MA: Jones & Bartlett.

Collaborative Alliance for Nursing Outcomes (CALNOC). (2013a). *Home page.* Retrieved July 30, 2013 from, http://calnoc.org.

Collaborative Alliance for Nursing Outcomes (CALNOC). (2013b). *Overview.* Retrieved July 30, 2013 from, http://www.calnoc.org/displaycommon.cfm?an=1.

Cummings, G. G., Midodzi, W. K., Wong, C. A., & Estabrooks, C. A. (2010). The contribution of hospital nursing leadership styles to 30-day patient mortality. *Nursing Research, 59*(5), 331–339.

Davies, B., Edwards, N., Ploeg, J., & Virani, T. (2008). Insights about the process and impact of implementing nursing guidelines on delivery of care in hospitals and community settings. *BMC Health Services Research, 8,* 29.

DeKeyser Ganz, F., & Berkovitz, K. (2012). Surgical nurses' perceptions of ethical dilemmas, moral distress and quality of care. *Journal of Advanced Nursing, 68*(7), 1516–1525.

Deyo, R. A. (1984). Measuring functional outcomes in therapeutic trials for chronic disease. *Controlled Clinical Trials, 5*(3), 223–240.

Deyo, R. A., & Carter, W. B. (1992). Strategies for improving and expanding the application of health status measures in clinical settings. *Medical Care, 30*(Suppl.), MS176–MS186.

Deyo, R. A., & Centor, R. M. (1986). Assessing the responsiveness of functional scales to clinical change: An analogy to diagnostic test performance. *Journal of Chronic Disease, 39*(11), 897–906.

Deyo, R. A., Taylor, V. M., Diehr, P., Conrad, D., Cherkin, D. C., Ciol, M., et al. (1994). Analysis of automated administrative and survey databases to study patterns and outcomes of care. *Spine, 19*(18), 2083S–2091S.

DiCenso, A., Martin-Misener, R., Bryant-Lukosius, D., Bourgeault, I., Kilpatrick, K., Donald, F., et al. (2010).

Advanced practice nursing in Canada: Overview of a decision support synthesis. *Canadian Journal of Nursing Leadership, 23*(special issue), 15–34.

Donabedian, A. (1976). *Benefits in medical care programs.* Cambridge, MA: Harvard University Press.

Donabedian, A. (1978). *Needed research in quality assessment and monitoring.* Hyattsville, MD: U.S. Department of Health, Education, and Welfare, Public Health Service, National Center for Health Services Research.

Donabedian, A. (1980). *Explorations in quality assessment and monitoring.* Ann Arbor, MI: Health Administration Press.

Donabedian, A. (1982). *The criteria and standards of quality.* Ann Arbor, MI: Health Administration Press.

Donabedian, A. (1987). Some basic issues in evaluating the quality of health care. In L. T. Rinke (Ed.), *Outcome measures in home care: Vol. I.* (p. 338). New York: National League for Nursing (Original work published in 1976.).

Donabedian, A. (1988). The quality of care: How can it be assessed? *Journal of the American Medical Association, 260*(12), 1743–1748.

Donabedian, A. (2005). Evaluating the quality of medical care. *The Milbank Quarterly, 83*(4), 691–729.

Doran, D. M. (Ed.). (2011). *Nursing outcomes: The state of the science.* (2nd ed.). Sudbury, MA: Jones & Bartlett.

Doran, D. M., Harrison, M., Laschinger, H. S., Hirdes, J., Rukholm, E., Sidani, S., et al. (2006a). Nursing sensitive outcomes data collection in acute care and long-term care settings. *Nursing Research, 55*(2S), S75–S81.

Doran, D., Harrison, M. B., Laschinger, H., Hirdes, J., Rukholm, E., Sidani, S., et al. (2006b). Relationship between nursing interventions and outcome achievement in acute care settings. *Research in Nursing & Health, 29*(1), 61–70.

Doran, D. M., Mildon, B., & Clarke, S. (2011). Toward a national report card in nursing: A knowledge synthesis. *Canadian Journal of Nursing Leadership, 24*(2), 38–57.

Doran, D. M., Regis, B., Hirdes, J. P., Baker, G. R., Poss, J. W., Li, X., et al. (2013). Adverse outcomes among home care clients associated with emergency room visit or pre-hospitalization: A descriptive study of secondary health databases. *BMC Health Services Research, 13,* 227.

Doran, D. M., Sidani, S., & Di Pietro, T. (2010). Nursing-sensitive outcomes. In J. S. Fulton, B. Lyon, & K. Goudreau (Eds.), *Foundations of clinical nurse specialist practices* (pp. 35–37). New York: Springer.

Doran, D. M., Sidani, S., Keatings, M., & Doidge, D. (2002). An empirical test of the Nursing Role

Effectiveness Model. *Journal of Advanced Nursing,* *38*(1), 29–39.

Edgar, D., Dawson, A., Hankey, G., Phillips, M., & Wood, F. (2010). Demonstration of the validity of the SF-36 for measurement of the temporal recovery of quality of life outcomes in burns survivors. *Burns,* *36*(7), 1013–1020.

Fasting, S., & Gisvold, S. E. (2003). Statistical process control methods allow the analysis and improvement of anesthesia care. *Canadian Journal of Anesthesia,* *50*(8), 767–774.

Feinstein, A. R., Josephy, B. R., & Wells, C. K. (1986). Scientific and clinical problems in indexes of functional disability. *Annals of Internal Medicine, 105*(3), 413–420.

Freedman, L. S., & Schatzkin, A. (1992). Sample size for studying intermediate endpoints within intervention trials or observational studies. *American Journal of Epidemiology, 136*(9), 1148–1159.

Gottman, J. M., & Rushe, R. H. (1993). The analysis of change: Issues, fallacies, and new ideas. *Journal of Consulting and Clinical Psychology, 61*(6), 907–910.

Graham, I. D., Bick, D., Tetroe, J., Straus, S. E., & Harrison, M. B. (2011). Measuring outcomes of evidence-based practice: Distinguishing between knowledge use and its impact. In D. Bick, & I. Graham (Eds.), *Evaluating the impact of implementing evidence-based practice* (pp. 18–37). Oxford, United Kingdom: Wiley-Blackwell.

Grove, S. K., Burns, N., & Gray, J. R. (2013). *The practice of nursing research: Appraisal, synthesis, and generation of evidence* (7th ed.). Philadelphia: Elsevier Saunders.

Guess, H. A., Jacobsen, S. J., Girman, C. J., Oesterling, J. E., Chute, C. G., Panser, L. A., et al. (1995). The role of community-based longitudinal studies in evaluating treatment effects. Example: Benign prostatic hyperplasia. *Medical Care, 33*(Suppl. 4), AS26–AS35.

Guyatt, G., Rennie, D., Meade, M. O., & Cook, D. J. (2008). *Users' guides to the medical literature: A manual for evidence-based practice* (2nd ed.). New York, NY: McGraw-Hill Medical.

Guyatt, G., Walter, S., & Norman, G. (1987). Measuring change over time: Assessing the usefulness of evaluative instruments. *Journal of Chronic Disease, 40*(2), 171–178.

Harris, C. W. (1967). *Problems in measuring change.* Madison, WI: University of Wisconsin Press.

Harris, M. R., & Warren, J. J. (1995). Patient outcomes: Assessment issues for the CNS. *Clinical Nurse Specialist, 9*(2), 82–86.

Hernandez, G., Fernandez, R., Luzon, E., Cuena, R., & Montejo, J. C. (2007). The early phase of the minute ventilation recovery curve predicts extubation failure better than the minute ventilation recovery time. *Chest, 131*(5), 1315–1322.

Herrmann, D. (1995). Reporting current, past, and changed health status: What we know about distortion. *Medical Care, 33*(Suppl. 4), AS89–AS94.

Howell, D. (2011). Psychological distress as a nurse-sensitive outcome. In D. M. Doran (Ed.), *Nursing outcomes: The state of the science* (pp. 285–358) (2nd ed.). Sudbury, MA: Jones & Bartlett.

Irvine, D. M., Sidani, S., & McGillis Hall, L. (1998). Linking outcomes to nurses' roles in health care. *Nursing Economic$, 16*(2), 58–64, 87.

Jaeschke, R., Singer, J., & Guyatt, G. H. (1989). Measurement of health status: Ascertaining the minimal clinically important difference. *Controlled Clinical Trials, 10*(4), 407–415.

Jefford, M., Stockler, M. R., & Tattersall, M. H. N. (2003). Outcomes research: What is it and why does it matter? *Internal Medicine Journal, 33*(3), 110–118.

Jenerette, C. M., & Murdaugh, C. (2008). Testing the theory of self-care management for sickle cell disease. *Research in Nursing & Health, 31*(4), 355–369.

Kirshner, B., & Guyatt, G. (1985). A methodological framework for assessing health indices. *Journal of Chronic Diseases, 38*(1), 27–36.

Kleib, M., Sales, A., Doran, D. M., Malette, C., & White, D. (2011). Nursing minimum data sets. In D. M. Doran (Ed.), *Nursing outcomes: The state of the science* (pp. 487–512) (2nd ed.). Sudbury, MA: Jones & Bartlett.

Knight, M. M. (2000). Cognitive ability and functional status. *Journal of Advanced Nursing, 31*(6), 1459–1468.

Kramer, M., Maguire, P., & Schmalenberg, C. (2006). Excellence through evidence: The what, when, and where of clinical autonomy. *Journal of Nursing Administration, 36*(10), 479–491.

Kutney-Lee, A., Sloane, D., & Aiken, L. (2013). Increase in the number of nurses with baccalaureate degrees is linked to lower rates of postsurgery mortality. *Health Affairs, 32*(3), 579–586.

Lake, E. T. (2006). Multilevel models in health outcomes research. Part I: Theory, design, and measurement. *Applied Nursing Research, 19*(1), 51–53.

Lee, T. H., & Goldman, L. (1989). Development and analysis of observational data bases. *Journal of the American College of Cardiology, 14*(Suppl. 3A), 44A–47A.

Leidy, N. K. (1991). Survey measures of functional ability and disability of pulmonary patients. In B. L. Metzger (Ed.), *Synthesis conference on altered functioning:*

Impairment and disability (pp. 52–79). Indianapolis: Nursing Center Press of Sigma Theta Tau International.

Loegering, L., Reiter, R. C., & Gambone, J. C. (1994). Measuring the quality of health care. *Clinical Obstetrics and Gynecology, 37*(1), 122–136.

Lohr, K. N. (1988). Outcome measurement: Concepts and questions. *Inquiry, 25*(1), 37–50.

Lynn, J., & Virnig, B. A. (1995). Assessing the significance of treatment effects: Comments from the perspective of ethics. *Medical Care, 33*(4), AS292–AS298.

Magnello, M. E. (2010). The passionate statistician. In S. Nelson, & A. M. Rafferty (Eds.), *Notes On Nightingale: The influence and legacy of a nursing icon* (pp. 115–129). Ithaca, NY: Cornell University Press.

Mark, B. A. (1995). The black box of patient outcomes research. *Image: Journal of Nursing Scholarship, 27*(1), 42.

McCauley, S. R., Hannay, H. J., & Swank, P. R. (2001). Use of the disability rating scale recovery curve as a predictor of psychosocial outcome following closed-headed injury. *Journal of the International Neuropsychology Society, 7*(4), 457–467.

McDonald, C. J., & Hui, S. L. (1991). The analysis of humongous databases: Problems and promises. *Statistics in Medicine, 10*(4), 511–518.

McGillis Hall, L., Doran, D., Baker, G. R., Pink, G. H., Sidani, S., O'Brien-Pallas, L., et al. (2003). Nurse staffing models as predictors of patient outcomes. *Medical Care, 41*(9), 1096–1109.

Merskey, H., & Bogduk, N. (1994). *Classification of chronic pain: Descriptions of chronic pain syndromes and definitions of pain terms* (2nd ed.). Seattle: IASP Press.

Mitchell, J. B., Bubolz, T., Pail, J. E., Pashos, C. L., Escarce, J. J., Muhlbaier, L. H., et al. (1994). Using Medicare claims for outcomes research. *Medical Care, 32*(Suppl. 7), JS38–JS51.

Mitchell, P. H., Ferketich, S., & Jennings, B. M. (1998). American Academy of Nursing Expert Panel on Quality Health Care: 1998 Quality Health Outcomes Model. *Image—Journal of Nursing Scholarship, 30*(1), 43–46.

Montalvo, I. (2007). *National Database of Nursing Quality Indicators (NDNQI).* Retrieved July 30, 2013, from, http://www.nursingworld.org/ojin.

Moore, J., & McQuestion, M. (2012). The clinical nurse specialist in chronic diseases. *Clinical Nurse Specialist, 26*(3), 149–163.

Moses, L. E. (1995). Measuring effects without randomized trials? Options, problems, challenges. *Medical Care, 33*(4), AS8–AS14.

National Database of Nursing Quality Indicators (NDNQI). (2013). *ANA's NQF-endorsed measure specifications: Guidelines for data collection on the American Nurses Association's national quality forum endorsed measures: Nursing care hours per patient day; skill mix; falls and falls with injury.* Retrieved July 30, 2013 from home page link at, http://www.nursingquality.org/FAQs.

National Quality Forum (NQF). (2013a). *About NQF.* Retrieved July 30, 2013 from, http://www.qualityforum.org/Measures_Reports_Tools.aspx.

National Quality Forum (NQF). (2013b). *National standards to evaluate health care quality based on how patients feel.* Retrieved July 30, 2013 from, http://www.qualityforum.org/News_And_Resources/Press_Releases/2013/National_Standards_to_Evaluate_Health_Care_Quality_Based_On_How_Patients_Feel.aspx.

Nelson, E. C., Landgraf, J. M., Hays, R. D., Wasson, J. H., & Kirk, J. W. (1990). The functional status of patients: How can it be measured in physicians' offices? *Medical Care, 28*(12), 1111–1126.

Oh, S. H., Park, E. J., Yin, Y., Piao, J., & Lee, S. (2013). Automatic delirium prediction system in Korean surgical intensive care unit. *Nursing in Critical Care.* http://dx.doi.org/10.1111/nicc.12048, Electronic publication ahead of print October 24, 2013.

Oncology Nursing Society (ONS). (2012). *About the ONS.* Retrieved July 30, 2013 from, http://www.ons.org/about.

Orem, D. (2001). *Nursing concepts of practice* (6th ed.). St Louis: Mosby.

Orwelius, L., Willebrand, M., Gerdin, L., Ekselius, L., Fredrikson, M., & Sjöberg, F. (2013). Long-term health-related quality of life after burns is strongly dependent on pre-existing disease and psychosocial issues and less due to the burn itself. *Burns, 39*(2), 229–235.

Patrick, D. L., & Deyo, R. A. (1989). Generic and disease-specific measures in assessing health status and quality of life. *Medical Care, 27*(Suppl. 3), S217–S232.

Sermeus, W., Delesie, L., Van den Heede, K., Diya, L., & Lesaffre, E. (2008). Measuring the intensity of nursing care: Making use of the Belgian nursing minimum data set. *International Journal of Nursing Studies, 45*(7), 1011–1021.

Setty, A. R., Curhan, G., & Choi, H. K. (2007). Smoking and the risk of psoriasis in women: Nurses' Health Study II. *American Journal of Medicine, 120*(11), 953–959.

Shi, L. (2008). *Health services research methods* (2nd ed.). Clifton Park, NY: Delmar Cengage Learning.

Sidani, S. (2011a). Self-care. In D. M. Doran (Ed.), *Nursing outcomes: The state of the science* (pp. 79–130) (2nd ed.). Sudbury, MA: Jones & Bartlett.

Sidani, S. (2011b). Symptom management. In D. M. Doran (Ed.), *Nursing outcomes: The state of the science* (pp. 131–199) (2nd ed.). Sudbury, MA: Jones & Bartlett.

Spence Laschinger, H., Gilbert, S., & Smith, L. (2011). Patient satisfaction as a nurse-sensitive outcome. In D. M. Doran (Ed.), *Nursing outcomes: The state of the science* (pp. 359–408) (2nd ed.). Sudbury, MA: Jones & Bartlett.

Spitzer, W. O. (1987). State of science 1986: Quality of life and functional status as target variables for research. *Journal of Chronic Disease, 40*(6), 465–471.

Stetler, C. B., & Caramanica, B. (2007). Evaluation of an evidence-based practice initiative: Outcomes, strengths, and limitations of a retrospective conceptually based approach. *Worldviews on Evidence-Based Nursing, 4*(4), 187–199.

Stewart, A. L., Greenfield, S., Hays, R. D., Wells, K., Rogers, W. H., Berry, S. D., et al. (1989). Functional status and well-being of patients with chronic conditions. *Journal of the American Medical Association, 262*(7), 907–913.

Stewart, B. J., & Archbold, P. G. (1992). Nursing intervention studies require outcome measures that are sensitive to change: Part 2. *Research in Nursing & Health, 16*(1), 77–81.

Stone, P. W., Mooney-Kane, C., Larson, E. L., Horan, T., Glance, L. G., Zwanziger, J., et al. (2007). Nurse working conditions and patient safety outcomes. *Medical Care, 45*(6), 571–578.

Swaen, G. M., & Meijers, J. M. (1988). Influence of design characteristics on the outcomes of retrospective cohort studies. *British Journal of Industrial Medicine, 45*(9), 624–629.

Tourangeau, A. E. (2011). Mortality rate: A nursing sensitive outcome. In D. M. Doran (Ed.), *Nursing outcomes: The state of the science* (pp. 409–437). (2nd ed.). Sudbury, MA: Jones & Bartlett.

Tourangeau, A. E., Doran, D. M., Hall, L. M., O'Brien Pallas, L., Pringle, D., Tu, J. V., et al. (2007). Impact of hospital nursing care on 30-day mortality for acute medical patients. *Journal of Advanced Nursing, 57*(1), 32–44.

Tourangeau, A. E. (2003). Modeling the determinants of mortality for hospitalized patients. *International Nursing Perspectives, 3*(1), 37–48.

Tracy, S., Schinco, M. A., Griffen, M. M., Kerwin, A. J., Devin, T., & Tepas, J. J. (2006). Urgent airway intervention: Does outcome change with personnel performing the procedure? *Journal of Trauma, 61*(5), 1162–1165.

Van den Heede, K., Sermeus, W., Diya, L., Clarke, S. P., Lesaffre, E., Vleugels, A., et al. (2009). Nurse staffing and patient outcomes in Belgian acute hospitals: Cross-sectional analysis of administrative data. *International Journal of Nursing Studies, 46*(7), 928–939.

Veatch, R. (1993). Justice and outcomes research: The ethical limits. *Journal of Clinical Ethics, 4*(3), 258–261.

Waltz, C. F., Strickland, O. L., & Lenz, E. R. (2010). *Measurement in nursing and health research* (4th ed.). New York: Springer.

Ware, J. R., & Sherbourne, J. E. (1992). The MOS, 36-item short-form health survey (SF-36). I. Conceptual framework and item selection. *Medical Care, 30*(6), 473–483.

World Health Organization (WHO). (2009). The conceptual framework for the International Classification for Patient Safety, *Version 1.0, 2007-2008*. Retrieved July 30, 2013 from, http://www.who.int/patientsafety/taxonomy/en.

Yoder, L., Xin, W., Norris, K., & Yan, G. (2013). Patient care staffing levels and facility characteristics in US hemodialysis facilities. *American Journal of Kidney Disease, 62*(6), 1130–1140.

GLOSSARY

A

Abstract (adjective) Expressed without reference to any specific instance.

Abstract (noun) Clear, concise summary of a study, usually limited to 100 to 250 words.

Acceptance rate The number or percentage of the subjects who agree to participate in a study. The percentage is calculated by dividing the number of subjects agreeing to participate by the number of subjects approached. For example, for a study in which 100 subjects are approached and 90 agree to participate, the acceptance rate is 90%: $90 \div 100 = 0.90 \times 100\% = 90\%$.

Accessible population Portion of the target population to which the researcher has reasonable access.

Accuracy Addresses the extent to which the instrument measures what it is supposed to in a study; comparable to validity.

Accuracy of a screening test Screening tests used to confirm a diagnosis are evaluated in terms of their ability to assess the presence or absence of a disease or condition correctly as compared with a gold standard.

Administrative data Data collected within clinical agencies; obtained by national, state, and local professional organizations and collected by federal, state, and local governmental agencies.

Administrative database Resource created by insurance companies, government agencies, and others not directly involved in providing patient care; contain standardized sets of data for enormous numbers of patients and providers

Algorithm Decision tree that provides a set of rules for solving a particular practice problem. Its development usually is based on research evidence and theoretical knowledge.

Alpha (α) Cutoff point used to determine whether the samples being tested are members of the same population or of different populations; alpha is commonly set at 0.05, 0.01, or 0.001.

Alternate forms reliability Degree of equivalence of two versions of the same paper and pencil instrument.

Analysis of covariance (ANCOVA) Statistical procedure in which a regression analysis is carried out before performing ANOVA; designed to reduce the variance within groups by partialing out the variance caused by a confounding variable.

Analysis of variance (ANOVA) Statistical test used to examine differences among two or more groups by comparing the variability between groups with the variability within each group.

Analyzing research reports Critical thinking skill that involves determining the value of a study by breaking the contents of a study report into parts and examining the parts for accuracy, completeness, uniqueness of information, and organization.

Anonymity Condition in which the subject's identity cannot be linked, even by the researcher, with his or her individual responses.

Applied research Scientific investigation conducted to generate knowledge that will directly influence clinical practice.

Assent to participate in research Affirmative agreement to participate in research by a child or adult with diminished autonomy.

Associative hypothesis Hypothesis that identifies variables that occur or exist together in the real world so that when one variable changes, the other changes.

Assumption Statement taken for granted or considered true, even though it has not been scientifically tested.

Attrition rate of a sample The percentage of subjects who drop out of a study before it is completed, creating a threat to the internal validity of the study. The attrition rate is calculated by dividing the number of subjects dropping out of a study by the original sample size. For example, if the sample size were 200 and 20 subjects dropped out of the study, then $20 \div 200 \times 100\% = 10\%$.

Authority Person with expertise and power who is able to influence the opinions and behaviors of others.

Autonomous agents Prospective subjects who are informed about a proposed study and who can voluntarily choose whether to participate.

B

Background for a problem Briefly identifies what we know about a problem area in a research study.

Basic (pure) research Scientific investigations for the pursuit of "knowledge for knowledge's sake" or for the pleasure of learning and finding truth.

Benchmarking Process of measuring outcomes from a health-care agency for comparison with identified national standards.

Beneficence, principle of Principle that encourages the researcher to do good and, "above all, do no harm."

Benefit-risk ratio Ratio considered by researchers and reviewers of research as they weigh potential benefits (positive outcomes) and risks (negative outcomes) of a study; used to promote the conduct of ethical research.

Best research evidence Produced by the conduct and synthesis of numerous, high-quality studies in a health-related area. The best research evidence is generated in the areas of health promotion, illness prevention, and the assessment, diagnosis, and management of acute and chronic illnesses.

Between-group variance A source of variation of the group means around the grand mean; determined by conducting analysis of variance statistical technique.

Bias Influence or action in a study that distorts the findings or slants them away from the true or expected.

Bibliographical database Compilation of citations.

Bimodal distribution Describes a data set in which two modes exist.

Bivariate analysis Statistical procedure in which the summary values from two groups of the same variable or two variables within a group are compared.

Bivariate correlation Measure of the extent of the linear relationship between two variables.

Borrowing Appropriation and use of knowledge from other disciplines to guide nursing practice.

Bracketing Qualitative research technique of suspending or setting aside what is known about an experience being studied.

Breach of confidentiality Accidental or direct action that allows an unauthorized person to have access to raw study data.

C

Case study In-depth analysis and systematic description of one patient or a group of similar patients to promote understanding of nursing interventions.

Causal hypothesis Hypothesis that states the relationship between two variables, in which one variable (independent variable) is thought to cause or determine the presence of the other variable (dependent variable).

Causality Relationship that includes three conditions: (1) there must be a strong correlation between the proposed cause and effect; (2) the proposed cause must precede the effect in time; and (3) the cause must be present whenever the effect occurs.

Chi-square test of independence Used to analyze nominal data to determine significant differences between observed frequencies within the data and frequencies that were expected.

Citation Information necessary to locate a reference. The citation for a journal article includes the author's name, year of publication, title, journal name, volume number, issue number, and page numbers.

Clinical database Database created by providers such as hospitals, HMOs, and healthcare professionals. The clinical data are generated as a result of routine documentation of care or in relation to a research protocol.

Clinical expertise A practitioner's knowledge, skills, and past experience in accurately assessing, diagnosing, and managing an individual patient's health needs.

Clinical importance Measure related to the practical relevance of the findings of a study.

Cluster sampling Sampling in which a frame is developed that includes a list of all the states, cities, institutions, or organizations (clusters) that could be used in a study; a randomized sample is drawn from this list.

Coding Way of indexing or identifying categories in qualitative data.

Coefficient of determination (R^2) Computed from a matrix of correlation coefficients; provides important information on multicolinearity. This value indicates the degree of linear dependencies among the variables.

Coefficient of multiple determination Statistical technique that involves the use of multiple independent variables to predict one dependent variable; represented by an R^2 statistic.

Coercion Overt threat of harm or excessive reward intentionally presented by one person to another to obtain compliance—for example, offering prospective subjects a large sum of money to participate in a dangerous research project.

Comparative descriptive design Design used to describe differences in variables in two or more groups in a natural setting.

Complete review Type of institutional review process for studies with risks that are greater than minimal. The review of a study is extensive or complete by an institutional review board.

Complex hypothesis Hypothesis that predicts the relationship (associative or causal) among three or more variables; thus, the hypothesis can include two (or more) independent and/or two (or more) dependent variables.

Complex search Search that combines two or more concepts or synonyms in one search. The concepts selected for search may be based on the results of previous searches.

Comprehending a source Process completed by reading and focusing on understanding the main points of an article or other sources.

Comprehending research reports Critical thinking process used in reading a research report, in which the focus is on understanding the major concepts and logical flow of ideas in a study.

Concept Term that abstractly describes and names an object or phenomenon, thus providing it with a separate identity or meaning.

Conceptual definition Definition that provides a variable or concept with connotative (abstract, comprehensive, theoretical) meaning; established through concept analysis, concept derivation, or concept synthesis.

Conceptual model Set of highly abstract, related constructs that broadly explains phenomena of interest, expresses assumptions, and reflects a philosophical stance.

Conclusion Synthesis and clarification of the meaning of study findings.

Concrete thinking Thinking that is oriented to and limited by tangible things or events observed and experienced in reality.

Conference proceedings Collection of papers presented for review, which are later published, of a conference of major professional organizations.

Confidence interval Probability of including the value of the population in an interval estimate.

Confidentiality Management of private data in research in such a way that only the researcher knows the subjects' identities and can link them with their responses.

Confirmatory analysis Analysis performed to confirm expectations regarding data expressed as hypotheses, questions, or objectives.

Confounding variables Variables that cannot be controlled; they may be recognized before the study is initiated or may not be recognized until the study is in process.

Consent form Written form, tape recording, or video recording used to document a subject's agreement to participate in a study.

Construct   Concept at very high levels of abstraction that has general meaning.

Construct validity   Measure of how well the conceptual and operational definitions of variables match each other; determines whether the instrument measures the theoretical construct that it purports to measure.

Content validity   Extent to which the method of measurement includes all the major elements relevant to the construct being measured.

Control   Writing of a prescription to produce the desired outcomes in practice; in research, the imposing of rules by the researcher to decrease the possibility of error and increase the probability that the study's findings are an accurate reflection of reality.

Control (or comparison) group   The group of elements or subjects not exposed to the experimental treatment in a study.

Convenience sampling   Including subjects in the study who happened to be in the right place at the right time, with the addition of available subjects, until the desired sample size is reached; also referred to as "accidental sampling."

Correlational design   Design used to examine relationships between or among two or more variables in a single group in a study.

Correlational research   Systematic investigation of relationships between two or more variables to explain the nature of relationships in the world; does not examine cause and effect.

Covered entity   Public or private entity that processes or facilitates the processing of health information.

Covert data collection   Data collection that occurs without subjects' knowledge or awareness.

Credibility   The confidence of the reader about the extent to which the researchers have produced results that reflect the views of the participants; similar to validity in the critical appraisal of quantitative studies.

Critical appraisal of qualitative studies   Examines how the integrity of the design and methods will affect the credibility and meaningfulness of the findings and their usefulness in clinical practice

Critical appraisal of research   Examination of the strengths, weaknesses, meaning, credibility, and significance of nursing studies in generating knowledge.

Cross-sectional design   Examination of a group of subjects simultaneously in various stages of development, levels of education, severity of illness, or stages of recovery to describe changes in a phenomenon across stages

Current sources   Sources published within 5 years prior to acceptance of a respective manuscript for publication.

D

Data   Information collected during a study.

Data analysis   Technique used to reduce, organize, and give meaning to data.

Data-based literature   Consists of research reports, both published reports in journals and books and unpublished reports such as theses and dissertations.

Data collection   Identification of subjects and the precise, systematic gathering of information (data) relevant to the research purpose or the specific objectives, questions, or hypotheses of a study.

Data use agreement   Agreement that limits how the data set with health information may be used and how it will be protected in research.

Deception   Misinforming subjects for research purposes. After a study is completed, subjects must be debriefed or informed of the true purpose and outcomes of a study so that areas of deception are clarified.

Decision theory   Theory based on assumptions associated with the theoretical normal curve; used in testing for differences between groups, with the expectation that all the groups are members of the same population. The expectation is expressed as a null hypothesis, and the level of significance (alpha) is often set at 0.05 before data collection.

Deductive reasoning   Reasoning from the general to the specific or from a general premise to a particular situation.

Degrees of freedom (df)   The freedom of a score's value to vary, given the values of other existing scores and the established sum of these scores ($df = N - 1$).

Demographic variables   Characteristics or attributes of subjects that are collected to describe the sample.

Dependability   Documentation of steps taken and decisions made during qualitative analysis.

Dependent groups   Subjects or observations selected for data collection that are in some way related to the selection of other subjects or observations. For example, when subjects in the control group are matched for age or gender with the subjects in the experimental group, these groups are dependent groups.

Dependent (response or outcome) variable   The response, behavior, or outcome that is predicted or explained in research; changes in the dependent variable are presumed to be caused by the independent variable.

Description   Identification of the characteristics of nursing phenomena or of the relationships among these phenomena.

Descriptive correlational design   Design used to describe variables and examine relationships that exist in a situation.

Descriptive design   Design used to identify a phenomenon of interest, identify variables within the phenomenon, develop conceptual and operational definitions of variables, and describe variables.

Descriptive research   Research that provides an accurate portrayal or account of the characteristics of a particular person, event, or group in real-life situations; research that is conducted to discover new meaning, describe what exists, determine the frequency with which something occurs, and categorize information.

Descriptive statistics   Statistics that allow the researcher to organize the data in ways that give meaning and facilitate insight, such as frequency distributions and measures of central tendency and dispersion.

Design   Blueprint for conducting a study; maximizes control over factors that could interfere with the validity of the findings.

Design validity   The probability that the study findings are an accurate reflection of reality.

Determining strengths and weaknesses in the studies   The second step in critically appraising studies to determine their quality. To complete this step, the researcher must have knowledge of what each step of the research process should be like from expert sources such as this text and other research sources and compare the study steps with these sources.

Digital object identifiers (DOIs)   These have become standard for the International Standards Organization (http://www.doi.org/), but have not yet received universal support.

Diminished autonomy   Condition of subjects whose ability to give informed consent voluntarily is decreased because of legal or mental incompetence, terminal illness, or confinement to an institution.

Direct measures   Concrete variables that can be measured objectively with a specific measurement strategy, such as using a scale to measure weight.

Directional hypothesis   Hypothesis stating the specific nature of the interaction or relationship between two or more variables.

Discomfort and harm   Phrase used to describe the degree of risk for a subject participating in a study. These levels of risk include no anticipated effects, temporary discomfort, unusual levels of temporary discomfort, risk of permanent damage, or certainty of permanent damage.

Dissertation   An extensive, usually original research project completed by a doctoral student as part of the requirements for a doctoral degree.

Distal outcome   An outcome removed from proximity to the care or a service received and that is more influenced by external (nontreatment) factors than is a proximal outcome.

Duplicate publication bias   Bias referring to studies with positive results might be published more than once.

Dwelling with the data   A phrase in qualitative data analysis used to indicate that the researcher spent considerable time reading and reflecting on the data.

E

Effect size   The degree to which the phenomenon studied is present in the population or to which the null hypothesis is false.

Electronic journals   Journals that are published and available on the Internet.

Elements in studies   Persons (subjects or participants), events, behaviors, or any other units examined in studies.

Eligibility criteria   See *Sampling criteria*.

Emic approach   Anthropological research approach to studying behaviors from within a culture.

Empirical literature   Knowledge derived from research. In other words, the knowledge is based on data from research (data-based).

Encyclopedia   An authoritative compilation of information on alphabetized topics that may provide background information and lead to other sources, but is rarely cited in academic papers and publications.

Environmental variables   Types of extraneous variables composing the setting in which a study is conducted.

Equivalence   Part of reliability testing. The comparison of two versions of the same paper and pencil instrument or of two observers measuring the same event.

Error in physiological measures   Error caused by environmental factors, variations in operation of equipment, machine instability and calibration, or misinterpreted electrical signals.

Ethical principles   Principles of respect for persons, beneficence, and justice relevant to the conduct of research.

Ethnographic research   Qualitative research methodology for investigating cultures. The research involves collection, description, and analysis of data to develop a theory of cultural behavior.

Ethnonursing research   Type of research that emerged from Leininger's Theory of Transcultural Nursing; focuses mainly on observing and documenting interactions with people to determine how daily life conditions and patterns influence human care, health, and nursing care practices.

Etic approach   Anthropological research approach to studying behavior from outside the culture and examining similarities and differences across cultures.

Evaluating the credibility and meaning of study findings   Determining the validity, credibility, significance, and meaning of the study by examining the relationships among the steps of the study, study findings, and previous studies

Evaluation phase   Step of a critical appraisal in which the reader examines the meaning, credibility, and significance of a study according to set criteria and compares it with previous studies conducted in the area.

Evidence-based guidelines   Patient care guidelines based on synthesized research findings from meta-analyses, integrative reviews of research, and extensive clinical trials supported by consensus from recognized national experts and affirmed by outcomes obtained by clinicians.

Evidence-based practice (EBP)   The conscientious integration of best research evidence with clinical expertise and patients' values and needs in the delivery of high-quality, cost-effective health care.

Evidence-based practice centers (EPCs)   Centers established to develop evidence reports and technology assessments on topics relevant to clinical, social science and behavioral, economic, and other healthcare organization and delivery issues, specifically those that are common, expensive, and/or significant for the Medicare and Medicaid population.

Evidence of validity from contrasting groups   Tested by identifying groups that are expected (or known) to have contrasting scores on the instrument.

Evidence of validity from convergence   Determined when a relatively new instrument is compared with an existing instrument(s) that measures the same construct. Both instruments are administered to a sample concurrently, and results are evaluated using correlational analyses. If the measures are highly positively correlated, the validity of each instrument is strengthened.

Evidence of validity from divergence   Correlational procedures performed with the measures of two opposite concepts. If the divergent measure (despair scale) is negatively correlational with the other instrument (hope scale), validity for each of the instruments is strengthened.

Exclusion sample criteria   Sampling criteria or characteristics that can cause a person or element to be excluded from the target population.

Exempt from review   Designation given to studies that have no apparent risks for the research subjects and thus are designated as exempt by an institutional review board.

Expedited review   Institutional review process for studies that have some risks, but the risks are minimal or no greater than those ordinarily encountered in daily life or during the performance of routine physical or psychological examinations.

Experiment   Procedure in which subjects are randomized into groups, data are collected, and statistical analyses are conducted to support a premise.

Experimental design   Design that provides the greatest amount of control possible to examine causality more closely.

Experimental (or treatment) group   Group of subjects receiving the experimental treatment.

Experimental research   An objective, systematic, controlled investigation to examine probability and causality among selected variables for the purpose of predicting and controlling phenomena.

Experimenter expectancy   Expectation of the researcher that can bias data. For example, experimenter expectancy occurs if a researcher expects a particular intervention to relieve pain.

Explained variance   Variation in values explained by the relationship between the two variables.

Explanation   Clarification of relationships among variables and identification of reasons why certain events occur.

Exploratory analysis   Examining the data descriptively to become as familiar as possible with it.

External validity   Concerned with the extent to which study findings can be generalized beyond the sample used in the study

Extraneous variables   Variables that exist in all studies and can affect the measurement of study variables and the relationships among these variables.

F

Fabrication in research   A form of scientific misconduct in research that involves making up results and recording or reporting them.

Factor   A category of several closely related variables that are considered together.

Factor analysis   Analysis that examines interrelationships among large numbers of variables and disentangles those relationships to identify clusters of variables that are most closely linked. Two common types of factor analysis conducted are exploratory and confirmatory.

False-negative   Outcome of a screening test indicating that a disease is not present when it is present.

False-positive   Outcome of a screening test indicating that a disease is present when it is not present.

Falsification of research   A type of scientific misconduct that involves manipulating research materials, equipment, or processes, or changing or omitting data or results, so that the research is not accurately represented in the research record.

Feasibility of a study   Suitability of a study determined by examining the time and money commitment, researcher's expertise, availability of subjects, facility, and equipment, cooperation of others, and study's ethical considerations.

Field notes   Notations recorded by the researcher while an observation is taking place.

Findings   The translated and interpreted results from a study.

Focus groups   Measurement strategy in which groups are assembled to obtain the participants' perceptions in focused areas in settings that are permissive and nonthreatening in a qualitative study.

Focused ethnography   An observation of an organizational culture for a short period of time

Forest plot   Type of diagram used to present the meta-analysis results of studies with dichotomous outcomes

Framework   Abstract, logical structure of meaning, such as a portion of a theory, that guides the development of the study, is tested in the study, and enables the researcher to link the findings to nursing's body of knowledge.

Frequency distribution   Statistical procedure that lists all possible measures of a variable and tallies each datum on the listing.

Funnel plots   Graphic representations of possible effect sizes (ESs) for interventions in selected studies.

G

Generalization   Extension of the implications of the findings from the sample or situation that was studied to a larger population or situation.

Going native   A complication of observation in which the researcher becomes a part of the culture and loses her or his ability to observe clearly.

Gold standard   The most accurate means of currently diagnosing a particular disease; serves as a basis for comparison with newly developed diagnostic or screening tests; also, a gold standard for managing patients' care that is linked to patient outcomes.

Grand Nursing Theory   Abstract, broad scope theory.

Grey literature   Studies that have limited distributions, such as theses and dissertations, unpublished research reports, articles in obscure journals, articles in some online journals, conference papers and abstracts, conference proceedings, research reports to funding agencies, and technical reports.

Grounded theory research   Inductive research technique based on symbolic interaction theory; conducted to discover the problems that exist in a social scene and the process that persons involved use to handle them. It involves formulation, testing, and redevelopment of propositions until a theory is developed.

Grouped frequency distribution Means of grouping continuous measures of data into categories.

Grove Model for Implementing Evidence-Based Guidelines in Practice In this model, nurses identify a practice problem, search for the best research evidence to manage the problem in their practice, and use an evidence-based guideline to manage the problem.

H

Health Insurance Portability and Accountability Act (HIPAA) Federal regulations implemented in 2003 to protect an individual's health information. The HIPAA Privacy Rule affects not only the healthcare environment but also the research conducted in this environment.

Heterogeneity Variations in study areas such as sample characteristics, sample size, design, types of interventions, outcome variables, and measurement methods.

Heterogeneous sample A sample in which subjects have a broad range of values being studied, which increases the representativeness of the sample and the ability to generalize from the accessible population to the target population.

Highly controlled setting Artificially constructed environment developed for the sole purpose of conducting research, such as a laboratory, research or experimental center, or test unit.

Highly sensitive test A screening test that indicates a true-positive test result for a large proportion of patients with the disease.

Highly specific test A screening test that indicates a true-negative test result for a large proportion of patients without the disease.

Historical research Narrative description or analysis of events that occurred in the remote or recent past.

Homogeneity A type of reliability testing used primarily with paper and pencil instruments or scales to address the correlation of each question to the other questions in the scale.

Homogeneous sample Sample in which subjects' scores on selected measurement methods in a study are similar, resulting in a limited or narrow distribution or spread of scores.

Human rights Claims and demands that have been justified in the eyes of an individual or by the consensus of a group of people and are protected in research.

Hypothesis Formal statement of the expected relationship between two or more variables in a specified population.

I

Identifying the steps of the research process The first step in critical appraisal. It involves understanding the terms and concepts in the report, as well as identifying study elements and grasping the nature, significance, and meaning of these elements.

Implications for nursing The meaning of research conclusions for the body of nursing knowledge, theory, and practice.

Implicit framework Rudimentary ideas for the framework of a theory or portions of a theory expressed in an introduction or in a literature review in which linkages among variables found in previous studies are discussed.

Inclusion sample criteria Those sampling criteria or characteristics that the subject or element must possess to be considered part of the target population.

Independent groups Study groups chosen so that the selection of one subject is unrelated to the selection of other subjects. For example, if subjects are randomly assigned to a treatment group or a comparison group, the groups are independent.

Independent (treatment or intervention) variable Treatment or intervention that is manipulated or varied by the researcher to cause an effect on the dependent variable.

Index Library resource that can be used to identify journal articles and other publications relevant to a topic.

Indirect measures or indicators Methods used with abstract concepts that are not measured directly; rather, indicators or attributes of the concepts are used to represent the abstraction and are measured in the study.

Individually identifiable health information (IIHI) "... any information, including demographic information collected from an individual that is created or received by healthcare provider, health plan, or healthcare clearinghouse; and related to past, present, or future physical or mental health condition of an individual, the provision of health care to an individual, or the past, present, or future payment for the provision of health care to an individual, and identifies the individual; or with respect to which there is a reasonable basis to believe that the information can be used to identify the individual" (U.S. Department of Health and Human Services, 2003, 45 CFR, Section 160.103).

Inductive reasoning Reasoning from the specific to the general, in which particular instances are observed and then combined into a larger whole or general statement.

Inference Generalization from a specific case to a general truth, from a part to the whole, from the concrete to the abstract, or from the known to the unknown.

Inferential statistics Statistics designed to address objectives, questions, and hypotheses in a study to allow inference from the study sample to the target population.

Informed consent Agreement by a prospective subject to participate voluntarily in a study after he or she has assimilated essential information about the study.

Institutional review Process of examining studies for ethical concerns by a committee of peers.

Institutional review board (IRB) A committee that reviews research to ensure that the investigator is conducting the research ethically.

Instrumentation Component of measurement in which specific rules are applied to develop a measurement device or instrument.

Integrative review of the literature Rigorous analysis and synthesis of results from independent quantitative and qualitative studies and theoretical and methodological literature to determine the current knowledge (what is known and not known) for a particular concept, measurement methods, or practice topic.

Integrative review of research Review conducted to identify, analyze, and synthesize the results from independent studies to determine the current knowledge (what is known and not known) in a particular area.

Intellectual critical appraisal of a study Careful examination of all aspects of a study to judge the strengths, weaknesses, meaning, credibility, and significance of the study based on previous research experience and knowledge of the topic.

Internal consistency Measures the extent to which all the items in an instrument consistently measure the construct.

Internal validity The extent to which the effects detected in the study are a true reflection of reality rather than the result of extraneous variables.

Interpretation Process whereby the researcher places the findings in a larger context and may link different themes or factors in the findings to each other.

Interpretation of research outcomes Process in which researchers examine the results from data analysis, form conclusions, consider the implications for nursing, explore the significance of the findings, generalize the findings, and suggest further studies.

Interrater reliability Comparison of two observers or two judges in a study

Interval-level measurement Measurement that uses interval scales, which have equal numerical distances between intervals and also follows the rules of mutually exclusive categories, exhaustive categories, and rank ordering, such as temperature.

Intervention Treatment or independent variable manipulated during the conduct of a study to produce an effect on the dependent or outcome variables.

Intervention fidelity Fidelity that includes the detailed description of the essential elements of the intervention and the consistent implementation of the intervention during the study.

Interview Structured or unstructured oral communication between the researcher and subject or study participant during which information is obtained for a study.

Intraproject sampling Additional sampling done during data collection and analysis to promote the development of quality study findings.

Intuition Insight or understanding of a situation or an event as a whole that usually cannot be logically explained.

Invasion of privacy Sharing private information with others without a person's knowledge or against his or her will.

Iowa Model of Evidence-Based Practice Provides direction for the development of EBP in a clinical agency. In a healthcare agency, there are triggers that initiate the need for change; the focus should always be on making changes based on the best research evidence.

J

K

Key informant Person in an ethnographic study with extensive knowledge and influence in a culture with whom a researcher may form a close bond.

Key words Major concepts or variables of a research problem or topic used to begin a search of a database.

Knowledge Information that is acquired in a variety of ways, is expected to be an accurate reflection of reality, and is incorporated and used to direct a person's actions.

L

Landmark studies Major projects generating knowledge that influence a discipline and sometimes society in general.

Levels of measurement Organized set of rules for assigning numbers to objects so that a hierarchy in measurement from low to high is established. The levels of measurement are nominal, ordinal, interval, and ratio.

Level of statistical significance Probability level at which the results of statistical analysis is judged to indicate a statistically significant difference between groups. The level of significance for most nursing studies is 0.05.

Likelihood ratios (LRs) Additional calculations that can help researchers determine the accuracy of diagnostic or screening tests, which are based on the sensitivity and specificity results.

Likert scale Scale designed to determine the opinions or attitudes of study subjects; contains a number of declarative statements, with a scale after each statement

Limitations Theoretical and methodological restrictions in a study that may decrease the generalizability of the findings.

Line of best fit Best reflection of the values on the scatterplot.

Literature All written sources relevant to the topic that the researcher has selected, including articles published in periodicals or journals, Internet publications, monographs, encyclopedias, conference papers, theses, dissertations, clinical journals, textbooks, and other books.

Literature review Review of theoretical and empirical sources to generate a picture of what is known and not known about a particular problem.

Location bias of studies Bias that can occur if studies are published in lower impact journals and indexed in less searched databases.

Longitudinal design Design that involves collecting data from the same subjects at different points in time; might also be referred to as repeated measures.

Low statistical power Statistical issue that increases the probability of concluding that there is no significant difference between samples when actually there is a difference (type II error).

M

Manipulation Moving around or controlling specific attributes of a treatment or intervention in a study.

Maps (or models) Diagrams that graphically express the concepts and relationships of theories or frameworks.

Mean The value obtained by summing all the scores and dividing the total by the number of scores being summed.

Mean difference A standard statistic that identifies the absolute difference between two groups.

Measurement Process of assigning numbers to objects, events, or situations in accordance with some rule.

Measurement error Difference between what exists in reality and what is measured by a research instrument.

Measure of central tendency Statistical procedure (mode, median, and mean) for determining the center of a distribution of scores.

Measure of dispersion Statistical procedure (range, difference scores, sum of squares, variance, and standard deviation) for examining how scores vary or are dispersed around the mean.

Median Score at the exact center of the ungrouped frequency distribution.

Mentorship Intense form of role modeling in which an expert nurse serves as a teacher, sponsor, guide, exemplar, and counselor for a novice nurse.

Meta-analysis Statistical analysis carried out to integrate and synthesize findings from completed studies to determine what is known and not known about a particular research area.

Meta-summary Synthesis of multiple primary qualitative studies to develop a description of current knowledge in an area.

Meta-synthesis Synthesis of qualitative research involving the critical analysis of primary qualitative studies and synthesis of findings into a new theory or framework for the topic of interest.

Methodological bias Bias related to design and data analysis problems in studies. For example, studies might have limitations related to the sample, intervention, outcome measurements, and analysis techniques that result in methodological bias.

Middle-range theories Theories that are relatively concrete and specific in focus; include a limited number of concepts and propositions. These theories are tested by empirical research.

Minimal risk Research subject's risk of harm anticipated in the proposed study that is not greater, considering probability and magnitude, than that ordinarily encountered in daily life or during the performance of routine physical or psychological examinations.

Mixed-methods approach Approach that offers investigators the ability to use the strengths of qualitative and quantitative research designs. Mixed-methods research is characterized as research that contains elements of qualitative and quantitative approaches

Mixed-methods systematic review Synthesis that includes various study designs, such as qualitative research and quasi-experimental, correlational, and descriptive quantitative studies

Mixed results Study results that include significant and non-significant findings.

Mode Numerical value or score that occurs with the greatest frequency in a distribution but does not necessarily indicate the center of the data set.

Model testing design Design that requires all concepts relevant to the model to be measured and the relationships among these concepts examined

Moderator, or facilitator Conductor of a focus group, who may or may not be the researcher.

Monographs Sources that usually are written once, such as books, booklets of conference proceedings, or pamphlets, and may be updated with a new edition.

Multicausality Recognition that a number of interrelated variables can cause a particular effect.

Multiple regression Extension of simple linear regression; more than one independent variable is analyzed.

N

Natural (field) setting Uncontrolled, real-life setting in which research is conducted, such as a subject's home, workplace, and school.

Necessary relationship Relationship in which one variable or concept must occur for the second variable or concept to occur.

Negative likelihood ratio The ratio of true-negative results to false-negative results,

Negative relationship Relationship in which one variable or concept changes (its value increases or decreases), and the other variable or concept changes in the opposite direction.

Network sampling Sampling technique that takes advantage of social networks and the fact that friends tend to have characteristics in common; subjects meeting the sample criteria are asked to assist in locating others with similar characteristics.

Nominal-level measurement The lowest of the four types of measurement categories. It is used when data can be organized into categories of a defined property that are exclusive and exhaustive but the categories cannot be rank-ordered, such as gender, ethnicity, marital status, and diagnoses.

Nondirectional hypothesis Hypothesis that states that a relationship exists but does not predict the exact nature of the relationship.

Nonequivalent comparison group design Design in which the control group is not selected by random means, such as the one-group post-test–only design, post-test–only design with nonequivalent groups, and one-group pretest–post-test design.

Nonexperimental design Descriptive and correlational design that focuses on examining variables as they naturally occur in an environment, not on the implementation of a treatment by the researcher.

Nonparametric analysis Analysis performed when variables are measured at the nominal and ordinal levels.

Nonprobability sampling Sampling in which not every element of the population has an opportunity for selection, such as convenience sampling, quota sampling, purposive sampling, and network sampling.

Nonsignificant results Results that are negative or contrary to the researcher's hypotheses; the results may accurately reflect reality or may be caused by study weaknesses.

Nontherapeutic research Research conducted to generate knowledge for a discipline; the results might benefit future patients but will probably not benefit the research subjects.

Normal curve   Symmetrical, unimodal, bell-shaped curve that is a theoretical distribution of all possible scores; no real distribution exactly fits the normal curve.

Null hypothesis (H0)   Hypothesis stating that no relationship exists between the variables being studied; a hypothesis used for statistical testing and for interpreting statistical outcomes.

Nurse's role in outcomes   The nurse's role in outcomes of a study has three subcomponents—nurse's" independent role, nurse's dependent role, and nurse's interdependent role. Independent role functions include assessment, diagnosis, nurse-initiated interventions, and follow-up care.

Nursing Care Report Card   Tool created by the American Nurses Association in 1994 to facilitate benchmarking or set a desired standard that would allow comparisons of hospitals in terms of their nursing care quality.

Nursing process   Subset of the problem-solving process. Steps include assessment, diagnosis, plan, implementation, evaluation, and modification.

Nursing research   Scientific process that validates and refines existing knowledge and generates knowledge that directly and indirectly influences clinical nursing practice.

Nursing-sensitive patient outcome (NSPO)   Outcome that is sensitive because it is influenced by nursing care decisions and actions. It may not be caused by nursing but is associated with nursing.

O

Observation   A fundamental method of gathering data for qualitative studies, especially ethnographic studies.

Observational measurement   Use of structured and unstructured observations to measure study variables.

Odds ratio (OR)   The ratio of the odds of an event occurring in one group, such as the treatment group, to the odds of it occurring in another group, such as the standard care group.

One-tailed test of significance   Analysis used with directional hypotheses, in which extreme statistical values of interest are thought to occur in a single tail of the normal curve.

Open-ended interview   Interview with a defined focus but no fixed sequence of questions. The questions addressed may change as the researcher gains insight from previous interviews and observations and respondents are encouraged to raise important issues not addressed by the researcher.

Operational definition   Description of how variables or concepts will be measured or manipulated in a study.

Ordinal-level measurement   Method whereby data are assigned to categories that can be ranked. To rank data, one category is judged to be (or is ranked) higher or lower, or better or worse, than another category. The intervals between the ranked data are not necessarily equal, such as ranking pain as mild, moderate, and severe.

Outcome reporting bias   Bias that occurs when study results are not reported clearly and with complete accuracy.

Outcomes research   Important scientific methodology developed to examine the end results of patient care. The strategies used in outcomes research are a departure from those used in traditional scientific endeavors; they incorporate evaluation research, epidemiology, and economic theory perspectives.

Outliers   Extreme scores or values caused by inherent variability, errors of measurement or execution, or error in identifying the variables important in explaining the nature of the phenomenon under study.

P

Paired (or dependent) groups   Subjects or observations selected for data collection which are related in some way to the selection of other subjects or observations.

Parametric analysis   Analysis of data for variables measured at the interval and ratio levels that are normally distributed. Interval and ratio levels of data are often included together because the analysis techniques are the same whether the data are at the interval or ratio level of measurement.

Paraphrasing   Clearly and concisely restating the ideas of an author in the researcher's own words.

Partially controlled setting   Environment that is manipulated or modified in some way by the researcher.

Participant   Individual who participates cooperatively in studies with researchers. Qualitative researchers use the term participants; quantitative researchers might call them subjects or participants.

Patient health outcomes   Outcomes based on the Nursing Role Effectiveness Model. The outcomes of the independent role are clinical and symptom control, freedom from complications, functional status and self-care, and knowledge of disease and its treatment, satisfaction, and costs.

Pearson product-moment correlation   Parametric test used to determine relationships among variables.

Peer-reviewed   Refers to publications for which scholars familiar with the topic of the research read the report and validate its accuracy and appropriateness of the methodology used in the study.

Percentage distributions   Percentage of the sample whose scores fall into a specific group and the number of scores in that group.

Periodicals   Literature sources such as journals that are published over time and are numbered sequentially for the years published.

Permission to participate in research   The agreement of parent(s) or guardian to the participation of their child or ward in research.

Personal experience   Knowledge gained through participation in rather than observation of an event, situation, or circumstance. Benner (1984) described five levels of experience in the development of clinical nursing knowledge and expertise: (1) novice, (2) advanced beginner, (3) competent, (4) proficient, and (5) expert.

Phenomenology   A philosophy and a group of research methods congruent with the philosophy.

Phenomenon (plural, phenomena)   An occurrence or a circumstance that is observed, something that impresses the observer as extraordinary, or something that appears to and is constructed by the mind.

Philosophies Rational, intellectual explorations of truths; principles of being, knowledge, or conduct.

Physiological measures Measurement methods used to quantify the level of functioning of living beings.

PICOS format Format used to formulate a relevant clinical question for a systematic review. Elements include population or participants of interest, intervention needed for practice, comparisons of interventions to determine the best for practice, outcomes needed for practice, and study design.

Pilot study Smaller version of a proposed study conducted to develop and refine the methodology, such as the treatment or intervention, instruments, or data collection process to be used in the larger study.

Plagiarism A type of scientific misconduct that appropriates another person's ideas, processes, results, or words without giving appropriate credit, including those obtained through confidential review of others' research proposals and manuscripts.

Population All elements (people, objects, events, or substances) that meet the sample criteria for inclusion in a study; sometimes referred to as a target population.

Population-based studies Important type of outcomes research that involves studying health conditions in the context of the community rather than the context of the medical system.

Positive likelihood ratio The ratio of the true-positive results to false-positive results. It is calculated by:

$$\text{Positive LR} = \text{sensitivity} \div (100\% - \text{specificity})$$

Positive relationship Relationship in which one variable changes (its value increases or decreases) and the second variable changes in the same direction.

Posthoc analyses Statistical techniques performed in studies with more than two groups to determine which groups are significantly different. For example, ANOVA may indicate significant differences among three groups, but the posthoc analyses indicate specifically which groups are different.

Power Probability that a statistical test will detect a significant difference or relationship that exists; power analysis is used to determine the power of a study.

Power analysis Technique used to determine the risk of a type II error so that the study can be modified to decrease the risk if necessary and ensure that the study has adequate sample size.

Practice theories Very specific theories developed to explain a particular element of practice. These theories can be generated through research and tested by research.

Precision Accuracy with which the population parameters have been estimated within a study; also used to describe the degree of consistency or reproducibility of measurements with physiological instruments.

Prediction Estimation of the probability of a specific outcome in a given situation that can be achieved through research.

Predictive correlational design Design developed to predict the value of one dependent variable based on values obtained for other independent variables; an approach to examining causal relationships between or among variables.

Premise Proposition or statement of the proposed relationship between two or more concepts.

Primary data Data collected for a particular study.

Primary source Source whose author originated or is responsible for generating the ideas published.

Principle of beneficence Ethical principle that encourages researchers to do good and, "above all, do no harm."

Principle of justice Ethical principle that states that human subjects should be treated fairly in terms of the benefits and risks of research.

Principle of respect for persons Ethical principle indicating that people should be treated as autonomous agents with the right to self-determination and the freedom to participate or not participate in research.

Privacy Freedom to determine the time, extent, and general circumstances under which private information will be shared with or withheld from others.

Probability Chance that a given event will occur in a situation; addresses the relative rather than the absolute causality of events.

Probability sampling Random sampling technique in which every member (element) of the population has a probability higher than zero of being selected for the sample, such as simple random sampling, stratified random sampling, cluster sampling, and systematic sampling.

Probability theory Theory addressing statistical analysis from the perspective of the extent of a relationship or the probability of accurately predicting an event.

Probe Query by the researcher to obtain more information from the participant about a particular question.

Problem-solving process Systematic identification of a problem, determination of goals related to the problem, identification of possible approaches to achieve those goals, implementation of selected approaches, and evaluation of goal achievement.

Problem statement Statement that concludes the discussion of a problem and indicates the gap in the knowledge needed for practice. The problem statement usually provides a basis for the study purpose.

Process Purpose, series of actions, and goal.

Proposition Abstract statements that further clarify the relationship between two concepts in theories.

Prospective cohort study An epidemiological study in which the researcher identifies a group of people at risk for experiencing a particular event and then follows them over time to observe whether or not the event occurs.

Proximal outcome An outcome close to the delivery of care.

Public library Library that serves the needs of the community in which it is located; usually contains few research reports.

Purposeful (or purposive) sampling Judgmental or selective sampling that involves the conscious selection by the researcher of certain participants or elements to include in a study. This sampling strategy is often used in qualitative research.

Q

Qualitative research Systematic, subjective methodological approach used to describe life experiences and give them meaning.

Qualitative research critical appraisal process   Three-part process that consists of (1) identifying the components of the qualitative research process in studies, (2) determining study strengths and weaknesses, and (3) evaluating the trustworthiness, credibility, and meaning of study findings.

Quality and Safety Education for Nurses (QSEN)   An initiative focused on developing the requisite knowledge, skills, and attitude (KSA) statements for each of the competencies for prelicensure and graduate education.

Quality of care   Outcome examined in the conduct of outcomes research.

Quantitative research   Formal, objective, systematic process used to describe variables, test relationships between them, and examine cause and effect interactions among variables.

Quantitative research process   Conceptualizing, planning, implementing, and communicating the findings of a quantitative research project.

Quasi-experimental design   Types of design developed to determine the effectiveness of interventions in quantitative quasi-experimental studies.

Quasi-experimental research   Type of quantitative research conducted to explain relationships, clarify why certain events happen, and examine causality between selected independent and dependent variables.

Questionnaire   Printed self-report form designed to elicit information that can be obtained through written or verbal responses of the subject.

Quota sampling   Convenience sampling technique with an added strategy to ensure the inclusion of subjects who are likely to be underrepresented in the convenience sample, such as women, minority groups, and undereducated persons.

R

Random assignment to groups   Procedure used to assign subjects randomly to a treatment or control group; subjects have an equal probability of being assigned to either group.

Random measurement error   Error that causes individual subjects' observed scores to vary haphazardly around their true scores.

Random sampling   Technique in which every member (element) of the population has a probability higher than zero for being selected for a sample, which increases the sample's representativeness of the target population.

Random variation   The expected difference in values that occurs when the researcher examines different subjects from the same sample.

Randomized controlled trial (RCT)   Classic means of examining the effects of various treatments in which the effects of a treatment are examined by comparing the treatment group with the nontreatment group.

Range   The simplest measure of dispersion. The range is determined by subtracting the lowest score from the highest score or just identifying the lowest and highest scores.

Rating scale   Scale that lists an ordered series of categories of a variable; assumed to be based on an underlying continuum.

Ratio-level measurement   The highest form of measurement; meets all the rules of other forms of measurement—mutually exclusive categories, exhaustive categories, ordered ranks, equally spaced intervals, and a continuum of values; also includes an absolute zero.

Readability level   Measurement focused on the study participants' ability to read and comprehend the content of an instrument or scale

Reading research reports   Process used to learn about research studies; skills used include skimming, comprehending, and analyzing the content of the report.

Reasoning   Processing and organizing ideas to reach conclusions; types of reasoning include problematic, operational, dialectic, and logistic.

Recommendations for further study   Suggestions provided by a study's researcher for ways to design a better study next time. Recommendations can include replications or repeating the design with a different or larger sample, using different measurement methods, or testing a new treatment.

Refereed journal   Journal that uses referees or expert reviewers to determine whether a manuscript will be accepted for publication.

Reference   A documentation of the origin of the cited quote or paraphrased idea that provides enough information for the reader to locate the original material.

Referencing   Comparing a subject's score against a standard; used in norm-referenced and criterion-referenced testing.

Refusal rate   The percentage of subjects who declined to participate in the study. The study should include their rationale for not participating. The refusal rate is calculated by dividing the number refusing to participate by the number of potential subjects approached. For example, if 100 subjects are approached and 15 refuse to participate, the refusal rate is $15 \div 100 = 0.15 \times 100\% = 15\%$.

Regression analysis   Statistical procedure used to predict the value of one variable using known values of one or more other variables.

Relational statement   Declaration that a relationship of some type exists between (or among) two or more concepts.

Relative advantage   Extent to which an innovation is perceived to be better than current practice.

Relevant studies   Investigations or studies that have a specific focus in a researcher's area of interest.

Reliability   Extent to which an instrument consistently measures a concept; three types of reliability are stability, equivalence, and homogeneity.

Reliability testing   Measure of the amount of random error in the measurement technique.

Replication studies   Studies that are reproduced or repeated to determine whether similar findings will be obtained.

Researcher-participant relationship   Relationship that has an impact on the collection and interpretation of data. The researcher creates a respectful relationship with each participant, which includes being honest and open about the purpose and methods of the study.

Representativeness Refers to the representativeness of a sample in a study or the degree to which the sample, accessible population, and target population are alike.

Research Diligent, systematic inquiry or investigation to validate and refine existing knowledge and generate new knowledge.

Research-based protocol Document providing clearly developed steps for implementing a treatment or intervention in practice that is based on findings from studies.

Research concepts The ideas, experiences, situations, or events that are investigated in qualitative research.

Research design Blueprint for conducting a study. It maximizes control over factors that could interfere with the validity of the findings and guides the planning and implementation of a study in a way that is most likely to achieve the intended goal.

Research hypothesis Alternative hypothesis to the null hypothesis; states that a relationship exists between two or more variables.

Research misconduct Intentional deviation from practices commonly accepted within the scientific community for proposing, conducting, or reporting research; may include fabrication, falsification, or plagiarism; does not include honest errors or honest differences in interpretation or judgment of data.

Research objective Clear, concise, declarative statement expressed to direct a study; focuses on identifying and describing variables and relationships among variables.

Research outcomes Conclusions of findings, generalization of findings, implications of findings for nursing, and suggestions for further study presented in the discussion section of the research report.

Research problem An area of concern in which there is a gap in the knowledge base needed for nursing practice. Research is conducted to generate essential knowledge to address the practice concern, with the ultimate goal of providing evidence-based practice. The research problem in a study needs to include significance, background, and problem statement.

Research process Process that requires an understanding of a unique language; involves rigorous application of a variety of research methods.

Research purpose Concise, clear statement of the specific goal or aim of the study. The purpose is generated from the problem.

Research question Concise interrogative statement developed to direct a study; focuses on describing variables, examining relationships among variables, and determining the differences between two or more groups.

Research report Report summarizing the major elements of a study and identifying the contributions of that study to nursing knowledge.

Research setting The site or location used to conduct a study.

Research topic Concept or broad problem area that provides the basis for generating numerous questions and research problems.

Research variables or concepts The qualities, properties, or characteristics identified in the research purpose and objectives or questions that are observed or measured in a study.

Researcher-participant relationship Relationship between the researcher and individual participants being studied in qualitative research.

Results Outcomes from data analysis that are generated for each research objective, question, or hypothesis; results can be mixed, nonsignificant, significant and not predicted, significant and predicted, or unexpected.

Retrospective cohort study An epidemiological study in which the researcher identifies a group of people who have experienced a particular event and study their outcomes.

Review of literature Summary of current theoretical and empirical sources to generate a picture of what is known and not known about a particular problem.

Review of relevant literature Review of current studies conducted to generate what is known and not known about a problem and to determine whether the knowledge is ready for use in practice.

Rigor Excellence in research; attained through the use of discipline, scrupulous adherence to detail, and strict accuracy.

Risk difference (RD) (or absolute risk reduction) The risk of an event in the experimental group minus the risk of the event in the control or standard care group.

Risk ratio, or relative risk (RR) The ratio of the risk of subjects in the intervention group to the risk of subjects in the control group for having a particular health outcome.

Role modeling Process of teaching less experienced professionals by demonstrating model behavior.

S

Sample Subset of the population that is selected for a study.

Sample attrition Withdrawal or loss of subjects from a study that can be expressed as the number of subjects withdrawing or a percentage. The percentage is the sample attrition rate; it is best if researchers include both the number of subjects withdrawing and the attrition rate. (See *Attrition rate of a sample*.)

Sample characteristics Demographic data analyzed to provide a picture of the sample.

Sample retention Number of subjects who remain in and complete a study.

Sample size Number of subjects, events, behaviors, or situations examined in a study.

Sampling Process of selecting a group of people, events, behaviors, or other elements that are representative of the population being studied.

Sampling, or eligibility, criteria List of the characteristics essential for inclusion or exclusion in the target population.

Sampling frame List of every member of the population; sampling criteria are used to define membership in the population.

Sampling method, or plan Strategies used to obtain a sample, including probability and nonprobability sampling techniques; also called a sampling plan.

Saturation of information Phenomenon that occurs when additional sampling provides no new information or there is redundancy of previously collected data. Sample size in a qualitative study is determined when saturation of data occurs.

Scale Self-report form of measurement composed of several items thought to measure the construct being studied; the subject responds to each item on the continuum or scale provided.

Scatterplot Diagram or figure showing the dispersion of scores on a variable from a study, or depicting the relationship of scores on one variable with scores on another variable. A scatterplot has two scales, horizontal (x-axis) and vertical (y-axis).

Scientific theory Theory that has been repeatedly tested through research with valid and reliable methods of measuring each concept and relational statement.

Secondary analysis Reanalysis of information or data that has previously been collected by another researcher or organization.

Secondary data Data collected from previous research, stored in a database, and used by other researchers to address their study purposes.

Secondary source Source whose author summarizes or quotes content from primary sources.

Semistructured interview Interview with a fixed set of questions and no fixed responses.

Sensitivity The proportion of patients with the disease who have a positive test result, or true-positive.

Sensitivity of physiological measures Amount of change of a parameter that can be measured precisely.

Setting Location for conducting research; can be natural, partially controlled, or highly controlled.

Significance of a research problem Indicates the importance of the problem to nursing and health care and to the health of individuals, families, and communities.

Significant and unpredicted results Results that are opposite of those predicted by the researcher; indicate that flaws are present in the logic of both the researcher and theory being tested.

Significant results Results that agree with those identified by the researcher.

Simple hypothesis Hypothesis stating the relationship (associative or causal) between two variables.

Simple linear regression Name of analysis procedure in which one independent variable is used to predict a dependent variable.

Simple random sampling Random selection of elements from the sampling frame for inclusion in a study.

Skewness Absence of symmetry in the curve formed by the distribution of scores; distribution can be positively or negatively skewed.

Skimming research reports Quickly reviewing a source to gain a broad overview of the content by reading the title, author's name, abstract or introduction, headings, one or two sentences under each heading, and discussion section.

Specific proposition Relational statement made in a narrow way, which makes the statement more concrete and testable.

Specificity The proportion of patients without the disease who have a negative test result, or true-negative.

Stability Type of measurement reliability that is concerned with the consistency of repeated measures; usually referred to as test-retest reliability.

Standard deviation Measure of dispersion calculated by taking the square root of the variance.

Standardized mean difference (SMD), or d A summary statistic that is reported in a meta-analysis when the same outcome is measured by different scales or methods.

Standardized mortality ratio (SMR) The observed number of deaths divided by the expected number of deaths and multiplied by 100. SMR is regarded as a measure of the relative risk of the studied group to die of a particular condition.

Standardized score Score used to express deviations from the mean (difference scores) in terms of standard deviation units, such as Z-score, in which the mean is 0 and the standard deviation is 1.

Standard of care Norm on which quality of care is judged.

Statements Express claims that compute to a theory; theories include existence and relational statements.

Statistical conclusion validity Extent to which the conclusions about relationships and differences drawn from statistical analyses reflect reality.

Statistical hypothesis, or null hypothesis (H0) Used for statistical testing and for interpreting statistical outcomes. Even if the null hypothesis is not stated, it is implied, because it is the converse of the research hypothesis.

Statistical significance Extent to which the results are probably not caused by chance.

Statistical techniques Analysis procedures used to examine, reduce, and give meaning to the numerical data gathered in a study.

Stetler Model of Research Utilization to Facilitate Evidence-Based Practice An initial model for research utilization in nursing to promote evidence-based practice for nursing; provides a comprehensive framework to enhance the use of research evidence by nurses to facilitate an EBP.

Stratified random sampling Technique used when the researcher knows some of the variables in the population that are critical to achieving representativeness; the sample is divided into strata or groups using these identified variables.

Structural variables Factors such as the organization of nursing care and nursing leadership that have effects on nursing practice and, in turn, on patient outcomes.

Structured interview Interview in which strategies are used that give the researcher increasing control over the content. An example is a questionnaire with structured responses.

Structured observational measurement Clear identification of what is to be observed; precise definition of how the observations are to be made, recorded, and coded.

Structure in outcomes Includes three subcomponents—nurse, organization, and patient.

Structures of care The elements of organization and administration that guide the processes of care.

Study validity   A measure of the truth or accuracy of the findings obtained from a study. The validity of a study's design is central to obtaining quality results and findings from a study

Subjects   Individuals participating in a study (those being studied), who are sometimes referred to as participants.

Substantive theory   Theory recognized within a discipline as being useful for explaining important phenomena.

Symbolic interaction theory   Explores how people define reality and how their beliefs are related to their actions.

Symmetrical   Term used to describe the normal curve, in which both sides of the curve are mirror images of each other.

Synthesis   Clustering and interrelating ideas from several sources to form a gestalt or a new, complete picture of what is known and not known in an area.

Systematic bias   See *Systematic variation*.

Systematic measurement error   Measurement error that is not random but occurs consistently in the same direction, such as a scale that inaccurately weighs subjects as being 3 pounds heavier than their actual weight.

Systematic review   Structured, comprehensive synthesis of quantitative and outcomes studies in a particular healthcare area to determine the best research evidence available for expert clinicians to use to promote evidence-based practice.

Systematic sampling   Selecting every kth (value determined by the researcher) individual from an ordered list of all members of a population, using a randomly selected starting point.

Systematic variation   Phenomenon that occurs when the selected subject's measurement values vary in some way from those of the population.

T

Target population   Population determined by the sampling criteria.

Tentative theory   Theory that is newly proposed, has had minimal exposure to critique by scholars in the discipline, and has undergone little testing.

Testable hypothesis   Hypothesis containing variables that can be measured or manipulated in the real world.

Test-retest reliability   Determination of the stability or consistency of a measurement technique by correlating the scores obtained from repeated measures.

Textbook   Book regarded as standard for the study of a particular subject.

Theoretical literature   Concept analyses, maps, theories, and conceptual frameworks that support a selected research problem and purpose.

Theoretical sampling   Sampling in which data are gathered from any individual study participant or group that can provide relevant information for theory generation.

Theory   Integrated set of defined concepts, existence statements, and relational statements that present a view of a phenomenon; can be used to describe, explain, predict, and control that phenomenon.

Therapeutic research   Research that provides a patient with an opportunity to receive an experimental treatment that might have beneficial results.

Thesis   Research project completed by a graduate student as part of the requirements for a master's degree.

Threats to design validity   Possible problems in a study's design that are organized into four categories—statistical conclusion validity, internal validity, construct validity, and external validity.

Time lag bias of studies   Time span between the generation of new knowledge through research and the use of this knowledge in practice.

Total variance   The combination of the within-group variance and between-group variance determined when conducting an analysis of variance statistical technique.

Traditions   Truths or beliefs based on customs and past trends.

Transcription   Written record created from an audio recording.

Transferable   Used to describe qualitative findings as they are applicable in other settings with similar participants.

Translational research   Evolving concept defined by the NIH as the translation of basic scientific discoveries into practical applications.

Trial and error   Approach with unknown outcomes used in an uncertain situation when other sources of knowledge are unavailable.

Triangulation   Use of two or more theories, methods, data sources, investigators, or analysis methods in a study.

True measure, or score   Score that would be obtained if no measurement error occurred (but there is always some measurement error).

True-negative   Negative test result that accurately indicates that a disease is not present.

True-positive   Positive test result that is an accurate identification of the presence of a disease.

Trustworthiness   Strength of a qualitative study determined by evaluating all study aspects.

***t*-test**   Parametric analysis technique used to determine significant differences between measures of two samples.

Two-tailed test of significance   Analysis technique used for a nondirectional hypothesis when the researcher assumes that an extreme score can occur in either tail of the normal curve.

Type I error   Error that occurs when the researcher concludes that the samples tested are from different populations (a significant difference exists between groups) when, in fact, the samples are from the same population (no significant difference exists between groups); the null hypothesis is rejected when it is true.

Type II error   Error that occurs when the researcher concludes that no significant difference exists between the samples examined when, in fact, a difference exists; the null hypothesis is regarded as true when it is false.

Typical descriptive design   Design used to examine and describe variables in a single sample.

U

Unexpected results   Study results indicating relationships between variables or differences among groups that were not hypothesized and not predicted from the framework being used.

Unexplained variance   Part of the variation between or among two or more variables that is the result of things other than the relationship.

Ungrouped frequency distribution   Means of identifying and displaying all numerical values obtained for a particular variable from the subjects studied.

Unstructured interview   Interview that is initiated with a broad question; subjects usually are encouraged to elaborate further on particular dimensions of a topic and often control the content of the interview.

Unstructured observation   Spontaneous observation and recording of what is seen; planning is minimal.

V

Validity   Extent to which an instrument accurately reflects the abstract construct (or concept) being examined.

Variables   Qualities, properties, or characteristics of persons, things, or situations that change or vary and are manipulated or measured in research.

Variance   Measure of dispersion in which the larger the variance, the larger the dispersion of scores. Variance is calculated as one of the steps in determining standard deviation.

Verification of information   Occurs when researchers are able to further confirm hunches, relationships, or theoretical models.

Visual analog scale   A 100-mm line, with right angle stops at either end, on which subjects are asked to record their response to a study variable.

Voluntary consent   Decision made by a prospective subject, of his or her own volition, without coercion or any undue influence, to participate in a study.

W

Within-group variance   Source of variation that reflects the individual scores in a group that vary from the group mean; determined by conducting analysis of variance.

X

x-axis   The horizontal scale of a scatterplot.

Y

y-axis   The vertical scale of a scatterplot.

Z

Z-score   Standardized score of the normal curve that is equivalent to the standard deviation of the normal curve.

INDEX

Note: Page numbers followed by *b* indicate boxes, *f* indicate figures and *t* indicate tables.

A

AAALAC. *see* American Association for Accreditation of Laboratory Animal Care (AAALAC)

AACN. *see* American Association of Colleges of Nursing (AACN)

Abstracts
critical appraisal of, 364
definition of, describing theories, 190
review of, to identify relevant studies, 179
section, in research reports, 51, 52*b*

Academic Center for Evidence-Based Nursing, website, 455

Academic Search Complete, as database for nursing literature reviews, 177*t*

Acceptance rates
adequacy of, 255*b*
of subjects, 253, 255*b*

Accessible population, 256*f*
definition of, 250
representativeness, 252–257

Accidental sampling. *see* Convenience sampling

Accuracy
of physiological measures, 289*t*, 292
and precision, in quantitative research, 36

Adaptation model, 195*t*

Administration, and nursing research, 3

Administrative data, collection of, 311

Administrative databases, 483

Advanced beginner stage, of nursing experience, 17

Advanced practice nurses (APNs)
safety and effectiveness of, 476, 477*t*
types of, 476

Advanced practice nursing, in outcomes research, 476

Advances in Nursing Science, 9*t*, 12, 50*t*

Adverse outcome, definition of, 472*t*

African American women, blood pressure in, 5, 6*f*

Age, as demographic variable, 157–158

Agency for Healthcare Policy and Research (AHCPR), on outcomes research, 9*t*, 13

Agency for Healthcare Research and Quality (AHRQ), 13, 143, 467, 473
developing evidence-based guidelines, 25

Agreement, data use, 106

AHCPR. *see* Agency for Healthcare Policy and Research (AHCPR)

AHRQ. *see* Agency for Healthcare Research and Quality (AHRQ)

Algorithms, 456, 458*f*
for identifying an appropriate analysis technique, 338, 339*f*

Alpha (α), 325

Alternate forms reliability, 289*t*, 290

American Association for Accreditation of Laboratory Animal Care (AAALAC), 124

American Association of Colleges of Nursing (AACN), on nursing research, 14, 25–26

American Association of Critical Care Nurses, research priorities of, 142

American Journal of Nursing, history of, 11

American Nurses Association (ANA)
National Database of Nursing Quality Indicators, 475*t*
Nursing Care Report Card, 474
on nursing research, 9*t*, 11, 25–26

American Nurses Credentialing Center (ANCC)
and Magnet Recognition Program, 363
website, 478

American Psychological Association (APA)
citation formatting, 185*t*
Publication Manual (2010), 184

American Recovery and Reinvestment Act, 473–474

ANA. *see* American Nurses Association (ANA)

Analysis of covariance (ANCOVA), 353
definition of, 353
uses for, 353

Analysis of data
on outcome research, 491
in qualitative studies, 391
strengths and weaknesses of, 393
in quantitative studies, strengths and weaknesses of, 374

Analysis of variance (ANOVA), 351–352
definition of, 351
interpreting results of, 351–352
research example of, 351*b*

ANCC. *see* American Nurses Credentialing Center (ANCC)

Ancestry searches, 432

ANCOVA. *see* Analysis of covariance (ANCOVA)

Animals, ethics of research use of, 123–125

Annual Review of Nursing Research, 9*t*, 13

Anonymity, 106–107

ANOVA. *see* Analysis of variance (ANOVA)

Anthropology, and ethnographic research, 74

APA. *see* American Psychological Association (APA)

Applied Nursing Research, 50

Applied Nursing Research and Nursing Science Quarterly, 12

Applied research, definition of, 35–36

Aquarobic exercise program, 230, 231*t*

Articles, 166
keywords for selecting, 178
obtain full-text copies of, 179–180
reading of, 180

Assent form, sample, 103*b*

Association of Women's Health, Obstetric, and Neonatal Nurse, website, 455

Associative hypotheses
versus causal, 149–150
definition of, 149

Assumptions
definition of
in quantitative research, 42
definition of conceptual model, 191

Authority, definition of, 16

Autonomous agents, definition of, 101

Autonomy, diminished, and informed consent competence, 101–104

B

Bachelor of Science in Nursing (BSN), roles of, in nursing research, 26

Basic research, definition of, 35

Bathing, research concerning, 301*b*

Beck Depression Inventory II, in predictive correlational design, 220*b*

Behavioral research, ethical conduct in, 98

Belmont Report, 98

Beneficence, principle of, 98, 108

Benefit-risk ratios
research example of, 121*b*
of a study, 119–121, 119*f*
definition of, 119–120

Best research evidence, 3–4, 21–22, 415, 461

Between-group variance, 351

Bias
definition of, 223
protection against, 212–213
in research design, 223

Bibliographic databases, 177

Bimodal distribution, 331–333, 333*f*